Endodontics

PRINCIPLES AND PRACTICE

FIFTH EDITION

Endodontics

PRINCIPLES AND PRACTICE

Mahmoud Torabinejad, DMD, MSD, PhD
Professor and Program Director
Department of Endodontics
School of Dentistry
Loma Linda University
Loma Linda, California

Richard E. Walton, DMD, MS
Professor Emeritus
Department of Endodontics
The University of Iowa
College of Dentistry
Iowa City, Iowa

Ashraf F. Fouad, BDS, DDS, MS
Department of Endodontics
Prosthodontics and Operative Dentistry
School of Dentistry
University of Maryland
Baltimore, Maryland

ELSEVIER

SAUNDERS

3251 Riverport Lane
St. Louis, Missouri 63043

ENDODONTICS: PRINCIPLES AND PRACTICE   ISBN: 978-1-4557-5410-6
Copyright © 2015 by Saunders, an imprint of Elsevier Inc.

Notices

Knowledge and best practice in this field are constantly changing. As new research and experience
broaden our understanding, changes in research methods, professional practices, or medical treatment may
become necessary.

Practitioners and researchers must always rely on their own experience and knowledge in evaluating
and using any information, methods, compounds, or experiments described herein. In using such
information or methods they should be mindful of their own safety and the safety of others, including
parties for whom they have a professional responsibility.

With respect to any drug or pharmaceutical products identified, readers are advised to check the most
current information provided (i) on procedures featured or (ii) by the manufacturer of each product to be
administered, to verify the recommended dose or formula, the method and duration of administration, and
contraindications. It is the responsibility of practitioners, relying on their own experience and knowledge
of their patients, to make diagnoses, to determine dosages and the best treatment for each individual
patient, and to take all appropriate safety precautions.

To the fullest extent of the law, neither the Publisher nor the authors, contributors, or editors, assume
any liability for any injury and/or damage to persons or property as a matter of products liability,
negligence or otherwise, or from any use or operation of any methods, products, instructions, or ideas
contained in the material herein.

Previous editions copyrighted 1989, 1996, 2002, 2009

ISBN: 978-1-4557-5410-6

Executive Content Strategist: Kathy Falk
Senior Content Development Specialist: Brian Loehr
Publishing Services Manager: Julie Eddy
Senior Project Manager: Richard Barber
Design Direction: Karen Pauls

Printed in China

Last digit is the print number: 9 8 7 6 5 4 3 2 1

Working together
to grow libraries in
developing countries

Book Aid International

www.elsevier.com • www.bookaid.org

Contributors

George Bogen, DDS
Lecturer
Department of Endodontics
Loma Linda University
Loma Linda, California
University of California
Los Angeles, California

Nestor Cohenca, DDS
Tenured Professor
Endodontics and Pediatric Dentistry
School of Dentistry
University of Washington
Seattle, Washington

Paul D. Eleazer, DDS
Professor, Chair, Program Director
Department of Endodontics
University of Alabama at Birmingham
Birmingham, Alabama

Ashraf F. Fouad, BDS, DDS, MS
Department of Endodontics
Prosthodontics and Operative Dentistry
School of Dentistry
University of Maryland
Baltimore, Maryland

Charles J. Goodacre, DDS
Professor
Restorative Dentistry
School of Dentistry
Loma Linda University
Loma Linda, California

Robert Handysides, DDS
Associate Dean for Academic Affairs
School of Dentistry
Loma Linda University
Loma Linda, California

Eric J. Herbranson, DDS, MS
Lecturer
Department of Endodontics
School of Dentistry
Loma Linda University
Loma Linda, California
Practitioner
San Leandro, California

Van T. Himel, DDS
Professor, Chair
Department of Endodontics
Louisiana State University
New Orleans, Louisiana

Graham Rex Holland, BDS, PhD
Professor
Department of Cariology
Restorative Sciences and Endodontics
School of Dentistry
University of Michigan
Ann Arbor, Michigan

Bradford R. Johnson, DDS, MHPE
Associate Professor, Director of Postdoctoral Endodontics
Department of Endodontics
University of Illinois at Chicago
Chicago, Illinois

James D. Johnson, DDS, MS
Chair, Advanced Program Director
Department of Endodontics
School of Dentistry
University of Washington
Seattle, Washington

William T. Johnson, DDS, MS
Richard D. Walton Professor and Chair
Department of Endodontics
College of Dentistry
The University of Iowa
Iowa City, Iowa

Bruce C. Justman, DDS
Clinical Associate Professor
Department of Endodontics
College of Dentistry
The University of Iowa
Iowa City, Iowa

Bekir Karabucak, DMD, MS
Associate Professor, Graduate Program Director
Department of Endodontics
School of Dental Medicine
University of Pennsylvania
Philadelphia, Pennsylvania

James C. Kulild, DDS, MS
Professor Emeritus
Department of Endodontics
University of Missouri
School of Dentistry
Kansas City, Missouri

Harold H. Messer, BDSc, MDSc, PhD
Professor Emeritus
Restorative Dentistry
School of Dental Medicine
University of Melbourne
Melbourne, Victoria, Australia

W. Craig Noblett, DDS
Assistant Clinical Professor
Division of Endodontics
Department of Preventive and Restorative Dental Sciences
San Francisco School of Dentistry
University of California
San Francisco, California
Private Practice
Berkeley, California

John M. Nusstein, DDS, MS
Associate Professor, Chair
Department of Endodontics
College of Dentistry
The Ohio State University
Columbus, Ohio

Ove A. Peters, DMD, MS, PhD
Professor, Co-Chair
Department of Endodontics
University of the Pacific
Arthur A. Dugoni School of Dentistry
San Francisco, California

Al Reader, DDS, MS
Professor, Program Director
Department of Endodontics
College of Dentistry
The Ohio State University
Columbus, Ohio

Eric M. Rivera, DDS, MS
Associate Professor, Chair, and Graduate Program Director
Department of Endodontics
School of Dentistry
University of North Carolina
Chapel Hill, North Carolina

Paul A. Rosenberg, DDS
Professor, Director of Advanced Education Program
Department of Endodontics
New York University
College of Dentistry
New York, New York

Ilan Rotstein, DDS
Professor, Chair
Department of Endodontics, Oral and Maxillofacial Surgery
    and Orthodontics
Ostrow School of Dentistry
University of Southern California
Los Angeles, California

Mohammad A. Sabeti, DDS, MA
Assistant Professor
Department of Endodontics
School of Dentistry
Loma Linda University
Loma Linda, California

Kent A. Sabey, DDS
Program Director
Advanced Education in Endodontics
Department of Endodontics
Louisiana State University
School of Dentistry
New Orleans, Louisiana

Shahrokh Shabahang, DDS, MS, PhD
Associate Professor
Department of Endodontics
School of Dentistry
Loma Linda University
Loma Linda, California

José F. Siqueira, Jr., DDS, MSc, PhD
Professor, Chair
Department of Endodontics and Molecular Microbiology
    Laboratory
Faculty of Dentistry
Estácio de Sá University
Rio de Janeiro, Brazil

Anthony J. Smith, BSc, PhD
Professor
Oral Biology
School of Dentistry
University of Birmingham
Birmingham, Great Britain

Mahmoud Torabinejad, DMD, MSD, PhD
Professor and Program Director
Department of Endodontics
School of Dentistry
Loma Linda University
Loma Linda, California

Richard E. Walton, DMD, MS
Professor Emeritus
Department of Endodontics
The University of Iowa
College of Dentistry
Iowa City, Iowa

Shane N. White, BDentSc, MS, MA, PhD
Professor
School of Dentistry
University of California
Los Angeles, California

Lisa R. Wilcox, DDS, MS
Adjunct Associate Professor
Department of Endodontics
College of Dentistry
The University of Iowa
Iowa City, Iowa

Anne E. Williamson, DDS, MS
Associate Professor, Director, Advanced Education in
   Endodontics
Department of Endodontics
College of Dentistry
The University of Iowa
Iowa City, Iowa

Preface

The primary objective of dentists has always been to relieve dental pain and prevent tooth loss. Despite this effort, many teeth develop caries, suffer traumatic injury, or are impacted by other diseases and disorders, often requiring endodontic care. Endodontics is a discipline of dentistry that deals with the morphology, physiology, and pathology of the human dental pulp and periapical tissues, as well as the prevention and treatment of diseases and injuries related to these tissues. Its scope is wide and includes diagnosis and treatment of pain of pulpal and/or periapical origin, vital pulp therapy, regenerative endodontic procedures, nonsurgical root canal treatment, retreatment of unsuccessful treatment, internal bleaching, and endodontic surgery. Ultimately, the primary goal in endodontics is to preserve the natural dentition. Root canal treatment is a well-tested procedure that has provided pain relief and has restored function and esthetics to patients. Millions of patients expect preservation of their natural dentition; if root canal treatment is necessary, they should be aware that the procedure is safe and has a high success rate if properly performed.

As with other dental specialties, the practice of endodontics requires two inseparable components: art and science. The *art* consists of executing technical procedures during root canal treatment. The *science* includes the basic and clinical sciences related to biological and pathological conditions that guide the art of endodontics through the principles and methods of evidence-based treatment. Evidence-based treatment integrates the best clinical evidence with the practitioner's clinical expertise and the patient's treatment needs and preferences. A principal objective of our textbook is to incorporate evidence-based information when available and when appropriate.

Because there are not enough endodontists to manage the endodontic needs of the public, general dentists must assist endodontists to preserve natural dentition. Their responsibility is to diagnose pulpal and periapical diseases and to perform noncomplicated root canal treatments. In fact, most of the endodontic procedures are performed by generalists. Our textbook, written specifically for dental students and general dentists, contains the information necessary for those who would like to incorporate endodontics in their practice. This includes diagnosis and treatment planning as well as management of pulpal and periapical diseases. In addition, the general dentist must be able to determine the case complexity and whether she or he can perform the necessary treatment or if referral is the better option.

Although many advances have been made in endodontics in the past decade, the main objectives of root canal therapy continue to be the removal of diseased tissue, the elimination of microorganisms, and the prevention of recontamination after treatment. This new edition of *Endodontics: Principles and Practice* has been systematically organized to simulate the order of procedures performed in a clinical setting. It contains information regarding normal structures, etiology of disease, diagnosis and treatment planning, local anesthesia, emergency treatment, root canal instruments, access preparations, cleaning and shaping, obturation, and temporization. In addition, it covers etiology, prevention, and treatment of accidental procedural errors, as well as treatment of inadequate root canal–treated teeth using nonsurgical and surgical approaches. A chapter is dedicated to the endodontic outcomes that provide guidelines regarding the assessment of outcomes of these procedures. In this edition we've included information on pulp and periapical stem cells, regenerative endodontic procedures, novel analyses of endodontic microflora, the use of cone beam CT in endodontics, the interaction of general dentists and endodontists, and systemic considerations in endodontics. Furthermore, a chapter discusses single tooth implant.

The other distinctive features of the new edition are (1) updated relevant and recent references, (2) information regarding new scientific and technological advances in the field of endodontics, (3) information regarding single tooth implant, and (4) a revised contents with new authors. The appendix provides colorized illustrations that depict the size, shape, and location of the pulp space within each tooth. There is also a website with video clips for selected procedures and an interactive version of the self-assessment questions. These features provide the reader with a textbook that is concise, current, and easy to follow in an interactive manner.

This textbook is not intended to include all background information on the art and science of endodontics. At the same time, it is not designed to be a "cookbook" or a preclinical laboratory technique manual. We have tried to provide the reader with the basic information to perform root canal treatment and to give the reader background knowledge in related areas. This textbook should be used as a building block for understanding the etiology and treatment of teeth with pulpal and periapical diseases; then the reader can expand her or his endodontic experiences with more challenging cases. Providing the best quality of care is the guiding light for treatment planning and performing appropriate treatment.

We thank the contributing authors for sharing their materials and experiences with our readers and with us. Their contributions improve the quality of life for millions of patients. We also express our appreciation to the editorial staff of Elsevier, whose collaboration and dedication made this project possible and Mohammad Torabinejad for editing and proofreading the manuscripts. In addition, we acknowledge our colleagues and students who provided cases and gave us constructive suggestions to improve the quality of our textbook. Because much of their material is incorporated into the new edition, we also would like to acknowledge the contributors to the fourth edition: Leif K. Bakland, Marie Therese Flores, Gerald N. Glickman, Gary R. Hartwell, Karl Keiser, Keith V. Krell, Ronald R. Lemon, Neville J. McDonald, Mary Rafter, Isabela N. Rôças, Asgeir Sigurdsson, James H.S. Simon, Henry O. Trowbridge, and Frank J. Vertucci.

Mahmoud Torabinejad
Richard E. Walton
Ashraf F. Fouad

Videos

Elsevier and Loma Linda University are pleased to provide these exciting videos that can be used as a teaching tool for the classroom or individual student use.

As you work through the textbook, you will find icons in the margin that direct you to videos on the website.

Chapter Review Questions

Chapter review questions can be found in an interactive format on the website.

As you work through the questions for each chapter, the program will provide a rationale for correct answer selections and a cross-reference to the textbook.

The program also keeps track of performance data for each chapter.

Please go to http://evolve.elsevier.com/torabinejad/endodontics/ to view the videos and review questions.

Video Contents

Contents

The biology of dental pulp and periradicular tissues

Graham Rex Holland, Mahmoud Torabinejad

CHAPTER OUTLINE

Development of the Dental Pulp
Anatomic Regions and Their Clinical Importance
Pulp Function
Morphology
Cells of the Dental Pulp
Extracellular Components

Blood Vessels
Innervation
Age Changes in the Dental Pulp and Dentin
Repair and Regeneration
Periradicular Tissues

LEARNING OBJECTIVES

After reading this chapter, the student should be able to:
1. Describe the development of pulp.
2. Describe the process of root development.
3. Recognize the anatomic regions of pulp.
4. List all cell types in the pulp and describe their function.
5. Describe both fibrous and non-fibrous components of the extracellular matrix of pulp.
6. Describe the blood vessels and lymphatics of pulp.

7. List the neural components of pulp and describe their distribution and function.
8. Discuss theories of dentin sensitivity.
9. Describe the pathway of efferent nerves from pulp to the central nervous system.
10. Describe the changes in pulp morphology that occur with age.
11. Describe the structure and function of the periradicular tissues.

The dental pulp is the loose connective tissue in the center of the tooth. The primary function of the pulp is to form and support the dentin that surrounds it and forms the bulk of the tooth. The pulp contains odontoblasts that not only form dentin, but also interact with dental epithelium early in tooth development to initiate the formation of enamel. The pulp remains vital throughout life and is able to respond to external stimuli. Both dentin and pulp contain nociceptive nerve fibers. Autonomic nerve fibers occur only in the pulp. When needed for repair, more dentin can be laid down and new odontoblasts differentiated.

The pulp is equipped with all the necessary peripheral components of the immune system and will react to foreign antigens, such as those presented by dental caries. Injury and foreign antigens lead to inflammation and pain. The good health of the pulp is important to the successful completion of restorative and prosthetic dental procedures. In restorative dentistry, for example, the size and shape of the pulp must be considered in determining cavity depth. The size and shape of the pulp depend on the tooth type (e.g., incisor, molar), the degree of tooth development related to the age of the patient, and any restorative procedures that may have been carried out on the tooth. When a tooth is injured, the stage of development the pulp influences the type of treatment rendered. Procedures routinely undertaken on a fully developed tooth are not always practicable for a tooth that is only partially developed, and special procedures are applied.

Because endodontics involves the diagnosis and treatment of diseases of the pulp and their sequelae, a knowledge of the biology of the pulp is essential for the development of an evidence-based treatment plan. This chapter presents an overview of the biology of the pulp and the periodontium as a fundamental component of the evidential base.

DEVELOPMENT OF THE DENTAL PULP

Early Development of Pulp

The tooth originates as a band of epithelial cells, the dental lamina (Fig. 1.1, *A*), on the surface of the embryonic jaws. Downgrowths from this band ultimately form the teeth. The stages of tooth formation are described by the shapes of these downgrowths. Initially, they look like the bud of a forming flower (bud stage, Fig. 1.1, *B*). The bud becomes invaginated at the cap stage (Fig. 1.1, *C*). The invagination deepens, and the bell stage is reached (Fig. 1.1, *D*). The bell-shaped downgrowth is the enamel organ. It is ectodermal in origin and will be responsible for amelogenesis. The tissue within the invagination ultimately becomes the dental pulp, known as the *dental papilla,* during the early stages of development. Before

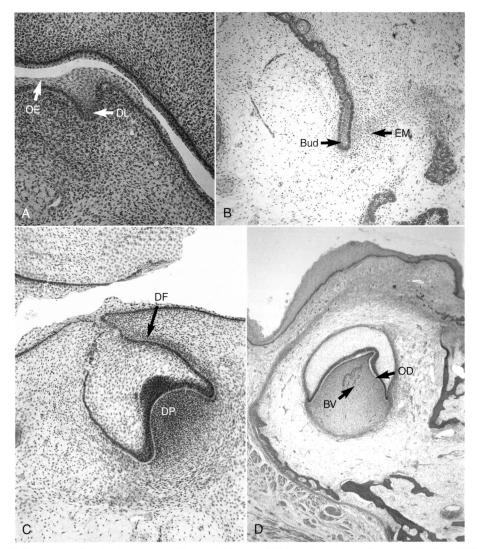

Fig. 1.1 **A,** Earliest stage of tooth development. The dental lamina *(DL)* invaginates from the oral epithelium *(OE).* **B,** Bud stage of tooth development. Ectomesenchyme *(EM)* is beginning to condense around the tooth germ. **C,** The cap stage of tooth development. The condensed ectomesenchyme within the invagination is the dental papilla *(DP).* The dental follicle *(DF)* is beginning to develop around the tooth germ. **D,** Early bell stage. The odontoblast layer *(OD)* and blood vessels *(BV)* are visible in the dental pulp. (Courtesy Dr. H. Trowbridge.)

that, the cells it contains differentiate. The papilla (and thus the pulp) is derived from cells that have migrated from the neural crest (ectomesenchymal cells) and mingled with cells of local mesenchymal origin.

During the bell stage, the inner layer of cells of the enamel organ differentiate into ameloblasts (Fig. 1.2, *A*). This is followed by the outer layer of cells of the dental papilla differentiating into odontoblasts (Fig. 1.2, *B*), which begin to lay down dentin in the late bell (or crown) stage (Fig. 1.2, *C*). From this point on, the tissue within the invagination is known as the *dental pulp.* A layer of tissue begins to differentiate around the enamel organ and dental papilla and forms the dental follicle, which later becomes the periodontal attachment. The combination of the enamel organ dental papilla/pulp and dental follicle is the tooth germ.

The histodifferentiation and morphodifferentiation of the tooth germ are genetically determined and executed by a group of growth factors, transcription factors, and other signaling molecules. Several of the genes controlling this process

have been identified. Disorder at this stage can lead to anodontia, amelogenesis imperfecta, odontogenesis imperfecta, and related defects. A substantial research effort has been underway for some years, with a long-term goal of using these molecules therapeutically in procedures such as apexogenesis and pulpal regeneration.

The differentiation of odontoblasts from undifferentiated ectomesenchymal cells is initiated and controlled by the ectodermal cells of the inner dental epithelium of the enamel organ. The ameloblasts synthesize growth factors and signaling molecules that pass into the basal lamina of the epithelium and from there to the preodontoblast. The cells beneath the forming odontoblasts remain as undifferentiated stem cells and retain the potential to differentiate.

Once the odontoblast layer has differentiated, the basal lamina of the inner dental epithelium that contained the signaling molecules disappears, and the odontoblasts, now linked to each other by tight junctions, desmosomal junctions, and gap junctions, begin to lay down dentin (see Fig. 1.2, *C*).[1]

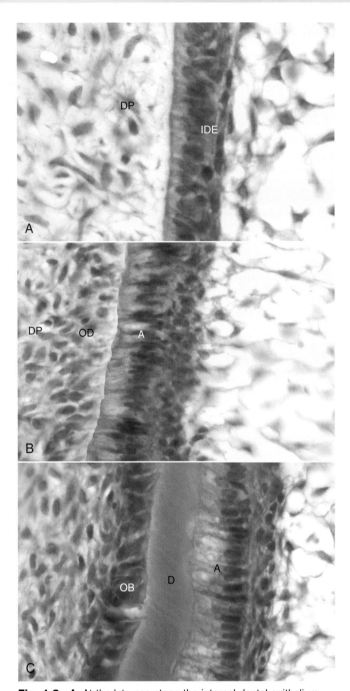

Fig. 1.2 **A,** At the late cap stage the internal dental epithelium *(IDE)* has differentiated into a layer of ameloblasts but has not laid down enamel. The outer layer of the dental papilla *(DP)* has not yet differentiated into odontoblasts. **B,** Slightly later than in Fig. 1.2, *A,* the outer cells of the dental papilla are beginning to become odontoblasts *(OD)* at the periphery of what now is the dental pulp *(DP).* The ameloblasts *(A)* are fully differentiated, but no enamel has formed yet. **C,** In the bell stage, the odontoblasts *(OB)* are laying down dentin *(D),* but the ameloblasts *(A)* have laid down little, if any, enamel. (Courtesy Dr. H. Trowbridge.)

Once dentin formation has begun, the cells of the inner dental epithelium begin responding to a signal from the odontoblasts and start to deposit enamel. This back-and-forth signal control is an example of epithelial-mesenchymal interaction, a key developmental process that has been heavily studied in the tooth germ model. Deposition of unmineralized dentin matrix

begins at the cusp tip and progresses in a cervical (apical) direction in a regular rhythm at an average of 4.5 µm/day.[2] Crown shape is genetically predetermined by the proliferative pattern of the cells of the inner dental epithelium. The first thin layer of dentin formed is called *mantle dentin.* The direction and size of the collagen fibers in mantle dentin, together with the mineralization pattern, differ from those in the subsequently formed circumpulpal dentin. Processes from the odontoblasts remain at least in the inner part of the dentinal tubules. A pattern of matrix formation followed by mineralization continues throughout dentin deposition. Between 10 and 50 µm of the dentin matrix immediately adjacent to the odontoblast layer remains unmineralized at all times and is known as *predentin.*

As crown formation occurs, nerves and blood vessels begin migrating into the pulp from the future root apex in a coronal direction. Both undergo branching and narrowing toward the odontoblast layer, and at a late stage, each forms plexuses beneath the layer with the nerves extending branches into the odontoblast layer and some of the dentinal tubules. Dentin formation continues throughout life in an incremental pattern marked by lines in the matrix and changes in direction of the tubules. The rate of deposition slows in adulthood but never completely stops. The rate can increase if the odontoblasts are stimulated by toxin molecules penetrating the dentin.

Root Formation

In the developing tooth, cells of the inner and outer dental epithelia meet at a point known as the *cervical loop.* This delineates the end of the anatomic crown and the site where root formation begins. Root formation is initiated by the apical proliferation of the two fused epithelia, now known as *Hertwig's epithelial root sheath.*[3] The function of the sheath is similar to that of the inner enamel epithelium during crown formation. It provides signals for the differentiation of odontoblasts and thus acts as a template for the root (Fig. 1.3, *A*). Cell proliferation in the root sheath is genetically determined; its pattern regulates whether the root will be wide or narrow, straight or curved, long or short, or single or multiple. Multiple roots result when opposing parts of the root sheath proliferate both horizontally and vertically. As horizontal segments of Hertwig's epithelial root sheath join to form the "epithelial diaphragm," the pattern for multiple root formation is laid down. This pattern is readily discernible when the developing root end is viewed microscopically (Fig. 1.3, *B*).

After the first dentin in the root has formed, the basement membrane beneath Hertwig's sheath breaks up and the innermost root sheath cells secrete a hyaline material over the newly formed dentin. After mineralization has occurred, this becomes the *hyaline layer of Hopewell-Smith,* which helps bind the soon-to-be-formed cementum to dentin. Fragmentation of Hertwig's epithelial root sheath occurs shortly afterward. This fragmentation allows cells of the surrounding dental follicle (the future periodontium) to migrate and contact the newly formed dentin surface, where they differentiate into cementoblasts and initiate acellular cementum formation (Fig. 1.4).[4] This cementum ultimately serves as an anchor for the developing principal fibers of the periodontal ligament (PDL). In many teeth, cell remnants of the root sheath persist in the periodontium in close proximity to the root after root development has been completed. These are the *epithelial cell rests of Malassez.*[5] Normally functionless, in the presence of **3**

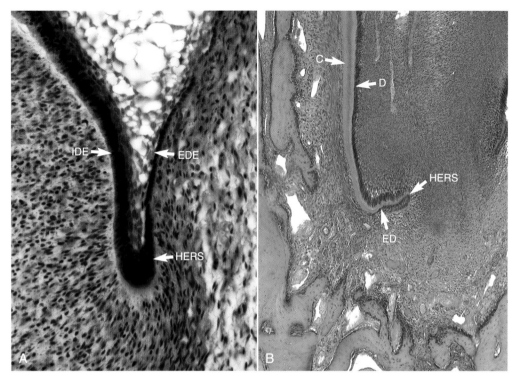

Fig. 1.3 A, The formation of Hertwig's epithelial root sheath *(HERS)* from the internal *(IDE)* and external *(EDE)* epithelia.
B, Hertwig's epithelial root sheath *(HERS)* has extended. Both dentin *(D)* and cementum *(C)* have been deposited. HERS has changed direction to form the epithelial diaphragm *(ED).*

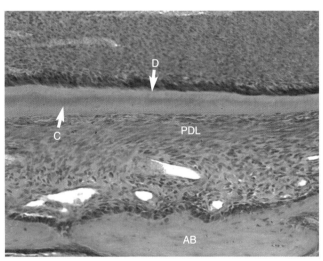

Fig. 1.4 Developing dentin *(D),* cementum *(C),* periodontal ligament *(PDL),* and alveolar bone *(AB).*

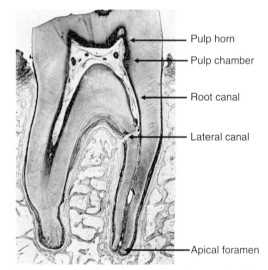

Fig. 1.5 Anatomic regions of the root canal system highlighting the pulp horn(s), pulp chamber, root canal, lateral canal, and apical foramen. The pulp, which is present in the root canal system, communicates with the periodontal ligament primarily through the apical foramen and the lateral canal(s). (Courtesy Orban Collection.)

inflammation they can proliferate and may under certain conditions give rise to a radicular cyst.[6]

Formation of Lateral Canals and Apical Foramen
Lateral Canals
Lateral canals (or, synonymously, accessory canals) are channels of communication between pulp and PDL (Fig. 1.5). They form when a localized area of root sheath is fragmented

before dentin formation. The result is direct communication between pulp and the PDL via a channel through the dentin and cementum that carries small blood vessels and, perhaps, nerves. Lateral canals may be single or multiple, large or small. They may occur anywhere along the root but are most common in the apical third. In molars, they may join the pulp chamber PDL in the root furcation. *Lateral canals are clinically significant; like the apical foramen, they represent pathways along which disease may extend from the pulp to periradicular tissues and from the periodontium to the pulp.*

Apical Foramen

The epithelial root sheath continues to extend until the full, predetermined length of the root is reached. As the epithelial root sheath extends, it encloses more of the dental pulp until only an apical foramen remains, through which pulpal vessels and nerves pass. During root formation, the apical foramen is usually located at the end of the anatomic root. When tooth development has been completed, the apical foramen is smaller and can be found a short distance coronal to the anatomic end of the root.[7] This distance increases later as more apical cementum is formed.

There may be one foramen or multiple foramina at the apex. Multiple foramina occur more often in multirooted teeth. When more than one foramen is present, the largest one is referred to as the *apical foramen* and the smaller ones as *accessory canals.* (Together they constitute the *apical delta.*) The diameter of the apical foramen in a mature tooth usually ranges between 0.3 and 0.6 mm. The largest diameters are found on the distal canal of mandibular molars and the palatal root of maxillary molars. Foramen size is unpredictable, however, and cannot be accurately determined clinically.

Formation of the Periodontium

Tissues of the periodontium develop from ectomesenchyme-derived tissue *(dental follicle)* that surrounds the developing tooth. After the mantle dentin has formed, enamel-like proteins are secreted into the space between the basement membrane and the newly formed collagen by the root sheath cells. This area is not mineralized with the mantle dentin but does mineralize later from the hyaline layer of Hopewell-Smith. After mineralization has occurred, the root sheath breaks down. This fragmentation allows cells from the follicle to proliferate and differentiate into cementoblasts, which lay down cementum over the hyaline layer. Bundles of collagen, produced by fibroblasts in the central region of the follicle *(Sharpey's fibers),* are embedded in the forming cementum and will become the principal fibers of the PDL.

At the same time, cells in the outermost area of the follicle differentiate into osteoblasts to form the bundle bone that will also anchor the periodontal fibers. Later, periodontal fibroblasts produce more collagen that binds the anchored fragments together to form the principal periodontal fibers that suspend the tooth in its socket. Loose, fibrous connective tissue carrying nerves and blood vessels remains between the principal fibers. Undifferentiated mesenchymal cells (tissue-specific stem cells) are plentiful in the periodontium and possess the ability to form new cementoblasts, osteoblasts, or fibroblasts in response to specific stimuli. Cementum formed after the formation of the principal periodontal fibers is cellular and plays a lesser role in tooth support. As with the development of the dental pulp, these processes are genetically predetermined and executed via signaling molecules. There is intense research in this area, because it promises truly biologic approaches to periodontal disease.

The blood supply to the periodontium is derived from the surrounding bone, gingiva, and branches of the pulpal vessels.[8] It is extensive and supports the high level of cellular activity in the area. The pattern of innervation is similar to that of the vasculature. The neural supply consists of small, unmyelinated sensory and autonomic nerves and larger myelinated sensory nerves. Some of the latter terminate as unmyelinated neural structures thought to be nociceptors and mechanoreceptors.

ANATOMIC REGIONS AND THEIR CLINICAL IMPORTANCE

The tooth has two principal anatomic divisions, root and crown, that join at the cervix *(cervical region).* The pulp space is similarly divided into coronal and radicular regions. In general, the shape and the size of the tooth surface reflect the shape and size of the pulp space. The coronal pulp is subdivided into the pulp horn(s) and pulp chamber (see Fig. 1.5). Pulp horns extend from the chamber into the cuspal region. In young teeth, they are extensive and may be inadvertently exposed during routine cavity preparation.

The pulp space becomes asymmetrically smaller after root growth is complete because of the slower production of dentin. There is a pronounced decrease in the height of the pulp horn and a reduction in the overall size of the pulp chamber. In molars, the apical-occlusal dimension is reduced more than the mesial-distal dimension. Excessive reduction of the size of the pulp space is clinically significant and can lead to difficulties in locating, cleaning, and shaping the root canal system (Fig. 1.6).

The anatomy of the root canal varies not only between tooth types, but also within tooth types. Although at least one canal must be present in each root, some roots have multiple canals of varying sizes. *Understanding and appreciating all aspects of root canal anatomy are essential prerequisites to root canal treatment.*

Variation in the size and location of the apical foramen influences the degree to which blood flow to the pulp may be compromised after a traumatic event. *Young, partially developed teeth have a better prognosis for pulp survival than teeth with mature roots* (Fig. 1.7).

Posteruptive deposition of cementum in the region of the apical foramen creates a disparity between the radiographic apex and the apical foramen. It also creates a funnel-shaped opening to the foramen that is often larger in diameter than the intraradicular portion of the foramen. The narrowest portion of the canal is referred to as the *apical constriction.* However, a constriction is not clinically evident in all teeth. The constriction coincides with the *cementodentinal junction* (CDJ). The level of the CDJ varies from root to root. One study estimated the junction to be located 0.5 to 0.75 mm coronal to the apical opening.[7] Theoretically, that is the point where the pulp terminates and the PDL begins, and it would be the ideal point for a procedure aimed at removing the pulp. However, clinically, it is not always possible to locate that point. Cleaning, shaping, and obturation of the root canal should terminate short of the apical foramen and remain confined to the canal to avoid unnecessary injury to the periapical tissues. *The determination of root length and the establishment of a working length are essential steps in root canal preparation. Radiographs and electronic apex locators are helpful in establishing the root length.*

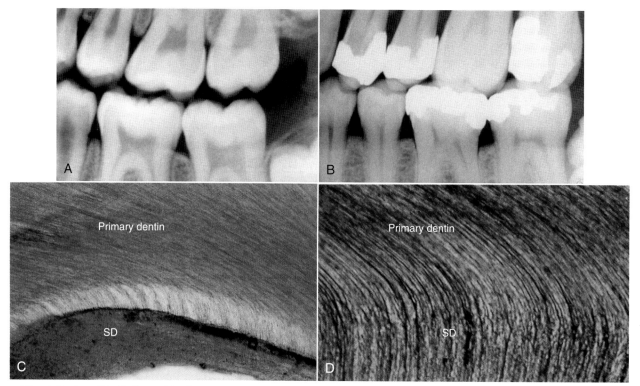

Fig. 1.6 **A** and **B,** Radiographic changes noted in the shape of the pulp chamber over time. The posterior bitewing radiographs were taken 15 years apart. The shapes of the root canal systems have been altered as a result of secondary dentinogenesis and by the deposition of tertiary dentin when deep restorations are present. **C,** Secondary dentin *(SD)*. Ground section at low power. **D,** Secondary dentin *(SD)* at high power.

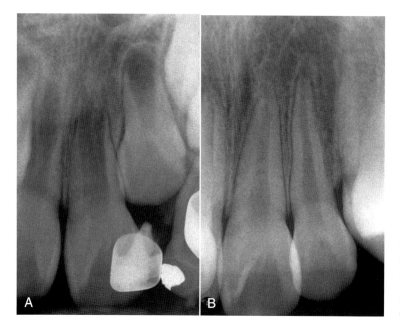

Fig. 1.7 Changes in the anatomy of the tooth root and pulp space. **A,** A small crown-to-root ratio, thin dentin walls, and divergent shape in the apical third of the canal are seen. **B,** Four years later, a longer root, greater crown-to-root ratio, smaller pulp space, and thicker dentin walls with a convergent shape are seen.

PULP FUNCTION

The pulp performs five functions, some formative and others supportive.

Induction

Pulp participates in the initiation and development of dentin.[9] When dentin is formed, it leads to the formation of enamel. These events are interdependent, in that enamel epithelium induces the differentiation of odontoblasts, and odontoblasts and dentin induce the formation of enamel. Such epithelial-mesenchymal interactions are the core processes of tooth formation.

Formation

Odontoblasts form dentin.[10] These highly specialized cells participate in dentin formation in three ways: (1) by synthesizing and secreting inorganic matrix, (2) by initially transporting inorganic components to newly formed matrix, and (3) by creating an environment that permits mineralization of the matrix. During early tooth development, primary dentinogenesis is a rapid process. After tooth maturation, when elongation of the root is complete, dentin formation continues at a much slower rate and in a less symmetric pattern *(secondary dentinogenesis)*. Odontoblasts can also form dentin in response to injury, which may occur in association with caries, trauma, or restorative procedures. In general, this dentin is less organized than primary and secondary dentin and mostly localized to the site of injury. This dentin is referred to as *tertiary dentin*. Tertiary dentin has two forms. *Reactionary* tertiary dentin is tubular, with the tubules continuous with those of the original dentin. It is formed by the original odontoblasts. *Reparative* dentin is formed by new odontoblasts differentiated from stem cells after the original odontoblasts have been killed. It is largely atubular (Fig. 1.8).

Nutrition

The pulp supplies nutrients that are essential for dentin formation and for maintaining the integrity of the pulp itself.

Defense

In the mature tooth, the odontoblasts form dentin in response to injury, particularly when the original dentin thickness has been reduced by caries, attrition, trauma, or restorative procedures. Dentin can also be formed at sites where its continuity has been lost, such as a site of pulp exposure. Dentin formation occurs in this situation by the induction, differentiation, and migration of new odontoblasts to the exposure site (Fig. 1.9).

Pulp also has the ability to process and identify foreign substances, such as the toxins produced by bacteria of dental caries, and to elicit an immune response to their presence.

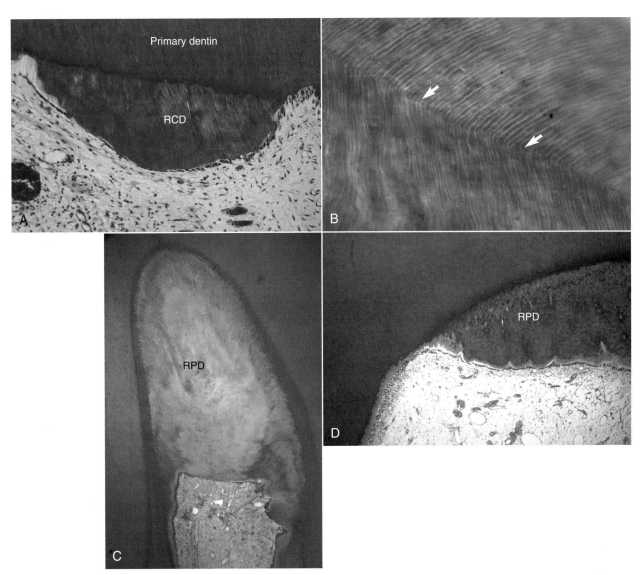

Fig. 1.8   A, Reactionary dentin *(RCD)* at low power. **B,** RCD at high power showing change in direction of tubules *(arrows)*.
C, Reparative dentin *(RPD)* at low power. **D,** RPD at high power. (Courtesy Dr. H. Trowbridge.)

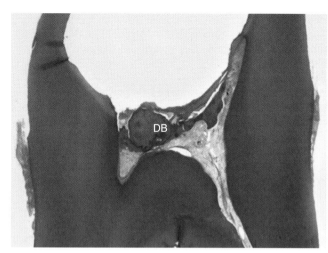

Fig. 1.9 Reparative dentin bridge *(DB)* formed over a cariously exposed pulp. (Courtesy Dr. H. Trowbridge.)

Sensation

Nerves in the pulp can respond to stimuli applied directly to the tissue or through enamel and dentin. Physiologic stimuli can only result in the sensation of pain. The stimulation of myelinated sensory nerves in the pulp results in fast, sharp pain. Activation of the unmyelinated pain fibers results in a slower, duller pain. Pulp sensation through dentin and enamel is usually fast and sharp and is transmitted by Aδ fibers *(narrow myelinated fibers)*.

MORPHOLOGY

Dentin and pulp are actually a single-tissue complex with a histologic appearance that varies with age and exposure to external stimuli.

Under light microscopy, a young, fully developed permanent tooth shows certain recognizable aspects of pulpal architecture. In its outer (peripheral) regions subjacent to predentin is the odontoblast layer. Internal to this layer is a relatively cell-free area *(zone of Weil)*. Internal to the zone of Weil is a higher concentration of cells (cell-rich zone). (These features are limited to the coronal pulp and are sometimes difficult to discern.) In the center is an area containing mostly fibroblasts and major branches of nerves and blood vessels referred to as the *pulp core* (Fig. 1.10).

CELLS OF THE DENTAL PULP

Odontoblasts

Odontoblasts are the characteristic cells of pulp. They form a single layer at its periphery, synthesize the matrix, and control the mineralization of dentin.[11] They produce collagen that becomes fibrous and three noncollagenous proteins in which the collagen fibers are embedded. In the coronal part of the pulp space, the odontoblasts are numerous (between 45,000 and 65,000/mm²), relatively large, and columnar in shape. In the cervical and midportion of the root, their numbers are lower and they appear flattened. The morphology of the cell reflects its level of activity; larger cells have a well-developed

synthetic apparatus and the capacity to synthesize more matrix. During their life cycle, they go through functional, transitional, and resting phases, all marked by differences in cell size and organelle expression.[12] Odontoblasts can continue at varying levels of activity for a lifetime. Some die by planned cell death (apoptosis), using an autophagic-lysosomal system as the volume of the pulp decreases.[12,13] Disease processes, principally dental caries, can kill odontoblasts, but if conditions are favorable, these cells can be replaced by new odontoblasts that have differentiated from stem cells. (Odontoblasts are end cells and as such do not undergo further cell division.)

The odontoblast consists of two major components, the cell body and the cell processes. The *cell body* lies subjacent to the unmineralized dentin matrix (predentin). One large *cell process* extends outward for a variable distance through a tubule in the predentin and dentin. Other, much smaller processes extend from the cell body and link odontoblasts to each other and possibly to fibroblasts. The cell body is the synthesizing portion of the cell and contains a basally located nucleus and a variety of organelles in the cytoplasm that are typical of a secreting cell. During active dentinogenesis, the endoplasmic reticulum and the Golgi apparatus are prominent, and there are numerous mitochondria and vesicles (Fig. 1.11).

Cell bodies are joined by a variety of membrane junctions, including gap junctions, tight junctions, and desmosomes. Each junction type has specific functions. Desmosomal junctions mechanically link the cells into a coherent layer. Gap junctions allow communication between cells in the layer. Tight junctions control the permeability of the layer. The secretory products of the odontoblasts are released through the cell membrane at the peripheral end of the cell body and through the cell process. The cell-to-cell junctions are specialized areas of the cell membrane. Other parts of the cell membrane are specialized to be *membrane receptors* to which signaling molecules can attach (as *ligands*) and thereby modify the behavior of the cell.

There are many types of membrane receptors. The type and number of receptors vary greatly between cell types and at different times of the cell's life. The odontoblast has several types of receptors on or within its cell membrane. Toll-like receptors (TLR2 and TLR4), when activated by components of gram-positive bacteria (lipoteichoic acid), cause the odontoblasts to release proinflammatory cytokines (Fig. 1.12). This indicates that the odontoblasts can act as antigen-recognition cells when bacterial products penetrate the dentin.[14] Other known receptors (e.g., TRPV1, capsaicin receptor, and TRK-1, vanilloid receptor) are thermosensitive and can sense heat- or cold-induced fluid movement in the tubules (Fig. 1.13).[15,16] Thus, the odontoblast has a role in the immune response and may act as a nociceptor.

Stem Cells (Preodontoblasts)

Newly differentiated odontoblasts develop after an injury that results in the death of existing odontoblasts. They develop from stem cells (also known as *undifferentiated mesenchymal cells*), which are present throughout the pulp, although densest in its core.[17] Under the influence of signaling molecules released in response to injury and cell death, these precursor cells migrate to the site of injury and differentiate into odontoblasts.[18] The key signaling molecules in this process are

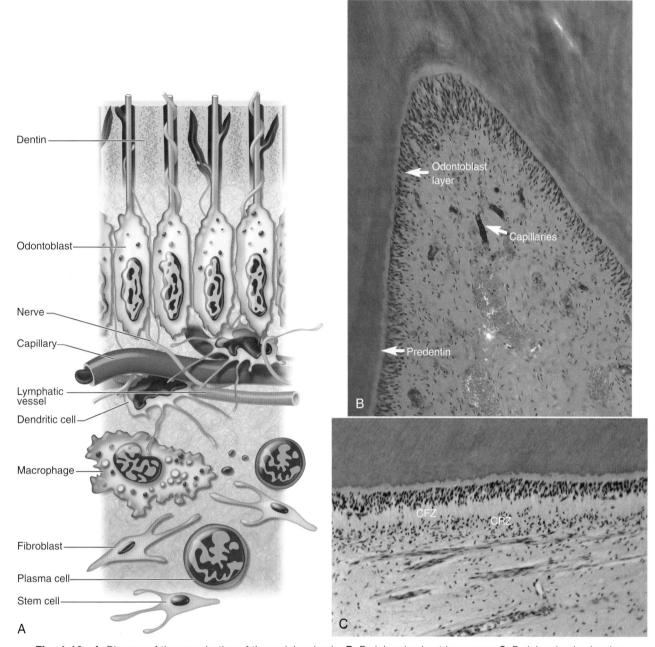

Fig. 1.10 **A,** Diagram of the organization of the peripheral pulp. **B,** Peripheral pulp at low power. **C,** Peripheral pulp showing cell-free zone *(CFZ)* and cell-rich zone *(CRZ).*

members of the bone morphogenetic protein (BMP) family and transforming growth factor β. These (and other) growth factors are embedded in dentin matrix, although their origin is unknown.

Dental pulpal stem cells (DSPC) can differentiate not only into odontoblasts, but also into other cell types, such as osteoblasts, adipocytes, cardiac muscle cells, and even neurons. These cells promise to be useful therapeutically in the regeneration of pulp and other tissues (Fig. 1.14).

Fibroblasts

Fibroblasts are the most common cell type in the pulp and are seen in greatest numbers in the coronal pulp. They produce and maintain the collagen and ground substance of the pulp

and alter the structure of the pulp in disease. As with odontoblasts, the prominence of their cytoplasmic organelles changes according to their activity. The more active the cell, the more prominent the organelles and other components necessary for synthesis and secretion. As do odontoblasts, these cells undergo apoptotic cell death and are replaced when necessary by the maturation of less differentiated cells.

Before immunocytochemistry and DNA/RNA analysis became available, simple techniques, such as hematoxylineosin staining, were used to identify cell types. However, they could not detect subtle differences between cell types. Using those methods, the majority of cells in loose connective tissues such as the pulp were designated as "fibroblasts." Certainly there are some main fibroblasts that synthesize and **9**

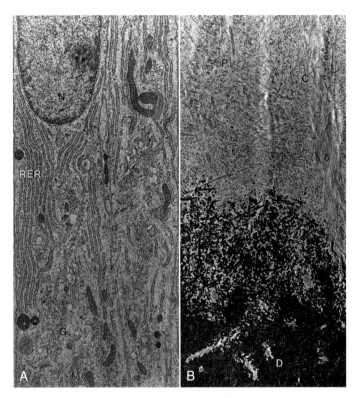

Fig. 1.11 A, Odontoblast cell body. The nucleus *(N)* is proximal, and the numerous organelles, such as rough endoplasmic reticulum *(RER)* and Golgi apparatus *(G),* which are responsible for synthesis of matrix components, occupy the central-distal regions. **B,** Predentin *(P)* shows the orientation of collagen *(C)* to the odontoblastic process, which is the secretory organ that extends through the predentin into the dentin *(D).* (Courtesy Dr. P. Glick and Dr. D. Rowe.)

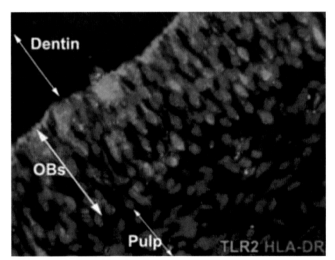

Fig. 1.12 The odontoblast layer, dentin, and subodontoblastic zone immunostained to label Toll-like receptors (TLR2) *(green)* and dendritic cells *(red)*. (Veerayutthwilai O, Byers MR, Darveau RP, Dale BA: Differential regulation of immune responses by odontoblasts, *Oral Microbiol Immunol* 2007: 22: 5-13, 2007.)

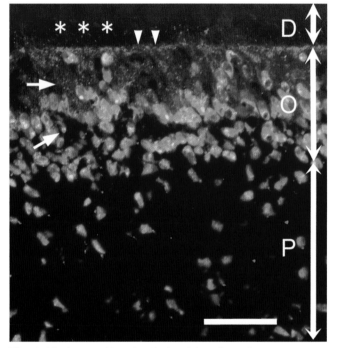

Fig. 1.13 Immunohistochemical staining of transient receptor potential vanilloid 1 (TRPV1) channels in rat odontoblasts that could induce electrical activity in the odontoblasts when stretched or compressed by fluid movement. Asterisks and arrowheads show TRPV1-positive staining (green) on odontoblast processes in the tubules and on the distal end of the odontoblastic cell membrane. The red stain indicates nuclei in all the cells present. TRPV1 staining is largely limited to the odontoblasts. D, Dentin; O, odontoblast layer; P, pulp. (Courtesy Dr. Y. Shibukawa.) (From Okumura R, Shima K, Muramatsu T, et al: The odontoblast as a sensory receptor cell? The expression of TRPV1 (VR-1) channels, Archives of Histology and cytology, 2005.)

secrete matrix components, but there is now a recognition of the heterogeneity of cells in the pulp.

Cells of the Immune System

The most prominent immune cells in the dental pulp are the dendritic cells.[19] These are antigen-presenting cells present most densely in the odontoblast layer and around blood vessels. They recognize a wide range of foreign antigens and, along with odontoblasts, initiate the immune response. Many other cells (e.g., macrophages and neutrophils) have antigen-presenting properties, but dendritic cells in the pulp, in terms

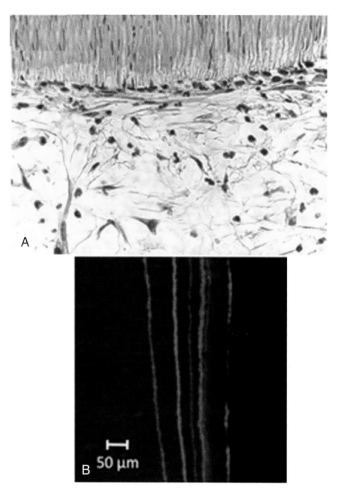

Fig. 1.14 Stem cells from exfoliated deciduous teeth (SHED) were placed on a scaffold in a tooth slice from which the pulp had been removed. The slice was then placed subcutaneously in a mouse and left for 32 days. **A,** The pulp and dentin were examined a month after placement. The stem cells differentiate into functional odontoblasts and endothelial cells (hematoxylin-eosin.) **B,** Once the stem cells differentiated into functional odontoblasts, they generated tubular dentin. This is demonstrated by injecting tetracycline intraperitoneally every 5 days and observing a section of the slice in a confocal microscope. The bright lines indicate areas where the tetracycline has been incorporated into the dentin. (From Sakai VT, Cordeiro MM, Dong Z, et al: *Advances in dental research: tooth slice/scaffold model of dental pulp tissue engineering*, Thousand Oaks, Calif., Jun 15, 2011, Sage Publishing.)

of numbers (estimated at 8% of the pulp) and position, are the most prominent in the pulp. Special stains are needed to recognize them histologically.

Macrophages in a resting form (histiocytes) and some T lymphocytes are also found in the normal pulp.[20]

EXTRACELLULAR COMPONENTS[21]

Fibers

The predominant collagen in dentin is type I; both type I and type III collagens are found within pulp in a ratio of approximately 55:45. Odontoblasts produce only type I collagen for incorporation into the dentin matrix, whereas fibroblasts produce both type I and type III. Pulpal collagen is present as fibrils that are 50 nm wide and several micrometers long. They form bundles that are irregularly arranged except in the periphery, where they lie approximately parallel to the predentin surface. The only noncollagenous fibers present in the pulp are tiny, 10 to 15 nm wide beaded fibrils of fibrillin, a large glycoprotein. Elastic fibers are absent from the pulp.

The proportion of collagen types is constant in the pulp, but with age there is an increase in the overall collagen content and an increase in the organization of collagen fibers into collagen bundles. Normally, the apical portion of pulp contains more collagen than the coronal pulp, facilitating pulpectomy with a barbed broach or endodontic file during root canal treatment.

Noncollagenous Matrix[22]

The collagenous fibers of the pulp are embedded in a histologically clear gel made up of glycosaminoglycans and other adhesion molecules. The glycosaminoglycans link to protein and other saccharides to form proteoglycans, a very diverse group of molecules. They are bulky hydrophilic molecules that, with water, make up the gel. At least six types of adhesion molecules have been detected in the pulp matrix. One of these, fibronectin is responsible for cell adhesion to the matrix.

Calcifications

Pulp stones or denticles (Fig. 1.15) were once classified as true or false, depending on the presence or absence of a tubular structure. This classification has been challenged, and a new nomenclature based on the genesis of the calcification has been suggested. Pulp stones have also been classified according to location. Three types of pulp stones have been described: *free stones,* which are surrounded by pulp tissue; *attached stones,* which are continuous with the dentin; and *embedded stones,* which are surrounded entirely by tertiary dentin.

Pulp stones occur in both young and old patients and may occur in one or several teeth. A recent radiographic (bitewing) survey of undergraduate dental students found that 46% of them had one or more pulp stones and that 10% of all the teeth contained a pulp stone. Pulp stones occur in normal pulps and in chronically inflamed pulps. They are not responsible for painful symptoms, regardless of size.

Calcifications may also occur in the form of diffuse or linear deposits associated with neurovascular bundles in the pulp core. This type of calcification is seen most often in aged, chronically inflamed, or traumatized pulp. Depending on shape, size, and location, pulp calcifications may or may not be detected on a dental radiograph (Fig. 1.16). *Large pulp stones are clinically significant, because they may block access to canals or the root apex during root canal treatment.*

BLOOD VESSELS

Mature pulp has an extensive and specialized vascular pattern that reflects its unique environment.[23] The vessel network has been examined using a variety of techniques, including India ink perfusion, transmission electron microscopy, scanning electron microscopy, and microradiography.

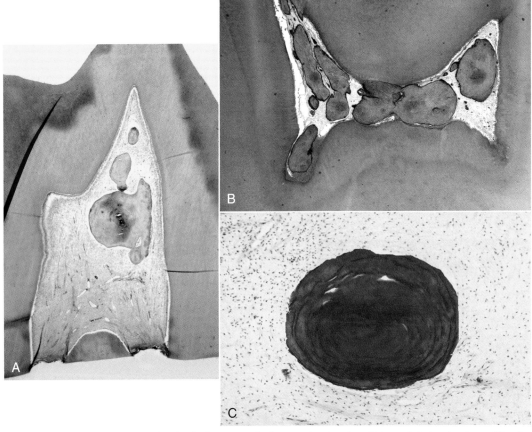

Fig. 1.15 **A,** Multiple stones in coronal pulp. **B,** Stones occluding a pulp chamber. **C,** Lamellated pulp stone. (Courtesy Dr. H. Trowbridge.)

Afferent Blood Vessels (Arterioles)

The largest vessels to enter the apical foramen are arterioles that are branches of the inferior alveolar artery, the superior posterior alveolar artery, or the infraorbital artery.

Once inside the radicular pulp, the arterioles travel toward the crown. They narrow, then branch extensively and lose their muscle sheath before forming a capillary bed (Fig. 1.17). The muscle fibers before the capillary bed form the "precapillary sphincters," which control blood flow and pressure. The most extensive capillary branching occurs in the subodontoblastic layer of the coronal pulp, where the vessels form a dense plexus (Fig. 1.18).[24] The loops of some of these capillaries extend between odontoblasts.[22] The exchange of nutrients and waste products takes place in the capillaries (Fig. 1.19).[25] There is an extensive shunting system composed of arteriovenous and venovenous anastomoses; these shunts become active after pulp injury and during repair.

Efferent Blood Vessels

Venules constitute the efferent (exit) side of the pulpal circulation and are slightly larger than the corresponding arterioles. Venules are formed from the junction of venous capillaries and enlarge as more capillary branches unite with them. They run with the arterioles and exit at the apical foramen to drain posteriorly into the maxillary vein through the pterygoid plexus or anteriorly into the facial vein.

Lymphatics[26,27]

Lymphatic vessels arise as small, blind, thin-walled vessels in the periphery of the pulp. They pass through the pulp to exit as one or two larger vessels through the apical foramen (Figs. 1.20 and 1.21). The lymphatic vessel walls are composed of an endothelium rich in organelles and granules. There are discontinuities in the walls of these vessels and in their basement membranes. This porosity permits the passage of interstitial tissue fluid and, when necessary, lymphocytes into the negative-pressure lymph vessel. The lymphatics assist in the removal of inflammatory exudates and transudates and cellular debris. After exiting from the pulp, some vessels join similar vessels from the PDL and drain into regional lymph glands (submental, submandibular, or cervical) before emptying into the subclavian and internal jugular veins. *An understanding of lymphatic drainage assists in the diagnosis of infection of endodontic origin.*

Vascular Physiology

The dental pulp, at least when young, is a highly vascular tissue. Capillary blood flow in the coronal region is almost twice that of the radicular region. Blood supply is regulated largely by the precapillary sphincters and their sympathetic innervation.[28] Other local factors and peptides released from sensory nerves also affect the vessels most prominently during inflammation.

As in other tissues, the volume of the vascular bed is much greater than the volume of blood that is normally passing through it. Only part of the vascular bed is perfused at any one time. This capacity allows for sizable local increases in blood flow in response to injury.

The factors that determine what passes in and out between the blood and the tissue include concentration gradients, osmosis, and hydraulic pressure. Concentration gradients vary along the capillary bed as oxygen, for example, diffuses out into the depleted tissue and carbon dioxide (CO_2) enters from high to low concentration. The hydraulic pressure in the pulpal capillaries falls from 35 mm Hg at the arteriolar end to 19 mm Hg at the venular end. Outside the vessel, the interstitial fluid pressure varies, but a normal figure would be 6 mm Hg.[29]

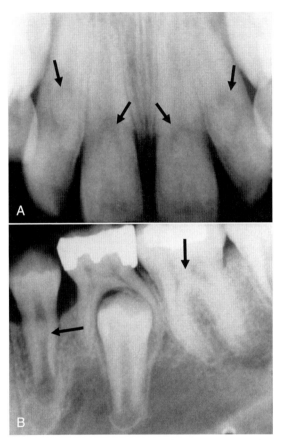

Fig. 1.16 Multiple pulp stones *(arrows)* in the pulp chamber and root canals of the anterior **(A)** and posterior **(B)** teeth of a young patient.

Vascular Changes During Inflammation[30]

When the dental pulp is injured, it responds in the same way as other connective tissues with a two-phase immune response. The initial immune response is nonspecific but rapid, occurring in minutes or hours. The second response is specific and includes the production of specific antibodies. Before the detailed nature of the immune response was known, the phenomenon associated with the response to tissue injury, including redness, pain, heat, and swelling, was known as *inflammation*. Although much more is now known about the response to injury at the cellular level, these "cardinal signs" remain important. Except for pain, they are all vascular in origin. Heat and redness are results of increased blood flow, and swelling results from increased formation of interstitial tissue fluid because of increased permeability of the capillaries. In other tissues, such as skin (in which inflammation was first described), the increased production of tissue fluid results in swelling. Because the dental pulp is within a rigid, noncompliant chamber, it cannot swell, and the increased interstitial fluid formation results in an increase in tissue fluid pressure.

At one time, it was thought that this rise in interstitial fluid pressure would spread rapidly and strangle vessels entering the root canal at the apical foramen. Closer study has revealed that this is not the case. Elevations in tissue fluid pressure remain localized to the injured area. A short distance from the injury, tissue fluid pressure is maintained within normal limits. As interstitial fluid pressure rises, the intraluminal (inside) pressure of the local capillaries increases to balance this so that the vessels remain patent. During the response to injury, the gradients by which nutrients and wastes leave and enter the capillaries change to allow greater exchange. At the same time these changes occur in the capillaries, lymphatic vessels become more heavily employed, removing excess tissue fluid and debris. In addition, anastomoses in the microvascular bed allow blood to be shunted around an area of injury, so that the oxygenation and nutrition of nearby uninjured tissue are not compromised. If the cause of the injury is removed, these processes gradually return the vasculature to normal and repair or regeneration can take place. If the injury persists and increases in size, this tissue necroses. This necrosis can remain localized as a pulpal abscess, although it more often spreads throughout the pulp. The necrosis extends as the toxins from the carious lesion diffuse through the tissue.

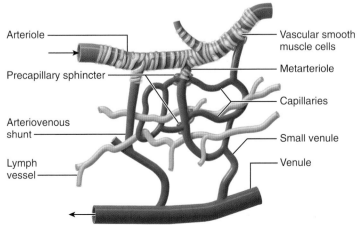

Fig. 1.17 Schematic of the pulpal vasculature. Smooth muscle cells that surround vessels and precapillary sphincters selectively control blood flow. Arteriovenous shunts bypass capillary beds.

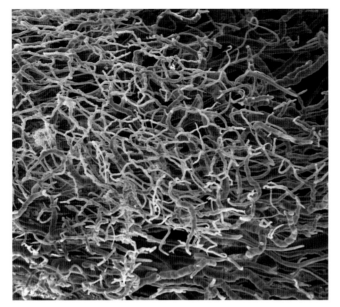

Fig. 1.18 The dense capillary bed in the subodontoblastic region is shown by resin cast preparation and scanning electron microscopy. (Courtesy Dr. C. Kockapan.)

The vascular changes seen in inflammation are largely mediated by local nerves. The sympathetic fibers through the precapillary sphincters can alter the pressure, flow, and distribution of blood. Sensory nerve fibers release a number of neuropeptides, most prominently calcitonin gene–related peptide (CGRP) and substance P. (These names are of historic origin and unrelated to the function of these molecules in this setting.) The release of these neuropeptides comes about through axon reflexes, whereby one branch of a sensory nerve stimulated by the injury causes the release of the peptides by another branch. This mechanism, in which excitation of sensory elements results in increased blood flow and increased capillary permeability, is known as *neurogenic inflammation.*

INNERVATION

The second and third divisions of the trigeminal nerve (V_2 and V_3) provide the principal sensory innervation to the pulp of maxillary and mandibular teeth, respectively. Mandibular premolars can also receive sensory branches from the mylohyoid nerve of V_3, which is principally a motor nerve. Branches from this nerve reach the teeth via small foramina on the lingual aspect of the mandible. Mandibular molars occasionally receive sensory innervation from the second and third cervical spinal nerves (C2 and C3). This can create difficulties in anesthetizing these teeth with an inferior dental block injection only.

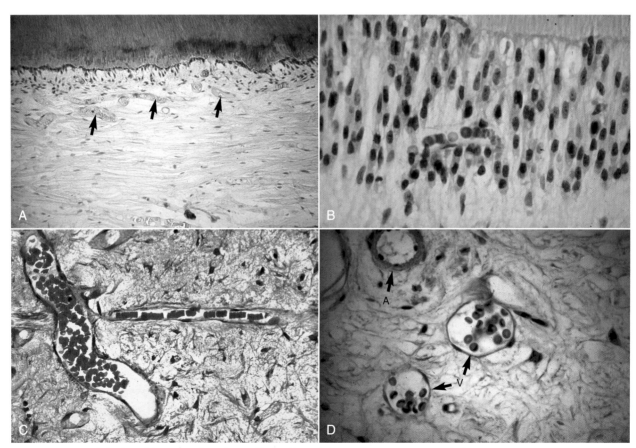

Fig. 1.19 **A,** Subodontoblastic capillary plexus. **B,** Capillary within the odontoblast layer. **C,** Branching capillaries in subodontoblastic plexus. **D,** Arteriole *(A)* and venules *(V)* in the peripheral pulp. (Courtesy Dr. H. Trowbridge.)

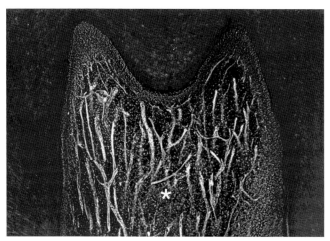

Fig. 1.20 Distribution of lymphatics. Scanning electron micrograph of secondary and back-scattered electrons after specific immune staining. (From Matsumoto Y, Zhang B, Kato S: *Microsc Res Tech* 56:50, 2002.)

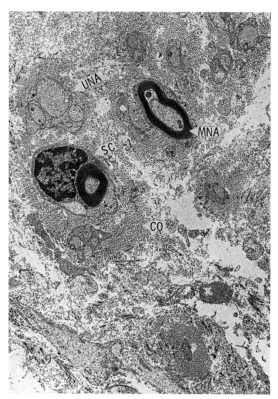

Fig. 1.22 Pulp nerves in region of the pulp core. A group of unmyelinated *(UNA)* and myelinated *(MNA)* nerve axons are shown in cross section. A Schwann cell *(SC)* associated with one of the myelinated axons is evident. Nerves are surrounded by collagen fibers *(CO)*.

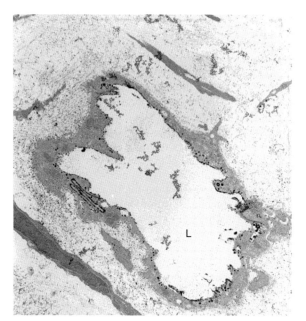

Fig. 1.21 Transmission electron micrograph of a lymphatic vessel *(L)* in the peripheral pulp. (From Matsumoto Y, Zhang B, Kato S: Lymphatic networks in the periodontal tissue and dental pulp as revealed by histochemical study, *Microsc Res Tech* 56:50, 2002.)

parasympathetic innervation of the pulp. This is not unusual. All tissues have an autonomic innervation, but not always from both divisions.

Neuroanatomy
Pulpal and Dentinal Nerves

Sensory nerves supplying the dental pulp contain both myelinated and unmyelinated axons (Fig. 1.22). The myelinated axons are almost all narrow, slow-conducting Aδ axons (1 to 6 µm in diameter) associated with nociception. A small percentage of the myelinated axons (1% to 5%) are faster-conducting Aβ axons (6 to 12 µm in diameter). In other tissues, these larger fibers can be proprioceptive or mechanoreceptive. Their role in the pulp is uncertain, but it is now known from other tissues that, in inflammation, these Aβ axons can be recruited to the pain system. Before they terminate, all the myelinated axons lose their myelin sheath and terminate as small, unmyelinated branches either below the odontoblasts, around the odontoblasts, or alongside the odontoblast process in the dentinal tubule (Fig. 1.23).[31] Beneath the odontoblast layer, these terminating fibers form the subodontoblastic plexus of Raschkow (Fig. 1.24).

The nerves that enter the dentinal tubules do not synapse with the process but remain in close proximity with it for part of its length. Approximately 27% of the tubules in the area of the pulp horn of a young, mature tooth contain an intratubular nerve. These nerves occur less often in the middle (11%) and cervical portions (8%) of the crown and not at all in the root.[32]

Cell bodies of trigeminal nerves are located in the trigeminal ganglion. Dendrites from these nerves synapse with neurons in the trigeminal sensory nucleus in the brainstem. Second-order neurons here travel to specific nuclei in the thalamus. Third-order neurons and their branches reach the sensory cortex and a number of other higher centers.

Pulp also receives sympathetic (motor) innervation from T1 and, to some extent, C8 and T2 via the superior cervical ganglion. These nerves enter the pulp space alongside the main pulp blood vessels and are distributed with them. They maintain the vasomotor tone in the precapillary sphincters, which control the pressure and distribution of blood. The presence of parasympathetic nerve fibers in the pulp has been controversial. The current consensus is that there is no

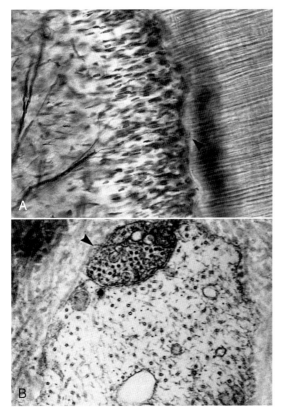

Fig. 1.23 **A,** Silver-stained section of pulp in a young human molar demonstrates arborization of nerves in the subodontoblastic region and a nerve *(arrow)* passing between odontoblasts into the predentin area. **B,** Transmission electron micrograph demonstrates an unmyelinated nerve axon *(arrow)* alongside the odontoblast process in the dentin tubule at the level of the predentin. (**A,** Courtesy Dr. S. Bernick.)

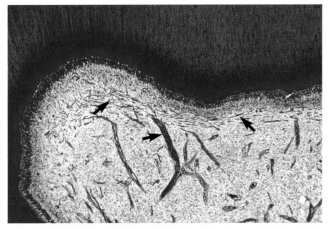

Fig. 1.24 Raschkow's subodontoblastic plexus *(arrows)* stained with silver.

Their incidence is higher in predentin than in mineralized dentin.

Developmental Aspects of Pulp Innervation

The types and relative number of nerves depend on the state of tooth maturity. Myelinated nerves enter the pulp at about the same time as unmyelinated nerves but in most instances do not form the subodontoblastic plexus of Raschkow until

some time after tooth eruption. As a result, there are significant variations in the responses of partially developed teeth to pulp vitality tests. *This undermines the value of stimulatory tests for determining pulp status in young patients, particularly after trauma.*

The number of pulpal nerves diminishes with age. The significance of this reduction in terms of responses to vitality testing is undetermined.

Pathways of Transmission from Pulp to Central Nervous System

Mechanical, thermal, and chemical stimuli initiate an impulse that travels along the pulpal axons in the maxillary (V_2) or mandibular (V_3) branches of the trigeminal nerve to the trigeminal (gasserian) ganglion, which contains the cell body of the neuron. Dendrites from the ganglion then pass centrally and synapse with second-order neurons in the trigeminal nuclear complex located at the base of the medulla and the upper end of the spinal cord. Most of the activity that originates in the dental pulp is conducted along axons that synapse with neurons in the spinal portion of the complex, most notably the subnucleus caudalis.

Many peripheral axons from different sites synapse on a single secondary neuron, a phenomenon known as *convergence.* Activity in a single synapse does not result in excitation of the second-order neuron. Activity in many synapses must summate to reach the threshold of the second-order neuron. The activation of the second-order neuron is also affected by fibers from the midbrain that belong to the endogenous opioid system. These, when active, reduce the activity of the second-order neurons. Thus, noxious input is modulated, explaining why the pain experience is not always closely related to the degree of peripheral noxious stimulation. Axons from the second-order neurons cross the midline and synapse in thalamic nuclei. From here, third-order neurons pass information to a variety of higher centers, the sensory cortex being only one of them. The distribution of noxious input centrally and the presence of a pain-modulating system descending from higher centers provide the broad framework for understanding and controlling pain. As a result of persistent noxious input, the properties of second-order neurons can change. These changes can be used to explain some of the complexities of diagnosing and treating pain as described in other sections of this text.

Theories of Dentin Hypersensitivity

Pain elicited by scraping or cutting of dentin or by the application of cold or hypertonic solutions to exposed dentin gives the impression that there may be a nerve pathway from the central nervous system to the dentinoenamel junction (DEJ). However, no direct pathway is present. The application of pain-producing substances, such as histamine, acetylcholine, or potassium chloride, to exposed dentin surface fails to produce pain. Eliciting pain from exposed dentin by heat or cold is not blocked by local anesthetics. At one time it was thought that dentin sensitivity was due to sensory nerves within the dentinal tubules.

Currently, two explanations for peripheral dentin sensitivity have broad acceptance (Fig. 1.25). One is that stimuli that are effective in eliciting pain from dentin cause fluid flow through the dentinal tubules.[33] This disturbance results in the activation of nociceptors in the inner dentin and peripheral pulp.

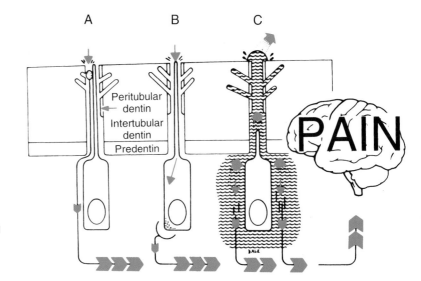

Fig. 1.25 Schematic drawing of theoretic mechanisms of dentin sensitivity. **A,** Classic theory (direct stimulation of nerve fibers in the dentin). **B,** Odontoblasts as a mediator between the stimuli and the nerve fibers. **C,** Fluid movement as proposed in hydrodynamic theory. (Modified from Torneck CD: Dentin-pulp complex. In Ten Cate AR, editor, *Oral histology,* ed 4, St Louis, 1994, Mosby.)

Several observations support this "hydrodynamic hypothesis." In experiments on extracted teeth, it has been shown that hot, cold, and osmotic stimuli cause fluid flow through dentin. In human subjects, the success of solutions in inducing pain is related to the osmotic pressure of the solution. Exposed dentin that is sensitive in patients has patent dentinal tubules.[34]

In exposed dentin that is not sensitive, the dentinal tubules are occluded. Substances and techniques that occlude dentinal tubules in sensitive dentin eliminate or reduce the sensitivity. A second explanation is that some substances can diffuse through the dentin and act directly on pulpal nerves. Evidence for this largely comes from animal experiments, which show that the activation of pulpal nerves is sometimes related to the chemical composition of a stimulating solution rather than its osmotic pressure. These are not mutually exclusive hypotheses; both may apply, and both should be addressed in treating sensitive dentin.

AGE CHANGES IN THE DENTAL PULP AND DENTIN

Secondary dentin is laid down throughout life. As a result, both the pulp chamber and root canals become smaller, sometimes to the point where they are no longer visible on radiographs. As age increases, more peritubular dentin is laid down, often completely occluding the dentinal tubules in the periphery (sclerotic dentin). As a result of these processes, the permeability of the dentin is reduced. The pulp tissue itself becomes less cellular and less vascular and contains fewer nerve fibers. Between the ages of 20 and 70, cell density decreases by approximately 50%. This reduction affects all cells, from the highly differentiated odontoblast to the undifferentiated stem cell.

REPAIR AND REGENERATION

The dental pulp can respond positively to external irritants, including the toxins released during dental caries. Inflammation is part of the response that leads to the formation of new dentin. This occurs in two forms: (1) tertiary response dentin, which is formed by the original odontoblasts and is tubular in structure, and (2) tertiary reparative dentin, which is formed after the original odontoblasts have been killed and is created by odontoblasts differentiated from stem cells. The type of dentin laid down is determined by the intensity of the stimulus.

Stem cells can be isolated from exfoliated deciduous teeth (known as "SHED" cells) and have been shown in an animal model to form new dentin and pulp in slices of tooth from which the pulp has been removed (Fig. 1.14).[35] This leads to the happy prospect that the pulp may be regenerated in pulpless teeth.

PERIRADICULAR TISSUES

The periodontium, the tissue surrounding and investing the root of the tooth, consists of the cementum, PDL, and alveolar bone (Fig. 1.26). These tissues originate from the dental follicle that surrounds the enamel organ; their formation is initiated when root development begins.[36] After the tooth has erupted, the cervical portion of the tooth is in contact with the epithelium of the gingiva, which, in combination with reduced dental epithelium on the enamel, forms the dentogingival junction. When intact, this junction protects the underlying periodontium from potential irritants in the oral cavity. The pulp and the periodontium form a continuum at sites along the root where blood vessels enter and exit the pulp at the apical foramen and lateral and accessory canals (Fig. 1.27).

Cementum

Cementum is a bonelike tissue that covers the root and provides attachment for the principal periodontal fibers. The several types of cementum that have been identified are as follows:

1. *Primary acellular intrinsic fiber cementum.* This is the first cementum formed, and it is present before principal periodontal fibers are fully formed. It extends from the cervical margin to the cervical third of the tooth in some

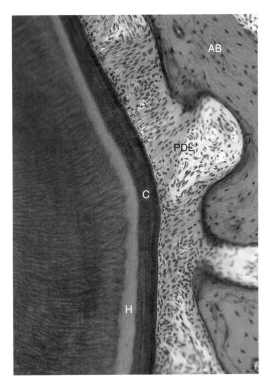

Fig. 1.26 Peripheral radicular dentin (*H*, hyaline layer), cementum *(C)*, periodontal ligament *(PDL)*, and alveolar bone *(AB)*.

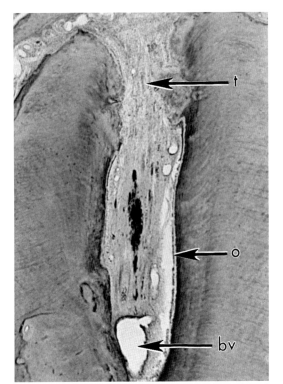

Fig. 1.27 Apical region of maxillary incisor showing apical foramen. *t*, Transitional tissue between periodontal ligament and pulp; *o*, odontoblasts; *bv*, blood vessel.

teeth and around the entire root in others (incisors and cuspids). It is more mineralized on the surface than near the dentin and contains collagen produced initially by cementoblasts and later by fibroblasts.

2. *Primary acellular extrinsic fiber cementum.* This is cementum that continues to be formed about the primary periodontal fibers after they have been incorporated into primary acellular intrinsic fiber cementum.

3. *Secondary cellular intrinsic fiber cementum.* This cementum is bonelike in appearance and only plays a minor role in fiber attachment. It occurs most often in the apical part of the root of premolars and molars.

4. *Secondary cellular mixed fiber cementum.* This is an adaptive type of cellular cementum that incorporates periodontal fibers as they continue to develop. It is variable in its distribution and extent and can be recognized by the inclusion of cementocytes, its laminated appearance, and the presence of cementoid on its surface.

5. *Acellular afibrillar cementum.* This is the cementum sometimes seen overlapping enamel, which plays no role in fiber attachment.

Cementum is similar to bone but harder and thus resists resorption during tooth movement. The junction between the cementum and the dentin (CDJ) that forms the apical constriction is ill defined and not uniform throughout its circumference. Biologic principles suggest that the most appropriate point to end a root canal preparation is at the junction of the pulp and periodontium, which occurs at the apical constriction. *Although many practitioners debate the probabilities and practicalities of achieving this goal, most agree that it is essential to measure canal length accurately and to restrict all procedures to a canal length that estimates this point as closely as possible.*

Although dentin is harder than bone and resorbs more slowly, it does resorb in periapical inflammatory lesions, often resulting in loss of the apical constriction. Occasionally, more rapid resorption of unknown cause is seen (idiopathic resorption), but this is often self-limiting.

Cementoenamel Junction
The junction of cementum and enamel at the cervix of the tooth varies in its arrangement even around a single tooth. Sometimes cementum overlies enamel and vice versa. When there is a gap between the cementum and the enamel, the exposed dentin may be sensitive.

Periodontal Ligament
As is dental pulp, the periodontal ligament is a specialized connective tissue.[36] Its function relates in part to the presence of specially arranged bundles of collagen fibers that support the tooth in the socket and absorb the forces of occlusion, preventing them from being transmitted to the surrounding bone. The PDL space is small, varying from an average of 0.21 mm in young teeth to 0.15 mm in older teeth. The uniformity of its width (as seen in a radiograph) is one of the criteria used to determine its health.

Lining the periodontal space are cementoblasts and osteoblasts. Interwoven between the principal periodontal fibers is a loose connective tissue that contains fibroblasts, stem cells, macrophages, osteoclasts, blood vessels, nerves, and lymphatics. Epithelial cell rests of Malassez are also present (Fig. 1.28). As already noted, these cells are of no known

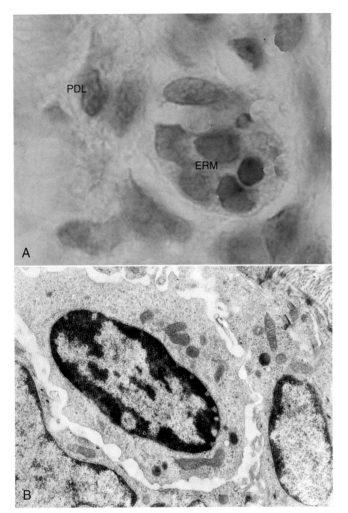

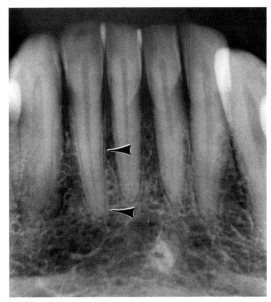

Fig. 1.29 Mandibular anterior teeth with normal, uniform periodontal ligament (PDL) space and identifiable lamina dura *(arrows)*. This usually, but not always, indicates the absence of periradicular inflammation.

Fig. 1.28 A, Epithelial rest of Malassez *(ERM)* in periodontal ligament *(PDL).* **B,** Transmission electron micrograph of epithelial rests. (From Cerri PS, Katchburian E: *J Periodont Res* 40:365, 2005.)

significance in the healthy periodontium, but during inflammatory states they can proliferate and give rise to cyst formation.

The vasculature of the periodontium is extensive and complex. Arterioles that supply the PDL arise from the superior and inferior alveolar branches of the maxillary artery in the cancellous bone. These arterioles pass through small openings in the alveolar bone of the socket, at times accompanied by nerves, and extend upward and downward throughout the periodontal space. They are more prevalent in posterior than anterior teeth. Other vessels arise from the gingiva or from dental vessels that supply the pulp. These latter vessels branch and extend upward into the periodontal space before the pulpal vessels pass through the apical foramen. The degree of collateral blood supply to the PDL and the depth of its cell resources impart an excellent potential for its repair subsequent to injury, a potential that is retained for life in the absence of systemic or prolonged local disease.

The periodontium receives both autonomic and sensory innervation. Autonomic nerves are sympathetics arising from the superior cervical ganglion and terminating in the smooth muscle of the periodontal arterioles. Activation of the sympathetic fibers induces constriction of the vessels. As in the pulp, there is no convincing evidence that a parasympathetic nerve supply exists.

Sensory nerves that supply the periodontium arise from the second and third divisions of the trigeminal nerve (V_2 and V_3). They are mixed nerves of large and small diameter. Unmyelinated sensory fibers terminate as nociceptive free endings. Large fibers are mechanoreceptors that terminate in special endings throughout the ligament but are in greatest concentration in the apical third of the periodontal space. These are highly sensitive, recording pressures in the ligament associated with tooth movement. They allow patients to identify teeth with acute periodontitis with some precision.

Alveolar Bone

The bone of the jaws that supports the teeth is referred to as the *alveolar process.* Bone that lines the socket and into which the principal periodontal fibers are anchored is referred to as the *alveolar bone proper* (bundle bone, cribriform plate). Alveolar bone is perforated to accommodate vessels, nerves, and investing connective tissues that pass from the cancellous portion of the alveolar process to the periodontal space. Despite these perforations, alveolar bone proper is denser than the surrounding cancellous bone and has a distinct opaque appearance when seen in periapical radiographs. On the radiograph, alveolar bone proper is referred to as *lamina dura* (Fig. 1.29). Its continuity is equated with periodontal health and its perforation with disease. Radiographic changes associated with periradicular inflammatory disease usually follow rather than accompany the disease. Significant bone loss is necessary before a radiographic image is seen.

Alveolar bone proper is principally lamellar and continually adapts to the stress of tooth movements. Because pressures are not constant, bone is constantly remodeling (by resorption and apposition).

REFERENCES

1. Koling A: Freeze fracture electron microscopy of simultaneous odontoblast exocytosis and endocytosis in human permanent teeth, *Arch Oral Biol* 32:153, 1987.
2. Kawasaki K, Tanaka S, Ishikawa T: On the daily incremental lines in human dentine, *Arch Oral Biol* 24:939, 1980.
3. Luan X, Ito Y, Diekwisch TGH: Evolution and development of Hertwig's epithelial root sheath, *Dev Dyn* 58:1167, 2006.
4. Hamamoto Y, Nakajima T, Ozawa H, et al: Production of amelogenin by enamel epithelium of Hertwig's root sheath, *Oral Surg Oral Med Oral Path Oral Radiol Endod* 81:703, 1996.
5. Cerri PS, Katchburian E: Apoptosis in the epithelial cells of the rests of Malassez of the periodontium of rat molars, *J Periodontal Res* 40:365, 2005.
6. Ten Cate AR: The epithelial cell rests of Malassez and genesis of the dental cyst, *Oral Surg Oral Med Oral Pathol* 34:956, 1972.
7. Kuttler Y: Microscopic investigation of root apices, *J Am Dent Assoc* 50:544, 1955.
8. Saunders RL: X-ray microscopy of the periodontal and dental pulp vessels in the monkey and in man, *Oral Surg Oral Med Oral Pathol* 22:503, 1966.
9. Lisi S, Peterkova R, Peterka M, et al: Tooth morphogenesis and pattern of odontoblast differentiation, *Connect Tissue Res* 44(suppl 1):167, 2003.
10. Lesot H, Lisi S, Peterkova R, et al: Epigenetic signals during odontoblast differentiation, *Adv Dent Res* 15:8, 2001.
11. Sasaki T, Garant PR: Structure and organization of odontoblasts, *Anat Rec* 245:235, 1996.
12. Couve E: Ultrastructural changes during the life cycle of human odontoblasts, *Arch Oral Biol* 31:643, 1986.
13. Franquin JC, Remusat M, Abou Hashieh I, et al: Immunocytochemical detection of apoptosis in human odontoblasts, *Eur J Oral Sci* 106(suppl 1):384, 1998.
14. Veerayutthwilai O, Byers MR, Pham T-T T, et al: Differential regulation of immune responses by odontoblasts, *Oral Microbiol Immunol* 22:5, 2007.
15. Magloire H, Maurin JC, Couble ML, et al: Dental pain and odontoblasts: facts and hypotheses, *J Orofac Pain* 24:335, 2010.
16. Sole-Magdalena A, Revuelta EG, Menenez-Diaz I, et al: Human odontoblasts express transient receptor protein and acid-sensing ion channel mechanosensor proteins, *Microsc Res Tech* 74:457, 2011.
17. Shi S, Bartold PM, Miura M, et al: The efficacy of mesenchymal stem cells to regenerate and repair dental structures, *Orthod Craniofac Res* 8:191, 2005.
18. Smith A: Vitality of the dentin-pulp complex in health and disease: growth factors as key mediators, *J Dent Ed* 67:678, 2003.
19. Jontell M, Bergenholtz G: Accessory cells in the immune defense of the dental pulp, *Proc Finn Dent Soc* 88:345, 1992.
20. Zhang J, Kawashima N, Suda H, et al: The existence of CD11c sentinel and F4/80 interstitial dendritic cells in dental pulp and their dynamics and functional properties, *Int Immunol* 18:1375, 2006.
21. Butler WT, Ritchie HH, Bronckers AL: Extracellular matrix proteins of dentine, *Ciba Found Symp* 205:107, 1997.
22. Linde A: Dentin matrix proteins: composition and possible functions in calcification, *Anat Rec* 224:154, 1989.
23. Kramer IRH: The vascular architecture of the human dental pulp, *Arch Oral Biol* 2:177, 1960.
24. Koling A, Rask-Andersen H: The blood capillaries in the subodontoblastic region of the human dental pulp, as demonstrated by freeze-fracturing, *Acta Odont Scand* 41:333, 1983.
25. Iijima T, Zhang J-Q: Three-dimensional wall structure and the innervation of dental pulp blood vessels, *Microsc Res Tech* 56:32, 2002.
26. Marchetti C, Poggi P, Calligaro A, et al: Lymphatic vessels in the healthy human dental pulp, *Acta Anat (Basel)* 140:329, 1991.
27. Matsumoto Y, Zhang B, Kato S: Lymphatic networks in the periodontal tissue and dental pulp as revealed by histochemical study, *Microsc Res Tech* 56:50, 2002.
28. Haug SR, Heyeraas KJ: Modulation of dental inflammation by the sympathetic nervous system, *J Dent Res* 85:488-495, 2006.
29. Heyeraas KJ, Berggreen E: Interstitial fluid pressure in normal and inflamed pulp, *Crit Rev Oral Biol Med* 10:328, 1999.
30. Kim S: Neurovascular interactions in the dental pulp in health and inflammation, *J Endod* 16:48-53, 1990.
31. Arwill T, Edwall L, Lilja J, et al: Ultrastructure of nerves in the dentinal-pulp border zone after sensory and autonomic nerve transection in the cat, *Acta Odont Scand* 31:273, 1973.
32. Lilja T: Innervation of different parts of predentin and dentin in young human premolars, *Acta Odont Scand* 37:339, 1979.
33. Brannstrom M, Astrom A: The hydrodynamics of the dentine: its possible relationship to dentinal pain, *Int Dent J* 22:219, 1972.
34. Holland GR: Morphological features of dentine and pulp related to dentine sensitivity, *Arch Oral Biol* 39(suppl 1):3S-11S, 1994.
35. Sakai VT, Zhang Z, Dong Z, et al: SHED differentiate into functional odontoblasts and epithelium, *J Dent Res* 89:791, 2010.
36. Cho MI, Garant PR: Development and general structure of the periodontium, *Periodontology 2000* 24:9, 2000.

Protecting the pulp and promoting tooth maturation

Ashraf F. Fouad, Anthony J. Smith

CHAPTER OUTLINE

Definitions
Iatrogenic Effects on the Dental Pulp
Protecting the Pulp from the Effects of Materials

Vital Pulp Therapies
The Open Apex

LEARNING OBJECTIVES

After reading this chapter, the student should be able to:

1. Describe pulp protection and pulp therapy.
2. Understand the special physiologic and structural characteristics of the pulp-dentin complex and how they affect the pulpal response to injury.
3. Describe the reparative mechanisms of the pulp, including immune responses and tertiary dentin formation.
4. Describe the effects of dental procedures and materials on the pulp.
5. Appreciate the significance of microleakage and smear layer on pulp response.
6. Describe the indications and procedures for vital pulp therapy.
7. Discuss the effects of pulpal injury in teeth with developing roots.
8. Describe diagnosis and case assessment of immature teeth with pulp injury.
9. Describe the techniques for vital pulp therapy (apexogenesis) and root-end closure (apexification).
10. Describe the prognosis for vital pulp therapy and root-end closure.
11. Describe the technique for pulp revascularization and the goals of regenerative endodontic therapy.
12. Recognize the potential of tissue engineering techniques in regenerating pulpal tissue.
13. Consider restoration of the treated immature tooth.

DEFINITIONS

Pulp Protection

Dental caries represents one of the principal challenges to the health of the dental pulp, although its treatment may well exacerbate the challenge. Cavity preparation and associated procedures, the toxicity of restorative materials and, significantly, the continuing challenge from leakage of bacteria and their products at the margins of restorations can contribute further damage to that caused by the original caries. This may tip the balance from a reversible to an irreversible pulpitis; it also highlights the importance of a holistic approach to management of dental caries, which aims to restore the functional integrity of the tooth while preserving its vitality and protect the pulp from further damage.

A fundamental consideration in pulp protection is the recognition that infection is a key driver of inflammation, which often determines the outcomes for pulp survival. Thus, the pulp always is likely to be inflamed when bacteria from dental caries are present, and their control should be a significant feature of any treatment planning. Even in teeth with white spot lesions and for which restorative procedures are not indicated, pulpal inflammation is frequently present (Fig. 2.1).[1]

When treatment plans are designed for patients who have several teeth with carious lesions, especially when lesions are extensive, a "triage" approach is preferable. In this approach, active caries is removed and good temporary restorations are placed at an early stage, allowing the pulp the maximum opportunity for recovery.

Vital Pulp Therapy

Maintenance of pulp vitality should always be the goal in treatment planning, and considerable interest is developing in the concept of regenerative endodontics for complete or partial pulp tissue regeneration. With mechanical exposure of the dental pulp by trauma or during cavity preparation, the pulp may be protected and its vitality maintained by immediately covering it (pulp capping) and placing a restoration, thereby avoiding root canal treatment. If the exposure is large or seriously contaminated, it may be possible to remove the more superficial diseased part of the pulp (pulpotomy), cap the remaining pulp, and place a restoration. This approach probably has the best prognosis in incompletely formed teeth (especially primary teeth) when the root has not yet reached its full length (apexogenesis); however, it can also be considered for fully formed and permanent teeth with reversible

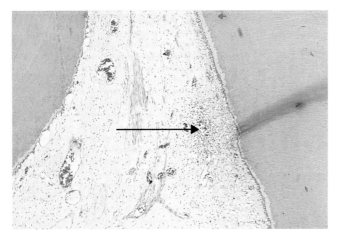

Fig. 2.1 Pulpal inflammation *(arrow)* at the base of the tubules beneath a white spot lesion in enamel.

pulpitis. In teeth with necrotic pulps and incomplete root formation, apical closure (but not root elongation) can be obtained by apexification. It is important to recognize, however, that pulp inflammation is a progressive disease, and the use of regenerative approaches to maintain pulp vitality requires a good understanding of the interplay of biologic factors influencing regenerative events, in addition to appropriate case selection. Such approaches may not be suitable for all cases, especially those showing deep pulp inflammation involving the radicular tissue, and the correlation of clinical symptoms with the pathophysiologic status of the dental pulp remains a significant challenge. In the future, tissue engineering may allow replacement of part or all of the pulp with new tissue[2,3] in the clinical setting.

Regeneration, Revascularization, and Revitalization

Pulp necrosis is clearly a terminal, irreversible pathosis of this tissue. In cases of pulp necrosis after complete tooth maturation, the tooth may survive in a state of normal health after root canal therapy. However, for the immature tooth, this treatment may be difficult to perform, and the tooth may be too weak to withstand normal function because of the thin dentinal wall and short root length. Therefore, techniques to control intracanal infection and induce regrowth of connective tissue that would then promote normal root maturation have been introduced in the past few years.[4] The use of the terms *revascularization, revitalization,* and *regeneration* to describe the result of these procedures has been open to some debate in the field. Most authors would use the term *revascularization* or *revitalization,* because animal studies have not shown that a functional dental pulp actually regenerates after these techniques.[5]

Table 2.1 presents the principal terms currently used in pulpal protection and vital pulp therapy.[6]

IATROGENIC EFFECTS ON THE DENTAL PULP

Local Anesthesia

When most local anesthetics containing vasoconstrictors are used in restorative dentistry, the blood flow to the pulp is reduced to less than half of its normal rate.[9] In the case of

Table 2.1 Definitions of the principal terms used in pulpal protection and vital pulp therapy

Term	Definition
Pulp cap	Treatment of an exposed vital pulp in which the pulpal wound is sealed with a dental material, such as calcium hydroxide or mineral trioxide aggregate (MTA), to facilitate the formation of reparative dentin and maintenance of a vital pulp.
Direct pulp cap	A dental material placed directly on a mechanical or traumatic vital pulp exposure.
Step-wise caries excavation	Incremental removal of caries over a period of time to allow pulpal healing and to minimize exposure[7]
Pulpectomy (pulp extirpation)	The complete surgical removal of the vital pulp.
Pulpotomy (pulp amputation)	Surgical removal of the coronal portion of a vital pulp as a means of preserving vitality of the remaining radicular portion; pulpotomy usually is performed as an emergency procedure for temporary relief of symptoms or as a therapeutic measure.
Partial pulpotomy (shallow pulpotomy; Cvek pulpotomy)	Surgical removal of a small diseased portion of vital pulp as a means of preserving the remaining coronal and radicular pulp tissues.
Apexification	Induction of a calcified or an artificial barrier in a root with an open apex or the continued apical development of an incompletely formed root in teeth with a necrotic pulp.
Apexogenesis	A vital pulp therapy procedure performed to enable continued physiologic development and formation of the root end; the term frequently used to describe vital pulp therapy that encourages the continuation of this process.
Pulp regeneration	The ability to recreate lost or damaged pulp tissue
Pulp revascularization	The restoration of blood supply in the pulp space
Pulp revitalization[8]	Recreation of vital connective tissue in the pulp space

From the American Association of Endodontists: *Glossary of endodontic terms,* Chicago, 2012, The Association.

lidocaine with epinephrine, this effect is entirely a result of the vasoconstrictor.[10] In procedures on teeth with pulps that are already compromised, this may be an additional stressor. A healthy pulp may survive episodes of ischemia lasting for 1 hour or longer. An already ischemic pulp subjected to severe injury may hemorrhage (blush) when subjected to trauma such as that associated with full crown preparation without the use of an adequate coolant.

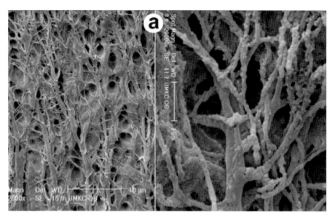

Fig. 2.2 Low- and high-power scanning electron microscopy (SEM) images of dentin after surface etching to reveal the intricate network of odontoblast processes and lateral branches permeating dentin matrix and facilitating communication by odontoblasts. (Lu Y, Xie Y, Zhang S, et al: DMP1-targeted Cre expression in odontoblasts and osteocytes, *J Dent Res* 86(4):320-325, 2007.)

Cavity/Crown Preparation

An appreciation of the cellular structure of the dentin-pulp complex is critical for cavity/crown preparation if further tissue injury is to be minimized and pulp vitality maintained. This is elegantly illustrated in Fig. 2.2, which demonstrates the intimate contact between odontoblasts, through their processes, and the dentin matrix, highlighting the communication between these cells and their environment.

Any surgical intervention to the dentin during cavity preparation may result in some degree of injury to the odontoblasts and their processes. Although this cannot be avoided during cavity preparation, it is important to recognize the consequences of such treatment and to minimize the extent of injury. It is also important to recognize that dentin matrix is not comprised simply of structural components (e.g., collagen and mineral); rather, it also contains a diverse mixture of biologically active molecules, including growth factors, cytokines, and other constituents. Both matrix dissolution during the carious process and the cutting and etching of the dentin during cavity preparation can lead to release of these molecules, with the consequent potential for stimulation of cellular responses in the pulp.[11]

Heat

Frictional heat is produced whenever a revolving bur or stone contacts tooth structure. Until the advent of the high-speed handpiece, enamel and dentin preparation involved heavy torque, low rotational speeds, and steel burs that were not cooled with water. Consequently, vital dentin was often scorched, and pulps were injured as a result of extreme heat (Fig. 2.3).[12]

Dentin is an effective insulator; for this reason, careful cutting with adequate cooling is less likely to damage the pulp unless the thickness of the dentin between preparation and pulp is less than 1 mm.[13] Even then, the inflammatory response may be mild (Fig. 2.4). The greatest amount of frictional heat is generated with a large diamond stone when teeth are prepared for a full crown, and the pulp is particularly at risk of injury. The heat generated may also have a desiccating effect by "boiling" away dentinal tubule fluid at the dentin surface.

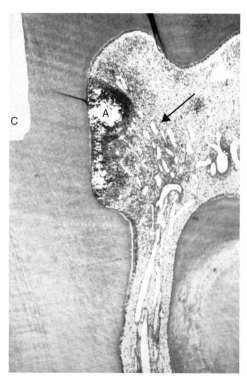

Fig. 2.3 Localized inflammation *(arrow)* and abscess *(A)* formation beneath a deep cavity preparation *(C)* without adequate coolant. (Courtesy Dr. H. Trowbridge.)

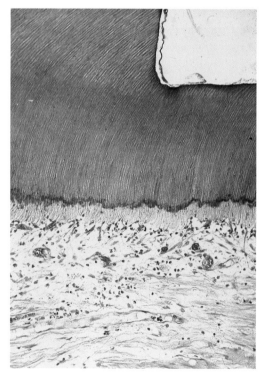

Fig. 2.4 Mild inflammation beneath a deep cavity preparation with adequate coolant. (Courtesy Dr. H. Trowbridge.)

The "blushing" of dentin during cavity or crown preparation is thought to be due to frictional heat resulting in vascular injury (hemorrhage) in the pulp.[14] The dentin takes on an underlying pinkish hue soon after the operative procedure, reflecting significant vascular injury. Crown preparation **23** performed without the use of a coolant leads to a marked reduction in pulpal blood flow, presumably because of vascular stasis and thrombosis. The amount of heat produced during cutting is determined by the sharpness of the bur, the amount of pressure exerted on the bur or stone, and the length of time the cutting instrument contacts the tooth structure. The safest way to prepare tooth structure is to make sure the bur-dentin interface is constantly wet.

The use of laser beams to fuse enamel and reduce the likelihood of carious invasion has been suggested.[15] Different lasers with different energy levels may also be used to remove caries. Lasers generate heat and increase the intrapulpal temperature. The heat generated varies with a number of parameters, but can be reduced by water cooling to a level similar to that for a water-cooled high-speed drill.[16]

Cavity Depth/Remaining Dentin Thickness

Dentin permeability increases exponentially with increasing cavity depth, because both the diameter and density of dentinal tubules increase with cavity depth (Fig. 2.5).[17] Thus the deeper the cavity, the greater the tubular surface area into which potentially toxic substances can penetrate and diffuse to the pulp. The length of the dentinal tubules beneath the cavity is also important. The farther substances diffuse, the more they are diluted and buffered by the dentinal fluid.

A remaining dentin thickness of 1 mm is often regarded as sufficient to shield the pulp from most forms of irritation. In noncarious teeth, tertiary reactionary dentin is formed most rapidly when the remaining dentin thickness is between 0.5 and 0.25 mm.[18] With a narrower remaining dentin thickness, odontoblast survival is compromised, and any regenerative response would likely involve reparative dentin formation by newly differentiated cells.[19]

The effects of remaining dentin thickness on cellular responses, however, are not only a function of the diffusion of noxious stimuli to the pulp. The morphology of the odontoblast processes is of a more tapered shape, with greater thickness near the cell body of the odontoblast.[20] Deeper cavity preparations sever the odontoblast processes in their regions of greater thickness; this affects the cell's attempts to restore its membrane integrity and increases the risk of a cell leaking its contents. Cells have well-developed mechanisms for responding to mechanical stress and repairing minor breaks in the integrity of their plasma membranes; however, failure of these mechanisms can lead to disease and loss of cell viability.[21]

Cavity Drying and Cleansing[12]

A prolonged blast of compressed air aimed onto freshly exposed vital dentin causes a rapid outward movement of fluid in patent dentinal tubules through strong capillary forces. Rapid outward flow of fluid in the dentinal tubules stimulates nociceptors in the dentin pulp, thus producing pain. Rapid outward fluid movement may also result in *odontoblast displacement* (Fig. 2.6).[22] Odontoblasts are dislodged from the odontoblast layer and drawn outward into the tubules, where they undergo autolysis and disappear. Providing the pulp has not been severely injured, displaced odontoblasts may be replaced by new cells derived from stem/progenitor cells deeper in the pulp. In this way, the odontoblast layer is reconstituted by "replacement" odontoblast-like cells capable of producing tertiary reparative dentin.[23] Although drying agents

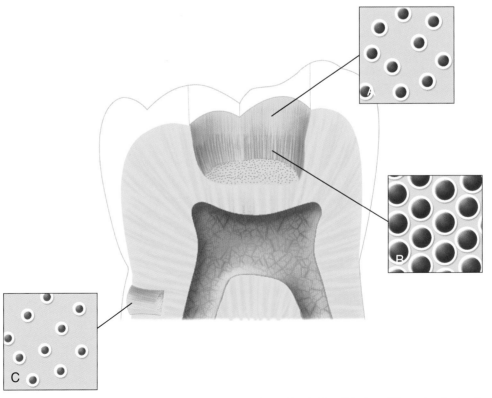

Fig. 2.5 Difference in size and number of tubules in the dentinal floor of a shallow **(A)**, deep **(B)**, and radicular dentin **(C)** cavity preparation. (From Trowbridge HO: *Dentistry* 82:22, 1982.)

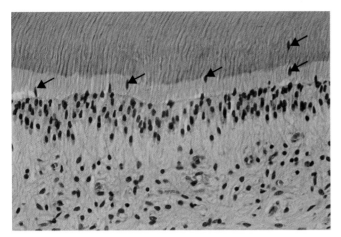

Fig. 2.6 Aspiration of odontoblasts *(arrows)* into dentinal tubules after desiccation of a cavity. (Courtesy Dr. H. Trowbridge.)

containing lipid solvents, such as acetone and ether, have been used to clean cavity floors, their rapid rate of evaporation can produce strong hydrodynamic forces in the tubules, causing odontoblast displacement. *Cavities should be dried with cotton pellets, and only short blasts of air should be carefully applied, rather than harsh chemicals.* Toxic antibacterial agents are not advisable for use on the cavity floor due to the risk of injury to the pulp or their limited broad-spectrum specificity to the microflora present. A new generation of antibacterial bonding agents for use with resin-bonded composites is emerging,[24-26] and such approaches may have merit in the control of residual bacteria. In contrast, use of antibacterial agents is of paramount importance to successful outcomes for root canal therapy, although even in the absence of vital pulp tissue within the root canal, care is required to avoid leakage of potent antibacterial agents into the periapical tissues, where they may compromise tissue vitality.

Etching Dentin/Smear Layer Removal[27-29]

Cutting dentin produces a smear layer on the cut surface consisting of fragments of microscopic mineral crystals and organic matrix debris, which may interfere with the adherence of adhesive restorative materials. Acidic cavity-cleansing products and chelating agents are often used to remove the smear layer, but their use is mainly justified only with the placement of an adhesive restoration. The smear layer does have one desirable property; by blocking the orifices of dentinal tubules, the smear plugs greatly decrease the permeability of dentin. Although the smear layer is largely impervious to bacteria, it is not a barrier to bacterial products. Complete dissolution of the smear layer opens the dentinal tubules, significantly increasing the permeability of dentin. If the dentin is left unsealed, the diffusion of irritants to the pulp may intensify and prolong the severity of pulpal reactions.

Traditionally, cavity etchants have been used based on their physicochemical properties of smear layer removal and cavity cleansing. It is now apparent, however, that they may also locally release some of the biologically active molecules contained within the dentin matrix.[30-32] Release of these molecules can signal the cellular responses, leading to stimulation of regenerative events[33]; therefore, it is important to consider the use of cavity etchants within this broader context. This has implications for the application time of these etchants,[33] which

reflects a compromise between achieving optimal smear layer removal and maximizing stimulation of regenerative cellular responses.

Other Restorative Procedures

Pulp damage may result from pinhole preparation or pin placement. Coolants do not reach the depth of the pin preparation. During pinhole preparation, there is always the risk of pulp exposure. Furthermore, friction-locked pins often produce microfractures that may extend to the pulp, subjecting the pulp to irritation and the effects of microleakage.[34,35]

Rubber-base and hydrocolloid materials do not injure the pulp. However, temperatures of up to 52°C have been recorded in the pulp during impression taking with modeling compound, and such temperatures may damage the pulp, especially if it is already inflamed.

Cooling is strongly recommended when provisional crowns are fabricated directly because of the exothermic reaction of autopolymerizing resins. *The temporary crown/cement should be left in place for a short period;* temporary cements are not stable and eventually wash out. Microleakage around temporary crowns is a common cause of postoperative sensitivity. During the cementation of crowns, inlays, and bridges, strong hydraulic forces may be exerted on the pulp as cement compresses the fluid in the dentinal tubules.

Continuous polishing of amalgam or other metallic restorations with rubber cups at high speeds causes a damaging temperature increase of up to 20°C. *Therefore, polishing with rubber wheels, points, or cups should be performed at low speeds using intermittent pressure and a coolant.*

The use of burs to remove metallic restorations can produce very high levels of frictional heat. A coolant, such as water spray or a combination of water and air, avoids a burn lesion in the pulp.

Postrestorative Hypersensitivity[36,37]

Many patients complain of hypersensitivity after a restorative procedure as a result of cumulative effects that irritate the pulp. Discomfort is usually of short duration. If the pain is prolonged, a preexisting pulpitis may have been exacerbated. If it is delayed in onset by days, the cause may be microleakage of bacterial irritants under a poorly sealed restoration. The absence of postoperative sensitivity after restoration with modern composites of both Class I and Class II preparations has been demonstrated in clinical studies, suggesting that variations in technique may be responsible for the anecdotal reports.[38,39] The use of hydroxymethacrylate/glutaraldehyde "desensitizer" does not reduce the incidence of sensitivity.[40] Self-etching, self-priming dentin bonding systems reduce the incidence of sensitivity after the restoration of deep carious cavities.[41,42]

One important clinical factor in the placement of resin restorations is the control of moisture. Applying a dental dam during the procedure is thought to help in moisture control. However, there are situations in which the restoration extends subgingivally. Proper moisture control for bonding of the restoration is difficult to achieve in these situations.

If pain is evoked by biting on a recently restored tooth, an intracoronal restoration may be exerting a strong shearing force on the dentin walls of the preparation. It is more likely to be caused by an injury to the periodontal ligament as a result of hyperocclusion. Hyperocclusion from an **25** extracoronal restoration does not injure the pulp but may cause a transient hypersensitivity.

Dental Materials
Microleakage[42-44]
The most important characteristic of any restorative material in determining its effect on the pulp is its ability to form a seal that prevents the leakage of bacteria and their products onto dentin and then into the pulp.

Cytotoxicity
Certain restorative materials are composed of chemicals that have the potential to irritate the pulp. However, when these materials are placed in a cavity, the intervening dentin usually neutralizes or prevents leachable ingredients from reaching the pulp in a high enough concentration to cause injury. For example, eugenol in zinc oxide–eugenol (ZnOE) is potentially irritating but very little can reach the pulp. Phosphoric acid is a component of silicate and zinc phosphate cements and was thought to be highly injurious to the pulp. However, the buffering capacity of dentin greatly limits the ability of hydrogen ions to reach the pulp. It is now clear that the problems that occurred after use of these materials were a result of their high degree of shrinkage and subsequent microleakage.[45]

Clearly, the thickness and permeability of dentin between a material and the pulp affect the response to the material. In addition, the penetration of some materials through dentin may be limited by the outward flow of fluid through the tubules, which is increased if the pulp is inflamed.[46] This factor has been overlooked in many in vitro studies investigating the passage of materials through dentin.

Many cytotoxicity studies examine isolated cell types in culture and do not take into account the immunocompetent cells present in the intact pulp. Materials may have a differential effect on these cells by either stimulating or inhibiting their activity.[47]

Materials are more toxic when they are placed directly on an exposed pulp. Cytotoxicity tests carried out on materials in vitro or in soft tissues may not predict the effect of these materials on the dental pulp. The toxicity of the individual components of a material may vary.[48,49] A set material may differ in toxicity from an unset material. The immediate pulpal response to a material is much less significant than the long-term response. A few days after placement, the pulp may show a strong inflammatory response. A few months later, the inflammatory response may subside and repair occurs. A good measure of long-term response is the thickness of tertiary dentin laid down by the affected pulp (Fig. 2.7).

Depth of Preparation
Deep cavity preparations are likely to destroy odontoblasts. These are replaced by new odontoblasts that often form an irregular, reparative dentin that has few tubules (see Figure 1-8, A). Deep preparations also limit the amount of dentin that separates the cavity from the pulp, thus increasing the deleterious effects of biologic and chemical irritants.[33]

Desiccation by Hygroscopy[50]
Some hygroscopic materials may cause injury by withdrawing fluid from dentin. However, the relationship between the hydrophilic properties of materials and their effect on the pulp

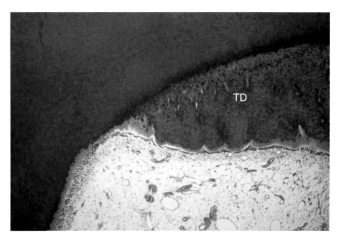

Fig. 2.7 Tertiary dentin *(TD)* formed under a deep preparation and irritating material. (Courtesy Dr. H. Trowbridge.)

is minimal. Moisture absorbed by materials is probably much less than that removed from dentin during cavity drying, which is a procedure that produces a small amount of pulpal inflammation.

Specific Materials
Zinc Oxide–Eugenol[18,51-53]
ZnOE has many uses in dentistry. It has a long history as a temporary filling material, cavity liner, cement base, and luting agent for provisional cementation of castings. Before the introduction of calcium hydroxide, ZnOE was the material of choice for direct pulp capping.

Eugenol, biologically the most active ingredient in ZnOE, is a phenol derivative and is toxic when placed in direct contact with tissue.[54] It also has antibacterial properties.[55] Eugenol's usefulness in pain control is attributed to its ability to block the transmission of nerve impulses.[56] Researchers have found that a thin mix of ZnOE significantly reduces intradental nerve activity when placed in a deep cavity preparation in cats' teeth; however, a dry mix of ZnOE has no effect.[57]

When included in cements to temporize crown preparation, some eugenol does reach the pulp, but the amounts are small and unrelated to remaining dentin thickness. "Desensitizing" agents do not seem to reduce the penetration.[42] The release of eugenol is by a hydrolytic mechanism, which depends on the presence of water. With little water available, release is low.[52,53]

The most important property of ZnOE is that it prevents microleakage of bacterial cells, thereby reducing hypersensitivity and providing antimicrobial properties.

Restorative Resins[58-60]
Early adhesive bonding and resin composite systems contract during polymerization, resulting in gross microleakage and bacterial contamination of the cavity. Bacteria on cavity walls and within axial dentin are associated with moderate pulpal inflammation. Over a period of time, some composites absorb water and expand; this tends to compensate for initial contraction. To limit microleakage and improve retention, enamel margins are beveled and acid etched to facilitate mechanical bonding. Compared with unfilled resins, the newer resin

composites present a coefficient of thermal expansion similar to that of tooth structure. With recently developed hydrophilic adhesive bonding composite systems, the problem of marginal leakage appears to have been diminished. A large, practice-based study has recently shown that the mean annual failure rate for resin-composite restorations was 2.9% and for amalgams it was 1.6%.[61]

Glass Ionomer Cements

Glass ionomer cements were originally used as esthetic restorative materials, but these cements are now being used as liners, luting agents, temporary restorative materials, and pulp capping agents (sometimes in conjunction with calcium hydroxide). The incidence of severe pulpal inflammation or necrosis caused by glass ionomer cement on exposed healthy pulps is similar to that for calcium hydroxide but greater than that for composite resins.[62] When placed in cavities in which the pulp is not exposed and the remaining dentin thickness is narrow (0.5 to 0.25 mm), both calcium hydroxide and composite resin show faster deposition of tertiary dentin than glass ionomer cements.[18]

When glass ionomer cements are used as a luting agent, the pulpal response is similar to that of polycarboxylate and zinc orthophosphate (ZnOP) cements.[63] Studies have shown that when glass ionomer cements are used with appropriate technique, the incidence of sensitivity is no greater than with other commonly used luting agents.[36]

Amalgam

Amalgam alloy is still a widely used material for restoring posterior teeth. Shrinkage during setting results in microleakage.[64] This microleakage decreases as corrosion products accumulate between restoration and cavity walls, and it can be reduced by the use of liners.[65] Amalgam is the only restorative material in which the marginal seal improves with time. Esthetics and public concern with the mercury content of amalgams have led to an accelerated use of composite resins as posterior restorative materials. Their use is more technique sensitive than amalgams. In deep cavities in posterior teeth, composites are associated with more pulpal injury than amalgams because of microleakage.[58] At least in part, this may be due to the difficulty with moisture control in some sites, as noted before.

Orthodontic Tooth Movement

Orthodontic tooth movement of a routine nature has not been considered to cause clinically significant changes in the dental pulp. Some experimental studies have reported vascular changes in the pulp after application of orthodontic forces[66,67]; these changes may be associated with the release of proangiogenic growth factors from pulp and dentin in response to these forces.[68] Modeling of external application of forces to the tooth has indicated that these forces may be transmitted to the pulp, leading to fibroblast proliferation and up-regulation of genes associated with cellular proliferation and extracellular matrix components.[69] Although these observations do not indicate a need to change current practice in orthodontics, advances in materials and approaches to orthodontic therapy may lead to application of greater forces at earlier stages during treatment than previously, with the consequent need to monitor carefully for pulp responses.

Vital Tooth Bleaching

The higher concentrations of peroxide used for professional, compared to vital, tooth bleaching place the pulp at greater risk of injury. Tooth sensitivity after bleaching treatment is commonly reported, although generally short lived, and there is little agreement on whether pulp responses to bleaching reflect the range of peroxide concentrations and treatment protocols used.[70] Overnight external bleaching of anterior teeth with 10% carbamide peroxide causes mild pulpitis, which is reversed within 2 weeks.[71] In vitro studies have shown that the principal bleaching agent, hydrogen peroxide, can reach the pulp[72] after application to the enamel. Whether this occurs in vivo is unclear, but caution should be adopted with the application of strong bleaching agents to vital tissues when these agents' oxidizing properties have the potential to cause appreciable cellular injury.

PROTECTING THE PULP FROM THE EFFECT OF MATERIALS

Cavity Varnishes, Liners, and Bases

A liner is routinely placed between restorative materials and the dentin, primarily to eliminate microleakage. In vitro studies suggest that most liners show some degree of leakage,[65] but it is unknown what level of dye leakage would relate to clinical problems. One 3-year clinical study[73] compared three common dentin treatments but found no recurrent caries around any of the restorations, including those in which no liner was used. All liners and bases reduce dentin permeability, but to different extents. Bases provide the greatest reduction, varnishes the least.[74]

Dentin is also an excellent thermal insulator of the pulp; additional insulation is rarely, if ever, needed. In fact, thick cement bases are no more effective than just a thin layer of varnish in preventing thermal sensitivity, indicating that postrestorative sensitivity is at least partly a result of microleakage.[75]

VITAL PULP THERAPIES

A primary goal in treatment of dental caries is maintenance of an intact, healthy pulp, which is preferable to root canal treatment or other endodontic procedures that are complex, expensive, and time-consuming and may compromise tooth survival unless performed under ideal conditions. For a deep carious lesion, indirect pulp capping, a procedure that avoids accidental pulp exposure during the removal of carious dentin, may be attempted. Invariably, this leaves some infected dentin, although risk analysis suggests this may be preferable to direct capping of carious pulp exposure, especially if lesion arrest can be achieved.[76] Another approach is to remove all carious dentin. If there is a carious exposure, the exposed pulp tissue is covered with a biocompatible liner (direct pulp capping). Traumatic pulp exposures tend to have a better prognosis than mechanical exposures during caries excavation or carious exposures due to the reduced infection risk. It is important, however, to consider not simply the extent of tissue involvement with caries, but also lesion activity and the rate of lesion progression. Some advocate a procedure involving either partial (pulpotomy) or complete (pulpectomy) surgical removal of inflamed pulp tissue; the remaining tissue is then covered with a dressing that aims to promote healing. The success rate for these procedures is variable; it depends on proper diagnosis and clinical judgment, but primarily on the status of the pulp before the procedure. A significant constraint on treatment planning is the lack of reliable or accurate diagnostic tools for clinical assessment of inflammation in the pulp. The terms *reversible* and *irreversible* pulpitis are frequently used to guide treatment approaches, but these simply reflect best clinical judgment and have no absolute diagnostic basis. Pulp sensibility is an important guide to case selection for vital pulp therapy. It is also a critical aspect of posttreatment monitoring, along with radiographic examinations.

Indirect Pulp Capping

In deep lesions, partial caries removal may reduce the risk of further pulp pathology, which can arise from exposure during complete caries removal, particularly in asymptomatic teeth. However, indirect pulp capping should be contemplated only if there are no clinical signs or symptoms of irreversible pulpitis. In a deep dentinal lesion, there is already a high likelihood of pulp involvement from the carious challenge, but it is the level of carious activity that is probably the greatest determinant of successful outcomes for indirect pulp capping. In slower progressing lesions or those in which caries has been either arrested or reduced in activity, a better prognosis is likely. The use of a step-wise technique for excavation of caries, in which caries is removed in increments over several visits rather than in one visit, reduces the risk of accidental mechanical exposure of the pulp and also may slow or arrest lesion development, leading to an improved prognosis for pulp vitality. Current evidence favors use of a step-wise excavation technique over indirect pulp capping.[7,77,78]

Direct Pulp Capping

Direct pulp capping is a procedure for treating an exposed pulp with a material to seal the exposure site and promote tissue repair and regeneration through reparative dentinogenesis, leading to dentin bridge formation. Calcium hydroxide has been used as a capping agent for nearly a century and highlights dentistry's position as a pioneer in regenerative medicine. However, outcome studies show that direct pulp capping of carious exposures with calcium hydroxide has an unfavorable long-term prognosis[79,80] Mineral trioxide aggregate (MTA) is increasingly finding favor for its easier handling properties and more predictable hard tissue barrier formation.[81] A clinical case series showed high success rates for MTA pulp capping when careful caries removal and hypochlorite disinfection were used.[82] A clinical outcomes study showed that pulp capping with MTA was significantly better than capping with calcium hydroxide.[83]

Considerations for direct pulp capping include traumatic exposure, accidental mechanical pulp exposure during cavity preparation, and exposure caused by caries. However, as with indirect pulp capping, the prognosis is heavily dependent on pulp vitality and the extent of infection and inflammation. Case selection for direct pulp capping should focus on asymptomatic teeth with no clinical signs or symptoms of irreversible pulpitis. The size of the exposure should be small, preferably less than 0.5 mm; hemorrhage should be adequately controlled; great care should be taken to avoid contamination of the area of exposure by using best clinical

practice, including a rubber dam; and a permanent restoration with a good marginal seal should be placed. The long-term success rate is high for direct pulp capping of small, clean, mechanical exposures but more controversial for carious exposures,[80,84] perhaps reflecting the importance of appropriate case selection for successful outcomes.

Pulpotomy

Pulpotomy represents an approach to vital pulp therapy in which infected coronal pulp is surgically excised, leaving intact the vital radicular pulp. It is an alternative to direct pulp capping when carious pulp exposures occur in deciduous and young permanent teeth and the inflammation may be restricted to the crown.[85] The pulp must be vital and asymptomatic.[86,87] All the carious dentin and the pulp to the level of the radicular pulp are removed.

An alternative approach is partial pulpotomy, which is based in part on the observation that inflammation is often localized to the more superficial region of the coronal pulp. High success rates have been reported for this approach.[88] Partial pulpotomy also allows elimination of much of the infected dentin debris after mechanical exposure of a deep carious lesion, thus reducing the infectious/inflammatory challenge such debris presents. After excision of 2 mm of the coronal pulp tissue, the technique is very similar to that for direct pulp capping, involving hemorrhage control, capping with calcium hydroxide or MTA, and use of a permanent restoration to provide a good marginal seal. Posttreatment follow-up should be the same as for any capping procedure, and teeth with immature roots should continue normal root development and apex formation and closure (Fig. 2.8).[89-93]

THE OPEN APEX[94,95]

An open apex is present in the developing root of immature teeth until apical closure occurs, approximately 3 years after eruption. In the absence of pulpal or periapical disease, such an open apex is normal. However, if the pulp becomes necrotic before root growth is complete, dentin formation ceases and root development is arrested. The resultant root is short with thin and consequently weakened dentin walls. The walls may diverge (Fig. 2.9), may be parallel, or may converge slightly, depending on the stage of root development. The apex is comparatively large and lacks constriction (Fig. 2.10). An open apex may also develop as a result of extensive resorption of a previously mature apex after orthodontic treatment or severe periapical inflammation (Fig. 2.11). The presence of an open apex presents significant challenges in the treatment of pulpal injury. When the apex is not closed, routine root canal procedures cannot be performed, and the results of treatment are unpredictable. Depending on the vitality of the affected pulp, several approaches are possible, such as apexogenesis (vital pulp therapy), apexification (root-end closure), and revascularization/revitalization.

Diagnosis and Case Assessment[96]

The importance of careful case assessment and accurate pulpal diagnosis in the treatment of immature teeth with pulpal injury cannot be overemphasized. Clinical assessment of pulpal status requires a thorough history of subjective

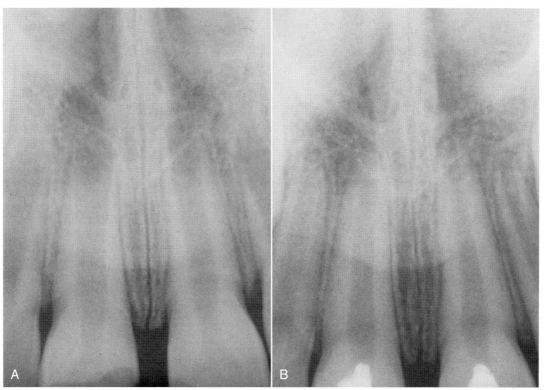

Fig. 2.8 Preoperative **(A)** and postoperative **(B)** radiographs demonstrate continued root development after pulpotomy procedures on both incisors. If these have good sealing restorations, the pulps should remain healthy; root canal treatment would be unnecessary.

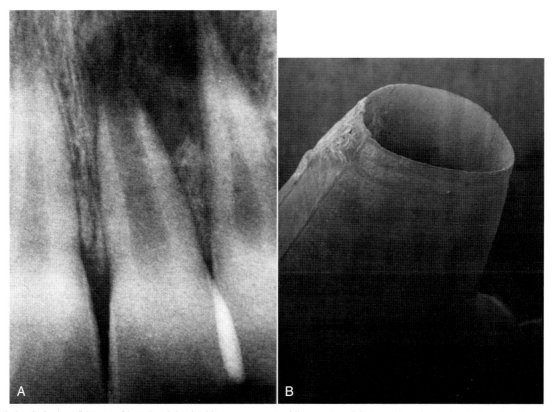

Fig. 2.9 **A,** Incisor (history of luxation injury) with an open apex (divergent walls), necrotic pulp, and apical pathosis. Root-end closure is indicated. **B,** Apical region of an immature central incisor extracted from a 7-year-old. Besides being open, the apical dentin walls are eggshell thin. These teeth are difficult to treat; long-term prognosis is questionable. (Courtesy Dr. L. Baldassari-Cruz.)

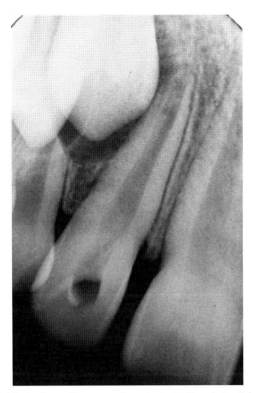

Fig. 2.10 Incisor with a necrotic pulp, but with substantial dentin formation and an open apex (parallel walls). An access opening has been made into the pulp chamber. Root-end closure with a barrier is indicated. Long-term prognosis is good.

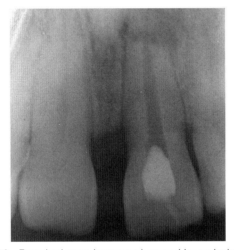

Fig. 2.11 Resorbed apex (now open) caused by periapical inflammation resulting from pulpal necrosis.

symptoms, careful clinical and radiographic examinations, and diagnostic tests (see Chapter 5).

Radiographic interpretation may be difficult in the case of the developing, immature root. A radiolucent area usually surrounds the apex of an immature root with a healthy pulp. It may be difficult to differentiate between this finding and a pathologic radiolucency resulting from a necrotic pulp. A radiolucent lesion tends to have a noncorticated, diffuse border. Also, comparison with the periapex of the contralateral tooth may be helpful. A radiograph is a two-dimensional picture of a three-dimensional situation; therefore, only the

mesiodistal aspect is seen in a routine radiograph. Frequently, the apex appears almost completely closed in this view but in actuality is wide open when observed from the proximal aspect (Fig. 2.12). In complex situations, cone beam computed tomography (CT) may be useful for diagnosis and treatment planning.

Unfortunately, a close correlation between the results of these individual tests and the actual histologic diagnosis of pulpal status does not exist. However, by combining the results of the history, clinical examination, and diagnostic tests, an accurate diagnosis of the pulpal and periapical condition can usually be established.

Treatment Planning

The major considerations in treatment planning are pulpal status and degree of root development (Fig. 2.13). If the pulpal diagnosis is reversible pulpitis, the appropriate treatment is vital pulp therapy, or apexogenesis, regardless of the degree of root development. Depending on the extent of pulp damage, pulp capping or shallow (partial) or conventional pulpotomy may be indicated.

If the diagnosis is irreversible pulpitis or pulpal necrosis, the appropriate treatment is determined by the degree of root development. If root development is complete and the apex is closed, conventional root canal therapy can be performed. However, when root development is incomplete, root-end closure must be induced before obturation. Alternatively, a regenerative procedure may be used, such as revascularization/revitalization of the pulp tissue.

In devising a treatment plan, the considerations are whether the tooth can be restored and the potential for root fracture because of the thin-walled roots. Patient compliance is important, particularly for the revascularization procedure. Treatment of the immature root by induced closure is no longer recommended, because long-term use of calcium hydroxide may weaken the root. Alternatives to induction of root-end closure include apical barrier techniques (single-visit apexification), revascularization, endodontic surgery, or extraction.

Apexogenesis[97-102]

Apexogenesis is defined as a vital pulp therapy procedure performed to encourage continued physiologic development and formation of the root end. The objective is to maintain the vitality of the radicular pulp; therefore, the pulp must be vital and capable of sustaining continued development, which is often the case when an immature tooth sustains a small coronal exposure after trauma. A small exposure can be treated by pulp capping. (The steps involved in pulp capping and apexogenesis with MTA can be viewed in Video 2.1.) 2-1

With more extensive pulpal exposures, an attempt is made to remove the inflamed tissue (partial pulpotomy), leaving the rest of the pulp intact. It has been demonstrated that, for up to 168 hours after the traumatic incident, inflammation is limited to the most superficial 2 mm of the pulp. Treatment in these cases is a shallow or partial pulpotomy (Cvek pulpotomy) in which only the superficial 2 to 4 mm of pulp is removed.

When there is a larger exposure, the pulp should be amputated at the level of the cervical constriction (conventional pulpotomy). With both pulpotomy techniques, the remaining pulp can be capped with a hard-set calcium hydroxide or, preferably, MTA.

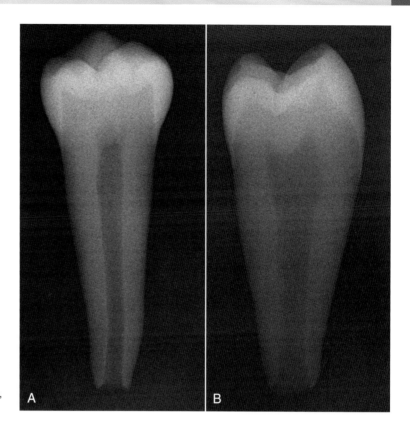

Fig. 2.12 **A,** The apex appears to be near parallel, as seen from the facial aspect. **B,** From the proximal aspect, the apical walls diverge.

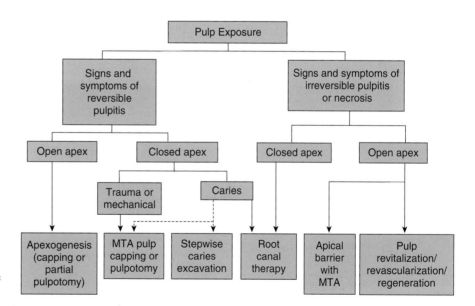

Fig. 2.13 Case selection decision tree in a young, healthy patient with asymptomatic pulp.

Technique

1. Anesthesia is obtained, and the rubber dam is placed.
2. The inflamed pulp tissue is removed. This may involve removal of the most superficial 2 to 4 mm of pulp (Cvek pulpotomy),[89,103-105] using a sharp round bur in a high-speed handpiece with water cooling, or removal of the entire coronal pulp to expose the radicular pulp (conventional pulpotomy) using a sharp spoon excavator.
3. Hemorrhage is controlled by pressure on a cotton pellet moistened with saline. Failure to achieve hemostasis may

indicate that inflamed tissue remains and that more pulp tissue must be removed.

4. The exposed pulp is rinsed with 1.25% sodium hypochlorite.
5. A material is placed over the amputated pulp. MTA is the preferred material, although hard-set calcium hydroxide traditionally has been widely used.[82,106-109] The tissue response to MTA is excellent, whereas there is always a zone of necrosis beneath calcium hydroxide.[86,97,110]

6. The MTA is prepared immediately before use by mixing the powder with sterile water or saline at a ratio of 3 : 1 on a glass or paper slab. The mixture is placed on the exposed pulp and patted in place with a moist cotton pellet. Because MTA sets in the presence of moisture over a 3-hour period, a wet cotton pellet is placed over the material and the rest of the cavity is filled with a temporary filling material. Alternatively, the entire cavity can be filled with white MTA and protected with a wet piece of gauze for 3 to 4 hours. The coronal 3 to 4 mm of MTA is removed, and a final restoration is placed immediately.

The primary goal of apexogenesis is to maintain pulp vitality, thus allowing dentin formation and root-end closure. Then the remaining primary odontoblasts can form dentin, increasing the thickness of the root dentin wall and making it less prone to fracture. The time required to produce a thicker root varies between 1 and 2 years, depending on the degree of root development at the time of the procedure. The patient should be recalled at 6-month intervals to determine the vitality of the pulp and the extent of apical maturation. Absence of symptoms does not indicate absence of disease. At each recall appointment, signs and symptoms are monitored, pulp vitality is tested, and radiographs are obtained to determine periapical status. One advantage of pulp capping and partial pulpotomy is the ability to test pulp vitality.

The ideal outcome of apexogenesis therapy is continued apical growth of the root with a normal apex (Fig. 2.14). Vital tissue may be maintained for long periods, often indefinitely. After pulp capping and partial pulpotomy, histologic examination of the pulp usually shows normal tissue. Therefore, histologic evidence does not support routine pulp extirpation

and root filling after apical closure. The success rate is lower after conventional pulpotomy; calcific metamorphosis is a common occurrence. When there is evidence of such calcification, it has been suggested that root canal therapy should be initiated. This is probably unwarranted, because calcific metamorphosis is not in itself pathologic. However, should the pulp become necrotic at some future date, the canals may not be negotiable and surgery would be necessary.

If it is determined that the pulp has become irreversibly inflamed or necrotic before root development is complete or if internal resorption is evident, the pulp is removed and apexification therapy is initiated.

Apexification[101,111]

Apexification is the induction of a calcific barrier (or the creation of an artificial barrier) across an open apex in a case involving pulp necrosis with or without a periapical lesion. Apexification involves removal of the necrotic pulp, followed by debridement of the canal and placement of an antimicrobial medicament (Fig. 2.15). In the past, much emphasis was placed on the type and properties of the medicament, and many materials have been proposed for induction of an apical barrier, although consensus for their use is lacking. However, it has been demonstrated that the critical factors in apical barrier formation are thorough debridement of the root canal system and establishment of a complete coronal seal.

Calcium hydroxide was accepted as the material for induction of an apical barrier in the past. Calcium hydroxide produces a multilayered, sterile necrosis accompanied by subjacent mineralization.[112] The cellular signaling of reparative events after calcium hydroxide application may be due to

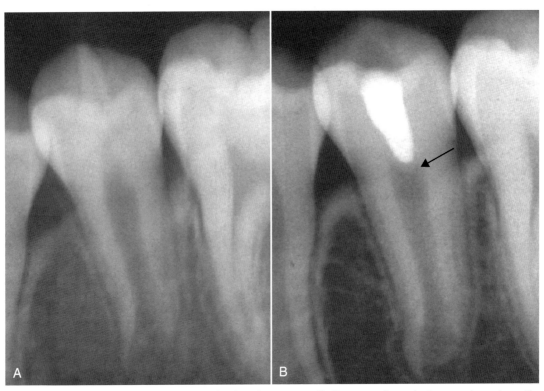

Fig. 2.14 **A,** Premolar with dens evaginatus resulting in pulp exposure. **B,** One year after pulpotomy and capping with mineral trioxide aggregate (MTA); note the evidence of a dentin barrier *(arrow)* and continued root development.

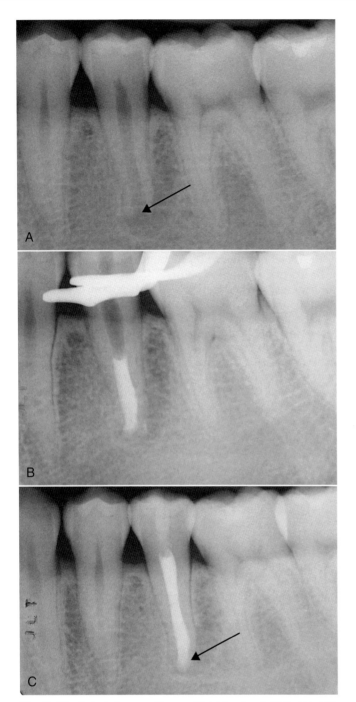

Fig. 2.15 Apical closure with an artificial barrier. **A,** Pulp necrosis with arrested root development and an open apex *(arrow)*. **B,** After cleaning and shaping, mineral trioxide aggregate (MTA) powder is compacted into the apical half. **C,** The coronal half is back-filled with gutta percha, and the access is restored with composite resin. MTA has formed an apical barrier *(arrow)*. (Courtesy Dr. A. Williamson.)

Technique

1. After isolation, a large access cavity is prepared to allow removal of all necrotic tissue.
2. Light debridement and irrigation with 1.25% sodium hypochlorite (NaOCl) are performed.
3. Working length is established, slightly short of the radiographic apex. Instrumentation beyond the apex is not advocated, because it may damage the tissue that ultimately forms the barrier.
4. Instrumentation is performed with gentle circumferential filing, starting with a relatively large file and progressing through the sizes. The objective is to maximize cleaning by disruption of microbial biofilms on the canal walls, followed by copious irrigation with sodium hypochlorite and minimal dentin removal.
5. Large paper points are used to dry the canal.
6. MTA is introduced into the canal as either a powder or paste (by mixing with sterile saline) and packed with endodontic pluggers or with the large end of the paper points.

MTA produces an artificial barrier against which an obturating material may be condensed. If calcium hydroxide were placed, it would allow the tissue to form a biologic barrier. After placement of the MTA barrier, a radiograph is made to confirm that the canal space close to the apex is adequately filled (see Fig. 2.15). A moist cotton pellet is placed in the canal to ensure setting, and a well-sealing temporary restoration is placed. The patient is recalled when the MTA has set (at least 24 hours) for obturation and placement of the permanent restoration.

Restoration After Apexification[112,117]

Because of the thin dentinal walls, there is a high incidence of root fracture in teeth after apexification. Restorative efforts should be directed toward strengthening the immature root. The use of newer dentin bonding techniques can significantly increase the resistance to fracture of these teeth, to levels close to those of intact teeth. The reinforcing effect of composite resin in teeth with large canal spaces, with or without a post, was shown in a bench top study.[117]

Success or Failure of Apexification

Failure can occur either during or after treatment. The most common cause of failure is bacterial contamination, usually caused by loss of the coronal restoration or inadequate debridement of the canal. After apparently successful treatment, all patients should be recalled at 12-month intervals for 4 years. At the recall appointment, the tooth should be carefully examined clinically and radiographically. Infected necrotic material trapped in the barrier may contribute to failures, particularly if treatment was not performed under strict aseptic conditions. A further cause of failure is an undetected root fracture. Studies have shown an overall success rate that is comparable to cases involving a mature apex and a preoperative periapical lesion.[118]

Tissue Engineering and Regenerative Endodontics

Currently, symptomatic teeth with clinical signs of irreversible pulpitis are unlikely to be successfully treated with vital pulp therapy, and root canal treatment is the probable fate of such teeth. However, significant recent advances in the fields

several mechanisms, although it has now become apparent that calcium hydroxide can release potent bioactive growth factors sequestered within dentin matrix.[113] However, the weakening of roots after long-term use of calcium hydroxide[114] and the favorable prognosis of an immediate MTA apical barrier led to the acceptance of the latter technique for apexification in recent years.[115,116]

of stem cell biology, regenerative medicine, and tissue engineering now provide a platform upon which regeneration of dentin-pulp or engineering of these tissues may become a clinical reality in the future. Already, we have proof-of-principle for such techniques in the laboratory,[2,3] although a number of challenges remain before these techniques are translated into everyday clinical practice.

Clinical translation of such techniques may take several different approaches, ranging from stimulating natural regeneration of the tissues, possibly with only partial removal of the existing pulp, to engineering an entire new pulp after loss of a necrotic pulp and sterilization of the pulp chamber. Natural tissue regeneration essentially reflects the body's natural wound healing processes, and stimulation of these processes may require a more modest change in traditional clinical practice to tip the balance in favor of tissue vitality rather than necrosis. Of fundamental importance is the creation of a conducive tissue environment for healing to take place, and control of infection and inflammation will be critical to achieving this goal. The close interplay between inflammation and regeneration is becoming apparent,[119,120] and opportunities for novel pharmaceutical approaches to control tissue events after injury may result in improved treatment outcomes. Although more ambitious, the engineering of new pulp tissue would greatly extend the clinician's treatment repertoire and allow teeth to preserve their biologic characteristics after restoration, a benefit not shared by current root canal treatment approaches. Most dental tissue regenerative and engineering strategies seek to mimic the molecular and cellular events occurring during tooth development,[3] and one of the most prominent features of development is the close temporospatial control of the sequence of events that results in a group of uncommitted stem cells in the embryo giving rise to the exquisite architecture of the tissues of the tooth. Clearly, such control mechanisms are complex and demand the interaction of three key elements:

- Stem/progenitor cells
- Molecular signals (also known as morphogens or growth factors) that induce morphogenesis/cellular differentiation and regulate matrix secretion by the differentiated cells
- A scaffold that provides a three-dimensional microenvironment for cell growth and differentiation

Designing and developing strategies for pulp engineering that can be readily translated into the clinic or dental office present a considerable challenge. However, exploiting the body's own stem cell sources and endogenous stores of signaling molecules sequestered within extracellular matrices may simplify the challenges. Considerable progress has been achieved recently in the identification of stem cell populations in dental pulp[121,122] and the migration of mesenchymal stem cells (MSCs) to sites of injury in teeth.[123] Promoting homing of stem cells to the pulp after injury[124] and identification of some of the molecular signals for cellular recruitment[125] may reduce the need to develop procedures for clinical transplantation of stem cells and their expansion in number, with the inherent risks of change in cell phenotype. The complex signaling mechanisms involved in differentiation of odontoblasts and other pulp cells likely involve a variety of molecular

signals, which may be difficult to mimic clinically. However, the components of the rich cocktail of growth factors and other bioactive molecules sequestered within dentin matrix are able to signal these differentiation events,[2,11] in addition to those involved in angiogenesis.[126] Strategies for local release of these signaling molecules may involve creation of acidic conditions through placement of an appropriate scaffold, such as polylactic acid; application of cavity-etching agents[31,32]; or pulp capping and use of restorative materials.[113,127] Clearly, we are now entering an exciting era in which more biologic approaches to the management of dental disease may allow tissue regeneration and engineering to become a clinical reality. Although very promising, these techniques must be proved clinically and must demonstrate that they provide a reliable and cost-effective alternative to currently available methods for treatment of pulp.

Regenerative endodontics currently refers to the techniques used to control infection and regenerate vital tissues within the pulp space of immature teeth for the purpose of promoting maturation of the root. This is also frequently referred to as revascularization or revitalization of the pulp tissue. The techniques involved in these procedures are mostly based on published case reports and case series, and are constantly being updated with new information on optimal disinfection protocols that would not interfere with stem cell viability and promote vital tissue growth. The American Association of Endodontists (AAE) has developed a web site that collects documentation on treated cases in a central database, and provides contemporary guidelines for clinicians on accepted protocols for regenerative endodontics.[128] As this textbook goes to press in 2014, the guidelines call for using a regenerative procedure in cases with pulp necrosis and an immature root apex, when the pulp space will not be utilized for the final restoration and with proper consent and explanation of treatment options.

Technique

The procedure is applied in two visits as follows:

In visit 1, following anesthesia and isolation, the necrotic pulp space is accessed and debrided with minimal instrumentation and copious irrigation with lower concentration of 1.5% sodium hypochlorite. A medicament of calcium hydroxide paste or an antibiotic mixture is placed and the tooth is temporarily sealed for 1 to 4 weeks. Minocycline is not recommended for anterior teeth because of tooth discoloration.

In visit 2, anesthesia is performed using 3% mepivacaine without vasoconstrictor to promote a blood clot formation. Following isolation, the medicament is removed using copious irrigation with 17% EDTA followed by drying. An endodontic instrument is then introduced 1 to 2 mm past the radiographic apex to induce a blood clot formation to a level that allows 3 to 4 mm of restorative material. A thin, resorbable collagen matrix is placed followed by white MTA or calcium hydroxide as capping material. MTA may also discolor the crown of anterior teeth. The tooth is then restored with a permanent restorative material.[128]

As noted before, this technique is constantly being updated and the reader is referred to the AAE web site for the latest changes.

REFERENCES

1. Brannstrom M, Lind PO: Pulpal response to early dental caries, *J Dent Res* 44(5):1045, 1965.
2. Cordeiro MM, Dong Z, Kaneko T, et al: Dental pulp tissue engineering with stem cells from exfoliated deciduous teeth, *J Endod* 34:962-969, 2008.
3. Smith AJ, Sharpe PT: Biological tooth replacement and repair. In Lanza R, Langer R, Vacanti J, editors: *Principles of tissue engineering*, ed 3, pp 1067-1079, St. Louis, 2007, Elsevier.
4. Banchs F, Trope M: Revascularization of immature permanent teeth with apical periodontitis: new treatment protocol? *J Endod* 30(4):196-200, 2004.
5. Wang X, Thibodeau B, Trope M, et al: Histologic characterization of regenerated tissues in canal space after the revitalization/revascularization procedure of immature dog teeth with apical periodontitis, *J Endod* 36(1):56-63, 2010.
6. American Association of Endodontists: *Glossary of endodontic terms*, Chicago, 2012, The Association.
7. Bjørndal L, Reit C, Bruun G, et al: Treatment of deep caries lesions in adults: randomized clinical trials comparing stepwise vs direct complete excavation, and direct pulp capping vs partial pulpotomy, *Eur J Oral Sci* 118(3):290-297, 2010.
8. Huang GT, Lin LM: Comments on the use of the term "revascularization" to describe root regeneration [letter to the editor], *J Endod* 34(5):511, 2008.
9. Ahn J, Pogrel MA: The effects of 2% lidocaine with 1:100,000 epinephrine on pulpal and gingival blood flow, *Oral Surg Oral Med Oral Path Oral Radiol Endod* 85(2):197, 1998.
10. Pitt Ford TR, Seare MA, McDonald F: Action of adrenaline on the effect of dental local anaesthetic solutions, *Endod Dent Traumatol* 9(1):31, 1993.
11. Smith AJ, Scheven BA, Takahashi Y, et al: Dentine as a bioactive extracellular matrix, *Arch Oral Biol* 57:109-121, 2012.
12. Mjor IA, Odont D: Pulp-dentin biology in restorative dentistry. Part 2. Initial reactions to preparation of teeth for restorative procedures, *Quintessence Int* 32(7):537, 2001.
13. Murray PE, Lumley PJ, Smith AJ: Preserving the vital pulp in operative dentistry. Part 3. Thickness of remaining cavity dentine as a key mediator of pulpal injury and repair responses [see comment], *Dent Update* 29(4):172, 2002.
14. Mullaney TP, Laswell HR: Iatrogenic blushing of dentin following full crown preparation, *J Prosthet Dent* 22(3):354, 1969.
15. Goodis HE, Fried D, Gansky S, et al: Pulpal safety of 9.6 micron TEA CO2 laser used for caries prevention, *Lasers Surg Med* 35(2):104, 2004.
16. Cavalcanti BN, Lage-Marques JL, Rode SM: Pulpal temperature increases with Er:YAG laser and high-speed handpieces, *J Prosthet Dent* 90(5):447, 2003.
17. Pashley DH, Pashley EL: Dentin permeability and restorative dentistry: a status report for the *American Journal of Dentistry*, *Am J Dent* 4(1):5, 1991.
18. Murray PE, About I, Lumley PJ, et al: Cavity: remaining dentin thickness and pulpal activity, *Am J Dent* 15(1):41, 2002.
19. About I, Murray PE, Franquin JC, et al: The effect of cavity restoration variables on odontoblast cell numbers and dental repair, *J Dent* 29(2):109, 2001.
20. Yamada T, Nakamura K, Iwaku M, et al: The extent of the odontoblast process in normal and carious human dentine, *J Dent Res* 62:798-802, 1983.
21. McNeil PL, Steinhardt RA: Plasma membrane disruption: repair, prevention and adaptation, *Ann Rev Cell Devel Biol* 19:697-731, 2003.
22. Stevenson TS: Odontoblast aspiration and fluid movement in human dentine, *Arch Oral Biol* 12(10):1149, 1967.
23. Smith AJ, Smith JG, Shelton RM, et al: Harnessing the natural regenerative potential of the dental pulp, *Dent Clin North Am* (2012). doi: 10.1016/j.cden.2012.05.011.

24. Imazato S, Kaneko T, Takahashi Y, et al: In vivo antibacterial effects of dentin primer incorporating MDPB, *Oper Dent* 29:369-375, 2004.
25. Zhang K, Melo MA, Cheng L, et al: Effect of quaternary ammonium and silver nanoparticle-containing adhesives on dentin bond strength and dental plaque microcosm biofilms, *Dent Mater* 28(8):842-852, 2012.
26. Cheng L, Zhang K, Melo MA, et al: Anti-biofilm dentin primer with quaternary ammonium and silver nanoparticles, *J Dent Res* 91(6):598-604, 2012.
27. de Souza Costa CA, do Nascimento AB, Teixeira HM: Response of human pulps following acid conditioning and application of a bonding agent in deep cavities, *Dent Mater* 18(7):543, 2002.
28. Baratieri LN, Ritter AV: Four-year clinical evaluation of posterior resin-based composite restorations placed using the total-etch technique, *J Esthet Restor Dent* 13(1):50, 2001.
29. Murray PE, Smyth TW, About I, et al: The effect of etching on bacterial microleakage of an adhesive composite restoration, *J Dent* 30(1):29, 2002.
30. Smith AJ, Smith G: Solubilisation of TGF-β1 by dentine conditioning agents, *J Dent Res* 77:1034, 1988.
31. Zhao S, Sloan AJ, Murray PE, et al: Ultrastructural localisation of TGF-β exposure in dentine by chemical treatment, *Histochem J* 32:489-494, 2000.
32. Galler KM, D'Souza RN, Federlin M, et al: Dentin conditioning codetermines cell fate in regenerative endodontics, *J Endod* 37:1536-1541. 2011.
33. Murray PE, Smith AJ, Garcia-Godoy F, et al: Comparison of operative procedure variables on pulpal viability in an ex vivo modelm, *Int Endod J* 41:389-400, 2008.
34. Felton DA, Webb EL, Kanoy BE, et al: Pulpal response to threaded pin and retentive slot techniques: a pilot investigation, *J Prosthet Dent* 66(5):597, 1991.
35. Knight JS, Smith HB: The heat sink and its relationship to reducing heat during pin-reduction procedures, *Oper Dent* 23(6):299, 1998.
36. Johnson GH, Powell LV, DeRouen TA: Evaluation and control of post-cementation pulpal sensitivity: zinc phosphate and glass ionomer luting cements, *J Am Dent Assoc* 124(11):38, 1993.
37. Silvestri AR Jr, Cohen SH, Wetz JH: Character and frequency of discomfort immediately following restorative procedures, *J Am Dent Assoc* 95(1):85, 1977.
38. Casselli DS, Martins LR: Postoperative sensitivity in Class I composite resin restorations in vivo, *J Adhes Dent* 8(1):53, 2006.
39. Sarrett DC, Brooks CN, Rose JT: Clinical performance evaluation of a packable posterior composite in bulk-cured restorations, *J Am Dent Assoc* 137(1):71, 2006.
40. Sobral MA, Garone-Netto N, Luz MA, et al: Prevention of postoperative tooth sensitivity: a preliminary clinical trial, *J Oral Rehabil* 32(9):661, 2005.
41. Unemori M, Matsuya Y, Akashi A, et al: Self-etching adhesives and postoperative sensitivity, *Am J Dent* 17(3):191, 2004.
42. Camps J, Dejou J, Remusat M, et al: Factors influencing pulpal response to cavity restorations, *Dent Mater* 16(6):432, 2000.
43. Bergenholtz G: Evidence for bacterial causation of adverse pulpal responses in resin-based dental restorations, *Crit Rev Oral Biol Med* 11(4):467, 2000.
44. Bergenholtz G: Effect of bacterial products on inflammatory reactions in the dental pulp, *Scand J Dent Res* 85(2):122, 1977.
45. Bergenholtz G, Cox CF, Loesche WJ, et al: Bacterial leakage around dental restorations: its effect on the dental pulp, *J Oral Pathol* 11(6):439, 1982.

46. Vongsavan N, Matthews RW, Matthews B: The permeability of human dentine in vitro and in vivo, *Arch Oral Biol* 45(11):931, 2000.
47. Jontell M, Hanks CT, Bratel J, et al: Effects of unpolymerized resin components on the function of accessory cells derived from the rat incisor pulp, *J Dent Res* 74(5):1162, 1995.
48. Al-Hiyasat AS, Darmani H, Milhem MM: Cytotoxicity evaluation of dental resin composites and their flowable derivatives, *Clin Oral Invest* 9(1):21, 2005.
49. Lonnroth EC, Dahl JE: Cytotoxicity of liquids and powders of chemically different dental materials evaluated using dimethylthiazol diphenyltetrazolium and neutral red tests, *Acta Odont Scand* 61(1):52, 2003.
50. Brannstrom M: The effect of dentin desiccation and aspirated odontoblasts on the pulp, *J Prosthet Dent* 20(2):165, 1968.
51. Camps J, About I, Gouirand S, et al: Dentin permeability and eugenol diffusion after full crown preparation, *Am J Dent* 16(2):112, 2003.
52. Hume WR: Influence of dentine on the pulpward release of eugenol or acids from restorative materials, *J Oral Rehabil* 21(4):469, 1994.
53. Hume WR: An analysis of the release and the diffusion through dentin of eugenol from zinc oxide–eugenol mixtures, *J Dent Res* 63(6):881, 1984.
54. Al-Nazhan S, Spangberg L: Morphological cell changes due to chemical toxicity of a dental material: an electron microscopic study on human periodontal ligament fibroblasts and L929 cells, *J Endod* 16(3):129, 1990.
55. Olasupo NA, Fitzgerald DJ, Gasson MJ, et al: Activity of natural antimicrobial compounds against *Escherichia coli* and *Salmonella enterica* serovar *Typhimurium*, *Lett Appl Microbiol* 37(6):448, 2003.
56. Brodin P: Neurotoxic and analgesic effects of root canal cements and pulp-protecting dental materials, *Endod Dent Traumatol* 4(1):1, 1988.
57. Trowbridge H, Edwall L, Panopoulos P: Effect of zinc oxide–eugenol and calcium hydroxide on intradental nerve activity, *J Endod* 8(9):403, 1982.
58. Whitworth JM, Myers PM, Smith J, et al: Endodontic complications after plastic restorations in general practice, *Int Endod J* 38(6):409, 2005.
59. Heys RJ, Heys DR, Fitzgerald M: Histological evaluation of microfilled and conventional composite resins on monkey dental pulps, *Int Endod J* 18(4):260, 1985.
60. Kitasako Y, Nakajima M, Pereira PN, et al: Monkey pulpal response and microtensile bond strength beneath a one-application resin bonding system in vivo, *J Dent* 28(3):193, 2000.
61. Kopperud SE, Tveit AB, Gaarden T, et al: Longevity of posterior dental restorations and reasons for failure, *Eur J Oral Sci* 120(6):539-548, 2012.
62. Murray PE, Hafez AA, Smith AJ, et al: Identification of hierarchical factors to guide clinical decision making for successful long-term pulp capping, *Quintessence Int* 34(1):61, 2003.
63. Heys RJ, Fitzgerald M, Hyeys DR, et al: An evaluation of a glass ionomer luting agent: pulpal histological response, *J Am Dent Assoc* 114(5):607, 1987.
64. Shimada Y, Seki Y, Sasafuchi Y, et al: Biocompatibility of a flowable composite bonded with a self-etching adhesive compared with a glass ionomer cement and a high copper amalgam, *Oper Dent* 29(1):23, 2004.
65. Morrow LA, Wilson NH: The effectiveness of four-cavity treatment systems in sealing amalgam restorations, *Oper Dent* 27(6):549, 2002.
66. Brodin P, Linge L, Aars H: Instant assessment of pulpal blood flow after orthodontic force application, *J Orofac Orthop* 57(5):306, 1996.

67. Nixon CE, Saviano JA, King GJ, et al: Histomorphometric study of dental pulp during orthodontic tooth movement, *J Endod* 19(1):13, 1993.

68. Derringer KA, Linden RW: Vascular endothelial growth factor, fibroblast growth factor 2, platelet-derived growth factor and transforming growth factor beta released in human dental pulp following orthodontic force, *Arch Oral Biol* 49(8):631, 2004.

69. Dhopatkar AA, Sloan AJ, Rock WO, et al: A novel in vitro culture model to investigate the reaction of the dentine-pulp complex to orthodontic force, *J Orthodont* 32:122-132, 2005.

70. Dahl JE, Pallesen U: Tooth bleaching: a critical review of the biological aspects, *Crit Rev Oral Biol Med* 14:292-304, 2003.

71. Fugaro JO, Nordahl I, Fugaro OJ, et al: Pulp reaction to vital bleaching, *Oper Dent* 29(4):363, 2004.

72. Gokay O, Tuncbilek M, Ertan R: Penetration of the pulp chamber by carbamide peroxide bleaching agents on teeth restored with a composite resin, *J Oral Rehabil* 27(5):428, 2000.

73. Baratieri LN, Machado A, Van Noort R, et al: Effect of pulp protection technique on the clinical performance of amalgam restorations: three-year results, *Oper Dent* 27(4):319, 2002.

74. Pashley DH, O'Meara JA, Williams EC, et al: Dentin permeability: effects of cavity varnishes and bases, *J Prosthet Dent* 53(4):511, 1985.

75. Piperno S, Barouch E, Hirsch SM, et al: Thermal discomfort of teeth related to presence or absence of cement bases under amalgam restorations, *Oper Dent* 7(3):92, 1982.

76. Fitzgerald M, Heys RJ: A clinical and histological evaluation of conservative pulpal therapy in human teeth, *Oper Dent* 16(3):101-112, 1991.

77. Hayashi M, Fujitani M, Yamaki C, et al: Ways of enhancing pulp preservation by stepwise excavation: a systematic review, *J Dent* 39:95-107, 2011.

78. Maltz M, Alves LS, Moura Mdos S, et al: Incomplete caries removal in deep lesions: a 10-year prospective study, *Am J Dent* 24:211-214, 2011.

79. Barthel CR, Rosenkranz B, Leuenberg A, et al: Pulp capping of carious exposures: treatment outcome after 5 and 10 years: a retrospective study, *J Endod* 26(9):525-528, 2000.

80. Al-Hiyasat AS, Barrieshi-Nusair KM, Al-Omari MA: The radiographic outcomes of direct pulp-capping procedures performed by dental students: a retrospective study, *J Am Dent Assoc* 137(12):1699-1705, 2006.

81. Nair PN, Duncan HF, Pitt Ford TR, et al: Histological, ultrastructural and quantitative investigations on the response of healthy human pulps to experimental capping with mineral trioxide aggregate: a randomized controlled trial, *Int Endod J* 41:128-150, 2008.

82. Bogen G, Kim JS, Bakland LK: Direct pulp capping with mineral trioxide aggregate: an observational study, *J Am Dent Assoc* 139(3):305-315, 2008.

83. Mente J, Geletneky B, Ohle M, et al: Mineral trioxide aggregate or calcium hydroxide direct pulp capping: an analysis of the clinical treatment outcome, *J Endod* 36(5):806-813, 2010.

84. Hilton TJ: Keys to clinical success with pulp capping: a review of the literature, *Oper Dent* 34:615-625, 2009.

85. Witherspoon DE, Small JC, Harris GZ: Mineral trioxide aggregate pulpotomies: a case series outcomes assessment, *J Am Dent Assoc* 137(5):610-618, 2006.

86. Percinoto C, de Castro AM, Pinto LMCP: Clinical and radiographic evaluation of pulpotomies employing calcium hydroxide and trioxide mineral aggregate, *Gen Dent* 54(4):258, 2006.

87. Rafter M: Vital pulp therapy: a review, *J Irish Dent Assoc* 47(4):115, 2001.

88. Mejare I, Cvek M: Partial pulpotomy in young permanent teeth with deep carious lesions, *Endod Dent Traumatol* 9:238-242, 1993.

89. Cvek M: A clinical report on partial pulpotomy and capping with calcium hydroxide in permanent incisors with complicated crown fracture, *J Endod* 4(8):232, 1978.

90. DeRosa TA: A retrospective evaluation of pulpotomy as an alternative to extraction, *Gen Dent* 54(1):37, 2006.

91. Fong CD, Davis MJ: Partial pulpotomy for immature permanent teeth, its present and future, *Pediatr Dent* 24(1):29, 2002.

92. Granath LE, Hagman G: Experimental pulpotomy in human bicuspids with reference to cutting technique, *Acta Odont Scand* 29(2):155, 1971.

93. Ward J: Vital pulp therapy in cariously exposed permanent teeth and its limitations, *Aust Endod J* 28(1):29, 2002.

94. Capurro M, Zmener O: Delayed apical healing after apexification treatment of non-vital immature tooth: a case report, *Endod Dent Traumatol* 15(5):244, 1999.

95. Kleier DJ, Barr ES: A study of endodontically apexified teeth, *Endod Dent Traumatol* 7(3):112, 1991.

96. American Academy of Pediatric Dentistry Council on Clinical Affairs Committee, Pulp Therapy Subcommittee: Guideline on pulp therapy for primary and young permanent teeth, *Pediatr Dent* 27(7 reference manual):130, 2005.

97. El-Meligy OAS, Avery DR: Comparison of mineral trioxide aggregate and calcium hydroxide as pulpotomy agents in young permanent teeth (apexogenesis), *Pediatr Dent* 28(5):399, 2006.

98. Kontham UR, Tiku AM, Damle SG, et al: Apexogenesis of a symptomatic mandibular first permanent molar with calcium hydroxide pulpotomy, *Quintessence Int* 36(8):653, 2005 [erratum appears in *Quintessence Int* 37(2):120, 2006].

99. Seo R, Maki K, Hidaka A, Higuchi M, et al: Long term radiographic study of bilateral second premolars with immature root treated by apexogenesis and apexification, *J Clin Pediatr Dent* 29(4):313, 2005.

100. Welbury R, Walton AG: Continued apexogenesis of immature permanent incisors following trauma, *Br Dent J* 187(12):643, 1999.

101. Webber RT: Apexogenesis versus apexification, *Dent Clin North Am* 28(4):669, 1984.

102. Tenca JI, Tsamtsouris A: Continued root end development: apexogenesis and apexification, *J Pedodont* 2(2):144, 1978.

103. Cvek M: Prognosis of luxated non-vital maxillary incisors treated with calcium hydroxide and filled with gutta-percha: a retrospective clinical study, *Endod Dent Traumatol* 8(2):45, 1992.

104. Cvek M, Cleaton-Jones PE, Austin JC, et al: Pulp reactions to exposure after experimental crown fractures or grinding in adult monkeys, *J Endod* 8(9):391, 1982.

105. Cvek M, Granath L, Cleaton-Jones P, et al: Hard tissue barrier formation in pulpotomized monkey teeth capped with cyanoacrylate or calcium hydroxide for 10 and 60 minutes, *J Dent Res* 66(6):1166, 1987.

106. Karabucak B, Li D, Lim J, et al: Vital pulp therapy with mineral trioxide aggregate, *Dent Traumatol* 21(4):240, 2005.

107. Shabahang S, Torabinejad M: Treatment of teeth with open apices using mineral trioxide aggregate, *Pract Periodontics Aesthet Dent* 12(3):315, quiz, 322; 2000.

108. Torabinejad M, Chivian N: Clinical applications of mineral trioxide aggregate, *J Endod* 25(3):197, 1999.

109. Witherspoon DE, Small JC, Harris GZ: Mineral trioxide aggregate pulpotomies: a case series outcomes assessment, *J Am Dent Assoc* 137(5):610, 2006.

110. Barrieshi-Nusair KM, Qudeimat MA: A prospective clinical study of mineral trioxide aggregate for partial pulpotomy in cariously exposed permanent teeth, *J Endod* 32(8):731, 2006.

111. Morse DR, O'Larnic J, Yesilsoy C: Apexification: review of the literature, *Quintessence Int* 21(7):589, 1990.

112. Finucane D, Kinirons MJ: Non-vital immature permanent incisors: factors that may influence treatment outcome, *Endod Dent Traumatol* 15(6):273, 1999.

113. Graham L, Cooper PR, Cassidy N, et al: The effect of calcium hydroxide on solubilisation of bio-active dentine matrix components, *Biomaterials* 27:2865-2873, 2006.

114. Andreasen JO, Farik B, Munksgaard EC: Long-term calcium hydroxide as a root canal dressing may increase risk of root fracture, *Dent Traumatol* 18(3):134-137, 2002.

115. Holden DT, Schwartz SA, Kirkpatrick TC, et al: Clinical outcomes of artificial root-end barriers with mineral trioxide aggregate in teeth with immature apices, *J Endod* 34(7):812-817, 2008.

116. Simon S, Rilliard F, Berdal A, et al: The use of mineral trioxide aggregate in one-visit apexification treatment: a prospective study, *Int Endod J* 40(3):186-197, 2007.

117. Katebzadeh N, Dalton BC, Trope M: Strengthening immature teeth during and after apexification, *J Endod* 24(4):256, 1998.

118. Mente J, Leo M, Panagidis D, et al: Treatment outcome of mineral trioxide aggregate in open apex teeth, *J Endod* 39(1):20-26, 2013.

119. Cooper PR, Takahashi Y, Graham LW, et al: Inflammation-regeneration interplay in the dentine-pulp complex, *J Dent* 38:687-697, 2010.

120. Cooper PR, Smith AJ: Molecular mediators of pulp inflammation and regeneration, *Endod Topics* 28:90-105, 2013.

121. Sloan AJ, Smith AJ: Stem cells and the dental pulp: potential roles in tissue regeneration, *Oral Dis* 13:151-157, 2007.

122. Huang GTJ, Gronthos S, Shi S: Mesenchymal stem cells derived from dental tissues vs those from other sources: their biology and role in regenerative medicine, *J Dent Res* 88:792-806, 2009.

123. Feng J, Mantesso A, De Bari C, et al: Dual origin of mesenchymal stem cells contributing to organ growth and repair, *Proc Natl Acad Sci U S A* 108:6503-6508, 2011.

124. Kim JY, Xin X, Moioli EK, et al: Regeneration of dental pulp-like tissue by chemotaxis-induced cell homing, *Tissue Eng Part A* 16:3023-3031, 2010.

125. Smith JG, Smith AJ, Shelton RM, et al: Recruitment of dental pulp cells by dentine and pulp extracellular matrix components, *Exp Cell Res* 318(18):2397-2406, 2012.

126. Zhang R, Cooper PR, Smith G, et al: Angiogenic activity of dentin matrix components, *J Endod* 34:26-30, 2011.

127. Tomson PL, Grover LM, Lumley PJ, et al: Dissolution of bio-active dentine matrix components by mineral trioxide aggregate, *J Dent* 35(7):636-642, 2007.

128. American Association of Endodontists: http://www.aae.org/publications-and-research/research/regenerative-database.aspx.

CHAPTER 3

Endodontic microbiology

José F. Siqueira, Jr., Ashraf F. Fouad

LEARNING OBJECTIVES

After reading this chapter, the student should be able to:
1. Understand the microbial etiology of apical periodontitis.
2. Describe the routes of entry of microorganisms to the pulp and periradicular tissues.
3. Recognize the different types of endodontic infections and the main microbial species involved in each one.
4. Understand the bacterial diversity within infected root canals.
5. Describe the factors involved with symptomatic endodontic infections.
6. Understand the ecology of the endodontic microbiota and the features of the endodontic ecosystem.
7. Discuss the role of microorganisms in the outcome of endodontic treatment.
8. Understand the development and implications of extraradicular infections.

MICROBIAL CAUSATION OF APICAL PERIODONTITIS

Apical periodontitis is an inflammatory disease of microbial etiology primarily caused by infection of the root canal system (Fig. 3.1).[1-3] The unequivocal role of microorganisms in the causation of apical periodontitis was established nearly 40 years ago, and a huge amount of new information about the microbiology of endodontic infections has emerged in the past decade. Endodontic infections usually develop after pulpal necrosis or in cases in which the pulp was removed for treatment. Although fungi, viruses and, more recently, Archaea have been found in endodontic infections, bacteria are the major microorganisms implicated in the etiology of apical periodontitis. Bacteria colonizing the root canal system contact the periradicular tissues via apical and lateral foramina. As a consequence of the encounter between bacteria and host defenses, inflammatory changes take place in the periradicular tissues and give rise to the development of apical periodontitis. Following pulp necrosis, bacteria can grow uninhibited by host defense mechanisms. They form polymicrobial biofilms that invade all complex anatomy of the root canal system and irritate the periradicular tissues.

The ultimate goal of endodontic treatment is either to prevent the development of apical periodontitis or to create adequate conditions for periradicular tissue healing. Taking into account the microbial etiology of apical periodontitis, the rationale for endodontic treatment is unarguably to eradicate the occurring infection or to prevent microorganisms from infecting or reinfecting the root canal or the periradicular tissues. The purpose of this chapter is to describe the microbiologic aspects of endodontic infections.

ROUTES OF ROOT CANAL INFECTION

Under normal conditions, the dental pulp and dentin are sterile and isolated from oral microorganisms by overlying enamel and cementum. There are situations in which the integrity of these protective layers is breached (e.g., as a result of caries, trauma-induced fractures and cracks, restorative procedures, scaling and root planing, attrition, or abrasion) or naturally absent (e.g., because of gaps in the cementoenamel junction at the cervical root surface). Occasionally, congenital anomalies of teeth, such as dens invaginatus, dens evaginatus, or palatal groove defects, result in spontaneous pulp exposures. As a consequence, the dentin-pulp complex is exposed to the oral environment and put at risk of infection by oral microorganisms. Microorganisms from subgingival biofilms associated with periodontal health or disease may also reach the pulp via dentinal tubules, or lateral and apical foramina, or possibly as a result of a systemic route.

Dentinal Tubules

Whenever dentin is exposed, the pulp is put at risk for infection as a consequence of the permeability of normal dentin,

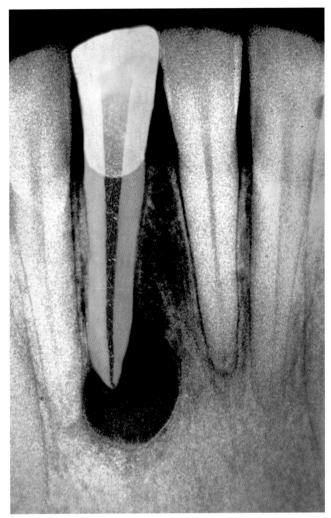

Fig. 3.1 Microorganisms infecting the root canal system are the major causative agents of the different forms of apical periodontitis.

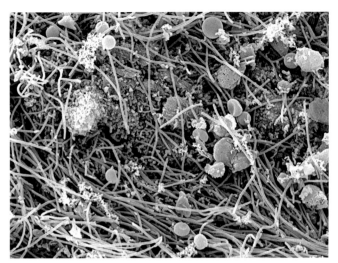

Fig. 3.2 Scanning electron micrograph showing bacteria in a carious lesion. Note the presence of different bacterial morphotypes.

which is dictated by its tubular structure. Dentin permeability is increased near the pulp because of the larger diameter and higher density of tubules.[4] Exposed dentin can be challenged by microorganisms present in carious lesions, in saliva bathing the exposed area, or in dental plaque formed onto the exposed area.

Dentinal tubules traverse the entire width of the dentin and have a conformation of inverted cones, with the smallest diameter in the periphery, near enamel or cementum (mean of 0.9 μm).[5] The smallest tubule diameter is entirely compatible with the cell diameter of most oral bacterial species, which usually ranges from 0.2 to 0.7 μm. Bacterial invasion of dentinal tubules occurs more rapidly in nonvital teeth than in vital ones.[6] In vital teeth, outward movement of dentinal fluid and the tubular contents influence dentinal permeability and can conceivably delay intratubular invasion by bacteria. Other factors, such as dentinal sclerosis beneath a carious lesion, reparative or reactionary dentin, smear layer, and intratubular accumulation of host defense molecules, such as antibodies, also limit or even impede bacterial progression to the pulp via dentinal tubules.[4] Thus, as long as the pulp is vital, dentinal exposure does not represent a significant route of pulpal infection, except when dentin thickness is considerably reduced;

then, dentin permeability is significantly increased. On the other hand, if the pulp is necrotic, exposed dentinal tubules can become true avenues for bacteria to reach and colonize the pulp.

Direct Pulp Exposure

Direct exposure of the dental pulp to the oral cavity is the most obvious route of endodontic infection. Caries is the most common cause of pulpal exposure, but microorganisms may also reach the pulp via direct pulpal exposure as a result of iatrogenic restorative procedures or trauma. There is a distinct difference, though, between the two processes of pulp exposure. Caries is a chronic disease that takes months to years to reach an exposure. Therefore, the pulp in the case of the carious exposure is exposed to biofilms containing high bacterial loads for a long period. The pulp in these cases is significantly inflamed and occasionally has an abscess formation at the site of the exposure,[7] even though the patient may be asymptomatic or mildly symptomatic. With mechanical exposure, however, only a few planktonic bacterial cells gain access to the pulp, particularly if a rubber dam is in place during preparation.

The reaction of the pulp, therefore, to the two types of exposure is widely different (see Chapter 2). The exposed pulp tissue develops direct contact with oral microorganisms from carious lesions, saliva, or plaque accumulated onto the exposed surface (Fig. 3.2). Almost invariably, exposed pulps undergo inflammation and necrosis and become infected. The time lapse between pulp exposure and infection of the entire canal is unpredictable, but it is usually a slow process.[8]

Periodontal Disease

In either normal or diseased periodontal tissues, microorganisms in subgingival biofilms could reach the pulp through dentinal tubules or lateral/furcal canals. As noted, the outward flow of dentinal fluid is protective of the pulp. However, pulpal necrosis as a consequence of periodontal disease develops only if the periodontal pocket reaches the apical foramen, leading to irreversible damage to the main blood vessels that penetrate through this foramen.[9] Once the pulp becomes necrotic, periodontal microorganisms can reach the root canal system via ramifications, exposed dentinal tubules, and apical foramina and establish an infectious process (see Chapter 7).

Anachoresis

Anachoresis is a process by which microorganisms are transported in the blood or lymph to an area of tissue damage, where they leave the vessel, enter the damaged tissue, and establish an infection. There is no clear evidence that this process represents a route for root canal infection. Research has shown that bacteria could not be recovered from unfilled root canals, when the bloodstream was experimentally infected, unless the root canals were overinstrumented during the period of bacteremia, with resulting injury to periodontal blood vessels and blood seepage into the canal.[10] Current evidence indicates that the main pathway of pulpal infection in traumatic injuries is from the gingival sulcus, through dentinal exposure as a result of enamel cracks[11] or the microvasculature of the traumatized periodontal ligament.[12]

MICROBIOTA OF ENDODONTIC INFECTIONS

Endodontic infections can be classified according to the anatomic location as intraradicular or extraradicular. Intraradicular infections can in turn be subdivided into three categories: primary, secondary, or persistent infection, depending on when the participating microorganisms established themselves in the root canal.

The composition of the microbiota may vary, depending on the different types of infection and different forms of apical periodontitis. Studies using culture-dependent approaches have allowed recognition of several candidate endodontic pathogens. More recently, with the advent of culture-independent molecular biology techniques, not only have the findings from culture studies been confirmed, but also a great deal of new information has been added to our knowledge of the microbiota associated with different types of endodontic infections. Molecular technology has enabled the recognition of new putative pathogens that had never been found in endodontic infections.[13] Moreover, many species that had already been considered putative pathogens because of their frequency of detection, as reported by culture-dependent methods, have been found in a similar or even higher prevalence by molecular approaches, strengthening these organisms' association with causation of apical periodontitis. As a consequence, the endodontic microbiota has been clearly redefined by molecular biology methods. The next sections discuss the main characteristics of the different types of endodontic infections.

Primary Intraradicular Infection

Microorganisms that initially invade and colonize the necrotic pulp tissue cause primary intraradicular infection. Participating microorganisms can be involved in the earlier stages of pulpal invasion, which culminate in inflammation and further necrosis, or they can be latecomers that take advantage of the environmental conditions in the canal after pulp necrosis. Primary infections are characterized by a mixed consortium composed of 10 to 30 bacterial species and 10^3 to 10^8 bacterial cells per canal.[2,13,14]

Sophisticated culture and molecular biology techniques have revealed the polymicrobial nature of endodontic infections, with a conspicuous dominance of obligate anaerobic bacterial species in primary infections. At a broader taxonomic level, endodontic bacteria fall into nine phyla, namely, Firmicutes, Bacteroidetes, Spirochaetes, Fusobacteria, Actinobacteria, Proteobacteria, Synergistetes, TM7, and SR1.[15] However, data from studies using advanced DNA sequencing technologies reveal that several other phyla may have been overlooked by previous identification techniques (see the following sections). Noteworthy is the high prevalence of as-yet-uncultivated species; about 40% to 66% of the endodontic microbiota is composed of bacteria that have yet to be cultivated and fully characterized.[16-18] In addition, bacterial profiles of the endodontic microbiota vary from individual to individual,[16,19] suggesting that apical periodontitis has a heterogeneous etiology in which multiple bacterial combinations can play a role in disease causation. Table 3.1 shows the bacterial genera commonly found in endodontic infections, and Fig. 3.3 shows the most prevalent bacterial taxa found in primary intraradicular infections associated with different forms of apical periodontitis.

Gram-Negative Bacteria

Gram-negative bacteria appear to be the most common microorganisms in primary endodontic infections. Species belonging to several genera of gram-negative bacteria have been consistently found in primary infections associated with different forms of apical periodontitis, including abscesses. These genera include *Dialister* (e.g., *D. invisus* and *D. pneumosintes*), *Fusobacterium* (e.g., *F. nucleatum*), *Porphyromonas* (e.g., *P. endodontalis* and *P. gingivalis*), *Prevotella* (e.g., *P. intermedia, P. nigrescens, P. baroniae* and *P. tannerae*), *Tannerella* (e.g., *T. forsythia*), and *Treponema* (e.g., *T. denticola* and *T. socranskii*).[16-18,20-36] Other gram-negative bacteria detected more sporadically in primary infections are shown in Table 3.1.

Gram-Positive Bacteria

Even though anaerobic gram-negative bacteria are reported to be the most common microorganisms in primary infections, several gram-positive bacteria have also been frequently detected in the endodontic mixed consortium, some of them in prevalence values as high as the most commonly found gram-negative species. The genera of gram-positive bacteria often found in primary infections include *Actinomyces* (e.g., *A. israelii*), *Filifactor* (e.g., *F. alocis*), *Olsenella* (e.g., *O. uli*), *Parvimonas* (e.g., *P. micra*), *Peptostreptococcus* (e.g., *P. anaerobius, P. stomatis*), *Pseudoramibacter* (e.g., *P. alactolyticus*), *Streptococcus* (e.g., *S. anginosus* group), and *Propionibacterium* (e.g., *P. propionicum* and *P. acnes*).[17,28,35-42] Other gram-positive bacteria found more sporadically in primary intraradicular infections are listed in Table 3.1.

As-Yet-Uncultivated Bacterial Phylotypes

Data from culture-independent molecular biology studies have indicated that several bacterial phylotypes can participate in endodontic infections. Phylotypes can be regarded as species that have not yet been cultivated and validly named and are known only by a 16S rRNA gene sequence. Uncultivated phylotypes have been frequently detected in samples from primary endodontic infections, including phylotypes

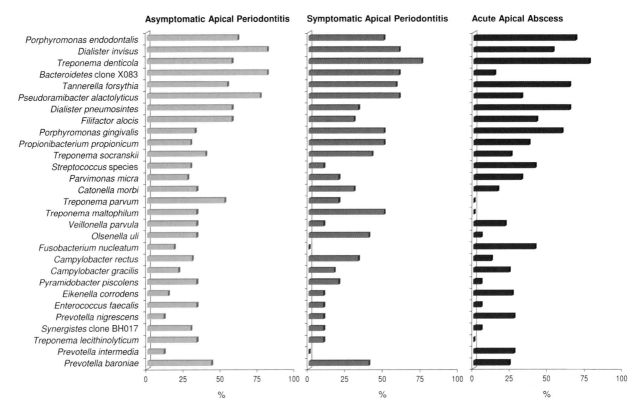

Fig. 3.3 Prevalence of bacteria detected in primary endodontic infections of teeth with different forms of apical periodontitis. Compilation of data from studies by one of the authors (Siqueira) using a molecular biology technique.

Table 3.1 Bacterial genera represented in endodontic infections

Gram-negative bacteria		Gram-positive bacteria	
Anaerobes	**Facultatives**	**Anaerobes**	**Facultatives**
Rods		*Rods*	
Dialister	Capnocytophaga	Actinomyces	Actinomyces
Porphyromonas	Eikenella	Pseudoramibacter	Corynebacterium
Tannerella	Haemophilus	Filifactor	Lactobacillus
Prevotella		Eubacterium	
Fusobacterium		Mogibacterium	
Campylobacter		Propionibacterium	
Pyramidobacter		Eggerthella	
Catonella		Olsenella	
Selenomonas		Bifidobacterium	
Centipeda		Slackia	
		Atopobium	
		Solobacterium	
		Lactobacillus	
Cocci		*Cocci*	
Veillonella	Neisseria	Parvimonas	Streptococcus
Megasphaera		Peptostreptococcus	Enterococcus
		Finegoldia	Granulicatella
		Peptoniphilus	
		Anaerococcus	
		Streptococcus	
		Gemella	
Spirilla			
Treponema			

belonging to the genera *Dialister, Prevotella, Solobacterium, Olsenella, Eubacterium,* and *Megasphaera;* the Lachnospiraceae family; and the Synergistetes phylum.[16-18,27,43-47] These phylotypes are previously unrecognized bacteria that may play a role in the pathogenesis of apical periodontitis. The fact that they have yet to be cultivated and phenotypically characterized does not mean that they are not important.

Complexity of Endodontic Polymicrobial Infections

For decades, the identification of endodontic microorganisms was performed using culturing techniques. There are advantages to being able to culture an organism, such as learning its growth requirements, virulence factors, and antibiotic sensitivity; this knowledge allows researchers to develop antimicrobial strategies. However, it appears that only about 10% of the human microbiome (i.e., the microbial communities that populate the human body) is cultivable.[48] Even with the advent of molecular techniques, studies sought first to identify known, cultivable bacteria with higher sensitivity than culturing and then to use techniques that relied on the cloning and sequencing of a few organisms per specimen. The latter techniques helped identify many organisms that have never been cultivated. The technology of molecular sequencing has advanced so rapidly that a massive amount of sequencing per specimen now is possible and affordable.[49] These technologies, which are referred to as "next-generation sequencing," or *pyrosequencing,* have allowed much greater depth of coverage in the identification of endodontic microorganisms.[50] Studies using pyrosequencing have revealed that endodontic infections may contain bacteria from 10 to 24 different phyla, with hundreds of taxa identified.[50-52] In addition, these studies can provide considerable information about the true differences in microbial diversity between acute and chronic infections[53] and about the transition of the microbiota from a healthy oral condition to an endodontic infection.[54]

Other Microorganisms in Endodontic Infections

Microorganisms other than bacteria occasionally have been found in endodontic infections. Fungi are eukaryotic microorganisms that have been only sporadically found in primary infections.[29,55] Archaea comprise a highly diverse group of prokaryotes, distinct from bacteria, with no known human pathogen. One study found methanogenic Archaea in 25% of the canals of teeth with chronic apical periodontitis,[56] but this relatively high prevalence was not confirmed by other studies.[57-59] Viruses are not cells but inanimate particles that have no metabolism on their own. Because viruses require viable host cells to infect and replicate themselves, they cannot survive in the root canal with necrotic pulp. Viruses have been reported to occur in the root canal only in teeth with vital pulps. For instance, the human immunodeficiency virus (HIV) has been detected in noninflamed vital pulps of patients who are HIV seropositive,[60] and some herpes viruses have been identified in both noninflamed and inflamed vital pulps.[61] Several herpes viruses have been found in inflamed periradicular tissues, including symptomatic apical periodontitis lesions[62] and abscesses.[63,64] The specific role of viruses in the pathogenesis of pulpitis and apical periodontitis, if any, remains to be elucidated.

Symptomatic Infections

It has been suggested that the probability of symptoms is increased when certain bacterial species are part of the infective endodontic microbiota.[2,16,22,41] Nevertheless, the same species can be found in asymptomatic cases with a prevalence comparable to that of symptomatic cases.[20,21,23,25,65] This raises the suspicion that factors other than the mere presence of a given putative pathogenic species can influence the development of symptoms. These factors include differences in virulence ability among strains of the same species; the number of occurring species and interactions among them that result in additive or synergistic pathogenic effects; the number of bacterial cells (load); the environmental cues regulating expression of virulence factors; host resistance; and concomitant herpes virus infection.[66] Association of some or all of these factors (rather than an isolated event) is likely to dictate the occurrence and intensity of symptoms.

Ecology of the Endodontic Microbiota

A root canal with necrotic pulp provides a space for bacterial colonization. It also gives bacteria a moist, warm, nutritious, and anaerobic environment that is mostly protected from host defenses because of the lack of active microcirculation in the necrotic tissue. Intuitively, the necrotic root canal might be considered a rather fertile environment for bacterial growth, and it might be realized that colonization should not be a difficult task for virtually every oral bacterial species. Although approximately 1,000 different bacterial taxa have been reported in the oral cavity,[67] and each individual's mouth can harbor about 100 to 200 taxa,[68] only a restricted assortment of these bacteria is found in an infected canal. This indicates that selective pressures must occur in the root canal system that favor the establishment of some species and inhibit others.[69] The key ecologic factors that influence the composition of the microbiota in the necrotic root canal include oxygen tension and redox potential, the type and amount of available nutrients, and bacterial interactions.

Oxygen Tension and Redox Potential

Root canal infection is a dynamic process, and different bacterial species apparently dominate at different stages of the infectious process. Early in the initial phases of the pulpal infectious process, facultative bacteria predominate.[70] After a few days or weeks, oxygen is depleted in the root canal as a result of pulp necrosis and consumption by facultative bacteria. An anaerobic milieu develops, with consequent low redox potential; this is highly conducive to the survival and growth of obligate anaerobic bacteria. With the passage of time, anaerobic conditions become even more pronounced, particularly in the apical third of the root canal, and as a consequence, anaerobes come to dominate the microbiota and outnumber facultative bacteria.

Available Nutrients

In the root canal system, bacteria can utilize the following as sources of nutrients: (1) the necrotic pulp tissue, (2) proteins and glycoproteins from tissue fluids and exudate that seep into the root canal system via apical and lateral foramina, (3) components of saliva that may coronally penetrate into the root canal, and (4) products of the metabolism of other bacteria. Because the largest amount of nutrients is available in the main canal, which is the most voluminous part of the root canal system, most of the infecting microbiota, particularly fastidious anaerobic species, is expected to be located in this region. At later stages of the infectious process, nutritional conditions favor the establishment of bacteria that metabolize peptides and amino acids.

Bacterial Interactions

The establishment of certain species in the root canal is also influenced by interactions with other species. Positive interactions (mutualism and commensalism) enhance the survival capacity of the interacting bacteria and increase the probability of certain species coexisting in the habitat. Negative interactions (competition and antagonism) limit population densities.

Apical Periodontitis as a Biofilm-Related Disease

A better understanding of the disease process and the development of effective antimicrobial therapeutic strategies depends on a knowledge of the anatomy of infection (i.e., the way microbial cells are distributed throughout the infected tissue). Bacteria in the root canal system may exist as planktonic (unattached) cells suspended in the fluid phase of the main root canal. However, the dominant pattern of bacterial colonization of the root canal system is through the formation of a biofilm that adheres to the root canal walls (Fig. 3.4).[71-75] Recognition of biofilms as the main form in which bacteria are found in endodontic infections permits apical periodontitis to be included among the biofilm-induced oral diseases, along with caries and marginal periodontitis.

Biofilm is the main form in which bacteria are found in nature; it can be defined as a sessile, multicellular microbial community characterized by cells that are firmly attached to a surface and enmeshed in a self-produced matrix of extracellular polymeric substances (EPS).[76,77] There are many advantages for bacteria in assuming the biofilm form, including improved communication among species, metabolic cooperation, and protection against exogenous threats. Bacterial

organization in multispecies biofilm communities results in collective pathogenic effects on the host.[78]

Biofilms are observed not only on the walls of the main canal; they can spread to apical ramifications, lateral canals, and isthmuses.[79-81] Dentinal tubules underneath biofilms covering the walls of the main apical canal are often invaded by bacteria from the bottom of the biofilm structure (Fig. 3.5). As noted previously, the diameter of dentinal tubules is large enough to permit penetration of most oral bacteria, and tubular infection is observed in most teeth with apical periodontitis lesions. Although shallow intratubular penetration is more common, bacterial cells can be observed reaching a depth of approximately 300 µm in some teeth (Fig. 3.6).[75] All these areas usually represent a challenge for proper disinfection, because they are difficult (or even impossible) to access with instruments and irrigants.

The larger the apical periodontitis lesion, the higher the prevalence of bacterial biofilms in the apical canal.[72] Because

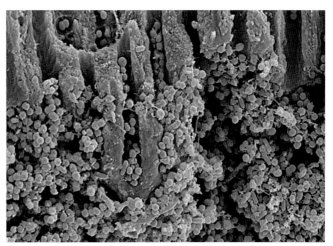

Fig. 3.5 Heavy infection of the root canal walls, mainly by cocci, but some small rods are also seen. Cocci are penetrating into dentinal tubules. (From Siqueira JF Jr, Rôças IN, Lopes HP: *Oral Surg Oral Med Oral Pathol Oral Radiol Endod* 93:174, 2002.)

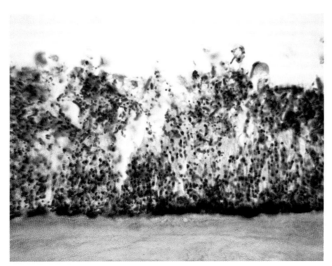

Fig. 3.4 Intracanal biofilms with predominance of cocci. Note the high concentration of cells at the bottom of the biofilm and in direct contact with the root canal wall. (From Ricucci D, Siqueira JF Jr: *J Endod* 36:1277, 2010.)

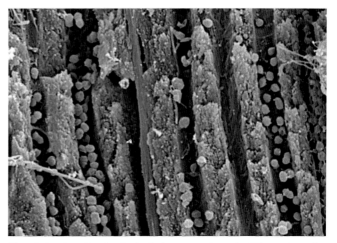

Fig. 3.6 Cocci in dentinal tubules approximately 300 µm from the main root canal. Dividing cells are seen within tubules. (From Siqueira JF Jr, Rôças IN, Lopes HP: *Oral Surg Oral Med Oral Pathol Oral Radiol Endod* 93:174, 2002.)

it takes time for apical periodontitis to develop and become visible on radiographs, large lesions can be assumed to represent a longstanding pathologic process caused by an even "older" intraradicular infection. In a longstanding infectious process, the involved bacteria may have had enough time and favorable conditions for adapting to the environment and establishing a mature and organized biofilm community. The fact that infected root canals of teeth with large lesions harbor a large number of cells and species, almost always organized into biofilms, may help explain why lesion size may influence the endodontic treatment outcome.[82,83]

Because the ideal outcome of endodontic treatment relies on elimination of the cause of apical periodontitis, effective antimicrobial strategies to eradicate endodontic infections should take into account the patterns of microbial colonization. Microorganisms present as planktonic cells in the main root canal can be easily eliminated with instruments and irrigants during treatment. Microorganisms present in biofilms adhering to the canal walls or located in isthmuses, lateral canals, or dentinal tubules are indisputably more difficult to eradicate and may require special therapeutic strategies.[79]

Persistent and Secondary Endodontic Infections

Persistent infections are caused by microorganisms from a primary infection that resisted intracanal antimicrobial procedures and managed to endure periods of nutrient deprivation in a prepared canal. Secondary infections are caused by microorganisms that were not present in the primary infection but that were introduced into the root canal system at some time during or after professional intervention. Entry can occur during treatment, between appointments, or even after root canal filling. Species involved in secondary infections can be oral or nonoral microorganisms, depending on the source of contamination. The main causes of microbial introduction in the canal *during treatment* include remnants of dental plaque, calculus, or caries on the tooth crown; leakage of the rubber dam; or contamination of endodontic instruments, irrigating solutions, or other intracanal medications. Microorganisms can enter the root canal system *between appointments* by loss or leakage of temporary restorative materials; fracture of the tooth structure; or through teeth left open for drainage. Microorganisms can penetrate the root canal system *after root canal filling* by loss or leakage of temporary or permanent restorative materials; preparation of posts or other intracanal restorations without the rubber dam; fracture of the tooth structure; recurrent decay that exposes the root canal filling material; or delay in the placement of permanent restorations.

For the most part, persistent and secondary infections are clinically indistinguishable. They can be responsible for several clinical problems, including persistent exudation, persistent symptoms, interappointment flare-ups, and failure of the endodontic treatment, characterized by a post-treatment apical periodontitis lesion. Secondary infections are suspected when a preoperative lesion heals after treatment and then recurs at a later time.

Most root canal–treated teeth with persistent apical periodontitis lesions have been demonstrated to harbor an intraradicular infection.[84-87] Microorganisms present in root canal–treated teeth can be "persisters" that survived the effects of intracanal disinfection procedures and were present in the canal at the root canal–filling stage (persistent infection), or

they can have infected the canal after filling as a result of coronal leakage (secondary infection). In fact, there is an increased risk of an adverse treatment outcome when microorganisms are present in the canal at the time of filling.[88,89] To exert pathogenicity and cause persistent apical periodontitis lesions, residual microorganisms must adapt to the modified environment induced by treatment, acquire nutrients, survive the antimicrobial effects of filling materials, reach critical numbers and exhibit virulence attributes sufficient to sustain periradicular inflammation, and have unrestrained access to the periradicular tissues.

Bacteria at the Root Canal–Filling Stage

Diligent antimicrobial treatment occasionally can fail to eradicate bacteria from root canals, with consequent selection of the most resistant segment of the microbiota. Gram-negative bacteria, which are common in primary intraradicular infections, are usually eliminated by endodontic treatment because they are very sensitive to strong oxidizing agents, such as sodium hypochlorite. Most studies on this subject have clearly revealed a higher occurrence of gram-positive bacteria (e.g., streptococci, lactobacilli, *Enterococcus faecalis*, *O. uli*, *Parvimonas micra*, *P. alactolyticus*, and *Propionibacterium* species) in both post-instrumentation and post-medication samples.[89-93] This gives support to the notion that gram-positive bacteria can be more resistant to antimicrobial treatment measures and have the ability to adapt to the harsh environmental conditions in instrumented and medicated canals. The presence of cultivable bacteria at the time of obturation has been shown in some studies to significantly reduce the chances of healing.[89,94] However, this finding does not appear to be universal.[95] Factors that influence whether residual bacteria affect long-term healing may involve the load and location of the residual bacteria, the extraradicular occurrence of bacteria, the quality of obturation, and the quality and integrity of postoperative restoration. Some studies have documented the presence of bacteria in apical periodontitis lesions in patients with persistent lesions[96,97] (see the following sections), although it is difficult to avoid contamination when sampling periradicular lesions during a surgical procedure.

Microbiota in Root Canal–Treated Teeth

The microbiota in root canal–treated teeth with post-treatment apical periodontitis lesions is composed of a more restricted group of microbial species than is seen in primary infections. Studies evaluating samples taken from retreatment cases have revealed that apparently well treated canals harbor up to five species, whereas canals with inadequate treatment can contain 10 to 30 species, a finding very similar to that for untreated canals.[85-87,98,99] Bacterial counts in treated canals range from 10^3 to 10^7 cell equivalents.[100-103]

E. faecalis is a facultative anaerobic gram-positive coccus that has been frequently found in root canal–treated teeth, with prevalence values ranging from 30% to 90% of cases.[19,85-87,101,103,104] Root canal–treated teeth are about nine times more likely to harbor *E. faecalis* than are teeth with a primary infection.[19] *Candida* species are fungi only sporadically found in primary infections, but detection frequencies in persistent and secondary infections range from 3% to 18% of cases.[55,85-87,102,104,105] Both *E. faecalis* and *C. albicans* have a series of attributes that may allow them to survive in treated **43** canals, including resistance to intracanal medications and the abilities to form biofilms, invade dentinal tubules, and endure long periods of nutrient deprivation.[106-110]

Despite the high prevalence of *E. faecalis* in the canals of teeth with post-treatment apical periodontitis, the organism's status as the main pathogen associated with treatment failure has been questioned, because if present, it is rarely the most dominant species in the bacterial community of treated canals.[98,103] In addition, it has been detected in root canal–treated teeth with no disease in a similarly high prevalence.[111,112] *Streptococcus* species, which are also frequently detected and in many cases are the dominant bacterial group, in addition to *P. alactolyticus, Propionibacterium* species, *F. alocis, T. forsythia, D. pneumosintes,* and *D. invisus,* can be involved in persistent and secondary intraradicular infections (Table 3.2).[27,85-87,103]

Table 3.2 Microorganisms detected in root canal–treated teeth associated with persistent apical periodontitis

Taxa	Frequency (%)*
Enterococcus faecalis	77
Pseudoramibacter alactolyticus	55
Propionibacterium propionicum	50
Filifactor alocis	48
Dialister pneumosintes	46
Bacteroidetes clone X083	44
Streptococcus spp.	23
Tannerella forsythia	23
Dialister invisus	14
Campylobacter rectus	14
Porphyromonas gingivalis	14
Treponema denticola	14
Fusobacterium nucleatum	10
Prevotella intermedia	10
Candida albicans	9
Campylobacter gracilis	5
Actinomyces radicidentis	5
Porphyromonas endodontalis	5
Parvimonas micra	5
Pyramidobacter piscolens	5
Olsenella uli	5

Data from Siqueira JF Jr, Rôças IN: *Oral Surg Oral Med Oral Pathol Oral Radiol Endod* 97:85, 2004; Siqueira JF Jr, Rôças IN: *J Clin Microbiol* 43:3314, 2005.
*Percentage of cases harboring each taxon.

Extraradicular Infections

Apical periodontitis develops in response to intraradicular infection, and in most situations it succeeds in preventing microorganisms from gaining access to the periradicular tissues. Nevertheless, in some specific circumstances, microorganisms can overcome this defense barrier and establish an extraradicular infection. Extraradicular infection is characterized by microbial invasion of and proliferation in the inflamed periradicular tissues and is almost invariably a sequel to intraradicular infection.

The most common form of extraradicular infection is the acute apical abscess (Fig. 3.7). However, another form of extraradicular infection has been associated with chronic infections and some cases of post-treatment apical periodontitis. This condition involves the establishment of microorganisms beyond the boundaries of the root canal, either by adherence to the apical external root surface in the form of biofilm structures[113] or by the formation of cohesive actinomycotic colonies in the body of the periradicular inflammatory lesion.[114] Extraradicular microorganisms have been discussed as one of the causes of persistence of apical periodontitis lesions in spite of diligent root canal treatment.[115]

Conceivably, the extraradicular infection can depend on or be independent of the intraradicular infection.[116] The question of whether the extraradicular infection is dependent on or independent of the intraradicular infection assumes special

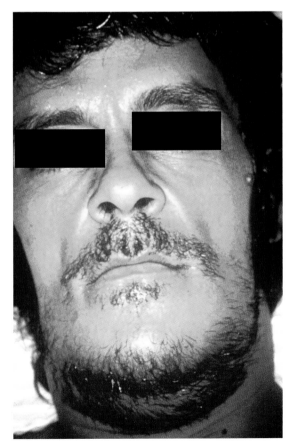

Fig. 3.7 Acute apical abscess with severe swelling. Cases such as this represent the most common form of extraradicular infection dependent on the intraradicular infection. (Courtesy Dr. Henrique Martins.)

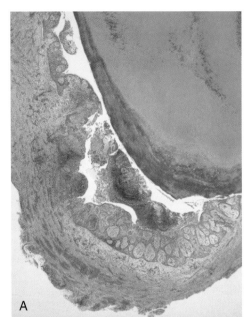

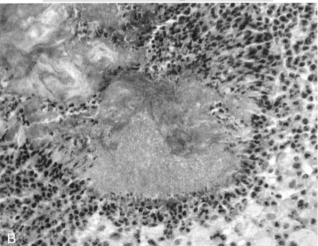

Fig. 3.8 Apical actinomycosis. **A,** Bacterial aggregate in an epithelialized apical periodontitis lesion, suggestive of actinomycosis. **B,** Higher magnification of the actinomycotic aggregate, which is surrounded by inflammatory cells. (Courtesy Dr. Domenico Ricucci.)

relevance from a therapeutic standpoint, because the former can be successfully managed by root canal therapy, whereas the latter can be treated only by endodontic surgery.

The presence of a sinus tract (fistula) usually indicates the extraradicular occurrence of bacteria. The fact that most sinus tracts close after proper root canal treatment suggests an extraradicular infection fostered by and dependent on the intraradicular infection. Also, the acute apical abscess, for the most part, is clearly dependent on the intraradicular infection. Once the intraradicular infection is properly controlled by root canal treatment or tooth extraction and drainage of pus is achieved, the extraradicular infection is handled by the host defenses and usually subsides. Apical actinomycosis is a pathologic entity caused by some *Actinomyces* species and *P. propionicum* and is the main example of an extraradicular infection supposedly independent of the intraradicular infection (Figure 3.8). However, there is no clear evidence in the literature that apical actinomycosis is actually independent of the intraradicular infection.[80]

It is still controversial whether asymptomatic apical periodontitis lesions can harbor bacteria for very long beyond initial tissue invasion. The incidence of extraradicular infections in untreated teeth is reportedly low.[71,72,117] Extraradicular biofilms are very infrequent and when present are virtually always associated with intraradicular biofilms.[72,118] This dependence of extraradicular infection on intraradicular infection is congruent with the high success rate of nonsurgical root canal treatment.[119] Even in root canal–treated teeth with recalcitrant lesions, in which a higher incidence of extraradicular bacteria has been reported, a high rate of healing after retreatment[119,120] indicates that the major cause of posttreatment disease is located within the root canal system, characterizing a persistent or secondary intraradicular infection.[85-87,104]

REFERENCES

1. Kakehashi S, Stanley HR, Fitzgerald RJ: The effects of surgical exposures of dental pulps in germ-free and conventional laboratory rats, *Oral Surg Oral Med Oral Pathol* 20:340-349, 1965.
2. Sundqvist G: *Bacteriological studies of necrotic dental pulps, odontological dissertation no 7,* Umea, Sweden, 1976, University of Umea.
3. Möller AJR, Fabricius L, Dahlén G, et al: Influence on periapical tissues of indigenous oral bacteria and necrotic pulp tissue in monkeys, *Scand J Dent Res* 89:475-484, 1981.
4. Pashley DH: Dynamics of the pulpo-dentin complex, *Crit Rev Oral Biol Med* 7:104-133, 1996.
5. Garberoglio R, Brännström M: Scanning electron microscopic investigation of human dentinal tubules, *Arch Oral Biol* 21:355-358, 1976.
6. Nagaoka S, Miyazaki Y, Liu HJ, et al: Bacterial invasion into dentinal tubules of human vital and nonvital teeth, *J Endod* 21:70-73, 1995.
7. Langeland K: Tissue response to dental caries, *Endod Dent Traumatol* 3:149-171, 1987.
8. Cvek M, Cleaton-Jones PE, Austin JC, et al: Pulp reactions to exposure after experimental crown fractures or grinding in adult monkeys, *J Endod* 8:391-397, 1982.
9. Langeland K, Rodrigues H, Dowden W: Periodontal disease, bacteria, and pulpal histopathology, *Oral Surg Oral Med Oral Pathol* 37:257, 1974.
10. Delivanis PD, Fan VS: The localization of blood-borne bacteria in instrumented unfilled and overinstrumented canals, *J Endod* 10:521-524, 1984.
11. Love RM, Jenkinson HF: Invasion of dentinal tubules by oral bacteria, *Crit Rev Oral Biol Med* 13:171-183, 2002.
12. Grossman LI: Origin of microorganisms in traumatized, pulpless, sound teeth, *J Dent Res* 46:551-553, 1967.
13. Siqueira JF Jr, Rôças IN: Exploiting molecular methods to explore endodontic infections. Part 2. Redefining the endodontic microbiota, *J Endod* 31:488-498, 2005.
14. Vianna ME, Horz HP, Gomes BP, et al: In vivo evaluation of microbial reduction after chemomechanical preparation of human root canals containing necrotic pulp tissue, *Int Endod J* 39:484-492, 2006.
15. Siqueira JF Jr, Rôças IN: Diversity of endodontic microbiota revisited, *J Dent Res* 88:969-81, 2009.
16. Sakamoto M, Rôças IN, Siqueira JF Jr, et al: Molecular analysis of bacteria in asymptomatic and symptomatic endodontic infections, *Oral Microbiol Immunol* 21:112-122, 2006.
17. Munson MA, Pitt-Ford T, Chong B, et al: Molecular and cultural analysis of the microflora associated with endodontic infections, *J Dent Res* 81:761-766, 2002.

18. Ribeiro AC, Matarazzo F, Faveri M, et al: Exploring bacterial diversity of endodontic microbiota by cloning and sequencing 16S rRNA, *J Endod* 37:922-926, 2011.

19. Siqueira JF Jr, Rôças IN, Rosado AS: Investigation of bacterial communities associated with asymptomatic and symptomatic endodontic infections by denaturing gradient gel electrophoresis fingerprinting approach, *Oral Microbiol Immunol* 19:363-370, 2004.

20. Haapasalo M, Ranta H, Ranta K, et al: Black-pigmented *Bacteroides* spp. in human apical periodontitis, *Infect Immun* 53:149-153, 1986.

21. Baumgartner JC, Watkins BJ, Bae KS, et al: Association of black-pigmented bacteria with endodontic infections, *J Endod* 25:413-415, 1999.

22. van Winkelhoff AJ, Carlee AW, de Graaff J: *Bacteroides endodontalis* and other black-pigmented *Bacteroides* species in odontogenic abscesses, *Infect Immun* 49:494-498, 1985.

23. Siqueira JF Jr, Rôças IN, Souto R, et al: Checkerboard DNA-DNA hybridization analysis of endodontic infections, *Oral Surg Oral Med Oral Pathol Oral Radiol Endod* 89:744-748, 2000.

24. Siqueira JF Jr, Rôças IN, Oliveira JC, et al: Molecular detection of black-pigmented bacteria in infections of endodontic origin, *J Endod* 27:563-566, 2001.

25. Fouad AF, Barry J, Caimano M, et al: PCR-based identification of bacteria associated with endodontic infections, *J Clin Microbiol* 40:3223-3231, 2002.

26. Vianna ME, Horz HP, Gomes BP, et al: Microarrays complement culture methods for identification of bacteria in endodontic infections, *Oral Microbiol Immunol* 20:253-258, 2005.

27. Siqueira JF Jr, Rôças IN: Uncultivated phylotypes and newly named species associated with primary and persistent endodontic infections, *J Clin Microbiol* 43:3314-3319, 2005.

28. Sundqvist G: Associations between microbial species in dental root canal infections, *Oral Microbiol Immunol* 7:257-262, 1992.

29. Lana MA, Ribeiro-Sobrinho AP, Stehling R, et al: Microorganisms isolated from root canals presenting necrotic pulp and their drug susceptibility in vitro, *Oral Microbiol Immunol* 16:100-105, 2001.

30. Baumgartner JC, Siqueira JF Jr, Xia T, et al: Geographical differences in bacteria detected in endodontic infections using polymerase chain reaction, *J Endod* 30:141-144, 2004.

31. Rôças IN, Siqueira JF Jr, Andrade AF, et al: Oral treponemes in primary root canal infections as detected by nested PCR, *Int Endod J* 36:20-26, 2003.

32. Siqueira JF Jr, Rôças IN: *Treponema* species associated with abscesses of endodontic origin, *Oral Microbiol Immunol* 19:336-339, 2004.

33. Baumgartner JC, Khemaleelakul SU, Xia T: Identification of spirochetes (treponemes) in endodontic infections, *J Endod* 29:794-797, 2003.

34. Foschi F, Cavrini F, Montebugnoli L, et al: Detection of bacteria in endodontic samples by polymerase chain reaction assays and association with defined clinical signs in Italian patients, *Oral Microbiol Immunol* 20:289-295, 2005.

35. Rôças IN, Siqueira JF Jr: Root canal microbiota of teeth with chronic apical periodontitis, *J Clin Microbiol* 46:3599-3606, 2008.

36. Siqueira JF Jr, Rôças IN: The microbiota of acute apical abscesses, *J Dent Res* 88:61-65, 2009.

37. Siqueira JF Jr, Rôças IN: Detection of *Filifactor alocis* in endodontic infections associated with different forms of periradicular diseases, *Oral Microbiol Immunol* 18:263-265, 2003.

38. Siqueira JF Jr, Rôças IN, Souto R, et al: *Actinomyces* species, streptococci, and *Enterococcus faecalis* in primary root canal infections, *J Endod* 28:168-172, 2002.

39. Fouad AF, Kum KY, Clawson ML, et al: Molecular characterization of the presence of *Eubacterium* spp and *Streptococcus* spp in endodontic infections, *Oral Microbiol Immunol* 18:249-255, 2003.

40. Rôças IN, Siqueira JF Jr: Species-directed 16S rRNA gene nested PCR detection of *Olsenella* species in association with endodontic diseases, *Lett Appl Microbiol* 41:12-16, 2005.

41. Gomes BP, Lilley JD, Drucker DB: Clinical significance of dental root canal microflora, *J Dent* 24:47-55, 1996.

42. Chu FC, Tsang CS, Chow TW, et al: Identification of cultivable microorganisms from primary endodontic infections with exposed and unexposed pulp space, *J Endod* 31:424-429, 2005.

43. Rôças IN, Siqueira JF Jr: Detection of novel oral species and phylotypes in symptomatic endodontic infections including abscesses, *FEMS Microbiol Lett* 250:279-285, 2005.

44. Siqueira JF Jr, Rôças IN, Cunha CD, et al: Novel bacterial phylotypes in endodontic infections, *J Dent Res* 84:565-569, 2005.

45. Rolph HJ, Lennon A, Riggio MP, et al: Molecular identification of microorganisms from endodontic infections, *J Clin Microbiol* 39:3282-3289, 2001.

46. Saito D, de Toledo LR, Rodrigues JLM, et al: Identification of bacteria in endodontic infections by sequence analysis of 16S rDNA clone libraries, *J Med Microbiol* 55:101-107, 2006.

47. Rôças IN, Siqueira JF Jr: Prevalence of new candidate pathogens *Prevotella baroniae, Prevotella multisaccharivorax* and as-yet-uncultivated Bacteroidetes clone X083 in primary endodontic infections, *J Endod* 35:1359-1362, 2009.

48. Relman DA: Microbial genomics and infectious diseases, *N Engl J Med* 365:347-357, 2011.

49. Siqueira JF Jr, Fouad AF, Rocas IN: Pyrosequencing as a tool for better understanding of human microbiomes, *J Oral Microbiol* 4: 10743 2012.

50. Siqueira JF Jr, Alves FR, Rocas IN: Pyrosequencing analysis of the apical root canal microbiota, *J Endod* 37:1499-1503, 2011.

51. Ozok AR, Persoon IF, Huse SM, et al: Ecology of the microbiome of the infected root canal system: a comparison between apical and coronal root segments, *Int Endod J* 45:530-541, 2012.

52. Li L, Hsiao WW, Nandakumar R, et al: Analyzing endodontic infections by deep coverage pyrosequencing, *J Dent Res* 89:980-984, 2010.

53. Santos AL, Siqueira JF Jr, Rocas IN, et al: Comparing the bacterial diversity of acute and chronic dental root canal infections, *PLoS One* 6:e28088, 2011.

54. Hsiao WW, Li KL, Liu Z, et al: Microbial transformation from normal oral microbiota to acute endodontic infections, *BMC Genomics* 13:345, 2012.

55. Egan MW, Spratt DA, Ng YL, et al: Prevalence of yeasts in saliva and root canals of teeth associated with apical periodontitis, *Int Endod J* 35:321-329, 2002.

56. Vianna ME, Conrads G, Gomes BPFA, et al: Identification and quantification of Archaea involved in primary endodontic infections, *J Clin Microbiol* 44:1274-1282, 2006.

57. Paiva SS, Siqueira JF Jr, Rocas IN, et al: Supplementing the antimicrobial effects of chemomechanical debridement with either passive ultrasonic irrigation or a final rinse with chlorhexidine: a clinical study, *J Endod* 38:1202-1206, 2012.

58. Rôças IN, Siqueira JF Jr: In vivo antimicrobial effects of endodontic treatment procedures as assessed by molecular microbiologic techniques, *J Endod* 37:304-310, 2011.

59. Siqueira JF Jr, Rôças IN, Baumgartner JC, et al: Searching for Archaea in infections of endodontic origin, *J Endod* 31:719-722, 2005.

60. Glick M, Trope M, Bagasra O, et al: Human immunodeficiency virus infection of fibroblasts of dental pulp in seropositive patients, *Oral Surg Oral Med Oral Pathol* 71:733-736, 1991.

61. Li H, Chen V, Chen Y, et al: Herpes viruses in endodontic pathoses: association of Epstein-Barr virus with irreversible pulpitis and apical periodontitis, *J Endod* 35:23-29, 2009.

62. Sabeti M, Simon JH, Slots J: *Cytomegalovirus* and Epstein-Barr virus are associated with symptomatic periapical pathosis, *Oral Microbiol Immunol* 18:327-328, 2003.

63. Ferreira DC, Paiva SS, Carmo FL, et al: Identification of herpes viruses types 1 to 8 and human papillomavirus in acute apical abscesses, *J Endod* 37:10-16, 2011.

64. Chen V, Chen Y, Li H, et al: Herpes viruses in abscesses and cellulitis of endodontic origin, *J Endod* 35:182-188, 2009.

65. Siqueira JF Jr, Rôças IN, Souto R, et al: Microbiological evaluation of acute periradicular abscesses by DNA-DNA hybridization, *Oral Surg Oral Med Oral Pathol Oral Radiol Endod* 92:451-457, 2001.

66. Siqueira JF Jr, Barnett F: Interappointment pain: mechanisms, diagnosis, and treatment, *Endod Topics* 7:93-109, 2004.

67. Dewhirst FE, Chen T, Izard J, et al: The human oral microbiome, *J Bacteriol* 192:5002-5017, 2010.

68. Paster BJ, Olsen I, Aas JA, et al: The breadth of bacterial diversity in the human periodontal pocket and other oral sites, *Periodontology* 2000 42:80-87, 2006.

69. Sundqvist G, Figdor D: Life as an endodontic pathogen: ecological differences between the untreated and root-filled root canals, *Endod Topics* 6:3-28, 2003.

70. Fabricius L, Dahlén G, Ohman AE, et al: Predominant indigenous oral bacteria isolated from infected root canals after varied times of closure, *Scand J Dent Res* 90:134-144, 1982.

71. Nair PNR: Light and electron microscopic studies of root canal flora and periapical lesions, *J Endod* 13:29-39, 1987.

72. Ricucci D, Siqueira JF Jr: Biofilms and apical periodontitis: study of prevalence and association with clinical and histopathologic findings, *J Endod* 36:1277-1288, 2010.

73. Ricucci D, Siqueira JF Jr, Bate AL, et al: Histologic investigation of root canal–treated teeth with apical periodontitis: a retrospective study from twenty-four patients, *J Endod* 35:493-502, 2009.

74. Molven O, Olsen I, Kerekes K: Scanning electron microscopy of bacteria in the apical part of root canals in permanent teeth with periapical lesions, *Endod Dent Traumatol* 7:226-229, 1991.

75. Siqueira JF Jr, Rôças IN, Lopes HP: Patterns of microbial colonization in primary root canal infections, *Oral Surg Oral Med Oral Pathol Oral Radiol Endod* 93:174-178, 2002.

76. Costerton JW: *The biofilm primer*, Berlin, 2007, Springer-Verlag.

77. Donlan RM, Costerton JW: Biofilms: survival mechanisms of clinically relevant microorganisms, *Clin Microbiol Rev* 15:167-193, 2002.

78. Siqueira JF Jr, Rôças IN: Community as the unit of pathogenicity: an emerging concept as to the microbial pathogenesis of apical periodontitis, *Oral Surg Oral Med Oral Pathol Oral Radiol Endod* 107:870-878, 2009.

79. Nair PN, Henry S, Cano V, et al: Microbial status of apical root canal system of human mandibular first molars with primary apical periodontitis after "one-visit" endodontic treatment, *Oral Surg Oral Med Oral Pathol Oral Radiol Endod* 99:231-252, 2005.

80. Ricucci D, Siqueira JF Jr: Apical actinomycosis as a continuum of intraradicular and extraradicular infection: case report and critical review on its involvement with treatment failure, *J Endod* 34:1124-1129, 2008.

81. Ricucci D, Siqueira JF Jr: Fate of the tissue in lateral canals and apical ramifications in response to pathologic conditions and treatment procedures, *J Endod* 36:1-15, 2010.

82. Chugal NM, Clive JM, Spangberg LS: A prognostic model for assessment of the outcome of endodontic treatment: effect of biologic and diagnostic variables, *Oral Surg Oral Med Oral Pathol Oral Radiol Endod* 91:342-352, 2001.

83. Ng YL, Mann V, Gulabivala K: A prospective study of the factors affecting outcomes of

nonsurgical root canal treatment. Part 1. Periapical health, *Int Endod J* 44:583-609, 2011.

84. Lin LM, Skribner JE, Gaengler P: Factors associated with endodontic treatment failures, *J Endod* 18:625-627, 1992.

85. Siqueira JF Jr, Rôças IN: Polymerase chain reaction–based analysis of microorganisms associated with failed endodontic treatment, *Oral Surg Oral Med Oral Pathol Oral Radiol Endod* 97:85-94, 2004.

86. Sundqvist G, Figdor D, Persson S, et al: Microbiologic analysis of teeth with failed endodontic treatment and the outcome of conservative re-treatment, *Oral Surg Oral Med Oral Pathol Oral Radiol Endod* 85:86-93, 1998.

87. Pinheiro ET, Gomes BP, Ferraz CC, et al: Microorganisms from canals of root-filled teeth with periapical lesions, *Int Endod J* 36:1-11, 2003.

88. Fabricius L, Dahlén G, Sundqvist G, et al: Influence of residual bacteria on periapical tissue healing after chemomechanical treatment and root filling of experimentally infected monkey teeth, *Eur J Oral Sci* 114:278-285, 2006.

89. Sjögren U, Figdor D, Persson S, et al: Influence of infection at the time of root filling on the outcome of endodontic treatment of teeth with apical periodontitis, *Int Endod J* 30:297-306, 1997.

90. Chu FC, Leung WK, Tsang PC, et al: Identification of cultivable microorganisms from root canals with apical periodontitis following two-visit endodontic treatment with antibiotics/steroid or calcium hydroxide dressings, *J Endod* 32:17-23, 2006.

91. Chavez de Paz LE, Molander A, Dahlen G: Gram-positive rods prevailing in teeth with apical periodontitis undergoing root canal treatment, *Int Endod J* 37:579-587, 2004.

92. Peters LB, van Winkelhoff AJ, Buijs JF, et al: Effects of instrumentation, irrigation and dressing with calcium hydroxide on infection in pulpless teeth with periapical bone lesions, *Int Endod J* 35:13-21, 2002.

93. Byström A, Sundqvist G: The antibacterial action of sodium hypochlorite and EDTA in 60 cases of endodontic therapy, *Int Endod J* 18:35-40, 1985.

94. Molander A, Warfvinge J, Reit C, et al: Clinical and radiographic evaluation of one- and two-visit endodontic treatment of asymptomatic necrotic teeth with apical periodontitis: a randomized clinical trial, *J Endod* 33:1145-1148, 2007.

95. Peters LB, Wesselink PR: Periapical healing of endodontically treated teeth in one and two visits obturated in the presence or absence of detectable microorganisms, *Int Endod J* 35:660-667, 2002.

96. Sunde PT, Olsen I, Debelian GJ, et al: Microbiota of periapical lesions refractory to endodontic therapy, *J Endod* 28:304-310, 2002.

97. Sunde PT, Olsen I, Gobel UB, et al: Fluorescence in situ hybridization (FISH) for direct visualization of bacteria in periapical lesions of asymptomatic root-filled teeth, *Microbiology* 149:1095-1102, 2003.

98. Rôças IN, Siqueira JF Jr, Aboim MC, et al: Denaturing gradient gel electrophoresis analysis of bacterial communities associated with failed endodontic treatment, *Oral Surg Oral Med Oral Pathol Oral Radiol Endod* 98:741-749, 2004.

99. Sakamoto M, Siqueira JF Jr, Rôças IN, et al: Molecular analysis of the root canal microbiota associated with endodontic treatment failures, *Oral Microbiol Immunol* 23:275-281, 2008.

100. Blome B, Braun A, Sobarzo V, et al: Molecular identification and quantification of bacteria from endodontic infections using real-time polymerase chain reaction, *Oral Microbiol Immunol* 23:384-390, 2008.

101. Sedgley C, Nagel A, Dahlen G, et al: Real-time quantitative polymerase chain reaction and culture analyses of *Enterococcus faecalis* in root canals, *J Endod* 32:173-177, 2006.

102. Peciuliene V, Reynaud AH, Balciuniene I, et al: Isolation of yeasts and enteric bacteria in root-filled teeth with chronic apical periodontitis, *Int Endod J* 34:429-434, 2001.

103. Rôças IN, Siqueira JF Jr: Characterization of microbiota of root canal–treated teeth with posttreatment disease, *J Clin Microbiol* 50:1721-1724, 2012.

104. Molander A, Reit C, Dahlen G, et al: Microbiological status of root-filled teeth with apical periodontitis, *Int Endod J* 31:1-7, 1998.

105. Möller AJR: Microbial examination of root canals and periapical tissues of human teeth, *Odontologisk Tidskrift* 74(suppl):1-380, 1966.

106. Haapasalo M, Ørstavik D: In vitro infection and disinfection of dentinal tubules, *J Dent Res* 66:1375-1379, 1987.

107. Distel JW, Hatton JF, Gillespie MJ: Biofilm formation in medicated root canals, *J Endod* 28:689-693, 2002.

108. Figdor D, Davies JK, Sundqvist G: Starvation survival, growth and recovery of *Enterococcus faecalis* in human serum, *Oral Microbiol Immunol* 18:234-239, 2003.

109. Sen BH, Safavi KE, Spangberg LS: Growth patterns of *Candida albicans* in relation to radicular dentin, *Oral Surg Oral Med Oral Pathol Oral Radiol Endod* 84:68-73, 1997.

110. Waltimo TM, Orstavik D, Siren EK, et al: In vitro susceptibility of *Candida albicans* to four disinfectants and their combinations, *Int Endod J* 32:421-429, 1999.

111. Kaufman B, Spangberg L, Barry J, et al: *Enterococcus* spp. in endodontically treated teeth with and without periradicular lesions, *J Endod* 31:851-856, 2005.

112. Zoletti GO, Siqueira JF Jr, Santos KR: Identification of *Enterococcus faecalis* in root-filled teeth with or without periradicular lesions by culture-dependent and -independent approaches, *J Endod* 32:722-726, 2006.

113. Tronstad L, Barnett F, Cervone F: Periapical bacterial plaque in teeth refractory to endodontic treatment, *Endod Dent Traumatol* 6:73-77, 1990.

114. Nair PNR, Schroeder HE: Periapical actinomycosis, *J Endod* 10:567-570, 1984.

115. Tronstad L, Sunde PT: The evolving new understanding of endodontic infections, *Endod Topics* 6:57-77, 2003.

116. Siqueira JF Jr: Periapical actinomycosis and infection with *Propionibacterium propionicum*, *Endod Topics* 6:78-95, 2003.

117. Siqueira JF Jr, Lopes HP: Bacteria on the apical root surfaces of untreated teeth with periradicular lesions: a scanning electron microscopy study, *Int Endod J* 34:216-220, 2001.

118. Subramanian K, Mickel AK: Molecular analysis of persistent periradicular lesions and root ends reveals a diverse microbial profile, *J Endod* 35:950-957, 2009.

119. Sjögren U, Hagglund B, Sundqvist G, et al: Factors affecting the long-term results of endodontic treatment, *J Endod* 16:498-504, 1990.

120. de Chevigny C, Dao TT, Basrani BR, et al: Treatment outcome in endodontics: the Toronto Study: phases 3 and 4—orthograde retreatment, *J Endod* 34:131-137, 2008.

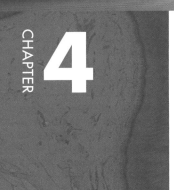

CHAPTER 4

Pulp and periapical pathosis

Mahmoud Torabinejad, Shahrokh Shabahang

LEARNING OBJECTIVES

After reading this chapter, the student should be able to:

1. Identify etiologic factors causing pulp inflammation.
2. Explain the mechanism of spread of inflammation in the pulp.
3. Explain why it is difficult for the pulp to recover from severe injury.
4. List specific and nonspecific mediators of pulpal inflammation.
5. Classify pulpal diseases and their clinical and histologic features.
6. Describe the mechanisms and explain the consequences of the spread of pulpal inflammation into periradicular tissues and the subsequent inflammatory and immunologic responses.

7. Classify periradicular lesions of pulpal origin.
8. Identify and distinguish between histologic features and clinical signs and symptoms of acute apical periodontitis, chronic apical periodontitis, acute and chronic apical abscesses (suppurative apical periodontitis), and condensing osteitis.
9. Describe the steps involved in repair of periradicular pathosis after successful root canal treatment.
10. Identify and describe, in general, nonendodontic pathologic lesions that may mimic endodontic periradicular pathosis.

IRRITANTS

Irritation of pulpal or periradicular tissues can result in inflammation. These irritants can be broadly classified as nonliving or living. Nonliving causes of inflammation may be mechanical, thermal, or chemical. Viable irritants include microorganisms and viruses.

Mechanical Irritants

Mechanical irritants, such as deep cavity preparations, removal of tooth structure without proper cooling, impact trauma, occlusal trauma, deep periodontal curettage, and orthodontic movement of teeth may lead to alterations in the underlying pulp. Transient changes, such as aspiration of odontoblasts into the dentinal tubules, are usually reversible in healthy pulps (Fig. 4.1). In typical clinical situations, however, the pulpal tissue is already inflamed due to the presence of caries or previous restorative procedures. If proper precautions are not taken, cavity or crown preparations may damage subjacent odontoblasts. The number of tubules per unit of surface area and the tubules' diameter increase closer to the pulp (Fig. 4.2).

As a result, dentinal permeability is greater closer to the pulp than near the dentinoenamel junction (DEJ) or cementodentinal junction (CDJ).[1] Therefore the potential for pulp irritation increases as more dentin is removed (i.e., as cavity preparation deepens and reaches closer to the pulp). Pulp damage is roughly proportional to the amount of tooth structure removed, in addition to the depth of removal.[2] Also, operative procedures without water coolant cause more irritation than those performed under water spray.[3] A study of the reactions and vascular changes occurring in experimentally induced acute and chronic pulpitis demonstrated increased permeability and dilation of blood vessels in the early stages of pulpitis.[4] Investigations in rodent models designed to determine the impact of heat generation on the dental pulp have shown that elevation of pulpal temperature above 42°C up-regulate heat shock proteins (HSPs).[5] HSP-70 plays a protective role, and its levels return to baseline within a few hours after removal of the heat stimulus.

Impact injuries with or without crown or root fractures may cause pulpal damage (see Chapter 11). The severity of trauma and degree of apical closure of the root are important factors

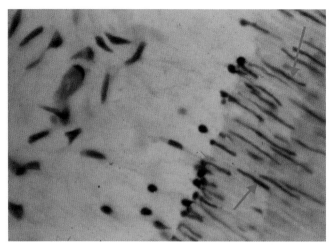

Fig. 4.1 Crown preparation through enamel and into 1 mm of dentin resulted in aspiration of odontoblasts *(arrows)* into the tubules and infiltration of the pulp by polymorphonuclear (PMN) leukocytes and lymphocytes. The specimen was taken 48 hours after crown preparation.

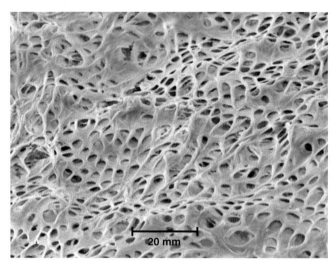

20 mm

Fig. 4.2 Photomicrograph illustration of numerous dentin tubules on the dentin wall adjacent to the canal lumen. The density of the tubules increases closer to the pulpal side of the dentin wall.

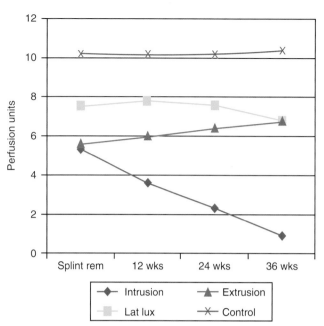

Fig. 4.3 Graphic representation of pulpal circulation subsequent to various types of luxation injuries to teeth. Pulp circulation is measured in perfusion units over a 36-week observation period.

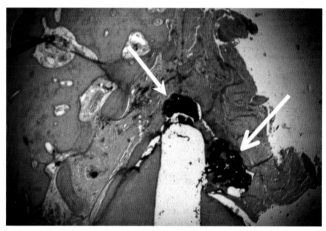

Fig. 4.4 Improper instrumentation and extrusion of filling materials into the periapical tissues causes periradicular inflammation *(arrows)*.

in the pulp's ability to recover. Teeth undergoing mild to moderate trauma and those with immature apices have a better chance of pulpal survival compared with those suffering severe injury or those with closed apices. Application of forces beyond the physiologic tolerance of the periodontal ligament (PDL) during orthodontic tooth movement results in disturbance of the blood and nerve supply of the pulp tissue.[6,7] The resulting changes include atrophy of cells and alteration of nerve axons. In addition, orthodontic movement may initiate resorption of the apex, usually without a change in vitality. Deep scaling and curettage may injure apical vessels and nerves, resulting in pulpal damage (see Chapter 7).

Periradicular tissues can be mechanically irritated and inflamed by impact trauma, hyperocclusion, endodontic procedures and accidents, pulp extirpation, overinstrumentation of root canals, perforation of the root, and overextension of the root canal filling materials. Intrusion injuries are more

likely to lead to pulp necrosis than are lateral or extrusion injuries (Fig. 4.3).[8] Mechanical irritation by instruments may occur during canal preparation. Inaccurate determination of canal length is usually the cause of overinstrumentation and the subsequent inflammation. In addition, lack of an adequate apical resistance form created during cleaning and shaping can cause overextension of filling materials into the periapical tissues, causing physical and chemical damage (Fig. 4.4).

Chemical Irritants

Chemical irritants of the pulp include various dentin cleansing, sterilizing, and desensitizing substances, in addition to some of the substances present in temporary and permanent restorative materials and cavity liners. Antibacterial agents, such as silver nitrate, phenol with and without camphor, and eugenol, have been used in an attempt to "sterilize" dentin after cavity preparations. The effectiveness of many of these products as dentin sterilizers is questionable,[9] and their cytotoxicity can cause inflammatory changes in the underlying dental pulp.[10] Other irritating agents include cavity cleansers, such as alcohol, chloroform, hydrogen peroxide, and various acids; chemicals present in desensitizers; cavity liners and bases; and temporary and permanent restorative materials.

Antibacterial irrigants used during cleaning and shaping of root canals, intracanal medications, and some compounds present in obturating materials are examples of potential chemical irritants of periradicular tissues. Most irrigants and medicaments are toxic and are not biocompatible.[11,12] Trevino and associates tested the impact of 17% ethylenediaminetetraacetic acid (EDTA) alone or in combination with sodium hypochlorite (NaOCl) or chlorhexidine on the viability of stem cells isolated from the apical papilla.[13] Their results showed that EDTA was best at supporting cell viability (89% cell survival), followed by the protocol using NaOCl (74% cell survival). In contrast, the addition of chlorhexidine led to absence of cell viability. EDTA has similar beneficial effects on dental pulp cells when used as a dentin conditioning agent.[14] When testing the impact of antimicrobial medications on dental pulp cells, researchers showed that calcium hydroxide and lower concentrations of antibiotic pastes are conducive to cell survival and proliferation, but more concentrated forms of antibiotic pastes have detrimental effects.[15]

Microbial Irritants

Although mechanical and chemical irritations are predominantly transient in nature, the most significant cause of inflammation is microbial. Microorganisms present in dental caries are the main source of irritation of the dental pulp and periradicular tissues. Carious dentin and enamel contain numerous species of bacteria, such as *Streptococcus mutans,* lactobacilli, and *Actinomyces* spp.[16] More recent studies using molecular techniques have implicated several other genera in the development of carious lesions, including *Veillonella, Bifidobacterium,* and *Propionibacterium* spp.[17]

Direct pulp exposure to microorganisms is not a prerequisite for pulpal response and inflammation. Microorganisms in caries produce toxins that penetrate into the pulp through tubules. Studies have shown that even small lesions in enamel are capable of attracting inflammatory cells in the pulp.[18,19] The initial reaction of the pulp to these irritants is mediated through the innate immune response. This early response to caries results in focal accumulation of chronic inflammatory cells such as macrophages, lymphocytes, and plasma cells.[20] As the decay progresses toward the pulp, the intensity and character of the infiltrate change. When actual exposure occurs, the pulp tissue is infiltrated locally by polymorphonuclear (PMN) leukocytes to form an area of liquefaction necrosis at the site of exposure (Fig. 4.5).[21] After pulp exposure, bacteria colonize and persist at the site of necrosis. Pulpal tissue may remain inflamed for long periods and may undergo eventual or rapid necrosis. This depends on several factors: (1) the virulence of the bacteria, (2) the ability to release inflammatory fluids to avoid a marked increase in intrapulpal pressure, (3) host resistance, (4) the amount of circulation and, an important factor, (5) lymphatic drainage. Yamasaki and associates created pulp exposures in rats and showed that necrosis extended gradually from the upper portion of the pulp to the apical portions.[22] A periapical lesion ensued after pulpal inflammation and necrosis.

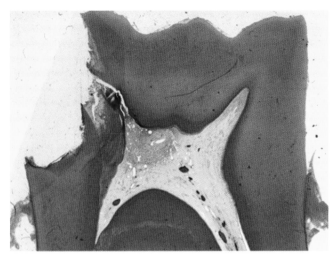

Fig. 4.5 A localized inflammatory reaction containing mainly polymorphonuclear leukocytes at the site of a carious pulpal exposure. The remainder of the coronal pulp is almost free of inflammatory cells. (Courtesy Dr. J.H. Simon.)

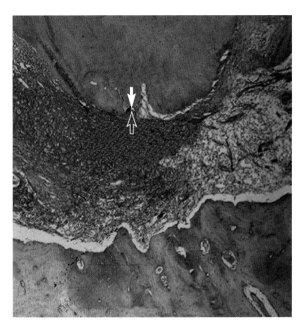

Fig. 4.6 Egress of irritants *(closed arrow)* from the root canal into the periapical tissue causes inflammation *(open arrow)* and replacement of normal periapical structures with a granulomatous tissue.

As a consequence of exposure to the oral cavity and to caries, pulp harbors bacteria and their byproducts. The dental pulp usually cannot eliminate these damaging irritants. At best, defenses temporarily impede the spread of infection and tissue destruction. If the irritants persist, the ensuing damage becomes extensive and spreads throughout the pulp. Subsequently, bacteria, or their byproducts, and other irritants from the necrotic pulp diffuse from the canal periapically, resulting in the development of inflammatory lesions (Fig. 4.6).

Bacteria play an important role in the pathogenesis of pulpal and periradicular pathoses. A number of investigations have established that pulpal or periradicular pathosis does not develop without the presence of bacterial contamination.[23-25]

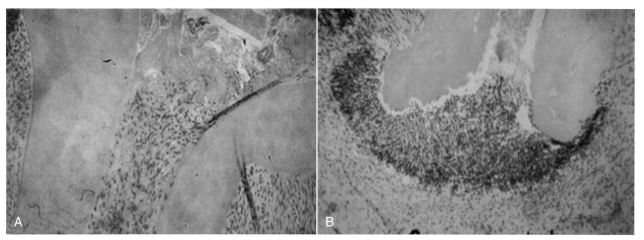

Fig. 4.7 **A,** No inflammation is seen in an exposed pulp *(P)* of a germ-free rat. Food particles and other debris *(D)* are packed into the chamber. **B,** Periapical lesion is apparent in a conventional rat after pulp exposure. (Courtesy Dr. H. Stanley.)

Kakehashi and associates created pulp exposures in conventional and germ-free rats.[23] This procedure in the germ-free rats caused only minimal inflammation throughout the 72-day investigation period. Pulpal tissue in these animals was not devitalized, but rather showed calcific bridge formation by day 14, with normal tissue apical to the dentin bridge (Fig. 4.7, *A*). In contrast, infection, pulpal necrosis, and abscess formation occurred by the eighth day in conventional rats (Fig. 4.7, *B*). Other investigators have examined the importance of bacteria in the development of periradicular lesions by sealing noninfected and infected pulps in the root canals of monkeys.[24] After 6 to 7 months, clinical, radiographic, and histologic examinations of teeth sealed with noninfected pulps showed an absence of pathosis in apical tissues, whereas teeth sealed with necrotic pulps containing certain bacteria showed periapical inflammation. The bacteriologic investigation by Sundqvist[25] examining the flora of human necrotic pulps supports the findings of Kakehashi and associates[23] and Möller and coworkers.[24] These studies examined previously traumatized teeth with necrotic pulps, with and without apical pathosis. Teeth without apical lesions were aseptic, whereas those with periapical pathosis had positive bacterial cultures.

Recent studies have shown a positive correlation between the presence of certain viruses and symptomatic apical pathoses.[26] Periapical lesions that contain cytomegalovirus (CMV) and Epstein-Barr virus (EBV) are more likely to be symptomatic than lesions that do not yield these viruses. Although a direct etiologic role has been suggested by some investigators,[27] this cause and effect relationship has yet to be demonstrated in experimental models.

Several mechanisms have been proposed for identification of bacteria as irritants by the immune system. Detection of these pathogens can occur via interaction between pathogen-associated molecular patterns (PAMPs) and specific receptors broadly identified as pattern recognition receptors (PRRs).[28] PRRs recognize PAMPs and initiate host defenses. G-protein coupled receptors and Toll-like receptors (TLRs) are part of the innate immune response and activate phagocytic functions to allow microbial ingestion. G-protein coupled receptors bind to chemokines, lipid mediators (e.g., platelet-activating factor, prostaglandin E2, and leukotriene B_4) or bacterial

Table 4.1 Examples of Toll-like receptors (TLRs) and associated activators

PAMP	PRR	Pathogen
LPS, Lipid A	TLR4	Gram-negative bacteria
Flagellin	TLR5	Bacteria, flagellum
dsRNA	TLR3	Virus
ssRNA	TLR7,8	Virus
CpG DNA	TLR9	Bacteria, DNA
PAMP	PRR	Pathogen

PAMP, Pathogen-associated molecular patterns; *PRR,* pattern recognition receptors.

proteins, causing extravasation of leukocytes and production of bactericidal substances. TLRs are transmembrane proteins that are expressed by cells of the innate immune system. These receptors recognize invading microbes and activate signaling pathways that launch immune and inflammatory responses to destroy the invaders. At least 13 TLRs have been discovered to date with different recognition abilities. Table 4.1 presents some of the currently identified TLRs and their specific interactions.

PULPAL PATHOSIS

Apart from anatomic configuration and diversity of inflicted irritants, pulp reacts to these irritants as do other connective tissues. A healthy pulp has tremendous capacity to repair itself and to heal; however, often, over time and with exposure to irritants, pulp tissue becomes compromised due to a state of inflammation or fibrosis. Pulpal injury results in cell death and inflammation. The degree of inflammation is proportional to the intensity and severity of tissue damage. Slight injuries, such as incipient caries or shallow cavity preparations, cause little or no inflammation in the pulp. In contrast, deep caries, **51** extensive operative procedures, or persistent irritants usually produce more severe inflammatory changes. Depending on the severity and duration of the insult and the host's capacity to respond, the pulpal response ranges from transient inflammation (reversible pulpitis) to irreversible pulpitis and then to total necrosis. These changes often occur without pain and without the knowledge of the patient or dentist.

Inflammatory Process

Dentin acts as a physical barrier against irrigants and prevents direct contact between inflammatory cells present in the pulp and the irritants, such as bacteria. Once the thickness of remaining dentin is less than 1.1 to 1.5 mm (e.g., due to caries), the number of inflammatory cells in the pulp increase.[29,30]

Irritation of the dental pulp results in the activation of a variety of biologic systems, such as nonspecific inflammatory reactions mediated by histamine, bradykinin, and arachidonic acid metabolites.[31] Also released are PMN lysosomal granule products (elastase, cathepsin G, and lactoferrin[32]; protease inhibitors (e.g., antitrypsin)[33]; and neuropeptides (e.g., calcitonin gene–related peptide [CGRP] and substance P [SP]).[34] Phagocytes are not required until direct contact between caries and pulp occurs[35]; in fact, as long as the dentin thickness remains greater than 2 mm, expression of genes related to PMNs is not up-regulated.[36]

Unlike connective tissue in other parts of the body, normal and healthy dental pulps lack mast cells. However, these cells are found in inflamed pulps (Fig. 4.8).[37] Mast cells contain histamine, leukotrienes, and platelet-activating factors. Physical injury to mast cells, or the bridging of two immunoglobulin E (IgE) molecules by an antigen on their cell surfaces, results in the release of histamine and/or other bioactive substances present in mast cell granules. The presence of histamine in the blood vessel walls and a marked increase in histamine levels indicate the importance of histamine in pulpal inflammation.[38]

Kinins, which cause many signs and symptoms of acute inflammation, are produced when plasma or tissue kallikreins contact kininogens. Bradykinin, SP, and neurokinin A have been identified in dental pulp tissue using high-performance

liquid chromatography.[39] In an in vitro study, bradykinin evoked immunoreactive CGRP (iCGRP) release from bovine dental pulps[35]; this activity is enhanced by prostaglandin E2 (PGE$_2$).[40] As a result of cellular damage, phospholipase A2 causes release of arachidonic acid from cell membranes. Metabolism of arachidonic acid results in the formation of prostaglandins, thromboxanes, and leukotrienes. Various arachidonic acid metabolites have been found in experimentally induced pulpitis.[41] The presence of these metabolites in inflamed pulps[42] indicates that arachidonic acid metabolites participate in inflammatory reactions of the dental pulp.

The dental pulp is densely innervated with sensory fibers containing immunomodulatory neuropeptides such as SP and CGRP. Studies have shown that denervation of the rat molar pulp, caused by axotomy of the inferior alveolar nerve, results in increased pulp tissue damage and a diminished infiltration of immunocompetent cells.[20] These findings indicate that pulpal nerves are protective in nature and that they may be involved in the recruitment of inflammatory and immunocompetent cells to the injured pulp.[20]

Mild to moderate pulpal injuries result in the sprouting of sensory nerves with an increase in iCGRP.[34,43] However, severe injuries have the opposite effect, resulting in either reduction or elimination of iCGRP and SP.[43] Experiments indicate that pulpal neuropeptides undergo dynamic changes after injury. In addition, recent studies have shown that stimulation of the dental pulp by caries results in the formation of various interleukins and recruitment of inflammatory cells to the site of injury.[44-46]

Immunologic Responses

Upon initial invasion of the pulp-dentin complex with microbial irritants, the innate immune system is activated. The innate immune system is immediately available and does not require a complicated method of selecting cells that react to the invaders and not the host, and there is no existence or development of memory. If the innate immune response is unable to eradicate the insult, the adaptive immune system is called into play with cellular and specific antibody responses.

Dendritic cells (DCs) are the master regulators of the immune system and are present in and scattered through normal pulp. In a healthy pulp, the odontoblasts are the cells in direct contact with the overlying dentin. When the pulp is irritated, the odontoblastic processes sense the invasion and elicit recruitment of DCs.[47] DCs phagocytose the invaders and present antigens to stimulate T lymphocytes.

In addition to nonspecific inflammatory reactions, immune responses also may initiate and perpetuate deleterious pulpal changes.[31] Potential antigens include bacteria and their byproducts within dental caries, which directly (or via the dentinal tubules) can initiate various types of reactions. Normal and uninflamed dental pulps contain immunocompetent cells, such as T and B (fewer) lymphocytes, macrophages, and a substantial number of class II molecule-expressing dendritic cells, which are morphologically similar to macrophages.[20] Elevated levels of immunoglobulins in inflamed pulps (Fig. 4.9) show that these factors participate in the defense mechanisms involved in protection of this tissue.[48] Arthus-type reactions do occur in the dental pulp.[49] In addition, the presence of immunocompetent cells, such as T lymphocytes, macrophages, and class II molecule-expressing cells appearing as dendritic cells (Fig. 4.10), in inflamed pulps

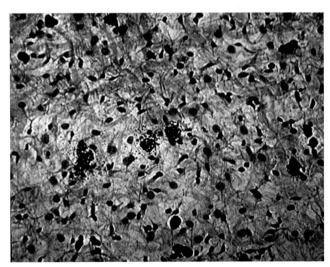

Fig. 4.8 Mast cells are readily visible as dark-stained cells in this inflamed human dental pulp.

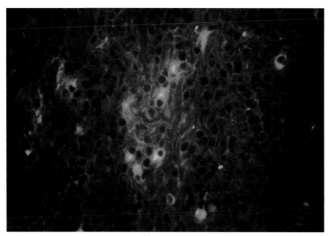

Fig. 4.9 Some plasma cells stain positively for IgM in inflamed human dental pulp, indicating immunologic activity.

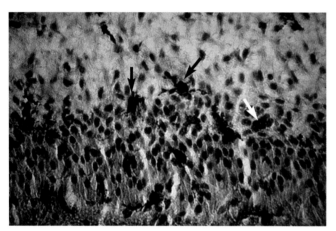

Fig. 4.10 Many dendritic cells *(arrows)* are present in an inflamed dental pulp. (Courtesy Dr. M. Jontell.)

indicates that delayed hypersensitivity reactions can also occur in this tissue.[20] Despite their protective mechanisms, immune reactions in the pulp can result in the formation of small necrotic foci and eventual total pulpal necrosis.

Lesion Progression

Mild injuries may not result in significant pulpal changes. However, moderate to severe injuries to the pulp result in localized inflammation[50] and the release of a high concentration of inflammatory mediators. An increase in protease inhibitors in moderately to severely inflamed pulps indicates the presence of natural modifiers.[33] As a consequence of the release of a large quantity of inflammatory mediators, increased vascular permeability, vascular stasis, and migration of leukocytes to the site of injury occur. Current research data show that the sensory neuropeptide, CGRP, is responsible for the increase in blood flow during pulpal inflammation.[51]

Elevated capillary pressure and increased capillary permeability move fluids from blood vessels into the surrounding tissues. If removal of fluids by venules and lymphatics does not coincide with the filtration of capillaries, an exudate forms. Pulp is encased in rigid surrounding tissues, forming

a low-compliance system; therefore, a small increase in tissue pressure causes passive compression and even complete collapse of the venules at the site of pulpal injury.[52] Pressure increases occur in small "compartmentalized" regions and progress slowly. Therefore, the dental pulp does not degenerate by extensive increases in pressure, with subsequent strangulation.[52,53]

Pain is often caused by several factors. The release of mediators of inflammation causes pain *directly* by lowering the sensory nerve threshold. These substances also cause pain *indirectly* by increasing both vasodilation in arterioles and vascular permeability in venules, resulting in edema and elevation of tissue pressure. This pressure acts directly on sensory nerve receptors.

Increased tissue pressure, the inability of the pulp to expand, and the lack of collateral circulation may result in pulpal necrosis and the development of subsequent periradicular pathosis.

CLASSIFICATION OF PULPAL DISEASES

Because there is little or no correlation between the histologic findings of pulpal pathosis and clinical symptoms,[54] the diagnosis and classification of pulpal diseases are based on clinical signs and symptoms rather than histopathologic findings. Pulpal conditions can be classified as normal pulp, reversible and irreversible pulpitis, hyperplastic pulpitis, necrosis, and previously treated pulp. Hard tissue responses include calcification and resorption.

Normal Pulp

A tooth with a normal pulp is clinically symptom free and responds normally to vitality tests. Such a tooth does not reveal any radiographic signs of pathosis.

Reversible Pulpitis

By definition, reversible pulpitis is a clinical condition associated with subjective and objective findings indicating the presence of mild inflammation in the pulp tissue. If the cause is eliminated, the inflammation reverses and the pulp returns to its normal state.

Mild or short-acting stimuli can cause reversible pulpitis, such as incipient caries, cervical erosion, or occlusal attrition; most operative procedures; deep periodontal curettage; and enamel fractures resulting in exposure of dentinal tubules.

Symptoms

Reversible pulpitis is usually asymptomatic. However, when present, symptoms usually follow a particular pattern. Application of stimuli, such as cold or hot liquids or air, may produce sharp, transient pain. Removal of these stimuli, which do not normally produce pain or discomfort, results in immediate relief. Cold and hot stimuli produce different pain responses in normal pulp.[55] When heat is applied to teeth with uninflamed pulp, the initial response is delayed; the intensity of pain increases as the temperature rises. In contrast, pain in response to cold in normal pulp is immediate; the intensity tends to decrease if the cold stimulus is maintained. Based on these observations, pulpal responses in both health and disease apparently result largely from changes in intrapulpal pressures.

Treatment

The removal of irritants and sealing and insulating the exposed dentin or vital pulp usually result in diminished symptoms and reversal of the inflammatory process in the pulp tissue (Fig. 4.11). Nevertheless, if irritation of the pulp continues or increases in intensity for the reasons stated earlier, moderate to severe inflammation develops, with resultant irreversible pulpitis and eventually pulpal necrosis.

Irreversible Pulpitis

Irreversible pulpitis may be classified as symptomatic or asymptomatic. It is a clinical condition associated with subjective and objective findings indicating the presence of severe inflammation in the pulp tissue. Irreversible pulpitis is often a sequel to and a progression from reversible pulpitis. Severe pulpal damage from extensive dentin removal during operative procedures or impairment of pulpal blood flow as a result of trauma or orthodontic movement of teeth may also cause irreversible pulpitis. Irreversible pulpitis is a severe inflammatory process that does not resolve, even if the cause is removed. The pulp is incapable of healing and slowly or rapidly becomes necrotic. Irreversible pulpitis can be symptomatic with spontaneous and lingering pain. It can also be asymptomatic, with no clinical signs and symptoms.

Symptoms

Irreversible pulpitis is usually asymptomatic. However, patients may report mild symptoms. Irreversible pulpitis may also be associated with intermittent or continuous episodes of spontaneous pain (with no external stimuli). Pain resulting from an irreversibly inflamed pulp may be sharp, dull, localized, or diffuse and can last anywhere from a few minutes up to a few hours. Localization of pulpal pain is more difficult than localization of periradicular pain and becomes more difficult as the pain intensifies. Application of external stimuli, such as cold or heat, may result in prolonged pain.

Accordingly, in the presence of severe pain, pulpal responses differ from those of uninflamed teeth or teeth with reversible pulpitis. For example, application of heat to teeth with irreversible pulpitis may produce an immediate response; also, occasionally with the application of cold, the response does not disappear and is prolonged. Application of cold in patients with painful irreversible pulpitis may cause vasoconstriction, a drop in pulpal pressure, and subsequent pain relief. Although it has been claimed that teeth with irreversible pulpitis have lower thresholds to electrical stimulation, Mumford found similar pain perception thresholds in inflamed and uninflamed pulps.[56]

Tests and Treatment

If inflammation is confined to the pulp and has not extended periapically, teeth respond within normal limits to palpation and percussion. The extension of inflammation to the PDL causes percussion sensitivity and allows better localization of pain. Root canal treatment or extraction is indicated for teeth with signs and symptoms of irreversible pulpitis.

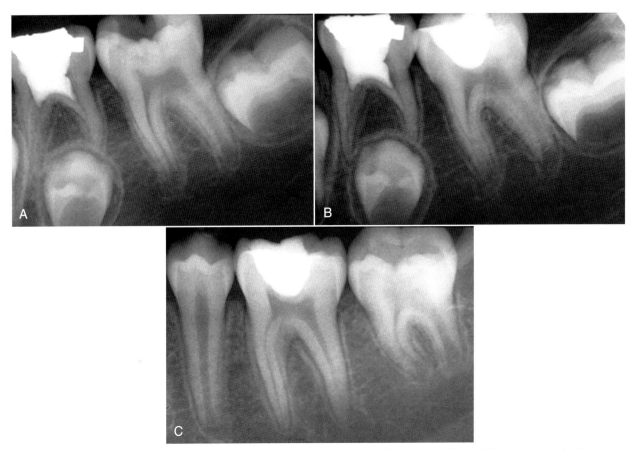

Fig. 4.11 **A,** Mechanically exposed pulp horns of a mandibular molar with signs of reversible pulpitis were capped with mineral trioxide aggregate. **B,** Immediate postoperative radiograph. **C,** Follow-up radiograph 5 years later shows no calcific metamorphosis in the pulp chamber, closure of apexes, and normal responses during clinical examination.

Hyperplastic Pulpitis

Hyperplastic pulpitis (pulp polyp) is a form of irreversible pulpitis that originates from overgrowth of a chronically inflamed young pulp onto the occlusal surface. It is usually found in carious crowns of young patients (Fig. 4.12, *A*). Ample vascularity of the young pulp, adequate exposure for drainage, and tissue proliferation are associated with the formation of hyperplastic pulpitis. Histologic examination of hyperplastic pulps shows surface epithelium overlying the inflamed connective tissue (Fig. 4.12, *B*). Cells of the oral epithelium are implanted and grow over the exposed surface to form an epithelial covering.

Hyperplastic pulpitis is usually asymptomatic. It appears as a reddish, cauliflower-like outgrowth of connective tissue into caries that has resulted in a large occlusal exposure. It is occasionally associated with clinical signs of irreversible pulpitis, such as spontaneous pain, in addition to lingering pain to cold and heat stimuli. The threshold to electrical stimulation is similar to that found in normal pulps. These teeth respond within normal limits when palpated or percussed. Hyperplastic pulpitis can be treated by pulpotomy, root canal treatment, or extraction.

Hard Tissue Changes Caused by Pulpal Inflammation

As a result of irritation, one of two distinct hard tissue changes may occur: calcification or resorption.

Pulp Calcification

Extensive calcification (usually in the form of pulp stones or diffuse calcification) occurs as a response to trauma, caries, periodontal disease, or other irritants. Thrombi in blood vessels and collagen sheaths around vessel walls are possible sources for these calcifications.

Another type of calcification is the extensive formation of hard tissue on dentin walls, often in response to irritation or death and replacement of odontoblasts. This process is called *calcific metamorphosis* (Fig. 4.13). As irritation increases, the amount of calcification may also increase, leading to partial or complete radiographic (but not histologic) obliteration of the pulp chamber and root canal.[57] A yellowish discoloration of the crown is often a manifestation of calcific metamorphosis. The pain threshold to thermal and electrical stimuli usually increases; often the teeth are unresponsive.

Palpation and percussion are usually within normal limits. In contrast to soft tissue diseases of the pulp, which have no radiographic signs and symptoms, calcification of pulp tissue is associated with various degrees of pulp space obliteration. A reduction in coronal pulp space followed by a gradual narrowing of the root canal is the first sign of calcific metamorphosis. This condition is not pathologic in nature and does not require treatment.

Internal (Intracanal) Resorption

Inflammation in the pulp may initiate resorption of adjacent hard tissues. The pulp is transformed into a vascularized

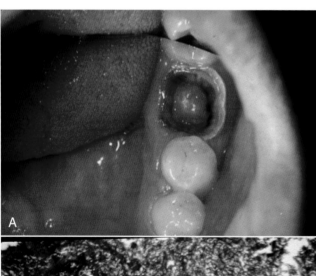
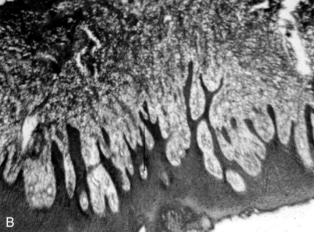

Fig. 4.12 **A,** Pulp polyp, also known as *hyperplastic pulpitis.* The involved tooth is usually carious with extensive loss of tooth structure; the pulp remains vital and proliferates from the exposure site. **B,** Histologic examination of hyperplastic pulpitis shows surface epithelium and underlying inflamed connective tissue.

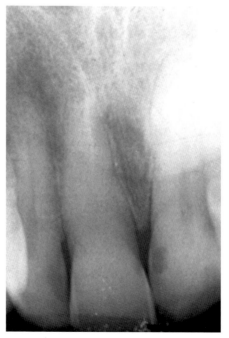

Fig. 4.13 Calcific metamorphosis does not represent pathosis per se and may occur with aging or low-grade irritation. It also may occur subsequent to a traumatic injury to the tooth.

inflammatory tissue with dentinoclastic activity; this condition leads to the resorption of the dentinal walls, advancing from its center to the periphery.[58] Most cases of intracanal resorption are asymptomatic. Advanced internal resorption involving the pulp chamber is often associated with pink spots in the crown.

Teeth with intracanal resorptive lesions usually respond within normal limits to pulpal and periapical tests. Radiographs reveal the presence of radiolucency with irregular enlargement of the root canal compartment (Fig. 4.14). Immediate removal of the inflamed tissue and completion of root canal treatment are recommended; these lesions tend to be progressive and eventually perforate to the lateral periodontium. When this occurs, pulp necrosis ensues, and treatment of the tooth becomes more difficult.

Pulpal Necrosis

As stated before, pulp is encased in rigid walls, it has no collateral blood circulation, and its venules and lymphatics collapse under increased tissue pressure. Therefore, irreversible pulpitis leads to liquefaction necrosis. If exudate produced during irreversible pulpitis is absorbed or drains through caries or through a pulp exposure into the oral cavity, necrosis is delayed; the radicular pulp may remain vital for a long time. In contrast, closure or sealing of an inflamed pulp induces rapid and total pulpal necrosis and periradicular pathosis.[59] In addition to liquefaction necrosis, ischemic necrosis of the pulp occurs as a result of traumatic injury from disruption of the blood supply. Necrotic pulp is a clinical condition associated with subjective and objective findings indicating death of the dental pulp.

Symptoms

Pulpal necrosis is usually asymptomatic but may be associated with episodes of spontaneous pain and discomfort or pain (from the periradicular tissues) on pressure. In teeth with necrotic pulps, pain provoked with application of heat is not due to an increase in intrapulpal pressure, as is the case in teeth with vital pulps. This pressure registers zero after heat application to teeth with necrotic pulps. It is commonly believed (but is unlikely) that applying heat to teeth with liquefaction necrosis causes thermal expansion of gases present in the root canal space, which provokes pain.[60] In fact, cold, heat, or electrical stimuli applied to teeth with necrotic pulps usually produce no response.

Tests and Treatment

By definition, the pulp of a tooth with necrotic pulp should be nonresponsive to vitality testing. However, various degrees of inflammatory response are possible, ranging from reversible pulpitis to necrosis in teeth with multiple canals, and this may occasionally cause confusion during testing for responsiveness. Furthermore, the effects of necrosis are seldom confined within canals. Because of the spread of inflammatory reactions to periradicular tissues, teeth with necrotic pulps are often sensitive to percussion. Sensitivity to palpation is an additional indication of periradicular involvement. Root canal treatment or extraction is indicated for these teeth.

Previously Initiated Root Canal Therapy

This condition represents a clinical diagnostic category in which the tooth has had either partial or complete endodontic therapy. The teeth in this category can be symptomatic or asymptomatic, depending on pulpal and periapical conditions. Completion of partial root canal therapy or retreatment of failed root canal treatment, endodontic surgery, or extraction is indicated for these teeth.

PERIAPICAL PATHOSIS

As a consequence of pulpal necrosis, pathologic changes can occur in the periradicular tissues. In contrast to pulp, periradicular tissues have an almost unlimited source of undifferentiated cells that participate in inflammation and repair. In addition, these tissues have a rich collateral blood supply and lymphatic drainage system. The interaction between the irritants emanating from the canal space and the host defense results in the activation of an extensive array of reactions to protect the host. Despite the benefits of this process, some of these reactions are associated with destructive consequences, such as periradicular bone resorption. Resorption of the bone provides a separation between the irritants and the bone, thereby preventing osteomyelitis. Depending on the severity of irritation, its duration, and the host response, periradicular pathoses may range from slight inflammation to extensive tissue destruction. The reactions involved are highly complex and are usually mediated both by nonspecific mediators of inflammation and by specific immune reactions (Fig. 4.15).[38]

Nonspecific Mediators of Periapical Lesions

Nonspecific mediators of inflammatory reactions include neuropeptides, fibrinolytic peptides, kinins, complement fragments, vasoactive amines, lysosomal enzymes, arachidonic acid metabolites, and various cytokines.[31] Neuropeptides have been demonstrated in inflamed periapical tissues of experimental animals, and it appears that these substances play a role in the pathogenesis of periradicular pathosis.[34]

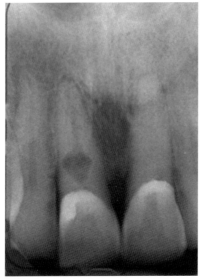

Fig. 4.14 Hard tissue resorption that causes disappearance of normal radiographic evidence of the root canal *usually* indicates an internal resorption defect.

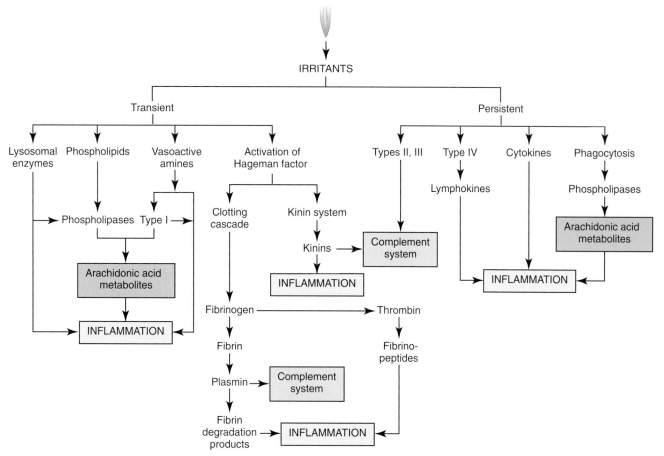

Fig. 4.15 Pathways of inflammation and bone resorption by nonspecific inflammatory mediators and specific immune reactions.

Severance of blood vessels in the PDL or bone during canal instrumentation can activate intrinsic and extrinsic coagulation pathways. Contact between the Hageman factor and the collagen of basement membranes, enzymes such as kallikrein or plasmin, or endotoxins from inflamed root canals activate the clotting cascade and the fibrinolytic system. Fibrinopeptides released from fibrinogen molecules and fibrin degradation products released during the proteolysis of fibrin by plasmin contribute to inflammation. Trauma to the periapical tissues during root canal treatment can also activate the kinin system and consequently the complement system. C3 complement fragments have been found in periradicular lesions.[38] Products released from the activated systems contribute to the inflammatory process and cause swelling, pain, and tissue destruction.

Mast cells are normal components of connective tissues and are present in a normal PDL. They are also found within periradicular lesions.[61] Physical or chemical injury causes the release of vasoactive amines (e.g., histamine), which are chemotactic for leukocytes and macrophages. In addition, lysosomal enzymes cause cleavage of C5 and generation of C5a, a potent chemotactic component, and liberation of active bradykinin from plasma kininogen.[31] Periradicular lesions show increased levels of lysosomal hydrolytic arylsulfatase A and B compared to normal tissues.[62] Significant levels of PGE_2 and leukotriene B_4 are also present in these lesions.[31] Other studies have confirmed these findings, demonstrating

cessation of symptoms subsequent to emergency cleaning and shaping.[63] With immunohistochemical staining, PGE_2, prostaglandin F2a (PGF_{2a}), and 6-keto-PGF_{1a} (a stable metabolite of prostaglandin I2 [PGI_2]) have been observed in inflamed pulp tissue and periradicular lesions.[64] Regions staining positive for prostaglandins gradually extend apically into areas of the pulp tissue that are not yet inflamed. Use of indomethacin, a prostaglandin inhibitor, experimentally reduces bone resorption, indicating that prostaglandins are also involved in the pathogenesis of periradicular lesions.[31,65]

Various cytokines, such as interleukins, tumor necrosis factors, and growth factors, are involved in the development and perpetuation of periradicular lesions.[44,66-69] Kawashima and Stashenko[68] examined the kinetics of expression of 10 cytokines in experimentally induced murine periapical lesions. Their results showed that a cytokine network is activated in the periapical tissues in response to root canal infections and that T helper 1–modulated proinflammatory pathways predominate during periapical bone resorption.

Specific Mediators of Periapical Lesions

In addition to the nonspecific mediators of inflammatory reactions, immunologic reactions participate in the formation and perpetuation of periradicular pathosis (see Fig. 4.16). Numerous potential antigens may accumulate in the necrotic pulp, including several species of microorganisms, their toxins, and altered pulp tissue. Root canals are a pathway for

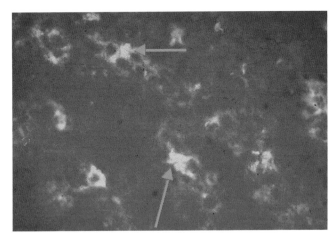

Fig. 4.16 Using the anticomplement immunofluorescence technique, immune complexes are identified *(arrows)* in human periapical lesions.

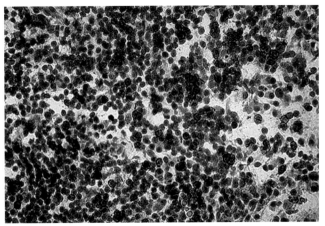

Fig. 4.17 T lymphocytes (red membrane cells) are identified in a human periapical lesion by an immunohistochemical technique.

sensitization.[31] The presence of potential antigens in root canals, IgE, and mast cells in pathologically involved pulp and periradicular lesions indicates that a type I immunologic reaction may occur.

Various classes of immunoglobulins have been found in inflamed lesions.[31,70] These include specific antibodies against a number of bacterial species in infected root canals.[71,72] In addition, numerous types of immunocompetent cells, such as antigen-presenting cells (Ia antigen-expressing nonlymphoid cells), macrophages,[73] PMN leukocytes, and B and T cells, have been found in human periradicular lesions.[74] The presence of immune complexes (Fig. 4.16) and immunocompetent cells (e.g., T cells; Fig. 4.17) indicates that various types of immunologic reactions (types II to IV) can initiate, amplify, or perpetuate these inflammatory lesions.[31]

Lesion Progression
As previously stated, bone resorption during periapical lesion formation allows bone to retreat from infection sites to prevent bacterial invasion of alveolar osseous tissues that could lead to the development of osteomyelitis.[75] A wide variety of factors have been implicated in the bone resorption observed in periapical lesion formation. Matrix metalloproteinases (MMPs) are a class of endopeptidases that significantly contribute to degradation of extracellular matrix components.[76] Elevated levels of MMPs have been reported in lesions isolated from animals[77] and humans.[78] MMP-9 (also known as *gelatinase-B*), in particular, which removes the collagenous layer from bone, has been isolated in chronic and acute lesions.[79]

Another key protein that plays a major role in bone resorption is nuclear factor-κB ligand (RANKL). RANKL binds to its receptor (RANK), resulting in osteoclast differentiation. This interaction is inhibited by osteoprotegerin (OPG), a decoy protein that binds to the receptor. Levels of RANKL and the ratio of RANKL to OPG both peak at 2 to 3 weeks, concurrent with the progression of periapical bone destruction.[80] RANKL production tapers off between weeks 4 and 8, whereas production of OPG increases during this time, creating a negative feedback loop that limits the amount of bone destruction caused by bacterial infection. The RANKL-RANK interaction is involved in both physiologic and pathologic bone resorption.[81] In periapical tissues, a significant increase in RANKL levels has been found in granulomatous lesions compared to healthy controls.[82,83]

CLASSIFICATION OF PERIAPICAL LESIONS

Periapical lesions have been classified on the basis of their clinical and histologic findings. As with pulpal disease, little correlation exists between the clinical signs and symptoms and duration of lesions and the histopathologic findings.[84] Because of these discrepancies and for convenience, these lesions are classified into six main groups: normal periapical tissues, symptomatic (acute) apical periodontitis, asymptomatic (chronic) apical periodontitis, condensing osteitis, acute apical abscess, and chronic apical abscess. Lesions associated with significant symptoms, such as pain or swelling, are referred to as acute (symptomatic), whereas those with mild or no symptoms are identified as chronic (asymptomatic).

Normal Periapical Tissues
The normal periapical tissue group represents a clinical and radiographic diagnostic category in which the tooth has normal periapical tissues and is not abnormally sensitive to percussion or palpation testing. The teeth in this category have normal lamina dura and periodontal ligament structures.

Symptomatic Apical Periodontitis
Etiology
The first extension of pulpal inflammation into the periradicular tissues is called *symptomatic apical periodontitis* (SAP). Eliciting irritants include inflammatory mediators from an irreversibly inflamed pulp or egress of bacterial toxins from necrotic pulps, chemicals (e.g., irrigants or disinfecting agents), restorations in hyperocclusion, overinstrumentation of the root canal, and extrusion of obturating materials. The pulp may be reversibly inflamed, irreversibly inflamed, or necrotic.

Signs and Symptoms
Clinical features of SAP are moderate to severe spontaneous discomfort, in addition to pain on biting or percussion. If SAP is an extension of pulpitis, its signs and symptoms include

responsiveness to cold, heat, and electricity. Cases of SAP caused by a necrotic pulp do not respond to vitality tests. Application of pressure by the fingertip or tapping with the butt end of a mirror handle (percussion) can cause marked to excruciating pain. SAP is not associated with an apical radiolucency. Occasionally there may be slight radiographic changes, such as a "widening" of the PDL space or a very small radiolucent lesion; however, usually there is a normal PDL space with an intact lamina dura.

Histologic Features

With SAP, PMN leukocytes and macrophages are visible within a localized area at the apical region of the pulp. At times there may be a small area of liquefaction necrosis (abscess). Bone and root resorption may be present histologically; however, resorption is usually not visible radiographically.

Treatment

Adjustment of occlusion (when there is evidence of hyperocclusion), removal of irritants or a pathologic pulp, or removal of periapical exudate usually results in relief.

Asymptomatic Apical Periodontitis
Etiology

Asymptomatic apical periodontitis (AAP) results from pulp necrosis and usually is a sequel to SAP.

Signs and Symptoms

By definition, AAP is a clinical, asymptomatic condition of pulpal origin associated with inflammation and destruction of periapical tissues. Because the pulp is necrotic, teeth with AAP do not respond to electrical or thermal stimuli. Percussion produces little or no pain. There may be slight sensitivity to palpation, indicating an alteration of the cortical plate of bone and extension of AAP into the soft tissues. Radiographic features range from interruption of the lamina dura (Fig. 4.18) to extensive destruction of periapical and interradicular tissues (Fig. 4.19).

Histologic Features

Histologically, AAP lesions are classified as either granulomas or cysts. A periapical *granuloma* consists of granulomatous tissue infiltrated by mast cells, macrophages, lymphocytes, plasma cells, and occasionally, PMN leukocytes (Fig. 4.20). Multinucleated giant cells, foam cells, cholesterol clefts, and epithelium are often found.

The apical (radicular) *cyst* has a central cavity filled with an eosinophilic fluid or semisolid material and is lined by stratified squamous epithelium (Fig. 4.21). The epithelium is surrounded by connective tissue containing all cellular elements found in the periapical granuloma. Therefore, an apical cyst is a granuloma that contains a cavity or cavities lined with epithelium. The origin of the epithelium is the remnants of Hertwig's epithelial sheath, the cell rests of Malassez. These cell rests proliferate in response to inflammatory stimuli. The actual genesis of the cyst is unclear.

The reported incidence of various classes of endodontic lesions is inconsistent. Variations may be due to sampling methods and the histologic criteria used for diagnosis. Nobuhara and del Rio examined periapical biopsies that were refractory to root canal treatment and showed most to be granulomas (59%), with some cysts (22%), a few scars (12%), and a scattering of other types of lesions (7%).[85] However, percentages such as these are misleading. Many lesions share combined features of granulomatous inflammatory lesions, cysts, and areas of scarring. The samples usually do not include abscesses, because their intact recovery is difficult during surgery. In fact, in the majority of cases, the entire lesion typically is not recovered for biopsy, and only fragments are obtained during curettage.

Treatment

Removal of inciting irritants (necrotic pulp) and complete obturation of the root canal system usually result in resolution of AAP (Fig. 4.22). There is no evidence that apical cysts resist resolution after adequate root canal treatment or extraction.

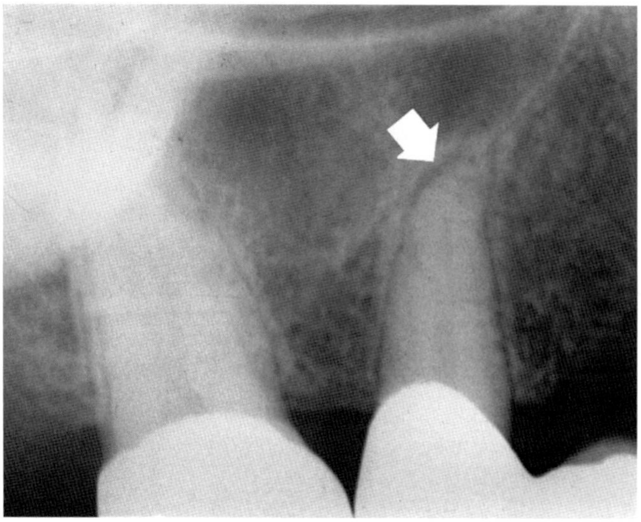

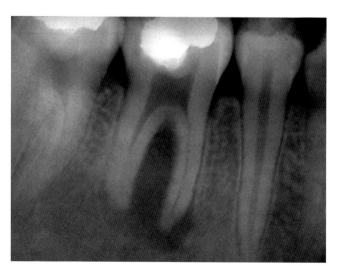

Fig. 4.18 After cementation of a three-unit bridge, the premolar developed clinical signs and symptoms of acute apical periodontitis. Radiograph shows a widened periodontal ligament space *(arrow)*.

Fig. 4.19 Chronic apical periodontitis. Extensive tissue destruction in the periapical area of a mandibular first molar has occurred as a result of pulpal necrosis. Lack of symptoms and the presence of a radiographic lesion are diagnostic.

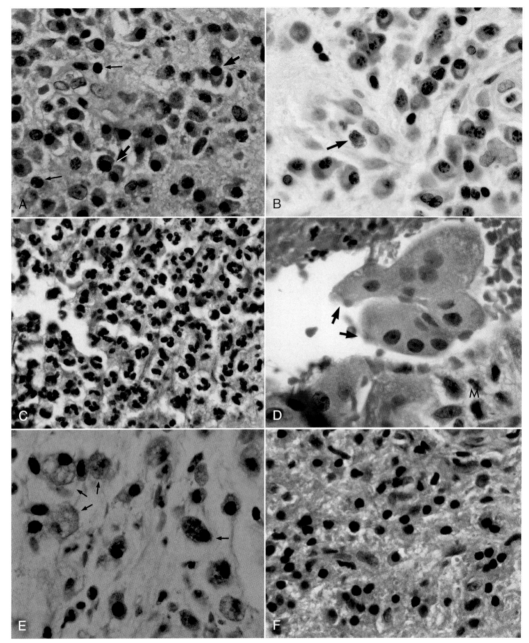

Fig. 4.20 **A,** Lymphocytes *(small arrows)*. Plasma cells *(large arrows)* have an eccentric nucleus with adjacent "clear zone" and a basophilic outer rim of cytoplasm. **B,** A plasma cell with an accumulation of immunoglobulins within the cytoplasm. **C,** Polymorphonuclear (PMN) leukocytes are concentrated in this field. They have multilobed nuclei, and many of them are degenerating and have disrupted cell walls. **D,** Giant cells *(arrows)* with multiple nuclei. Macrophages *(M)* with lighter-stained nuclei and diffuse cytoplasm. **E,** Macrophages *(arrows)* are larger and often have ingested material, as indicated by a "foamy" cytoplasm in these cells. **F,** Lymphocytes, with their densely basophilic nuclei, dominate this field. (Courtesy Dr. C. Kleinegger.)

Condensing Osteitis
Etiology

Condensing osteitis, a variant of asymptomatic apical periodontitis, represents an increase in trabecular bone in response to persistent irritation. The irritant diffusing from the root canal into periradicular tissues is the main cause of condensing osteitis. This lesion is usually found around the apices of mandibular posterior teeth, which show a probable cause of pulp inflammation or necrosis. However, condensing osteitis can occur in association with the apex of any tooth.

Signs and Symptoms

Depending on the cause (pulpitis or pulpal necrosis), condensing osteitis may be either asymptomatic or associated with pain. Pulp tissue of teeth with condensing osteitis may or may not respond to electrical or thermal stimuli. Furthermore, these teeth may or may not be sensitive to palpation or percussion. Radiographically, the presence of a diffuse, concentric arrangement of radiopacity around the root of a tooth is pathognomonic (Fig. 4.23). Histologically, there is an increase in irregularly arranged trabecular bone and inflammation.[86]

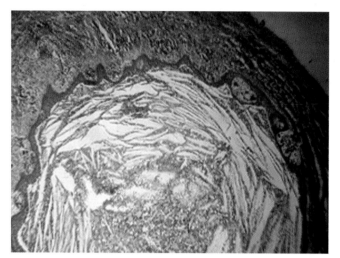

Fig. 4.21 A region of human apical cyst consists of a central cavity filled with eosinophilic material (EM) and a wall lined with epithelium.

Root canal treatment, when indicated, may result in the complete resolution of condensing osteitis.[87] Condensing osteitis is often confused with enostosis (sclerotic bone), a nonpathologic entity.

Acute Apical Abscess
Etiology
Acute apical abscess (AAA) is a localized (Fig. 4.24, A) or diffuse (Fig. 4.24, B) liquefaction lesion of pulpal origin that destroys periradicular tissues and a severe inflammatory response to microbial and nonbacterial irritants from a necrotic pulp.

Signs and Symptoms
AAA is characterized by rapid onset and spontaneous pain. Depending on the severity of the reaction, patients with AAA usually have moderate to severe discomfort and/or swelling. There often is no swelling if the abscess is confined to bone. In addition, they occasionally have systemic manifestations of an infective process, such as elevated temperature, malaise, and leukocytosis. Because these findings are only observed in association with a necrotic pulp, electrical or thermal stimulation produces no response. However, these teeth are usually painful to percussion and palpation. Depending on the degree of hard tissue destruction inflicted by irritants, radiographic features of AAA range from no changes to widening of the PDL space to an obvious radiolucent lesion.

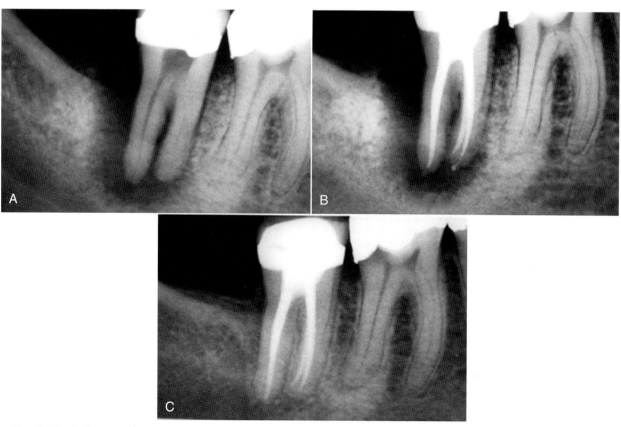

Fig. 4.22 **A,** Preoperative radiograph of a second molar with pulpal necrosis and evidence of chronic apical periodontitis. **B,** Postoperative radiograph of the tooth. **C,** Postoperative radiograph 2 years after root canal therapy shows complete resolution of the periradicular pathosis.

Histologic Features

Histologic examination of AAA usually shows a localized destructive lesion of liquefaction necrosis containing numerous disintegrating PMN leukocytes, debris, and cell remnants and an accumulation of purulent exudate (see Fig. 4.24, *C*). Surrounding the abscess is granulomatous tissue; therefore, the lesion is best categorized as an abscess within a granuloma. Notably, the abscess often does not communicate directly with the apical foramen; frequently an abscess does not drain through an accessed tooth.

Removal of the underlying cause, release of pressure (drainage where possible), and routine root canal treatment lead to resolution of most cases of AAA.

Chronic Apical Abscess

The chronic apical abscess (CAA) is an inflammatory lesion of pulpal origin characterized by the presence of a long-standing lesion that has resulted in an abscess that drains to a mucosal (sinus tract) or skin surface.

Etiology

CAA has a pathogenesis similar to that of AAA. It also results from pulpal necrosis and is usually associated with chronic apical periodontitis that has formed an abscess. The abscess has "burrowed" through bone and soft tissue to form a sinus tract stoma on the oral mucosa (Fig. 4.25, *A*) or sometimes onto the facial dermis. The histologic findings in these lesions are similar to those found in SAP (Fig. 4.25, *B*). CAA may also drain through the periodontium into the sulcus and may mimic a periodontal abscess or pocket (see Chapter 7).

Signs and Symptoms

Because drainage exists, CAA is usually asymptomatic, except when there is occasional closure of the sinus pathway, which can cause pain. Clinical, radiographic, and histopathologic features of CAA are similar to those described for AAP. An additional feature is the sinus tract, which may be lined

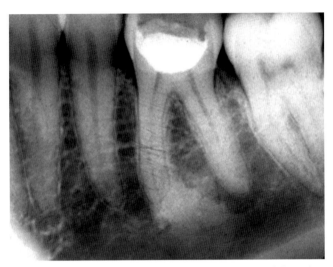

Fig. 4.23 Condensing osteitis. Chronic inflammation of the pulp of the first molar has resulted in radiopacity of periapical tissue.

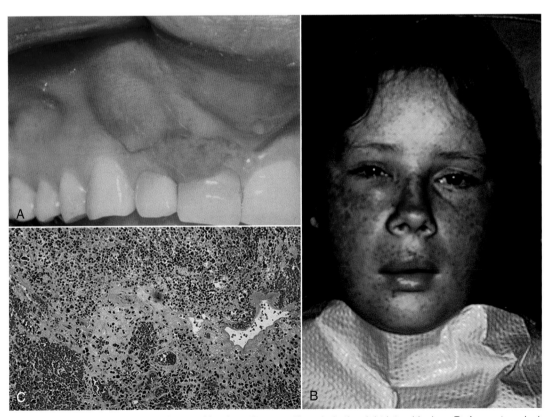

Fig. 4.24 A, Localized vestibular swelling resulting from the necrotic pulp in the right lateral incisor. **B,** An acute apical abscess (AAA) has created diffuse facial swelling. **C,** Histologic examination of the AAA shows edematous tissue heavily infiltrated by degenerating PMN leukocytes.

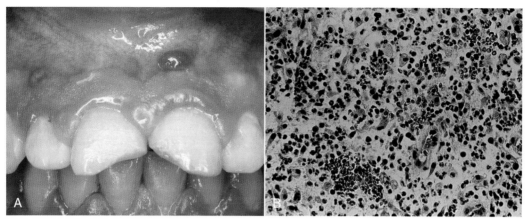

Fig. 4.25 **A,** Sinus tract stoma associated with a necrotic pulp in the left central incisor. **B,** Histologic examination of the periapical tissue shows numerous lymphocytes, plasma cells, and macrophages (foam cells).

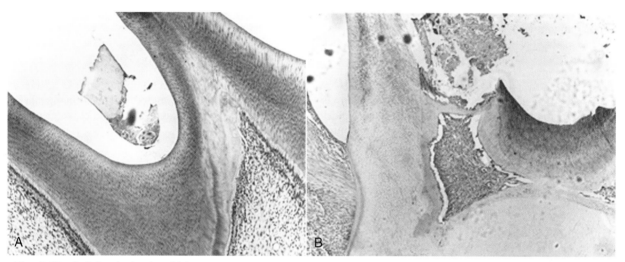

Fig. 4.26 **A,** Sclerotic dentin, which appears as an irregularly organized, mineralized tissue and stains lighter than normal tubular dentin with antibody against dentin sialoprotein (DSP). **B,** Dentin bridge; also, secondary dentin, deposited along canal wall after a pulp capping procedure, which shows a tubular structure and stains similarly to the primary dentin with antibody against DSP.

partially or completely by epithelium surrounded by inflamed connective tissue.[88]

HEALING OF PULP AND PERIAPICAL TISSUES

Regeneration is a process by which altered tissues are completely replaced by tissues native to their original architecture and function. Repair is a process by which altered tissues are not completely restored to their original structures. Histologic examination of most tissue sections in experimental animals and humans shows that healing of periradicular lesions after root canal therapy is by repair rather than regeneration of the periradicular tissues. Inflammation and healing are not two separate entities; in fact, they constitute part of one process in response to tissue injury. On the molecular and cellular levels, they are inseparable. Inflammation dominates the early events after tissue injury, shifting toward healing after the early responses have subsided. However, for convenience and to simplify the complex inflammatory-resorptive process, they are studied as two separate entities.

Extent of Healing

The level of healing is proportional to the degree and extent of tissue injury and the nature of tissue destruction. When injury to the underlying tissues is slight, little repair or regeneration is required. On the other hand, extensive damage requires substantial healing (see Fig. 4.22). In other words, pulp and periradicular repair ranges from a relatively simple resolution of an inflammatory infiltrate to considerable reorganization and repair of a variety of tissues.

Process of Pulp Healing

In the absence of irritants, a healthy pulp has tremendous capacity to heal. Andelin and associates used immunostaining with dentin sialoprotein (DSP) to determine the type of tissue that forms after pulp capping procedures.[89] DSP is present in both bone and dentin but is expressed at an approximately 400-fold higher level in dentin than in bone.[90] Andelin's study showed that, depending on the capping material used, dentin healing may occur through regeneration of dentin (identified through heavy DSP staining; Fig. 4.26, *A*) or through repair with an amorphous mineralized scar tissue (light DSP staining; Fig. 4.26, *B*). This study also showed that formation of ectopic bone may occur in the presence of certain materials (e.g. bone morphogenic protein-7). This finding may be an indication that the pulpal stem cells may differentiate into different specialized cells, depending on the signal received. Mild injury to the pulp and endothelial cells stimulates stem cell recruitment, and proliferation of dental stem cells can be stimulated by platelet-derived growth factor BB (PDGF-BB), vascular endothelial growth factor (VEGF), insulin-like growth factor 1 (IGF-1) and transforming growth factor β1 (TGF-β1).[91] On the other hand, prolonged injury (e.g., as seen in microbial infections) results in stem cell apoptosis and impairment of these cells' function and ability to repair the pulp.[92]

Process of Periapical Healing
The sequence of events leading to resolution of periapical lesions has not been studied extensively. Based on the processes involved in the repair of extraction sites,[93] after removal of irritants, inflammatory responses decrease and tissue-forming cells (fibroblasts and endothelial cells) increase; and finally, tissue organization and maturation ensue. Bone that has resorbed is replaced by new bone; resorbed cementum and dentin are repaired by cellular cementum. The PDL, which is the first tissue affected, is the last to be restored to normal architecture. Histologic examination of healing of periapical lesions shows evidence of healing in the form of cementum deposition, increased vascularity, and increased fibroblastic and osteoblastic activities.[94] Studies have shown that some cytokines play an important role during healing of periapical lesions.[95,96]

Some lesions do not completely regain all of the original structures. Variations are seen in different fiber or bone patterns. These may be obvious radiographically with a widened lamina dura or altered bony configuration. Certain factors, such as the size of the defect or the extent of injury to the underlying stroma, may affect complete regeneration of the original tissue architecture. Boyne has shown that these critical-sized defects do not heal unless stimulated by inductive factors such as bone morphogenetic proteins.[97]

Factors Influencing Healing
Other factors that may affect the healing of periapical lesions include inherent host factors (e.g., leukopenia, impairment of blood supply, inadequate nutrition), corticosteroids, and other systemic diseases. For instance, patients with insulin-dependent diabetes mellitus have a significantly lower healing rate after root canal therapy of teeth with apical lesions than do nondiabetic patients.[98] Uncontrolled hyperglycemia may also affect pulp healing. In a pulp capping model using streptozotocin-induced diabetes in rats, Garber and coworkers found significant impairment of dentin bridge formation compared to normal rats.[99] Impairment of dentin bridge formation was directly correlated with the amount of pulp inflammation.

NONENDODONTIC PERIRADICULAR PATHOSIS

Differential Diagnosis
A number of radiolucent and radiopaque lesions of nonendodontic origin simulate the radiographic appearance of endodontic lesions. Because of their similarities, dentists must use their knowledge and perform clinical tests in a systematic manner to arrive at an accurate diagnosis and avoid critical mistakes. Pulp vitality tests are the most important aids in differentiating between endodontic and nonendodontic lesions. Teeth associated with radiolucent periradicular lesions have necrotic pulps and therefore generally do not respond to vitality tests. In contrast, lesions of nonpulpal origin usually do not affect the blood or nerve supply to adjacent tooth pulp; therefore, the vitality (responsiveness) of these teeth remains unaffected.

Unfortunately, many clinicians rely solely on radiographs for diagnosis and treatment, without obtaining a complete history of the signs and symptoms and performing clinical tests. Many nonendodontic radiolucencies (including those resulting from pathoses and those with normal morphology) mimic endodontic pathoses and vice versa. To avoid grievous mistakes, all relevant vitality tests, radiographic examinations, clinical signs and symptoms, and details of the patient history should be used.

Normal and Pathologic Entities
Most radiographic changes arise from pathologic changes in the pulp. However, other radiographic variations, such as anatomic variations, in addition to benign and malignant lesions, may simulate the appearance of periradicular lesions.[100]

Normal Structures
Anatomic variations include large marrow spaces adjacent to the apices of teeth, submandibular fossae, maxillary sinus, apical dental papillae of developing teeth, nasopalatine foramen, mental foramen (Fig. 4.27), and lingual depressions in the mandible. Associated teeth respond to vitality tests and show no clinical signs and symptoms of any disease process. In addition, by changing the cone angulation, the location of

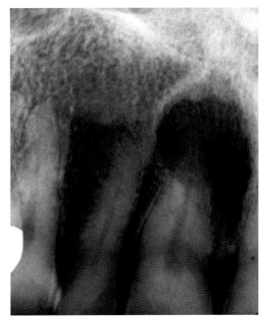

Fig. 4.27 Incisive foramen simulating a periapical lesion of pulpal origin. Pulp test results are within normal limits, indicating that this radiolucency could not be endodontic pathosis.

these radiolucent lesions can be altered relative to their original positions and to the root apices.

Nonendodontic Pathoses

Benign lesions with radiographic appearances similar to periradicular lesions include (but are not limited to) the initial stages of periapical cemental dysplasia (Fig. 4.28), early stages of monostotic fibrous dysplasia, ossifying fibroma, primordial cyst, lateral periodontal cyst, dentigerous cyst, median maxillary or mandibular cyst, bone cyst, central giant cell granuloma, central hemangioma, hyperparathyroidism, myxoma, and ameloblastoma. Usually (but not always), radiographically, the lamina dura around the root apices is intact, and responses to pulp tests are normal. The final diagnosis of these lesions is often based on surgical biopsy and histopathologic examination.

Malignant lesions that may simulate periapical lesions of pulpal origin and are often metastatic include lymphoma (Fig. 4.29), squamous cell carcinoma, osteogenic sarcoma, chondrosarcoma, and multiple myeloma. Unlike endodontic lesions, these lesions are usually associated with rapid and extensive hard tissue (bone and tooth) destruction. Ordinarily, the teeth in the affected region remain responsive to vitality tests, although occasionally the pulps or sensory nerves are disrupted and nonresponsive. For a more complete list and description of lesions that may mimic the radiographic appearance of endodontic lesions of pulpal origin, an oral pathology text should be consulted.[100]

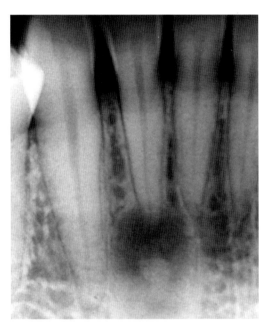

Fig. 4.28 A periapical radiolucency in the early stages of cementoma can simulate a periapical lesion of pulpal origin. However, the pulps' responses are within normal limits.

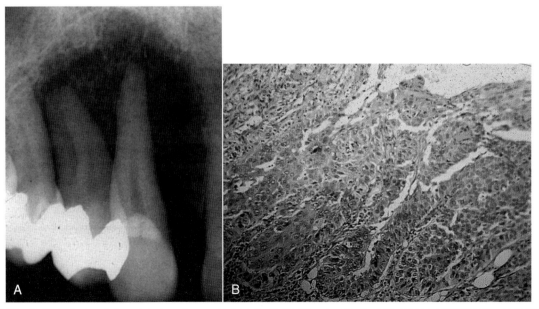

Fig. 4.29 **A,** Periapical radiolucent lesion of nonpulpal origin. **B,** Positive results of vitality tests and histologic examination of the tissue confirmed a diagnosis of carcinoma.

REFERENCES

1. Garberoglio R, Brannström M: Scanning electron microscopic investigation of human dentinal tubules, *Arch Oral Biol* 21:355, 1976.
2. Zach L, Cohen G: Biology of high speed rotary operative dental procedures. I. Correlation of tooth volume removed and pulpal pathology (abstract), *J Dent Res* 37:67, 1958.
3. Hamilton AI, Kramer IR: Cavity preparation with and without water spray: effects on the human dental pulp and additional effects of further dehydration of the dentine, *Br Dent J* 123:281, 1967.
4. Takahashi K: Changes in the pulpal vasculature during inflammation, *J Endod* 16:92, 1990.
5. Amano T, Muramatsu T, Amemiya K, et al: Responses of rat pulp cells to heat stress in vitro, *J Dent Res* 85(5):432-435, 2006.
6. Kayhan F, Kucukkeles N, Demirel D: A histologic and histomorphometric evaluation of pulpal reactions following rapid palatal expansion, *Am J Orthod Dentofacial Orthop* 117:465, 2000.
7. Taspinar F, Akgul N, Simsek G, et al: The histopathological investigation of pulpal tissue following heavy orthopaedic forces produced by rapid maxillary expansion, *J Int Med Res* 31:1971, 2003.
8. Strobl H, Haas M, Norer B, et al: Evaluation of pulpal blood flow after tooth splinting of luxated permanent maxillary incisors, *Dent Traumatol* 20:36, 2004.
9. Messer HH, Chen RS: The duration of effectiveness of root canal medicaments, *J Endod* 10:240, 1984.
10. Langeland K: Management of the inflamed pulp associated with deep carious lesion, *J Endod* 7:169, 1981.
11. Masillamoni C, Kettering J, Torabinejad M: The biocompatibility of some root canal medicaments and irrigants, *Int Endod J* 14:115, 1981.
12. Bowden JR, Ethunandan M, Brennan PA: Life-threatening airway obstruction secondary to hypochlorite extrusion during root canal treatment, *Oral Surg Oral Med Oral Pathol Oral Radiol Endod* 101:402, 2006.
13. Trevino EG, Patwardhan AN, Henry MA, et al: Effect of irrigants on the survival of human stem cells of the apical papilla in a platelet-rich plasma scaffold in human root tips, *J Endod* 1109, 2011.
14. Galler KM, D'Souza RN, Federlin M, et al: Dentin conditioning codetermines cell fate in regenerative endodontics, *J Endod* 37:1536, 2011.
15. Ruparel NB, Teixeira FB, Ferraz CCR, et al: Direct effect of intracanal medicaments on survival of stem cells of the apical papilla, *J Endod* 38:1372, 2012.
16. McKay GS: The histology and microbiology of acute occlusal dentine lesions in human permanent molar teeth, *Arch Oral Biol* 21:51, 1976.
17. Aas JA, Griffen AL, Dardis SR, et al: Bacteria of dental caries in primary and permanent teeth in children and young adults, *J Clin Microbiol* 46:1407, 2008.
18. Brannström M, Lind P: Pulpal response to early dental caries, *J Dent Res* 44:1045, 1965.
19. Baume L: Dental pulp conditions in relation to carious lesions, *Int Dent J* 20:309, 1970.
20. Jontell M, Okiji T, Dahlgren U, et al: Immune defense mechanisms of the dental pulp, *Crit Rev Oral Biol Med* 9:1790, 1998.
21. Lin L, Langeland K: Light and electron microscopic study of teeth with carious pulp exposures, *Oral Surg Oral Med Oral Pathol* 51:2926, 1981.
22. Yamasaki M, Kumazawa M, Kohsaka T, et al: Pulpal and periapical tissue reactions after experimental pulpal exposure in rats, *J Endod* 20:13, 1994.
23. Kakehashi S, Stanley H, Fitzgerald R: The effects of surgical exposures of dental pulps in germ-free and conventional laboratory rats, *Oral Surg Oral Med Oral Pathol* 20:340, 1965.

24. Möller ÅJR, Fabricius L, Dahlén G, et al: Influence on periapical tissues of indigenous oral bacteria and necrotic pulp tissue in monkeys, *Scand J Dent Res* 89:475, 1981.
25. Sundqvist G: Bacteriological studies of necrotic dental pulps, odontol doctoral dissertation no 7, Umeå, Sweden, 1976, University of Umeå.
26. Slots J, Nowzari H, Sabeti M: Cytomegalovirus infection in symptomatic periapical pathosis, *Int Endod J* 37:519, 2004.
27. Slots J, Sabeti M, Simon JH: Herpesviruses in periapical pathosis: an etiopathogenic relationship? *Oral Surg Oral Med Oral Pathol Oral Radiol Endod* 96:327, 2003.
28. Janeway CA Jr, Medzhitov R: Innate immune recognition, *Annu Rev Immunol* 20:197, 2002.
29. Reeves R, Stanley HR: The relationship of bacterial penetration and pulpal pathosis in carious teeth, *Oral Surg Oral Med Oral Pathol* 22:59, 1966.
30. Izumi T, Kobayashi I, Okamura K, et al: Immunohistochemical study on the immunocompetent cells of the pulp in human non-carious and carious teeth, *Arch Oral Biol* 40:609, 1995.
31. Torabinejad M: Mediators of acute and chronic periradicular lesions, *Oral Surg Oral Med Oral Pathol* 78:511, 1994.
32. Rauschenberger CR, McClanahan SB, Pederson ED, et al: Comparison of human polymorphonuclear neutrophil elastase, polymorphonuclear neutrophil cathepsin-G, and alpha 2-macroglobulin levels in healthy and inflamed dental pulps, *J Endod* 20:546, 1994.
33. McClanahan SB, Turner DW, Kaminski EJ, et al: Natural modifiers of the inflammatory process in the human dental pulp, *J Endod* 17:589, 1991.
34. Byers M, Taylor P, Khayat B, et al: Effects of injury and inflammation on pulpal and periapical nerves, *J Endod* 16:78, 1990.
35. Hahn CL, Liewehr FR: Innate immune responses of the dental pulp to caries, *J Endod* 33:643, 2007.
36. McLachlan JL, Sloan AJ, Smith AJ, et al: S100 and cytokine expression in caries, *Infect Immun* 72:4102, 2004.
37. Zachrisson BU, Skogedal O: Mast cells in inflamed human dental pulp, *Scand J Dent Res* 79:488, 1971.
38. Torabinejad M, Eby WC, Naidorf IJ: Inflammatory and immunological aspects of the pathogenesis of human periapical lesions, *J Endod* 11:479, 1985.
39. Goodis H, Saeki K: Identification of bradykinin, substance P, and neurokinin A in human dental pulp, *J Endod* 23:201, 1997.
40. Goodis HE, Bowles WR, Hargreaves KM: Prostaglandin E2 enhances bradykinin-evoked iCGRP release in bovine dental pulp, *J Dent Res* 79:1604, 2000.
41. Lessard GM, Torabinejad M, Swope D: Arachidonic acid metabolism in canine tooth pulps and the effects of nonsteroidal anti-inflammatory drugs, *J Endod* 12:146, 1986.
42. Cohen JS, Reader A, Fertel R, et al: A radioimmunoassay determination of the concentrations of prostaglandins E2 and F2 alpha in painful and asymptomatic human dental pulps, *J Endod* 11:330, 1985.
43. Grutzner E, Garry M, Hargreaves K: Effect of injury on pulpal levels of immunoreactive substance P and immunoreactive calcitonin gene-related peptide, *J Endod* 18:553, 1992.
44. Barkhordar R, Hayashi C, Hussain M: Detection of interleukin-6 in human dental pulp and periapical lesions, *Endod Dent Traumatol* 15:26, 1999.
45. Huang GT, Potente AP, Kim JW, et al: Increased interleukin-8 expression in inflamed human dental pulps, *Oral Surg Oral Med Oral Pathol Oral Radiol Endod* 88:214, 1999.
46. Rauschenberger CR, Bailey JC, Cootauco CJ: Detection of human IL-2 in normal and inflamed dental pulps, *J Endod* 23:366, 1997.

47. Yoshiba N, Yoshiba K, Nakamura H, et al: Immunohistochemical localization of HLA-DR-positive cells in unerupted and erupted normal and carious human teeth, *J Dent Res* 75:1585, 1996.
48. Nakanishi T, Matsuo T, Ebisu S: Quantitative analysis of immunoglobulins and inflammatory factors in human pulpal blood from exposed pulps, *J Endod* 21:131, 1995.
49. Bergenholtz G, Ahlstedt S, Lindhe J: Experimental pulpitis in immunized monkeys, *Scand J Dent Res* 85:3966, 1977.
50. Proctor ME, Turner DW, Kaminski EJ, et al: Determination and relationship of C-reactive protein in human dental pulps and in serum, *J Endod* 17:265, 1991.
51. Berggreen E, Heyeraas K: The role of sensory neuropeptides and nitric oxide on pulpal blood flow and tissue pressure in the ferret, *J Dent Res* 78:1535, 1999.
52. Van Hassel HJ: Physiology of the human dental pulp, *Oral Surg Oral Med Oral Pathol* 32:126, 1971.
53. Heyeraas KJ: Pulpal, microvascular, and tissue pressure, *J Dent Res* 64(spec no):585, 1985.
54. Johnson RH, Dachi SF, Haley JV: Pulpal hyperemia: a correlation of clinical and histologic data from 706 teeth, *J Am Dent Assoc* 81:108, 1970.
55. Bender IB: Pulpal pain diagnosis: a review, *J Endod* 26:175, 2000.
56. Mumford JM: Pain perception threshold on stimulating human teeth and the histological condition of the pulp, *Br Dent J* 123:427, 1967.
57. Kuyk JK, Walton RE: Comparison of the radiographic appearance of root canal size to its actual diameter, *J Endod* 16:528, 1990.
58. Walton RE, Leonard LA: Cracked tooth: an etiology for "idiopathic" internal resorption? *J Endod* 12:167, 1986.
59. Walton RE, Garnick JJ: The histology of periapical inflammatory lesions in permanent molars in monkeys, *J Endod* 12:49, 1986.
60. Mumford JM: *Orofacial pain: aetiology, diagnosis and treatment*, ed 3, New York,1982, Churchill Livingstone.
61. Perrini N, Fonzi L: Mast cells in human periapical lesions: ultrastructural aspects and their possible physiopathological implications, *J Endod* 11:1972, 1985.
62. Aqrabawi J, Schilder H, Toselli P, et al: Biochemical and histochemical analysis of the enzyme arylsulfatase in human lesions of endodontic origin, *J Endod* 19:335, 1993.
63. Shimauchi H, Takayama S, Miki Y, et al: The change of periapical exudate prostaglandin E2 levels during root canal treatment, *J Endod* 23:755, 1997.
64. Miyauchi M, Takata T, Ito H, et al: Immunohistochemical detection of prostaglandins E2, F2 alpha, and 6-keto-prostaglandin F1 alpha in experimentally induced periapical inflammatory lesions in rats, *J Endod* 22:635, 1996.
65. Anan H, Akamine A, Hara Y, et al: A histochemical study of bone remodeling during experimental apical periodontitis in rats, *J Endod* 17:332, 1991.
66. Lim GC, Torabinejad M, Kettering J, et al: Interleukin 1-beta in symptomatic and asymptomatic human periradicular lesions, *J Endod* 20:225, 1994.
67. Tyler LW, Matossian K, Todd R, et al: Eosinophil-derived transforming growth factors (TGF-alpha and TGF-beta 1) in human periradicular lesions, *J Endod* 25:619, 1999.
68. Kawashima N, Stashenko P: Expression of bone-resorptive and regulatory cytokines in murine periapical inflammation, *Arch Oral Biol* 44:55, 1999.
69. Stashenko P, Teles R, D'Souza R: Periapical inflammatory responses and their modulation, *Crit Rev Oral Biol Med* 9:4981, 1998.

70. Torres JO, Torabinejad M, Matiz RA, et al: Presence of secretory IgA in human periapical lesions, *J Endod* 20:87, 1994.

71. Baumgartner J, Falkler W Jr: Reactivity of IgG from explant cultures of periapical lesions with implicated microorganisms, *J Endod* 17:207, 1991.

72. Kettering JD, Torabinejad M, Jones SL: Specificity of antibodies present in human periapical lesions, *J Endod* 17:213, 1991.

73. Metzger Z: Macrophages in periapical lesions, *Endod Dent Traumatol* 16:1, 2000.

74. Matsuo T, Ebisu S, Shimabukuro Y, et al: Quantitative analysis of immunocompetent cells in human periapical lesions: correlations with clinical findings of the involved teeth, *J Endod* 18:4970, 1992.

75. Wang CY, Stashenko P: Characterization of bone-resorbing activity in human periapical lesions, *J Endod* 19:107, 1993.

76. Paula-Silva FW, da Silva LA, Kapila YL: Matrix metalloproteinase expression in teeth with apical periodontitis is differentially modulated by the modality of root canal treatment, *J Endod* 36:231, 2010.

77. Matsui H, Yamasaki M, Nakata K, et al: Expression of MMP-8 and MMP-13 in the development of periradicular lesions, *Int Endod J* 44:739, 2011.

78. de Paula-Silva FW, D'Silva NJ, da Silva LA, et al: High matrix metalloproteinase activity is a hallmark of periapical granulomas, *J Endod* 35:1234, 2009.

79. Buzoglu HD, Unal H, Ulger C, et al: The zymographic evaluation of gelatinase (MMP-2 and -9) levels in acute and chronic periapical abscesses, *Oral Surg Oral Med Oral Pathol Oral Radiol Endod* 108:121, 2009.

80. Kawashima N, Suzuki N, Yang G, et al: Kinetics of RANKL, RANK and OPG expressions in experimentally induced rat periapical lesions, *Oral Surg Oral Med Oral Pathol Oral Radiol Endod* 103:707, 2007.

81. Saidenberg Kermanac'h N, Bessis N, Cohen-Solal M, et al: Osteoprotegerin and inflammation, *Eur Cytokine Netw* 13:144, 2002.

82. Sabeti M, Simon J, Kermani V, et al: Detection of receptor activator of NF-κβ ligand in apical periodontitis, *J Endod* 31:17, 2005.

83. Vernal R, Dezerega A, Dutzan N, et al: RANKL in human periapical granuloma: possible involvement in periapical bone destruction, *Oral Dis* 12:283, 2006.

84. Morse DR, Seltzer S, Sinai I, et al: Endodontic classification, *J Am Dent Assoc* 94:685, 1977.

85. Nobuhara WK, del Rio CE: Incidence of periradicular pathoses in endodontic treatment failures, *J Endod* 19:315, 1993.

86. Maixner D, Green TL, Walton R: Histologic examination of condensing osteitis (abstract), *J Endod* 18:196, 1992.

87. Hedin M, Polhagen L: Follow-up study of periradicular bone condensation, *Scand J Dent Res* 79:436, 1971.

88. Baumgartner J, Picket A, Muller J: Microscopic examination of oral sinus tracts and their associated periapical lesions, *J Endod* 10:146, 1984.

89. Andelin WE, Shabahang S, Wright K, et al: Identification of hard tissue after experimental pulp capping using dentin sialoprotein (DSP) as a marker, *J Endod* 29:646, 2003.

90. Qin C, Brunn JC, Cadena E, et al: Dentin sialoprotein in bone and dentin sialophosphoprotein gene expressed by osteoblasts, *Connect Tissue Res* 44:179(suppl 1), 2003.

91. Leprince JG, Zeitlin BD, Tolar M, et al: Interactions between immune system and mesenchymal stem cells in dental pulp and periapical tissues, *Int Endod J* 45:689, 2012.

92. Kobayashi C, Yaegaki K, Calenic B, et al: Hydrogen sulfide causes apoptosis in human pulp stem cells, *J Endod* 37:479, 2011.

93. Amler M: The time sequence of tissue regeneration in human extraction wounds, *Oral Surg Oral Med Oral Pathol* 27:309, 1969.

94. Fouad A, Walton R, Rittman B: Healing of induced periapical lesions in ferret canines, *J Endod* 19:123, 1993.

95. Danin J, Linder LE, Lundqvist G, et al: Tumor necrosis factor-alpha and transforming growth factor-beta₁ in chronic periapical lesions, *Oral Surg Oral Med Oral Pathol Oral Radiol Endod* 90:514, 2000.

96. Leonardi R, Lanteri E, Stivala F, et al: Immunolocalization of CD44 adhesion molecules in human periradicular lesions, *Oral Surg Oral Med Oral Pathol Oral Radiol Endod* 89:480, 2000.

97. Boyne PJ: Application of bone morphogenetic proteins in the treatment of clinical oral and maxillofacial osseous defects, *J Bone Joint Surg Am* 83A(suppl 1):S146, 2001.

98. Fouad A, Burleson J: The effect of diabetes mellitus on endodontic treatment outcome: data from an electronic patient record, *J Am Dent Assoc* 134:43, 2003.

99. Garber SE, Shabahang S, Escher AP, et al: The effect of hyperglycemia on pulpal healing in rats, *J Endod* 35:60, 2009.

100. Eversole L: *Clinical outline of oral pathology*, ed 2, Philadelphia, 1984, Lea & Febiger.

Diagnosis, treatment planning, and systemic considerations

Richard E. Walton, Ashraf F. Fouad

CHAPTER OUTLINE

Diagnosis
Treatment Planning

Systemic Considerations

LEARNING OBJECTIVES

After reading this chapter, the student should be able to:

1. Recognize that diagnosis of and treatment planning for pulpal and periapical conditions should be part of a broader examination and treatment plan.
2. Integrate the endodontic diagnosis and treatment plan into an overall treatment plan.
3. Understand the importance of the medical and dental history to endodontic diagnosis.
4. Address the correct questions regarding the history and symptoms of the present complaint.
5. Describe clearly to the patient the diagnostic procedure to be followed.
6. Conduct an intraoral examination of both soft and hard tissues that focuses on determining the pulpal and periapical health.
7. Apply, interpret, and understand the limitations of vitality tests.
8. Know when and how to use special approaches, such as a test cavity, and selective anesthesia.
9. Interpret diagnostic radiographs.
10. Understand the mechanisms of pain and how variable the pain experience can be.
11. Understand and detect when pain is referred and when hyperalgesia and allodynia are present.
12. Consolidate all data from the history, symptoms, examination, and tests to form a diagnosis of pulpal and periapical conditions, using appropriate terminology.
13. Identify conditions for which root canal treatment is indicated and contraindicated.
14. Recognize the indications for adjunctive treatments, such as vital pulp therapy, bleaching, root amputation,

endodontic surgery, intentional replantation, autotransplantation, hemisection, apexification, orthodontic extrusion, and retreatment.
15. Identify problems that require treatment modifications, such as operative complications, cracked tooth, periodontal problems, isolation difficulties, restorability, strategic value, patient management, medical complications, abnormal root or pulp anatomy, impact trauma, and restricted opening.
16. Design an endodontic treatment plan that is integrated into the overall treatment plan.
17. Present the patient with the preferred treatment plan and any alternatives and explain its development from diagnostic data.
18. Discuss the prognosis of any suggested treatment.
19. Classify potential complications of endodontic procedures.
20. Identify which procedures are ordinarily not within the graduating dentist's realm of training or experience and which patients should be considered for referral.
21. Recognize the various ways endodontic pathosis and systemic disease interact and also some of the mechanisms of such interactions.
22. Identify the effects of diabetes mellitus, smoking, genetic predisposition, irradiation, sickle cell disease, and viral infections on the pathogenesis of endodontic pathosis and endodontic treatment outcomes.
23. Determine the potential for acute and chronic endodontic infections to cause or contribute to systemic disease, including cardiovascular disease.

Three processes separate the professional from the non-professional: (1) diagnosis, (2) treatment planning, and (3) problem solving. Expanded-duty assistants can obtain information and perform tests, but only the dentist can interpret the findings, establish a diagnosis, and design the appropriate treatment plan.

Endodontic diagnosis and treatment occur in two basic scenarios. In the first scenario, the emergency patient presents with pain and possibly swelling or with displaced, fractured, or avulsed teeth. The second scenario is part of the restorative treatment plan when pulpal or periapical disease is detected but without symptoms. In the first case, urgent treatment is needed to relieve pain, prevent the spread of infection, and immobilize avulsed or loosened teeth. In the second scenario, definitive endodontic treatment is carried out as part of a comprehensive treatment plan. Once an emergency has been relieved, the first scenario becomes the second scenario.

In both scenarios a thorough history and examination that lead to a diagnosis are essential to provide appropriate and effective care (Fig. 5.1). *The key to effective treatment is accurate diagnosis.* The key to accurate diagnosis is an understanding of the pathologic processes occurring in the affected tissue (see Chapters 1, 3, and 4).

Diagnosis is the science of recognizing disease by means of signs, symptoms, and tests. Often, diagnosis is straightforward; sometimes it is not. The basic steps in the diagnostic process are as follows:

1. Chief complaint
2. History (medical and dental)
3. Oral examination
4. Data analysis (leading to differential diagnosis)
5. Treatment plan

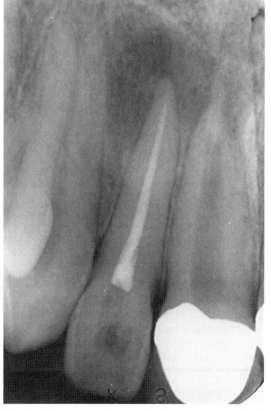

Fig. 5.1 In this case, a reliance on "clinical experience" rather than on adequate tests resulted in the wrong treatment. The dentist relied on a radiograph only (no tests) and concluded that the lateral incisor was the painful problem tooth. After treatment, with no change in the level of pain, the patient was referred for root-end surgery. Examination of preoperative and postoperative radiographs, in addition to clinical test results, showed that treatment had been performed on a tooth with normal pulp. The central incisor was found to have pulp necrosis and an acute apical abscess. Immediate pain relief followed root canal treatment on the correct tooth.

A limited number of possible diagnoses exists for conditions of the pulp and periapical conditions (Table 5.1). These diagnoses are:

- Pulpal diagnoses
  - Normal
  - Reversible pulpitis
  - Irreversible pulpitis
    - Asymptomatic
    - Symptomatic
  - Necrosis
- Periapical diagnoses
  - Normal
  - Symptomatic apical periodontitis
  - Asymptomatic apical periodontitis
  - Acute apical abscess
  - Chronic apical abscess
  - Condensing osteitis

The pathosis of these conditions is described in Chapter 4.

Although diagnosis is a science, it is an imperfect science, and sometimes a detailed, definitive diagnosis is difficult or impossible. Importantly *significant pulpal or periapical pathosis is frequently without marked symptoms at present or in the past.*[1] The clinician must be alert for other indicators of pathosis that require careful examination.

Pain as a presenting symptom is obviously a key concern both of the patient having the experience and of the dentist, who is eager to resolve the pain. Unfortunately, this symptom often leads to a misdiagnosis, because pain is often referred from its true origin to another site. In addition, pulpal pathosis is frequently painless.[2] A well-known example is appendicitis; the pain seems to originate from the region of the navel, which is a long way from the diseased organ. A similar phenomenon occurs in the mouth; pain may be referred from one tooth to another. In addition, pain that arises from the temporomandibular joint and associated musculature, from sinus infections, and even from cardiac problems[3] may refer to the teeth. The mechanism of referral is discussed later, but diagnosis of a painful condition in the orofacial region must begin with consideration of these complicating factors.

Other pathologic conditions, such as neuralgia, multiple sclerosis, myocardial ischemia, or psychiatric disorders, may produce the same symptoms. *A thorough understanding of the complicated, multifactorial, and versatile nature of pain is essential to an accurate diagnosis and then successful treatment.*

DIAGNOSIS

Chief Complaint

The chief complaint is the first information obtained and is usually volunteered by the patient. Patients express their complaint in their own words, which should be recorded in the chart as such. This, after all, is why the patient seeks treatment, and the patient will judge the outcome of treatment by whether the problem, as he or she saw it, was managed. To gain the patient's confidence, the clinician must pay attention to the chief complaint. When this confidence has been achieved, the patient will be able understand that diagnosis requires a thorough and methodical approach, and he or she can cooperate in this approach.

Table 5.1 Diagnostic terminology

	Symptoms	Radiographic	Pulp tests	Periapical tests
Pulpal				
Normal	None of any significance	No periapical changes	Responds	Not sensitive
Reversible	May or may not have slight symptoms to thermal stimulus	No periapical changes	Responds	Not sensitive
Irreversible Asymptomatic	Similar to reversible (diagnosed by caries excavation to reveal exposure)	None or slight periapical changes	Responds to pulp tests	No pain
Irreversible Symptomatic	Severe pain to thermal stimulus; also may have spontaneous pain	None or slight or slight periapical changes. One exception: occasional condensing osteitis	May have severe pain With thermal; often spontaneous pain	Often painful
Necrotic	None to thermal stimulus Other symptoms (see Periapical, below)	See Periapical, below	No response	Depends on periapical status
Periapical				
Normal	None of significance	No significant changes	Response or no response (depends on pulp status)	Not sensitive
Symptomatic apical periodontitis	Significant pain on mastication or pressure	No significant changes, or May show radiolucency	Response or no response (depends on pulp status)	Pain on percussion or palpation
Asymptomatic apical periodontitis and apical cyst	None to mild	Apical radiolucency	No response	None to mild on percussion or palpation
Acute apical abscess	Swelling and significant pain	Usually a radiolucent lesion	No response	Pain on percussion or palpation
Chronic apical abscess	Draining sinus tract or parulis	Usually a radiolucent lesion	No response	Not sensitive
Condensing osteitis	Varies (depends on pulp or periapical status)	Increased trabecular bone density	Response or no response (depends on pulp status)	May or may not have pain on percussion or palpation

Importantly, there are many facial pains are not of odontogenic origin. These may be easily confused with tooth pain by both the patient and the dentist.

Health History
Health and Medical History
Whether the patient is returning to the practice or has filled out a new health questionnaire, the medical history is reviewed with the patient directly; this is recorded in the clinical record. Patients who seek and require endodontic treatment are older, on average, and have a higher incidence and more complex profile of systemic medical problems.[4] Some conditions are of concern in diagnosing endodontic problems. For example, acute respiratory infections, particularly of the maxillary sinus, often produce toothache-like symptoms. Stress commonly leads to neuromuscular pain in the masticatory apparatus, with a presentation that includes tooth pain.

Although no medical conditions contraindicate endodontic treatment, there are some conditions that can reduce the patient's ability to respond to treatment.[4] Acquired immunodeficiency syndrome (AIDS) clearly compromises the immune system, as may hepatitis.[5,6] Drugs used to prevent the rejection of transplants and grafts, in addition to those used to combat glucocorticosteroid deficiency and serious allergies, may have a similar effect. The incidence of type II diabetes is increasing rapidly in the general population and may affect the pathogenesis or healing of endodontic pathosis (see below, Diabetes Mellitus). Patients with active ischemic heart disease may need special consideration, which should be based on a consultation with their cardiologist.[7,8]

Other factors related to therapeutics may complicate diagnosis. Bisphosphonates are a factor to consider in diagnosis and treatment planning (this is discussed under systemic considerations).

A more frequent concern is that patients who have experienced pain and/or swelling may already be taking antibiotics and analgesics that can mask signs and symptoms.

Antibiotic Prophylaxis

In 2007 an update on the guidelines for antibiotic prophylaxis was released by a task force of the American Heart Association, with input from the American Dental Association.[9] These recommendations greatly reduce the indications for coverage to a limited number of cardiac conditions, which include (1) artificial heart valve, (2) previous history of infective endocarditis, (3) incomplete or repaired congenital heart tissue repair, and (4) some heart transplants. In these patients, the regimen is 2 g of amoxicillin given 30 to 60 minutes before surgery for adults. The dosage for children is 50 mg/kg. For allergic patients, a good choice is clindamycin 600 mg 30 to 60 minutes before the procedure.

The American Association of Orthopedic Surgeons, in conjunction with the American Dental Association, recently updated the guidelines for prophylaxis in joint replacement patients.[10] Patients considered to be at risk include those who have had joint replacements within the past year, particularly those who are immunocompromised or immunosuppressed, those with hemophilia or insulin-dependent diabetes, and those who have had previous joint prosthesis infections. The most recent guidelines state that there is no evidence that dental procedures are directly responsible for instances of artificial joint infections, that local oral antimicrobials should be considered in the prevention of periprosthetic joint infections, and that good oral hygiene measures should be maintained.[11] If antibiotics are indeed indicated, the same regimen is recommended as for cardiac patients.

Endodontic procedures considered to be a risk in patients with cardiac conditions or joint prostheses include instrumentation beyond the apex, periapical surgery, or other procedures that may produce bleeding, such as aggressive rubber dam placement or incision for drainage.

Dental History

Endodontic problems usually have a history (Fig. 5.2). Recent trauma is obviously relevant, as are recent restorations and previous treatment for temporomandibular dysfunction. A longer overview may indicate the type of treatment that would be most appropriate. A patient with a poorly maintained dentition and several missing teeth may not be an ideal candidate for endodontic treatment and subsequent restorative procedures.

History of the Present Complaint

After the patient has explained why he or she is seeking care (and this has been recorded in the patient's own words), details must be established through methodical questioning. There are a limited number of complaints of endodontic consequence. The patient may have more than one complaint. Pain and swelling, for example, often occur together. The most common complaints are as follows:

- Pain
- Swelling
- Broken tooth
- Loose tooth
- Tooth discoloration
- Bad taste

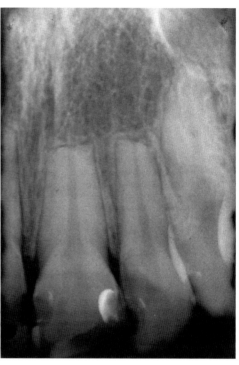

Fig. 5.2 Short roots, an absence of pathosis in the periapical tissues, and a history of orthodontics indicate that resorption is due to tooth movement in the past.

If there are two or more concurrent complaints, such as pain and swelling, then the history of each complaint must be obtained.

Pain is the most obvious and most important. Understanding the physiology of pain and the anatomy of nociceptive pathways is essential to the diagnosis and treatment of painful conditions.[12] A brief synopsis of pain mechanisms is presented here. Boxes 5.1 and 5.2 present the key elements in list form.

Pain is a multifactorial experience subject to modulation. The basic mechanism of nociception is well established. The pulp is innervated largely by nociceptive fibers, either Aδ (fast conducting; sharp pain) or C fibers (slow conducting; dull, throbbing pain). During inflammation, the C fibers dominate, and pulpal pain is characteristically dull, throbbing, and poorly localized. The periodontal ligament (PDL) has a much greater large-fiber innervation than does the pulp, and many of these fibers are mechanosensitive, which explains why pain from the tooth is more easily localized when inflammation has spread into the supporting tissues. First-order nociceptive fibers connect with second-order neurons in the dorsal horn of grey matter in the spinal cord or in its equivalent in the brainstem, the subnucleus caudalis of the trigeminal system. This is a key relay; it is here that much of the modulation of pain takes place. Through endogenous opioid mechanisms, descending tracts from midbrain areas can reduce or prevent the activity from traveling further centrally. The degree to which this mechanism is involved is variable, but much of the affective/motivational component of the pain experience is explained by descending modulation. This explains why similar levels of tissue damage may be related to very different levels of pain.

Box 5.1   What Is Pain?

- An unpleasant sensory and emotional experience associated with actual or potential tissue damage or described in terms of such damage.
- A dedicated "pain system" includes *nociceptors* (receptors preferentially sensitive to a noxious stimulus), small-diameter fibers, tracts, and central processing areas.
- Noxious stimuli activate nociceptors, but this activation does not inevitably result in pain.
- Activity in pain pathways can be modulated upward or downward, both peripherally and centrally. In particular, descending opioid influences can facilitate or impede the transmission of activity from first-order neurons to higher centers, thus reducing the pain experience.
- Affective, motivational, and cultural factors contribute substantially to the pain experience.
- *Hyperalgesia* (an increased response to a stimulus that is normally painful), *allodynia* (pain from a stimulus that does not normally provoke pain), and *spontaneous pain* (pain without a stimulus) result from both peripheral and central changes after inflammation or injury. Central changes may persist after peripheral injury has resolved.
- Pain may be acute or chronic. Acute pain arises from inflammation or injury to the pulp and periapex. Acute pain is protective. It leads to avoidance and escape to prevent or minimize tissue damage. When it continues, it forces an injured area to be rested. Chronic pain is nonprotective. It may continue long after an injury has healed or may not be associated with an injury. Trigeminal neuralgia and long-term pain of unknown origin are types of chronic pain.

Box 5.2   What Is Central Sensitization?

- Prolonged nociceptive input leads to functional alterations in the subnucleus caudalis, the spinal dorsal horn, and probably the thalamus.
- Lower thresholds (hyperalgesia)
- Wider receptive fields
- Spontaneous activity
- Recruitment of nonpain fibers (allodynia)
- A major change is the up-regulation of N-methyl-D-aspartate (NMDA) receptors on the second-order neuron.

Box 5.3   What Are Key Features of Referred Pain?

- Common occurrence
- Never crosses the midline
- Can be referred from other teeth or extraoral structures
- Anesthetizing the true origin reduces or eliminates the pain.

Box 5.4   Case: Pain Referred to Muscles of Mastication

Complaint
Moderately severe but continuous dull ache in left lower jaw

History
The pain has lasted several weeks and is most severe in the morning. It is not intensified by hot and cold stimuli and is relieved temporarily by mild analgesics. A three-unit mandibular-posterior bridge had been placed a few months earlier. There was neither recent acute infection nor trauma. The referring dentist had completed root canal treatment on the premolar abutment with no change in symptoms.

Examination
No visible or palpable intraoral soft tissue abnormalities are present. All teeth on the left side respond within normal limits to vitality tests and percussion. Radiographs show no lesions in mineralized tissues. Discomfort is not relieved by an inferior alveolar nerve block. Palpation of the left masseter muscle shows it to be acutely tender, particularly on the anterior border. Occlusal examination shows imbalances and premature contacts on the left side. Injecting a local anesthetic into the tender region of the muscle relieves the pain.

Diagnosis
Acute myofascial pain in the left masseter muscle after dental treatment

Etiology
Afferents from the muscle (probably in tendons or fascia) converge on the same second-order neuron in the brainstem trigeminal nucleus as periodontal afferents from the mandibular abutment teeth. The higher centers to which the second-order neuron projects are unable to differentiate between the two inputs. The higher nerve centers "assume" that the new input (from the muscle) originates from the same site as the original input (the teeth).

Sustained and continuous noxious input may cause changes in the second-order neurons, reducing their threshold and increasing their receptive fields.[13,14] These are elements of central sensitization, a group of changes that contribute to the presentation of long-term and chronic pain (see Box 5.2). Central sensitization explains the nature of hyperalgesia, allodynia, and spontaneous pain. Once sensitized, these second-order neurons may be activated by inputs from multiple areas converging on them; this is the phenomenon of *referred pain* (Box 5.3).

With referred pain, the pain originating in a tooth can seem to come from another tooth or another area, even outside the mouth.[2,15-19] It also allows teeth to appear painful when the true origin of the pain is in another tooth, in the neuromuscular system (Box 5.4), in the upper respiratory tract, or even in cardiac muscle.

When neurons from several teeth or other structures converge on a second-order neuron that is sensitized, non-nociceptive levels of activity from these structures may induce firing and activity in the higher levels of the pain system. The higher centers may then identify this as painful activity in these areas. The reverse is also true. For example, painful input from the maxillary sinus may seem to originate from a tooth (Box 5.5).

The Pain Referral Phenomenon

The pain referral phenomenon must be taken into account when making a diagnosis.[15,18,19] The identification and location of an injured tooth should be straightforward in the early stages of the injury, when activity in nociceptors predominates. Identification of the source is more complex in the longer term, when modulation can modify the presentation by the referral of pain (Box 5.6).

Box 5.5   What Are Indicators of a Difficult Diagnosis?

- Patient cannot localize the pain, or the site seems to vary.
- No local dental cause for the pain can be identified.
- Pain is spontaneous or intermittent and not necessarily related to an initiating stimulus.
- Stimulation of a suspected tooth does not reproduce the symptoms.
- A suspected tooth shows no clear etiology (caries, fracture).
- More than one tooth seems to be involved.
- Symptoms are bilateral.
- Selective anesthesia fails to localize the source of pain.

Box 5.6   Case: Psychogenic Pain

Complaint
A 45-year-old woman was seen with a continuous, moderate, dull, and occasionally severe ache from bilateral temporomandibular joints and molars. Discomfort began with the onset of marital problems and financial hardship. Root canal treatment of a molar provided temporary relief, as did occlusal splint therapy and pharmacologic treatment for depression. However, the discomfort returned.

Examination
Clinical and radiographic examinations of teeth show no abnormalities. Treatment appears successful. Palpation of the temporomandibular joints reveals no abnormality. Further questioning reveals extended emotional stress after marital break-up.

Diagnosis
Orofacial pain of psychogenic origin (tentative)

Etiology
Pain originates from higher nerve centers and is probably entirely affective. Various forms of treatment are only transiently effective, because they affect higher central nervous system centers.

Treatment
Long-term relief depends on removal of the emotional problems sustaining the central nervous system changes or on the patient adopting suppressive strategies. A careful, nonjudgmental explanation of psychogenic pain was given to the patient. In particular, the contribution of both organic and psychological components to the pain experience was described. Clearly, the patient was experiencing pain, but because no organic cause was evident, interventional dental treatment would not bring long-term relief. The prescription of antidepressants by a physician is virtually always a component of treatment.

When pain is one of the complaints, the following questions should be asked:

1. When did the pain begin?
2. Where is the pain located?
3. Is the pain always in the same place?
4. What is the character of the pain (short, sharp, long lasting, dull, throbbing, continuous, occasional)?
5. Does the pain prevent sleeping or working?
6. Is the pain worse in the morning?
7. Is the pain worse when you lie down?
8. Did or does anything initiate the pain (trauma, biting)?
9. Once initiated, how long does the pain last?
10. Is the pain continuous, spontaneous, or intermittent?

11. Does anything make the pain worse (hot, cold, biting)? Does anything make the pain better (cold, analgesics)?

It is also frequently useful to ask the patient to quantify the amount of pain on a scale of 0 to 10, with 0 being no pain and 10 being the most excruciating pain imaginable. This quantification not only gives the practitioner an idea about the urgency and severity of the problem, but also allows comparison of the pain from visit to visit, particularly if there is residual pain after treatment.

If the complaint is swelling or includes swelling, there is a similar list of questions:

1. When did the swelling begin?
2. How quickly has the swelling increased in size?
3. Where is the swelling located?
4. What is the nature of the swelling (soft, hard, tender)?
5. Is there drainage from the swelling?
6. Is the swelling associated with a loose or tender tooth?

If a fractured tooth is part of the complaint, the time and nature of the trauma should be determined, particularly whether other teeth were involved in the trauma even though they were not visibly damaged. Was there any injury to the lips or gingiva? Similarly, with a loose or discolored tooth, the time when it was first noticed should be recorded, along with the history of any trauma that might be involved and whether the tooth was recently restored. A bad taste can result from a number of causes but often is from purulence draining through a sinus tract from a chronic periapical or periodontal abscess.

After thorough questioning that elicits reliable answers, the clinician should be able to generate a tentative diagnosis from the history. This is really a hypothesis that the objective component of the examination will test. The astute clinician's mind remains open to other possibilities.

Nonodontogenic Pain

Pain in the lower face, particularly in the regions of the jaws, is commonly believed by both the patient and the dentist to be tooth related. Furthermore, the assumption is often that there is significant pulp and/or periapical pathosis that requires root canal treatment. Thus, the first approach is to try to identify an offending tooth with the idea that treatment is required. Frequently, this is not the case. In fact, often this pain is neither odontogenic nor related to any oral tissues. Furthermore, there may be no pathosis or any identifiable etiology. These pains often are inconsistent with nerve patterns and "wander" to different structures; they have different descriptors, such as *atypical facial pain, nonodontogenic toothache, atypical odontalgia, persistent dental pain,* and *psychogenic pain.*[20] Unfortunately, attempts to try to resolve these pains with local treatment or even with analgesics are unsuccessful; the pain persists, much to the distress of both the patient and the dentist.[21] When patients present with these unusual pain patterns, the generalist should consider referral to an endodontist, who rules in or rules out an endodontic etiology (see Chapter 6). Often, these patients are further referred to a dental pain clinic or to a neurologist, who examines the patient for neurologic disorders.

Objective Examination

Extraoral and intraoral tissues are examined, tested, and compared with other teeth and soft tissues for pathosis.

Extraoral Examination

General appearance, skin tone, facial asymmetry, swelling, discoloration, redness, extraoral scars or sinus tracts, and lymphadenopathy are indicators of physical status. A careful extraoral examination helps to identify the cause of the patient's complaint and also the presence and extent of an inflammatory reaction in the oral cavity or even at an extraoral site (Fig. 5.3).

Intraoral Examination
Soft Tissue

Soft tissue examination includes a thorough visual, digital, and probing examination of the lips, oral mucosa, cheeks, tongue, periodontium, palate, and muscles. These tissues are evaluated, and abnormalities are noted. Alveolar mucosa and attached gingiva are examined for the presence

of discoloration, inflammation, ulceration, and sinus tract formation. Sinus tracts are common. A stoma (parulis) usually indicates the presence of a necrotic pulp and chronic apical abscess (Fig. 5.4) and sometimes a periodontal abscess. Gutta-percha placed in the sinus tract occasionally assists in tactile and radiographic localization of the source of these lesions. Probing determines the presence of deep, isolated periodontal defects that may be endodontic in origin (Fig. 5.5).

Dentition

Teeth are examined with a mirror and an explorer for discolorations, fractures, abrasions, erosions, caries, failing restorations, or other abnormalities. A discolored crown is often pathognomonic of pulpal pathosis or is the sequela of earlier root canal treatment. Although in some cases the diagnosis is

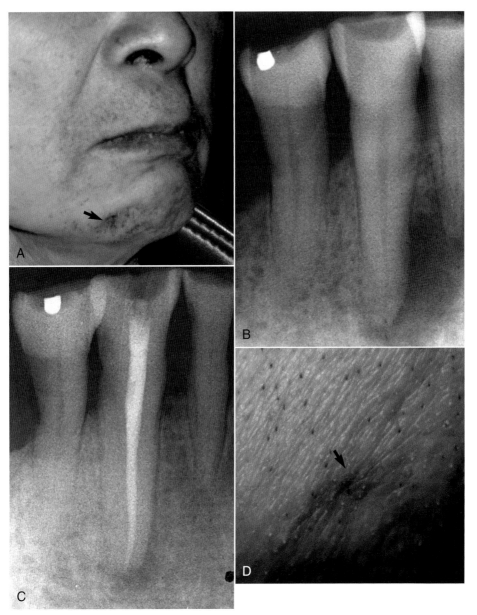

Fig. 5.3 Extraoral sinus tract. **A,** This surface lesion *(arrow)* was misdiagnosed and treated unsuccessfully by a dermatologist for several months. Fortunately, the patient's dentist recognized it as a draining sinus tract; the source was a mandibular anterior tooth. **B,** The pulp was necrotic because of severe attrition with pulp exposure. After proper root canal treatment only, **(C),** the sinus tract and surface lesion resolved completely (**D,** *arrow*).

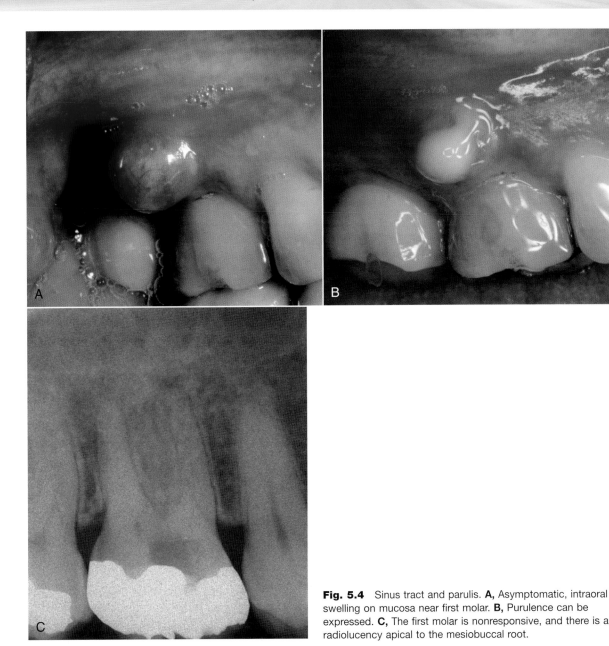

Fig. 5.4 Sinus tract and parulis. **A,** Asymptomatic, intraoral swelling on mucosa near first molar. **B,** Purulence can be expressed. **C,** The first molar is nonresponsive, and there is a radiolucency apical to the mesiobuccal root.

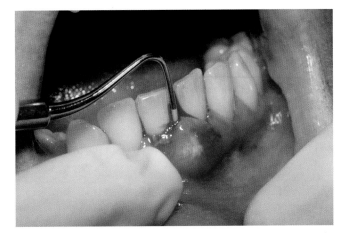

Fig. 5.5 Periodontal probing reveals a deep defect. Pulp necrosis suggests that this lesion is endodontic and not periodontic.

very likely known at this stage of examination, a prudent diagnostician should never proceed with treatment before performing appropriate confirmatory clinical and radiographic examinations.

Clinical Tests

There are a number of special tests that can be applied to individual teeth suspected of pathologic change. These tests have inherent limitations; some cannot be used on each tooth, 5-3 and the test results themselves may be inconclusive. The data they provide must be interpreted carefully and in conjunction with all the other information available. Importantly, these are *not* tests of *teeth;* they are tests of a patient's *response* to a variety of applied stimuli, which can be highly variable.

Control Teeth

When using any test, it is important to include control (comparison) teeth of a similar type to the suspect tooth or teeth. **75**

Tests on these teeth educate the patient on what response to expect and provide a "calibrated" baseline for the responses to tests on suspected teeth. The patient should not be told whether the tooth being tested is a control or a suspect tooth. A patient may not respond in the same way or to the same extent when tests are repeated. The first application of the test is the most significant.

The tests used fall into two groups: percussion and palpation, which reflect the condition of the supporting tissues, and vitality tests, which provide information on the condition of the pulp.

Percussion and Palpation of Supporting Tissues

Percussion is performed by different means. One way is tapping on the incisal or occlusal surface of the tooth with the end of a mirror handle held either parallel or perpendicular to the crown. This should be preceded by gentle digital pressure to detect teeth that are very tender and should *not* be tapped with the mirror handle. If a painful response is obtained, this may indicate the presence of periapical inflammation. *Periapical inflammation* may show a sharp pain. An additional approach, useful if the patient complains of pain on chewing, is the biting test, in which the patient bites down on a cotton swab between each tooth in turn (Fig. 5.6).

Both neighboring teeth and contralateral control teeth should also be percussed. Teeth adjacent to the diseased tooth often show some tenderness because of the local spread of cytokines and neuropeptides that lower the pain threshold.

At the same time the tooth is percussed, its mobility should be estimated by placing a finger lightly on the lingual surface of the tooth and pushing on the facial surface with the end of the mirror handle. The degree of movement can be visualized and felt. A healthy periodontium allows movement of only a fraction of a millimeter. Increased mobility is usually the result of periodontal disease, but in teeth with periapical inflammation, the tooth may have some mobility. This movement reduces after the periapical problem resolves.

Palpation is firm pressure on the mucosa overlying the apex. As does percussion, palpation determines how far the inflammatory process has extended periapically. A painful response to palpation indicates periapical inflammation.

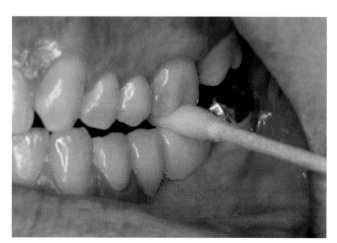

Fig. 5.6 Biting test. Firm pressure on a cotton swab that produces definite pain is a good indicator of apical periodontitis.

Pulp Vitality Tests

Vitality tests are an important, often critical, component of the examination. Studies comparing the histologic condition of the pulp to the results of vitality tests have shown that there is only a limited correlation between the two. As a consequence, the results of these tests require very careful interpretation. There are several types of vitality tests, and each can be applied by a variety of techniques. Not all tests are appropriate for every case, nor are all tests equally reliable. There are five basic types of vitality tests. Four apply either a cold, hot, electrical, or dentin stimulus to the tooth, and the patient's verbal response is recorded. The fifth attempts to measure pulpal blood flow, on the principle that blood flow increases in inflamed tissue and is not present with necrotic pulp. Selecting which tests to use is based on the patient's complaint and the test's reliability; it should be the one that reproduces the stimulus that causes the complaint.

An electric pulp test, conducted correctly, usually determines whether there is vital tissue within the tooth.[22] It cannot determine whether that tissue is inflamed, nor can it indicate whether there is partial necrosis. The cold test can also detect vital tissue. Prolonged pain provides an indication of irreversible inflammation, although not very accurately. The heat test is the least reliable. Measuring blood flow or presence is difficult under routine conditions, but as the technology improves, this technique may become more useful.

Selecting the Appropriate Pulp Test

Selection of the appropriate pulp test depends on the situation.[2] Additional meaningful information is collected when stimuli similar to those that the patient reports provoke pain are used during clinical tests. When cold (or hot) food or drink initiates a painful response, a cold (or hot) test is conducted in place of other vitality tests. Replication of the *same* symptoms in a tooth often indicates the offender. Overall, electrical stimulation is similar to cold (refrigerant) in identifying pulp necrosis[23]; heat is best used when this is the chief complaint.

When other tests are inconclusive or cannot be used and a necrotic pulp is suspected, dentin stimulation with a *test cavity* is helpful. For example, a tooth with a porcelain-fused-to-metal crown often cannot be tested accurately by standard thermal or electrical tests. After careful subjective examination and an explanation of the nature of the test to the patient, an access preparation without anesthesia is started. With a vital pulp, the surface of the restoration or the enamel can be penetrated without too much discomfort. If the pulp is vital, there will be a sudden sensation of pain when dentin is reached. In contrast, if discomfort or pain is absent, the pulp is probably necrotic; the procedure may be continued.

Cold Tests Three methods are generally used for cold testing: frozen water (ice), carbon dioxide (CO_2) ice (dry ice), and refrigerant. CO_2 ice requires special equipment (Fig. 5.7), whereas refrigerant in a spray can is more convenient (Fig. 5.8). Regular ice delivers less cold and is not as effective as refrigerant or CO_2 ice. One study found that refrigerant sprayed on a large cotton pellet was the most effective in reducing temperature within the chamber under full-coverage restorations.[24] Overall, refrigerant spray and CO_2 ice are equivalent for pulp testing.[25]

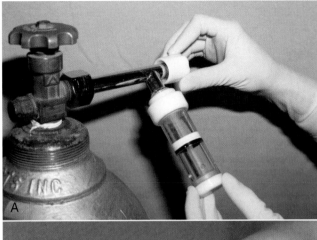

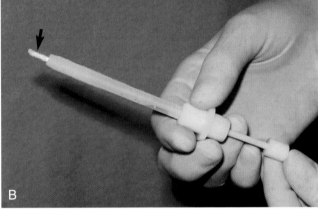

Fig. 5.7 Carbon dioxide ice testing. **A,** A carbon dioxide tank and special "ice maker" are required. **B,** A carbon dioxide ice stick is formed *(arrow)*. The stick is held in gauze and touched to the facial surfaces of suspect and control teeth. This technique can be used in teeth with various types of restorations. (Courtesy Dr. W. Johnson.)

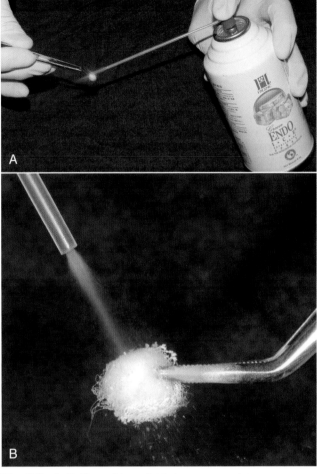

Fig. 5.8 **A,** Refrigerant is available in a pressured can. **B,** Refrigerant sprayed on a large cotton pellet is convenient and effective for determining pulp responsiveness.

After the tooth has been isolated with cotton rolls and dried, a CO_2 ice stick or large cotton pellet[26] saturated with refrigerant is applied. This stimulus over a vital pulp usually results in sharp, brief pain. This short response may occur regardless of pulp status (normal or reversible or irreversible pulpitis). However, an intense and prolonged response is usually taken to indicate irreversible pulpitis. In contrast, necrotic pulps do not respond. A *false-negative* response is often obtained when cold is applied to teeth with calcific metamorphosis, whereas a *false-positive* response may result if cold contacts gingiva or is transferred to adjacent teeth with vital pulps.

Cold is more effective on anterior than posterior teeth. Lack of a response to cold on a posterior tooth indicates that another type of vitality test (electrical) should be included. Surprisingly, gingival recession and attachment loss decrease the sensitivity to cold testing.[27]

Heat Tests Teeth are best isolated by a rubber dam to prevent false-positive responses. Various techniques and materials are used. The best, safest, and easiest technique is to rotate a dry rubber prophy cup to create frictional heat (Fig. 5.9) or to apply hot water. Gutta-percha heated in a flame can be applied to the facial surface of the tooth after first coating

the surface of the crown with petroleum jelly. A flame-heated instrument is difficult to control, and its use is best avoided. Battery-powered devices are better controlled and deliver heat safely and effectively.[28]

Heat is not used routinely but is helpful when the major symptom is heat sensitivity and the patient cannot identify the offending tooth. After applying heat, the temperature is gradually increased until pain is elicited. As with cold, a sharp and nonlingering pain response indicates a vital (not necessarily normal) pulp.

Electrical Pulp Testing[29,30] All the electrical pulp testers currently available produce a high-frequency electrical current with an amperage that can be changed. These testers are also *monopolar,* which means that the current flows from the probe through the tooth and then through the patient back to the testing unit. Thus nerves in any part of the pulp are stimulated.

Electrical pulp testers with digital readouts are popular (Fig. 5.10). These testers are not inherently superior to other electrical testers but are more user-friendly. High readings usually indicate necrosis. Low readings indicate vitality. Testing of normal control teeth establishes the approximate

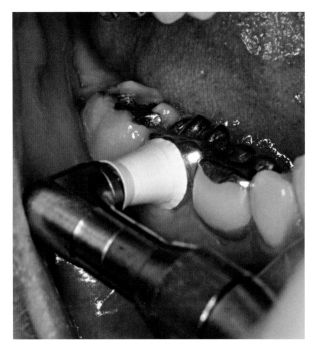

Fig. 5.9 A prophy cup run at high speed without lubricant generates controlled heat for pulp testing.

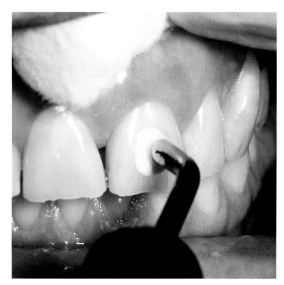

Fig. 5.11 The tooth surface is carefully scrubbed, dried, and isolated. A small spot of conductive medium is placed on the electrode, which is applied to the tooth structure.

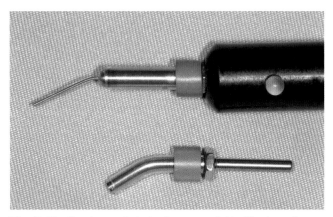

Fig. 5.10 Two types of electrodes are available. The lower is a conventional tip. The upper is a "minitip," which is useful when small areas of tooth structure are available for electrode contact.

5-9

boundary between the two conditions. The exact number of the reading is of no significance and does not reflect subtle degrees of vitality, nor can any electrical pulp tester indicate inflammation.[30]

All electrical pulp testers are used in a similar manner. It is important to clean, dry, and isolate the teeth. The surface is scrubbed with a cotton roll, isolated with the same roll, and dried thoroughly with the air syringe. A small amount of toothpaste is placed on the electrode. The electrical circuit is completed by using a lip clip or having the patient touch the metal handle. The electrode is placed on the facial or lingual surface (Fig. 5.11), and the level of current is gradually increased to detection. The electrical pulp tester is not infallible and may produce false-positive or false-negative responses 10% to 20% of the time.[31] Small canals, in particular, may lead to a false-negative response.[29]

Significance of Thermal Tests

An exaggerated and lingering response after hot or cold application is an indication of irreversible pulpitis. Absence of response in conjunction with other tests, compared with the results on control teeth, usually indicates pulpal necrosis.

One test alone is seldom conclusive for the presence or absence of pulpal or periapical disease. Two or more pulp tests are more likely to be accurate. The data obtained from vitality testing must be processed in conjunction with the history of the complaint, the intraoral examination, and radiographs. Cold testing with CO_2 snow or refrigerant was shown to have a sensitivity (ability to detect pulp necrosis that is verified clinically) of 75% and specificity (ability to identify a normal pulp) of 92%. The sensitivity of an electrical pulp test (EPT) was 92%, and the specificity was 75%.[25] Therefore, it is clear that the two tests are complementary and thus can help the practitioner reach an accurate determination of the vitality of the pulp.

Blood Flow Determination

Instruments that detect pulp circulation are part of a developing technology that is likely to produce new approaches for determining the presence of vital pulp tissue and possibly the extent of any inflammation present.[32-34] Sensors are applied to the enamel surface, usually on both the facial and lingual nerves. Blood flow is shown by beams of light (dual wavelength spectrophotometry),[35] pulse oximetry,[36,37] or laser Doppler flowmetry.[35] Blood components are demonstrated by detecting oxyhemoglobin levels in blood or pulsations in the pulp. These approaches are still more experimental than clinically practical, and the devices are expensive. As the technology improves and becomes less costly, and more experience is gained, these devices' use as sensitive pulp testers in the future is likely.

Periodontal Examination

Periapical and periodontal lesions may mimic each other and therefore require differentiation (see Chapter 7). It is also important to establish the periodontal health of the tooth or teeth as part of overall treatment planning.

Probing

Probing is an important clinical test that is often overlooked and underused for diagnosing periapical lesions. Bone and periodontal soft tissue destruction are induced by both periodontal disease and periapical lesions and may not be easily detected or differentiated radiographically.

A probe helps to determine the tissue attachment levels (periodontal). Also, the probe may penetrate into an inflammatory periapical lesion that extends cervically. Probing is a diagnostic aid that has prognostic value. The prognosis for a tooth with a necrotic pulp that induces cervically extending periapical (endodontic) inflammation is good after adequate root canal treatment. However, the outcome of root canal treatment on a tooth with severe periodontal disease usually depends on the success of periodontal treatment. Probing depths should be recorded for future comparison.

Mobility

The mobility test partially determines both the status of the PDL and the prognosis. Teeth with extreme mobility usually have little periodontal support. Occasionally an extensive periapical lesion may alter the periodontal support markedly; mobility usually decreases dramatically after successful root canal treatment.

Radiographic Examination

Radiographs are essential for the examination of mineralized tissue. Their value, however, is often overestimated. During an examination, clinicians often study a radiograph first and do little in the way of a visual and digital examination. This is a mistake. The logical place for radiographic observation is after the full history and direct examination. Then the data derived are interpreted as part of the overall examination, rather than as a replacement for the history and exam. Conventional radiographs are compressed, two-dimensional images in which much detail may be hidden by superimposition. This limitation can be reduced by making more than one radiograph at different angles. Recent advances in technology allow three-dimensional (3D) techniques, such as cone beam computed tomography (CBCT), to aid in the diagnosis of complex cases.

Radiographs allow the evaluation of carious lesions, defective restorations, root canal treatments, abnormal pulpal and periapical appearances, malpositioned teeth, the relationship of the neurovascular bundle and maxillary sinuses to the apexes, and any bone loss from periodontal disease. They may also reveal structural changes and bony disease unrelated to the pulp (Fig. 5.12).

Periapical Lesions

The primary value of radiographs in endodontic diagnosis is to determine the health of the periapical tissues. Inflammation results in bone resorption and creation of a radiolucent area (a "lesion") around the apex; it is important to recognize, however, that lesions develop before they are visible on a radiograph.[38] In addition, some radiolucencies may be either normal or pathoses of nonendodontic origin. Periapical lesions of endodontic origin usually have four characteristics: (1) the lamina dura is absent apically; (2) the lucency remains at the

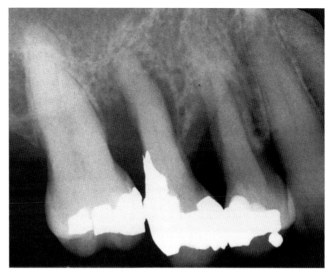

Fig. 5.12 Horizontal and vertical bone loss is evident in this quadrant. All teeth are responsive to vitality tests; therefore, the resorptive defects represent a severe periodontal condition and not pulp or apical pathosis. Root canal treatment is not indicated.

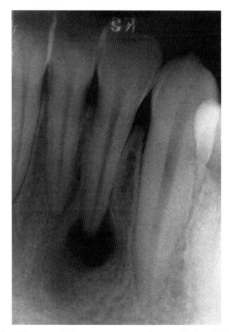

Fig. 5.13 Characteristic appearance of an endodontic lesion. This radiograph shows loss of lamina dura and a hanging-drop appearance. This patient had a history of trauma. A film made at a different angle would show the lesion remaining at the apex. (Courtesy Dr. L. Wilcox.)

apex in radiographs made at different cone angles; (3) the lucency tends to resemble a hanging drop; and (4) the tooth usually shows an injury that caused the pulp necrosis (Fig. 5.13).

A sizable radiolucency in the periapical region of a tooth with a vital pulp is *not* endodontic in origin and is either a normal structure or nonendodontic pathosis.

Radiopaque changes also occur.[39-45] Condensing osteitis is a reaction to pulp or periapical inflammation and results in an increase in the density of bone. It has a diffuse, **79** circumferential, medullary pattern with indistinct borders (Fig. 5.14). The well-circumscribed, more homogeneous normal structure that occurs commonly in the mandibular posterior region is enostosis (or sclerotic bone); this is a non-pathologic condition. Similarly, tori may sometimes be seen over the roots of maxillary molars. Contrary to popular belief, a radiopaque (corticated) margin on a lesion does not necessarily indicate a cyst.[46,47]

New radiographic technology permits early detection of bony changes, allowing new approaches to differential diagnosis.[48,49] Digital subtraction radiography "reads" subtle early changes in periapical bone resorption. Magnetic resonance imaging demonstrates changes in resorptive lesions in relation to hard and soft tissue structures.[50] Studies are beginning to show some benefits for clinical application.

Undoubtedly, these or similar devices will prove even more useful in the future.

Pulpal Lesions

An inflamed pulp with dentinoclastic activity may show abnormally altered pulp space enlargement and is pathognomonic of internal resorption (Fig. 5.15). Extensive diffuse calcification in the chamber may indicate long-term, low-grade irritation (not necessarily from irreversible pulpitis). Dentin formation that radiographically "obliterates"[51] the canals (usually in patients with a history of trauma) does not indicate pathosis (Fig. 5.16). These teeth ordinarily require no treatment, but when treatment is necessary, they can be managed with reasonable success. Pulp stones are discrete, calcified bodies found occasionally in pulp chambers and are

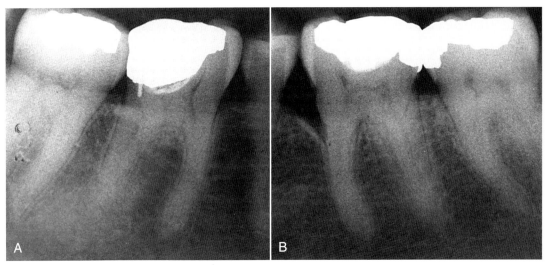

Fig. 5.14 Condensing osteitis. **A,** Diffuse trabeculation surrounds the distal root apex. **B,** This contrasts with the contralateral molar, which demonstrates a normal, sparse trabecular pattern.

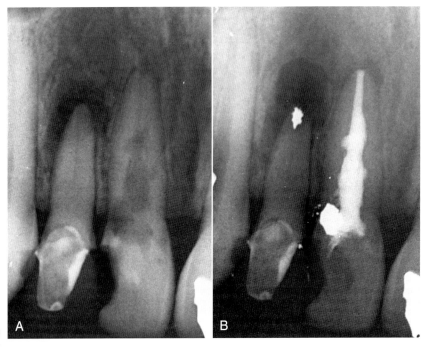

Fig. 5.15 Differing pulp responses to injury. **A,** Central incisor shows extensive, perforating internal resorption; the lateral incisor has calcific metamorphosis. **B,** These problems are managed with special techniques and both surgical and nonsurgical treatment.

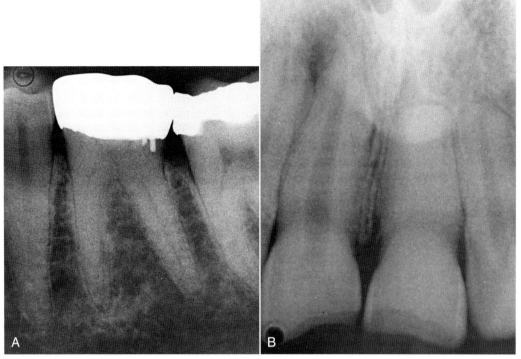

Fig. 5.16 Calcific metamorphosis. **A,** This lesion resulted from repeated insults from caries and restorations. **B,** This dentin formation ("obliteration") resulted from trauma and irritation to the pulp. Neither the lesion in **A** nor that in **B** represents pathosis. Occasionally, apical pathosis does develop, presenting a treatment challenge. (**B** courtesy Dr. L. Wilcox.)

sometimes visible on radiographs. They are of no pathologic significance, although one study correlated their presence with cardiovascular disease.[52] Usually they do not block access to the root canals during treatment.

Additional Diagnostic Procedures

After subjective and objective examinations and clinical tests have been completed, it is usually possible to make an accurate diagnosis and create a reasonable treatment plan. However, if special circumstances still prevent a definitive diagnosis, additional tests, such as *caries removal, selective anesthesia, the bite test,* and *transillumination,* are options.

Caries Removal

Determining the depth of caries penetration is necessary in some situations for definitive pulp diagnosis. A common clinical situation is the presence of deep caries on radiographs with no significant history or presenting symptoms and a pulp that responds to clinical tests. All other findings are normal. The final definitive test is complete caries removal to establish pulp status. Pulp exposure by soft caries without significant symptoms is considered asymptomatic irreversible pulpitis; nonexposure is usually reversible pulpitis.

Selective Anesthesia

Selective anesthesia is somewhat useful in localizing a painful tooth when the patient cannot identify the offender (usually between arches). If a mandibular tooth is suspected, a mandibular block confirms at least the region if the pain disappears after the injection. Selective anesthesia of individual teeth is not useful in the mandible. The PDL injection often anesthetizes several teeth. However, it is marginally more effective in the maxilla.

Bite Test

When the patient presents with sharp, brief pain on biting, a Tooth Slooth or cotton swab is used to attempt to reproduce the symptom (see Fig. 5.6). These are applied to different cusps of different teeth until the patient recognizes the same type of pain that he or she feels with eating. This is usually indicative of a crack, which may be hidden underneath a large occlusal restoration.

Transillumination

Transillumination helps identify longitudinal crown fractures, because a fracture does not transmit the light. This test produces contrasting vertical dark and light segments of the tooth at the fracture site (see Chapter 8 for more information). 5-13

Reaching a Diagnosis

The process of conducting the history and examination takes much longer to describe than to conduct, particularly if an organized format is followed to record it. A sequence of subjective and objective tests ensures that nothing is omitted and that the various phases are carried out to provide an accessible record of conditions at the first appointment. Once all data have been obtained and assembled, they must be processed and interpreted.

The findings are arranged in a rational order to arrive at both a pulpal and a periapical diagnosis (see Table 5.1). This process is summarized in Fig. 5.17. Consistency in all findings does not always occur because of the limitations of the **81**

<table>
<tr>
<td>

1. SUBJECTIVE FINDINGS

Chief Complaint:

Significant Medical History:

History of Tooth (mark all
   appropriate):
  1 Trauma
  2 Caries
  3 Carious exposure
  4 Mechanical exposure
  5 Restoration
  6 Pulp cap (direct or indirect)
  7 Pulpotomy
  8 Root canal treatment
  9 Other _____

Reaction to Thermal Stimulus:
  0 None   1 Short
               2 Continuous

Reaction to Mastication:
  0 None   1 Mild-Moderate
               2 Severe

Nature of Pain (mark all
   appropriate):
  0 None   2 Diffuse
  1 Spontaneous 3 Localized

Duration of Pain:
  4 Short   5 Prolonged

**2. OBJECTIVE SIGNS AND
TESTS**
(include suspect and
control teeth)

Tooth No.: ___ ___ ___ ___
Pulp testing
  (+, −, NA) ___ ___ ___ ___
  EPT   ___ ___ ___ ___
  Thermal ___ ___ ___ ___
    Short   ___ ___ ___ ___
    Prolonged ___ ___ ___ ___
  Dentin
  stimulation ___ ___ ___ ___

</td>
<td>

*Periapical
  tests* (none
  [0], mild-
  mod [+],
  severe [++] ___ ___ ___ ___
  Percussion ___ ___ ___ ___
  Palpation ___ ___ ___ ___
Swelling (if present):
  Intraoral   Localized
  Extraoral   Diffuse

Sinus Tract:
  0 Absent   1 Present

**Caries excavation necessary for
diagnosis?** Yes No
  Result: Exposure No exposure

**Periodontal Status of Suspected
Tooth:**
  0 Normal
  1 Excessive mobility
  2 Significant periodontitis
  3 Significant probing depths
  Record   M: D:
  If not normal, describe findings:
  _____
  _____

Evidence of Cracks/Fractures:
  0 Yes   1 No   2 NA
  If yes, explain _____

**3. RADIOGRAPHIC
FINDINGS**

0 Normal
1 Apical radiolucency
2 Apical root resorption
3 Apical radiopacity
4 Furcal radiolucency
5 Other _____

4. DIAGNOSIS

Pulp
  1 Normal
  2 Reversible pulpitis
  3 Irreversible pulpitis
  4 Necrotic pulp
  5 NA

</td>
<td>

Periradicular
  6 Normal periapical
  7 Symptomatic apical periodontitis
  8 Asymptomatic apical periodontitis
  9 Chronic apical
    abscess
 10 Acute apical abscess
 11 Condensing ostitis
 12 Nonendodontic pathosis

**5. OTHER RADIOGRAPHIC
OR CLINICAL FINDINGS
AFFECTING DIAGNOSIS
AND/OR TREATMENT**
(anatomy, isolation,
calcifications, etc.)

_____
Adjacent teeth? _____
Referral needed? _____
If yes, why? _____

**6. ETIOLOGY OF PULP AND
PERIAPICAL PATHOSIS**

_____
_____
_____

7. PRETREATMENT PROGNOSIS
(include endodontic,
periodontic, restorative)

0 Favorable
1 Questionable
2 Unfavorable
If unfavorable, why? _____
_____
_____

8. TREATMENT PLAN

Endodontic:
Urgent/emerg. care: _____
_____
Definitive care: _____
_____
Periodontic: _____
_____
Restorative: _____
_____

</td>
</tr>
</table>

Fig. 5.17   Sample form used for diagnosis and treatment planning.

diagnostic techniques available and because of variations in patient responses.

The Difficult Diagnosis

Fortunately, on most occasions, if there is a thorough and methodical approach to the history and examination, the diagnosis of endodontic conditions is fairly straightforward. Some cases are more challenging and may require referral to a specialist.[53] The source of the patient's pain is often difficult to localize. This occurs most often with inflamed pulp tissue. Once the inflammation has reached the periodontium, with its heavy supply of mechanoreceptors, localization is more obvious. Thus, in some cases it may be necessary to treat the patient symptomatically and wait until the source of the pain becomes clear. This is especially important if more than one tooth in the area may be responsible for the patient's symptoms.

The astute clinician is always alert to the possibility that the source of the pain may be nonodontogenic. Atypical tooth-related pain is not uncommon. Some findings are particularly suggestive of a difficult diagnosis. Box 5.5 lists factors that require approaching a case with more caution. In fact, if the findings in Box 5.5 are present, there may be no significant pathosis, or none at all, and treatment would not be indicated.

In addition to diagnosing pathoses and determining what treatment is indicated, the approach used must fit into the patient's expectations. To choose the correct approach, the practitioner must know the indications for and contraindications to treatment and recognize conditions that make treatment difficult. This knowledge, combined with the diagnosis, determines the treatment plan.

TREATMENT PLANNING

The decision on whether a tooth requires endodontic therapy follows directly from the diagnosis (see Table 5.1). Once the need for endodontic treatment has been established, in the majority of cases the choice of procedures is straightforward, and the technique should be intracoronal (sometimes described as "conventional," "orthograde," or "nonsurgical" root canal treatment). There are indications for a surgical (retrograde) approach when coronal access to the canal system in the apical root is impossible. The difficulty of intracoronal procedures varies considerably but should be assessed before the general practitioner considers undertaking the treatment. Once the decision has been made that treatment is needed and that the practitioner will perform it, the patient's overall treatment plan should be considered and the positioning of endodontic treatment determined. If a patient is in pain or is swollen, immediate resolution of these symptoms is imperative even if the ultimate disposition of the case is referral to a specialist (see Chapter 6; endodontic emergencies are considered in Chapter 10).

Patients are interested in the number of appointments it will take to complete the procedure. The available evidence suggests that, overall, single and multiple appointments have the same success rate and the same level of post-treatment complications.[54-60] Most patients prefer single-appointment treatment; some select multiple appointments, depending on the circumstances.[61] However, some situations require more than a single appointment. Some conditions are complex or time-consuming. Related to this, and most important, are patient management and the tolerance level of the patient and the operator. If fatigue or frustration on the part of either occurs, the appointment is terminated, a temporary filling is placed, and another appointment is scheduled.

Another situation is the patient with severe periapical symptoms or persistent canal exudation. These are often emergencies, and the tolerance level of the patient may be low. Also, flare-ups between appointments occur more often in these situations and are considerably more difficult to manage if the canals have been obturated.

Restorability
Restorability must be determined before definitive treatment is initiated. This usually requires complete removal of restorations and caries to identify whether the tooth is salvageable and to determine how it is to be restored.[62]

Specific Treatments
Pulpitis
Normal or Reversible Pulpitis
Root canal treatment is not indicated (unless it is done as an elective procedure for restorative purposes). In patients with reversible pulpitis, the cause is usually removed and restoration follows.

Irreversible Pulpitis
Root canal treatment with total pulp removal (pulpectomy) is the treatment of choice with irreversible pulpitis. In emergency situations and when apexogenesis is being attempted, partial pulp removal (pulpotomy) may be indicated. Intracanal medications are not beneficial for pain control but may be used to prevent bacterial contamination of the residual pulp. If a patient refuses root canal treatment (or it is impractical), permanent pulpotomy is an option and preferable to extraction. However, the long-term success rate has not been determined for pulpotomies, although short-term success has been shown to be comparable to that for root canal treatment.[63,64]

Necrosis
Root canal treatment or extraction is indicated when necrosis is present.

Periapical Diagnosis
Normal
No special treatment approach is required.

Symptomatic Apical Periodontitis
With a diagnosis of symptomatic apical periodontitis, the inflamed pulp or necrotic tissue is removed. After the cause of the disease process is removed, inflammation resolves. If there is an abscess within bone (no swelling), drainage is attempted in conjunction with canal debridement.

Asymptomatic Apical Periodontitis
Treatment for asymptomatic apical periodontitis is the same as that for symptomatic apical periodontitis. The size of the lesion seen on radiograph is of little concern. Lesions of different sizes heal after appropriate treatment (Fig. 5.18).

Acute Apical Abscess
The basic treatment for acute apical abscess is the same as for the preceding conditions, with the addition that drainage of the abscess is attempted either through the tooth or by incision of the soft tissue. Occasionally, such drainage cannot be achieved, so resolution of symptoms is slow.

Chronic Apical Abscess
The basic treatment for chronic apical abscess is the same as for the previous diagnoses except that drainage has already been established naturally. The sinus tract usually resolves a few days to a month after debridement and obturation. If the sinus tract persists, there may have been a misdiagnosis and the lesion is a periodontal abscess. Calcium hydroxide should be placed in the canal (or canals) and in the access cavity, which is always closed between appointments.

Condensing Osteitis
Condensing osteitis requires no special treatment. Because it occurs with different pulp conditions, treatment varies. Condensing osteitis resolves in approximately 50% of teeth after *successful* root canal treatment. There is no apparent problem if the condensing osteitis does *not* resolve; no further treatment is required unless there are other findings that indicate failure.

Extraction as an Alternative to Endodontic Therapy

At times, the only definitive alternative is extraction, which may be indicated by coexisting severe periodontal disease, by cost factors, and perhaps for strategic reasons in an overall treatment plan. If pain has been present, persuading the patient that some treatment is needed is not difficult. He or she may opt for extraction; the negative sequelae of this self-destructive decision must be explained first.

Patients who are asymptomatic may not be as easily guided toward definitive treatment. Again, the best approach is to advise the patient that disease is present and that treatment is most successfully performed now. Otherwise, disease is likely to progress to a point where symptoms occur and treatment will be more difficult or will have a less favorable prognosis (Fig. 5.19).

Treatment Planning Considerations
Diagnosis

Appropriate treatment follows accurate diagnosis. Many procedures are done inappropriately (or not done) because of diagnostic errors. The endodontist is experienced, and the generalist may be unfamiliar with a particular problem. *Referred pain is a good example of a condition that often presents the practitioner with a significant diagnostic challenge.* Unless a definitive diagnosis is obtained, no treatment should be rendered and the patient should be referred (see Box 5.6).

Endodontic-Periodontal Status

If there is doubt about whether the problem is endodontic or periodontal (or has another cause), the patient should be referred. Differential diagnosis of periodontal and endodontic lesions is discussed in Chapter 7.

Resorption

Resorption may be either internal or external. Perforating resorptions (pulp-periodontal communication) are often complex. Tooth resorption, whether internal or external, is high risk and should be referred for evaluation and treatment (Fig. 5.20).

Limited internal resorption may not present treatment complications, but external apical resorption may drastically alter the geometry of the apex or the root surface. Extensive apical or root surface resorption is best referred.

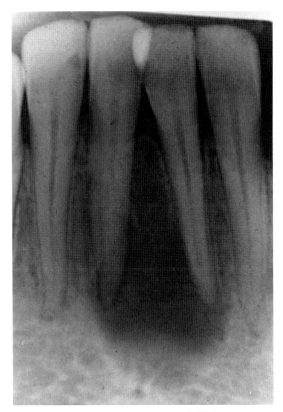

Fig. 5.18 Because of its size, this lesion is likely to be an apical radicular cyst. The lesion is related to pulp necrosis in the left central incisor. Although superimposed over the apex of the adjacent incisor, the pulp is not affected and therefore does not require treatment. Proper root canal treatment of the left incisor would lead to resolution without surgery.

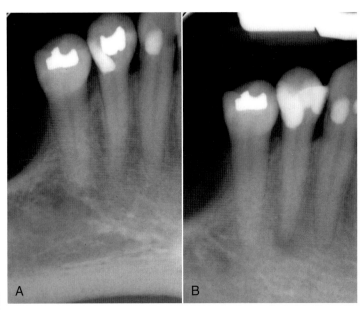

A   B

Fig. 5.19 **A,** The mandibular right first premolar was excavated and had a carious pulp exposure (the diagnosis was asymptomatic irreversible pulpitis). The patient declined endodontic treatment. **B,** Eight months later the tooth had pulp necrosis and asymptomatic apical periodontitis, resulting in a worse prognosis than the original diagnosis.

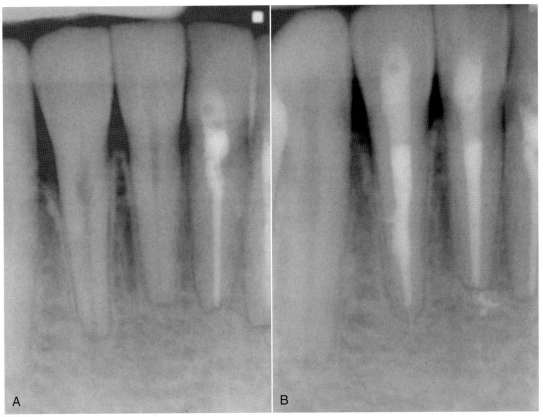

Fig. 5.20 **A,** Complexity caused by trauma. The lateral and central incisors had undergone previous treatment. The other central incisor is symptomatic, with percussion sensitivity and nonresponsiveness to pulp testing. The adjacent lateral shows internal resorption *(arrow)* that is asymptomatic. Care must be taken to completely clean and shape the irregular canal system, as is demonstrated in the postoperative image. **B,** This situation exhibits a high degree of difficulty.

Radiographs

Diagnostic and treatment films of good quality are critical. Patient characteristics, such as gagging, and oral anatomy (e.g., shallow palatal vault, large and narrow dental arches), may hinder the acquisition of quality radiographs.

Procedural Difficulties
Health and Medical History

General practitioners may treat patients who require premedication and patients with medical complications that affect diagnosis and treatment. However, the severity of the condition (or conditions) must be evaluated. In patients with more serious disorders, an endodontist may best provide treatment. Specialist care is generally more expedient and offers better prevention and management of complications during treatment (see Chapter 6).

Physical Limitations

If the patient cannot be suitably reclined or if the mouth opening is limited, referral should be considered.

Restorative Considerations

Severe caries or fractures from trauma may render the tooth difficult to isolate or restore.

Anatomy
Pulp Chamber

As the tooth ages, pulp chamber space decreases. Chamber size and pulp stones, in addition to the extent of calcifications in the canal system, must be considered.

Canal Calcification (Calcific Metamorphosis)

Secondary and perhaps tertiary dentin formation leads to narrowing of the canals, sometimes to an extent that they are not visible radiographically (Figures 5.21 and 5.22).

Root Curvature

Canals are rarely straight, although they may appear straight on a facial radiograph. Curvature factors include the direction, severity, and number of curves. "Recurvatures" of the mesial roots of mandibular molars, in which the apices bend toward each other, are especially common. Bayonet (S-shaped) curves are difficult to negotiate and prepare (Figures 5.23 and 5.24).

Number of Canals

A good rule is to always expect "extra" canals or roots unless the preoperative film clearly shows a distinct number of canals; the reality is that more may exist (Fig. 5.25). There **85**

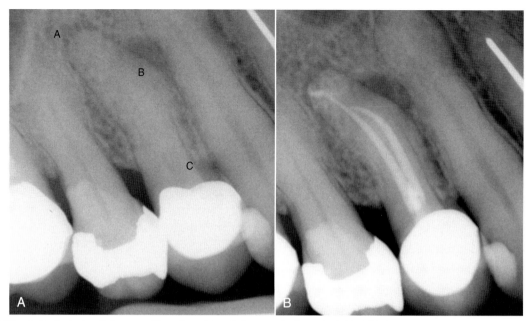

Fig. 5.21 **A,** Periapical radiolucency *(A)* and mesial radiolucency in the apical third *(B)*. The canals are calcified, the root is narrow, and there is a hint of a significant mesial concavity in the coronal third *(C)*. The tooth is also crowned, which increases access complexity. This is considered a high-risk case. **B,** Postoperatively, the mesial radiolucency resulted from the buccal root exiting several millimeters shorter than the palatal root, with a significant distal curvature. The practitioner must be prepared to manage the unexpected should problems arise during treatment.

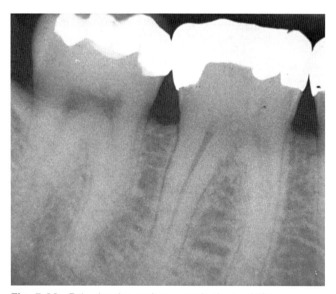

Fig. 5.22 Pulp chamber and root canals show calcific metamorphosis; this situation is rated as extreme risk.

are difficulties with multiple canals. For example, many mandibular incisors have two root canals, and mandibular premolars may have multiple canals. A significant percentage of mandibular first molars have two canals in the distal root, and mesiobuccal roots of maxillary molars often have two canal systems.

Root Length
Very short or very long roots may be a challenge to treat.

Tooth Location
Generally, second and third molars, especially maxillary molars, are difficult to manage, particularly in a patient with limited opening. Buccally positioned maxillary second molars are associated with a variety of treatment problems. Rotated, tipped, or crowded teeth may complicate isolation and access; they also may inhibit adequate cleaning and shaping or obturation and are difficult to restore. Maxillary second molars requiring root canal treatment should be strongly considered for extraction, particularly if the tooth is not important functionally. Because of these negative factors, long-term survival is compromised.

Degree of Apical Closure
The size of the apical opening correlates with the treatment difficulty of the situation. Recently erupted teeth with immature apices are complicated and often require special procedures. The outcome and duration of treatment are unpredictable; these are difficult to manage (see Chapters 2 and 6).

Unusual Anatomy
Different tooth forms often present treatment difficulties (Fig. 5.26).

SYSTEMIC CONSIDERATIONS

Dentists are members of the health team whose role ultimately is to ensure that the patient's health, including oral health, is maintained at an optimal level. Over the past two to three decades, the close relationship between oral health and systemic health has gained a lot of attention, and many advances in this area have been achieved. In the early part of the twentieth century, endodontic infections were thought to be a focus of infection that may lead to a variety of ailments and chronic diseases in the body. However, more recently, a direct relationship to that effect has not been proved. The available

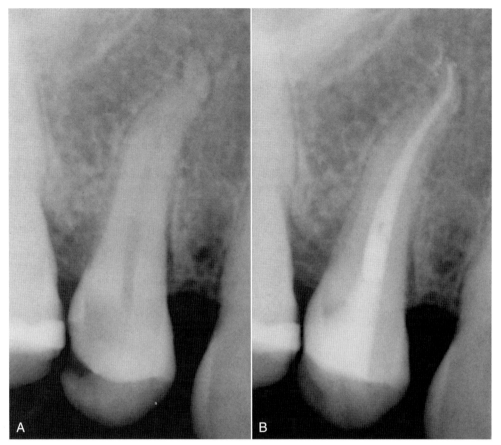

Fig. 5.23 **A,** Dilaceration in the apical third. The degree and location of curvature strongly suggest caution and consideration of referral. **B,** Note in the postoperative radiograph that the apical third curvature has been maintained.

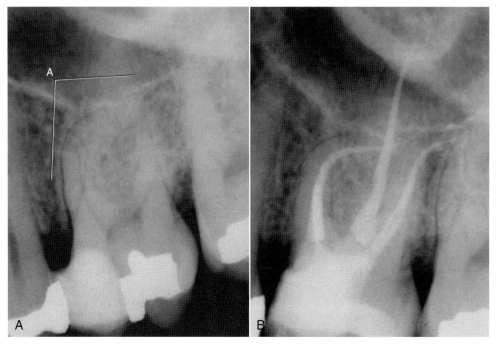

Fig. 5.24 **A,** Extreme curvature of the mesiobuccal root. Because of the nearly 90-degree curve *(A)*, this situation falls into the extreme risk category, and the patient should be considered for referral. **B,** Note the curvature of the distobuccal root in the postoperative radiograph.

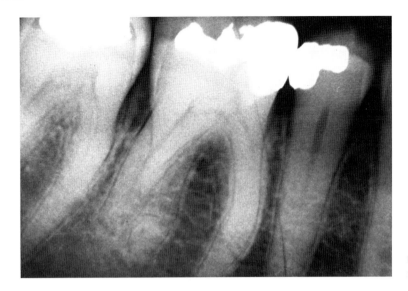

Fig. 5.25 Mandibular molar with an "extra" distolingual root; this situation is rated as high risk.

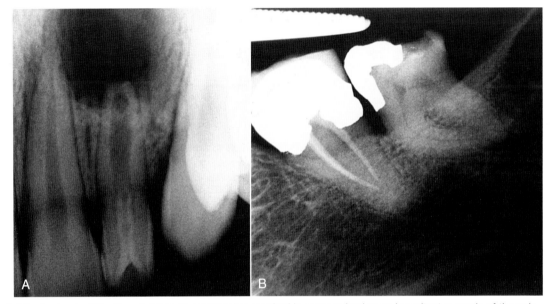

Fig. 5.26 Anatomic difficulties. **A,** Dens invaginatus has resulted in communication and resultant necrosis of the pulp. Incomplete dentin formation and an irregular internal form make these teeth anatomically difficult to clean, shape, and obturate. The size of the lesion does not contraindicate nonsurgical treatment. **B,** A severely curved root and the posterior position make treatment for this third molar difficult.

evidence on the relationship between endodontic pathosis and systemic disease is presented here.

With regard to the relationship between endodontic pathosis and systemic disease, the practitioner needs to be aware of three factors: systemic diseases that mimic endodontic pain or periapical radiolucency, as noted before; systemic diseases that may accelerate or potentiate pulpal pathosis or influence treatment outcomes; and conditions in which the endodontic infection may initiate or contribute to an infection in a distant site.

Systemic Diseases that May Influence Endodontic Pathosis or Its Treatment

Patients with medical conditions that compromise their immune response may have a less favorable endodontic treatment outcome. In a study by Marending and associates,[65] patients who had any of a group of eight such systemic conditions were found to have significantly reduced chances of healing. Studies such as these raise concern about the interaction of systemic disease with endodontic healing, but they do not help identify a mechanism or pathway for this interaction. The effects of a number of specific diseases are considered next.

Diabetes Mellitus

Diabetes mellitus is one of the most important chronic diseases that affects humans worldwide. In the United States, about 26 million individuals (8% of the population) are diabetic, and more alarmingly, one third of them are not aware that they are diabetic.[66] The percentage of diabetics rises to about 27% of all people over age 65.[66] Diabetes is not curable, and it has serious complications, including cardiovascular disease, renal disease, blindness, limb amputations, and periodontal disease, making it a huge societal cost burden.

It is generally known that diabetics have a higher prevalence of teeth with periapical lesions.[67-70,73] The longitudinal treatment outcome is generally no different between diabetics and nondiabetics.[71-73] However, if the outcomes of cases with and without preoperative periapical lesions are separated, a notable difference is observed. In cases with preoperative lesions, diabetics are significantly less likely to have successful treatment than nondiabetics, especially when controlling for a number of other confounding factors.[72] More recently, it was shown that in cases with preoperative lesions that were adequately treated endodontically, the area of the residual lesions 2 to 4 years after treatment correlated significantly with the degree of glycemia of both diabetics and nondiabetics, as measured by the hemoglobin A1c test.[74] This is consistent with older observations that healing of periapical lesions correlated with postprandial glycemia at the time of treatment.[75]

There are several reasons diabetics may have compromised healing, particularly those with higher glycemic rates and with preoperative endodontic infection. These individuals may select for specific microorganisms that may be more virulent.[76] They may have a variant of inflammatory cells, such as monocytes, characterized by excessive secretion of inflammatory mediators, including bone resorptive cytokines, which are critical for the development of periapical lesions.[77] The increased glycemia may also spontaneously result in excessive production of advanced glycation end-products (AGEs). AGEs interact with their receptors (RAGEs), resulting in the production of bone resorptive mediators,[78] which may lead to persistence of the periapical lesions.

Hypertension

Hypertension is a sign of cardiovascular disease that may indicate a variety of underlying conditions and comorbidities, including diabetes. Hypertension appears to be associated with reduced survival (meaning continued presence of the tooth in the mouth) of endodontically treated teeth. In a study of the Indian Health Service in two U.S. states, 4,500 patients were examined.[79] It was found that patients who had diabetes and/or hypertension had a significantly reduced chance of retention of endodontically treated teeth within a period of 10 years. In another cohort that included more than 49,000 teeth followed for about 2 years, it was also shown that the presence of diabetes and/or hypertension resulted in significant reduction in tooth retention.[80] It is noteworthy, however, that the study of tooth survival in the absence of exact endodontic diagnosis and assessment of periapical health is confounded by the fact that diabetes and cardiovascular diseases are also associated with periodontal disease, which may have played an important role in the loss of these teeth.

Risk for Osteoradionecrosis or Osteonecrosis of the Jaw

Patients who have undergone radiation therapy for the treatment of malignancies in the craniofacial area are at risk of osteoradionecrosis at the site of a surgical procedure such as tooth extraction. Therefore, many of these patients have teeth that would ordinarily not be amenable to treatment but that are retained with endodontic treatment to avoid the risk of osteoradionecrosis. A report documented the treatment outcome in 22 patients treated endodontically after having received 5,000 cGy irradiation in the area within the preceding 6 months.[81] After a mean of 19 months, successful treatment was found in 91% of the patients, which was consistent with treatment averages for normal patients in other studies. However, treatment of patients who have undergone radiation therapy is frequently complicated by fibrotic tissues that do not permit adequate mouth opening (Fig. 5.27); also, dry mouth results in recurrent caries, compromising the prognosis.

Over the past decade, it has been recognized that patients undergoing bisphosphonate therapy may be at risk for bisphosphonate-related osteonecrosis of the jaw (BRONJ). This risk is greater in patients receiving intravenous (IV) bisphosphonates, particularly if more than one agent is used simultaneously, and the risk increases with the duration of bisphosphonate use and with surgical procedures such as extractions.[82] Although rare, BRONJ may occur after

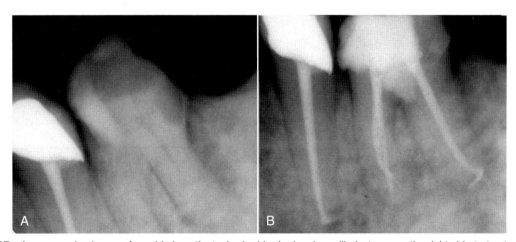

Fig. 5.27 A compromised case of an elderly patient who had had a hemimandibulectomy on the right side to treat oral cancer, together with radiation therapy; this resulted in severe restriction in mouth opening. The patient could open her mouth only about 15 mm at the incisors, making the introduction of radiographic sensors, mirrors, and dental instruments very difficult. **A,** A poor-quality preoperative radiograph shows a previous restoration that compromised pulp health and led to a periradicular lesion. **B,** Treatment was attempted to prevent osteoradionecrosis and save the tooth for function. Complications arose in the furcation area, because the clinician was unable to use the mirror and the handpiece together for access preparation.

endodontic treatment[83] or endodontic surgery.[84] When nonsurgical endodontic treatment is performed on a patient receiving IV bisphosphonates, care should be taken not to injure the soft tissue. For example, the clamps should be carefully placed to avoid injury to the soft tissues and alveolar bone.

Oral bisphosphonates pose a much lower risk of BRONJ. Endodontic outcomes are no different between patients taking oral bisphosphonates and other patients.[85]

Viral Infections
HIV/AIDS
When the human immunodeficiency virus (HIV) was first identified, practitioners were concerned that patients with HIV infection would be so compromised that severe complications would ensue with endodontic disease and/or endodontic treatment, particularly in patients whose CD4+ cell count had dropped below 200/mL. However, a cohort study of patients with AIDS who had received various oral health procedures documented that the patients did not appear to suffer any undue pain or infection with endodontic treatment.[86] In addition, 1 year after treatment, no difference was seen in the outcomes of treatment between patients who were HIV positive and those who were not infected with the virus.[87]

Herpes Viruses
There are many different types of herpes viruses that affect humans. These include varicella zoster virus (VZV), which causes herpes zoster infection; human herpes viruses (HHV1-8); human cytomegalovirus (CMV); and Epstein-Barr virus (EBV).

Herpes zoster infections frequently represent a diagnostic dilemma, because after the herpetic blisters heal, the patient may suffer from postherpetic neuralgia, which mimics endodontic pain. Careful documentation of the medical history and diagnostic tests should help the practitioner identify this condition and make the right decisions and/or referrals. However, herpes zoster infection may also induce spontaneous pulpal pathosis.[88-90]

Periapical lesions in patients infected with CMV and/or EBV, but not herpes simplex viruses, are larger and more painful.[91,92] In addition, irreversible pulpitis or acute endodontic infections may be associated with a higher incidence of EBV or the HHV pathogens.[93-95] However, it is not yet conclusively known whether the viral association potentiates the development of more aggressive forms of endodontic pathosis or whether the findings of the small studies available were merely coincidental.

Sickle Cell Anemia
Sickle cell anemia is characterized by a congenital abnormality of red blood cells that results in deficient oxygenation of the blood. A milder form of the disease, known as *sickle cell trait,* results from homozygous transmission of the affected gene. Oral findings of sickle cell anemia include the radiographic "stepladder" trabecular pattern of bone, enamel hypomineralization, calcified canals, increased overbite, and overjet.[96] An older case series showed the spontaneous development of pulpal pathosis in some noncarious teeth in patients with sickle cell anemia.[97] More recently, it was shown that patients with sickle cell anemia have a significantly higher incidence of orofacial pain than controls and have pulp

necrosis in 6% of their teeth that have no other apparent etiologies, compared with none in the controls.[98]

Smoking
The oral health problems of smoking, including the increase in periodontal disease, mucositis, and oral premalignant and malignant lesions, have been well documented. More recently, there has been an interest in the association of smoking with pulpal and periapical diseases. Smoking is also associated with a high prevalence of periapical lesions[99-101] and with incident root canal treatment as a marker of pulpal and periapical diseases.[102] The incidence of root canal treatment is also increased with the duration of smoking and reduced in smokers who stopped smoking more than 9 years before the evaluation time. Smoking was also shown to increase the incidence of pain and/or swelling after endodontic surgery.[103]

Genetic Predisposition
There are many diseases today that have been linked to specific variants of genes, thus allowing physicians to provide the patient with an accurate risk assessment for disease incidence and the likely disease progression and outcome of treatment. For example, it has been known for some time that individuals who have a genetic polymorphism of the gene that encodes for interleukin-1β (IL-1β) may have increased manifestation of some diseases, including periodontal disease.[104] More recently, several gene polymorphism associations have been made with endodontic treatment outcomes. Thus IL-1β allele 2 was found to be associated with reduced healing after endodontic treatment.[105] Another study investigated the gene polymorphism variants IL-1α (1 or 2), IL-1β (1 or 2), FcγRIIA (R131 or H131), and FcγRIIIB (NA1 or NA2).[106] FcγR is a receptor that allows monocytes and macrophages to recognize antibodies bound to antigens and phagocytose them (a process called opsonization); it therefore represents a critical step in the host response. It was found that allele H131 of the FcγRIIa gene and a combination of this allele with allele NA2 of the FcγRIIIb gene were significantly associated with less favorable treatment outcomes.[106] It is noteworthy, however, that these associations do not prove causation and that studies with large sample sizes are needed to confirm these initial findings.

Endodontic Disease May Initiate or Contribute to Systemic Diseases
The oral cavity is the first component of the digestive system and has a large component of the human microbiome (see Chapter 3). The diversity of microorganisms in the mouth is related to its exposure to dietary and environmental factors and to the unique characteristics of the oral environment. Deleterious effects of these microorganisms are prevented by an intact mucosal lining, which is capable of a formidable immune response, and by oral hygiene measures that limit the progression of oral microbial biofilms. The dental pulp is protected from bacteria by intact enamel and dentin, whereas the periodontium is protected by periodontal attachment and sulcular epithelium. With marginal periodontitis or pulpal pathosis, these barriers are absent, and the oral microflora may have free access to the periodontium or periapical tissues; in this way, microorganisms that are normally commensals become pathogenic.

Acute Endodontic Infections

There is no doubt that bacteria from acute endodontic infections can cause bacteremia and can migrate to local lymph nodes and fascial spaces. Case reports have documented the association of acute endodontic infections with brain abscess,[107-110] mediastinitis,[111-113] and fatal necrotizing fasciitis.[114] In fact, it was recently reported that about 8,000 patients in the United States are hospitalized annually for periapical abscesses, many of whom have comorbid conditions such as diabetes or hypertension.[115] Therefore, it is essential for the practitioner to obtain adequate diagnostic data for patients with acute endodontic infections and to treat the patients appropriately. Patients with abscesses should have their temperature measured, and they must be evaluated for lymphadenopathy, malaise, and fascial space infection. These patients should receive prompt and complete elimination of local irritants, including drainage of the swelling. Those with a fascial space infection (cellulitis) also should be treated with adjunctive antibiotics and, most important, should be monitored carefully until their condition improves.

Chronic Endodontic Infections

The evidence for the presence of bacteria in periapical lesions, and their escape systemically, in chronic endodontic infections is less conclusive. Animal[116,117] and human[118,119] studies show that this is infrequent in primary lesions (Fig. 5.28). There is evidence that the number of bacteria in persistent periapical lesions after unsuccessful treatment may be much higher.[120,121] If present in the periapical area, bacteria may form a biofilm and may migrate slowly to different sites to contribute to some chronic diseases.

One way to investigate this potential for bacteria in chronic infections to travel from the endodontic environment to participate in the pathogenesis of systemic disease is to determine the epidemiologic associations between the two forms of disease. One report associated periapical lesion-years (the number of years with a periapical lesion) and incident coronary heart disease in men younger than age 40.[122] Another study of patients with myocardial infarction (MI) showed a significantly higher number of patients with missing teeth and teeth with periapical lesions in the MI

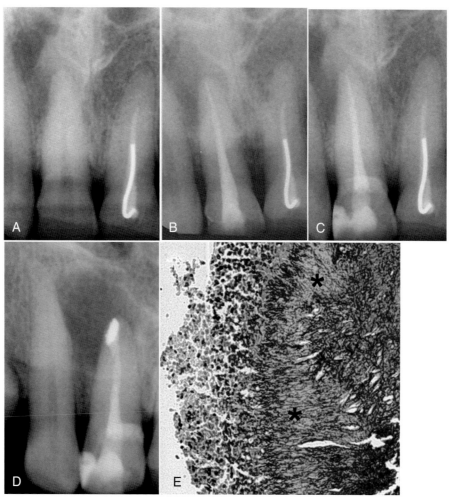

Fig. 5.28 Periapical actinomycosis. **A,** Preoperative radiograph shows tooth #8 presenting with signs of pulp necrosis and chronic apical abscess. **B,** Root canal treatment was completed. **C,** Recall in 6 months revealed a persistent sinus tract. **D,** Root-end surgery was completed, and tissues were submitted for biopsy. **E,** Biopsy result revealed actinic filaments (*) surrounded by a severe inflammatory reaction. (Courtesy Dr. Blythe Kaufman.)

group compared with controls.[123] An additional large cohort study of health professional men showed that the presence of coronary heart disease was significantly associated with the presence of one or more root canal–treated teeth (as a marker of pulpal and periapical disease).[124] Clearly, these association studies, despite having relatively large samples, do not prove causation, because the associated variables may be related to other, untested environmental, dietary, or genetic factors. However, they raise questions about the interrelationship of these different diseases, warranting further animal and human studies. Interventional studies would be required to prove causation, and these are clearly difficult to perform, given the ethical problems involved.

REFERENCES

1. Niederman R, Clarkson J, Richards D: The Affordable Care Act and evidence-based care, *J Am Dent Assoc* 142:364-367, 2011.
2. Michaelson PL, Holland GR: Is pulpitis painful? *Int Endod J* 35:829-832, 2002.
3. Kreiner M, Okeson JP: Toothache of cardiac origin, *J Orofac Pain* 13:201-207, 1999.
4. Walton RE: Endodontic considerations in the geriatric patient, *Dent Clin North Am* 41:795-816, 1997.
5. Murray CA, Saunders WP: Root canal treatment and general health: a review of the literature, *Int Endod J* 33:1-18, 2000.
6. Suchina JA, Levine D, Flaitz CM, et al: Retrospective clinical and radiologic evaluation of nonsurgical endodontic treatment in human immunodeficiency virus (HIV) infection, *J Contemp Dent Pract* 7:1-8, 2006.
7. Findler M, Galili D, Meidan Z, et al: Dental treatment in very high risk patients with active ischemic heart disease, *Oral Surg Oral Med Oral Pathol* 76:298-300, 1993.
8. Niwa H, Sato Y, Matsuura H: Safety of dental treatment in patients with previously diagnosed acute myocardial infarction or unstable angina pectoris, *Oral Surg Oral Med Oral Pathol Oral Radiol Endod* 89:35-41, 2000.
9. Wilson W, Taubert KA, Gewitz M, et al: Prevention of infective endocarditis: guidelines from the American Heart Association—a guideline from the American Heart Association Rheumatic Fever, Endocarditis and Kawasaki Disease Committee; the Council on Cardiovascular Disease in the Young; the Council on Clinical Cardiology; the Council on Cardiovascular Surgery and Anesthesia; and the Quality of Care and Outcomes Research Interdisciplinary Working Group, *J Am Dent Assoc* 138:739-745, 47, 2007.
10. American Academy of Orthopaedic Surgeons/American Dental Association: AAOS/ADA guidelines for management of patients with artificial joint replacement. Available at: www.ada.org/2157.aspx?currentTab=2#replace. Accessed October 8, 2013.
11. Watters W III, Rethman MP, Hanson NB, et al: Prevention of orthopaedic implant infection in patients undergoing dental procedures, *J Am Acad Orthop Surg* 21:180-189, 2013.
12. Lund JP: *Orofacial pain: from basic science to clinical management—the transfer of knowledge in pain research to education,* Chicago, 2000, Quintessence.
13. Hu B, Chiang CY, Hu JW, et al: P2X receptors in trigeminal subnucleus caudalis modulate central sensitization in trigeminal subnucleus oralis, *J Neurophysiol* 88:1614-1624, 2002.
14. Torneck CD, Kwan CL, Hu JW: Inflammatory lesions of the tooth pulp induce changes in brainstem neurons of the rat trigeminal subnucleus oralis, *J Dent Res* 75:553-561, 1996.
15. Ehrmann EH: The diagnosis of referred orofacial dental pain, *Aust Endod J* 28:75-81, 2002.
16. Reeh ES, elDeeb ME: Referred pain of muscular origin resembling endodontic involvement: case report, *Oral Surg Oral Med Oral Pathol* 71:223-227, 1991.
17. Silverglade D: Dental pain without dental etiology: a manifestation of referred pain from otitis media, *ASDC J Dent Child* 47:358-359, 1980.
18. Wright EF, Gullickson DC: Identifying acute pulpalgia as a factor in TMD pain, *J Am Dent Assoc* 127:773-780, 1996.
19. Wright EF, Gullickson DC: Dental pulpalgia contributing to bilateral preauricular pain and tinnitus, *J Orofac Pain* 10:166-168, 1996.
20. Baad-Hansen L: Atypical odontalgia: pathophysiology and clinical management, *J Oral Rehab* 35:1-11, 2008.
21. Benjamin P: Pain after routine endodontic therapy may not have originated from the treated tooth: a critical summary, *J Am Dent Assoc* 142:1383, 2011.
22. Miller SO, Johnson JD, Allemang JD, et al: Cold testing through full-coverage restorations, *J Endod* 30:695-700, 2004.
23. Chen E, Abbott PV: Evaluation of accuracy, reliability, and repeatability of five dental pulp tests, *J Endod* 37:1619-1623, 2011.
24. Jones VR, Rivera EM, Walton RE: Comparison of carbon dioxide versus refrigerant spray to determine pulpal responsiveness, *J Endod* 28:531-533, 2002.
25. Weisleder R, Yamauchi S, Caplan DJ, et al: The validity of pulp testing: a clinical study, *J Am Dent Assoc* 140:1013-1017, 2009.
26. Jones DM: Effect of the type carrier used on the results of dichlorodifluoromethane application to teeth, *J Endod* 25:692-694, 1999.
27. Rutsatz C, Baumhardt SG, Feldens CA, et al: Response of pulp sensibility test is strongly influenced by periodontal attachment loss and gingival recession, *J Endod* 38:580-583, 2012.
28. Bierma MM, McClanahan S, Baisden MK, et al: Comparison of heat-testing methodology, *J Endod* 38:1106-1109, 2012.
29. Myers JW: Demonstration of a possible source of error with an electric pulp tester, *J Endod* 24:199-200, 1998.
30. Petersson K, Söderström C, Kiani-Anaraki M, et al: Evaluation of the ability of thermal and electrical tests to register pulp vitality, *Endod Dent Traumatol* 15:127-131, 1999.
31. Rosenberg RJ: Using heat to assess pulp inflammation, *J Am Dent Assoc* 122:77-78, 1991.
32. Emshoff R, Moschen I, Strobl H: Use of laser Doppler flowmetry to predict vitality of luxated or avulsed permanent teeth, *Oral Surg Oral Med Oral Pathol Oral Radiol Endod* 98:750-755, 2004.
33. Evans D, Reid J, Strang R, et al: A comparison of laser Doppler flowmetry with other methods of assessing the vitality of traumatised anterior teeth, *Endod Dent Traumatol* 15:284-290, 1999.
34. Sasano T, Onodera D, Hashimoto K, et al: Possible application of transmitted laser light for the assessment of human pulp vitality. Part 2. Increased laser power for enhanced detection of pulpal blood flow, *Dent Traumatol* 21:37-41, 2005.
35. Akpinar KE, Er K, Polat S, et al: Effect of gingiva on laser Doppler pulpal blood flow measurements, *J Endod* 30:138-140, 2004.
36. Radhakrishnan S, Munshi AK, Hegde AM: Pulse oximetry: a diagnostic instrument in pulpal vitality testing, *J Clin Pediatr Dent* 26:141-145, 2002.
37. Schnettler JM, Wallace JA: Pulse oximetry as a diagnostic tool of pulpal vitality, *J Endod* 17:488-490, 1991.
38. Tanomaru-Filho M, Jorge EG, Duarte MA, et al: Comparative radiographic and histological analyses of periapical lesion development, *Oral Surg Oral Med Oral Pathol Oral Radiol Endod* 107:442-447, 2009.
39. Bender IB, Mori K: The radiopaque lesion: a diagnostic consideration, *Endod Dent Traumatol* 1:2-12, 1985.
40. Caliskan MK, Türkün M, Oztop F: Histological evaluation of a tooth with hyperplastic pulpitis and periapical osteosclerosis, *Int Endod J* 30:347-351, 1997.
41. Eversole LR, Stone CE, Strub D: Focal sclerosing osteomyelitis/focal periapical osteopetrosis: radiographic patterns, *Oral Surg Oral Med Oral Pathol* 58:456-460, 1984.
42. Marmary Y, Kutiner G: A radiographic survey of periapical jawbone lesions, *Oral Surg Oral Med Oral Pathol* 61:405-8, 1986.
43. Monahan R: Periapical and localized radiopacities, *Dent Clin North Am* 38:113-136, 1994.
44. Purton DG, Chandler NP: Sclerotic bone lesions: report of three cases, *N Z Dent J* 93:14-16, 1997.
45. Stheeman SE, Mileman PA, van't Hof MA, et al: Diagnostic confidence and the accuracy of treatment decisions for radiopaque periapical lesions, *Int Endod J* 28:121-128, 1995.
46. Ricucci D, Mannocci F, Pitt Ford TR: A study of periapical lesions correlating the presence of a radiopaque lamina with histological findings, *Oral Surg Oral Med Oral Pathol Oral Radiol Endod* 101:389-394, 2006.
47. Shrout MK, Hall JM, Hildebolt CE: Differentiation of periapical granulomas and radicular cysts by digital radiometric analysis, *Oral Surg Oral Med Oral Pathol* 76:356-361, 1993.
48. de Paula-Silva FW, Wu MK, Leonardo MR, et al: Accuracy of periapical radiography and cone-beam computed tomography scans in diagnosing apical periodontitis using histopathological findings as a gold standard, *J Endod* 35:1009-1012, 2009.
49. Holtzmann DJ, Johnson WT, Southard TE, et al: Storage-phosphor computed radiography versus film radiography in the detection of pathologic periradicular bone loss in cadavers, *Oral Surg Oral Med Oral Pathol Oral Radiol Endod* 86:90-97, 1998.
50. Idiyatullin D, Corum C, Moeller S, et al: Dental magnetic resonance imaging: making the invisible visible, *J Endod* 37:745-752, 2011.
51. McCabe PS, Dummer PM: Pulp canal obliteration: an endodontic diagnosis and treatment challenge, *Int Endod J* 45:177-197, 2012.
52. Edds AC, Walden JE, Scheetz JP, et al: Pilot study of correlation of pulp stones with cardiovascular disease, *J Endod* 31:504-506, 2005.
53. Krell K, Walton R: *Odontalgia: diagnosing pulpal, periapical and periodontal pain,* Hagerstown, Md, 1976, Harper & Row.
54. Glennon JP, Ng YL, Setchell DJ, et al: Prevalence of and factors affecting postpreparation pain in patients undergoing two-visit root canal treatment, *Int Endod J* 37:29-37, 2004.
55. Inamoto K, Kojima K, Nagamatsu K, et al: A survey of the incidence of single-visit endodontics, *J Endod* 28:371-374, 2002.

56. Kvist T, Molander A, Dahlén G, et al: Microbiological evaluation of one- and two-visit endodontic treatment of teeth with apical periodontitis: a randomized, clinical trial, *J Endod* 30:572-576, 2004.

57. Peters LB, Wesselink PR: Periapical healing of endodontically treated teeth in one and two visits obturated in the presence or absence of detectable microorganisms, *Int Endod J* 35:660-667, 2002.

58. Roane JB, Dryden JA, Grimes EW: Incidence of postoperative pain after single- and multiple-visit endodontic procedures, *Oral Surg Oral Med Oral Pathol* 55:68-72, 1983.

59. Sathorn C, Parashos P, Messer HH: Effectiveness of single- versus multiple-visit endodontic treatment of teeth with apical periodontitis: a systematic review and meta-analysis, *Int Endod J* 38:347-355, 2005.

60. Spangberg LS: Evidence-based endodontics: the one-visit treatment idea, *Oral Surg Oral Med Oral Pathol Oral Radiol Endod* 91:617-618, 2001.

61. Vela KC, Walton RE, Trope M, et al: Patient preferences regarding one-visit versus two-visit root canal therapy, *J Endod* 38:1322-1325, 2012.

62. Abbott PV: Assessing restored teeth with pulp and periapical diseases for the presence of cracks, caries and marginal breakdown, *Aus Dent J* 49, 2004; 49(1):33-9

63. Asgary S, Eghbal MJ: A clinical trial of pulpotomy vs root canal therapy of mature molars, *J Dent Res* 89:1080-1085, 2010.

64. McDougal RA, Delano EO, Caplan D, et al: Success of an alternative for interim management of irreversible pulpitis, *J Am Dent Assoc* 135:1707-1712, 2004.

65. Marending M, Peters OA, Zehnder M: Factors affecting the outcome of orthograde root canal therapy in a general dentistry hospital practice, *Oral Surg Oral Med Oral Pathol Oral Radiol Endod* 99:119-124, 2005.

66. National Institute of Diabetes and Digestive and Kidney Disease: National diabetes statistics fact sheet: general information and national estimates on diabetes in the United States, 2000. Bethesda, Md, 2012, US Department of Health and Human Services, National Institutes of Health. http://www2.niddk.nih.gov/Accessed October 20, 2012.

67. Britto LR, Katz J, Guelmann M, Heft M: Periradicular radiographic assessment in diabetic and control individuals, *Oral Surg Oral Med Oral Pathol Oral Radiol Endod* 96:449-452, 2003.

68. Falk H, Hugoson A, Thorstensson H: Number of teeth, prevalence of caries and periapical lesions in insulin-dependent diabetics, *Scand J Dent Res* 97:198-206, 1989.

69. Lopez-Lopez J, Jane-Salas E, Estrugo-Devesa A, et al: Periapical and endodontic status of type 2 diabetic patients in Catalonia, Spain: a cross-sectional study, *J Endod* 37:598-601, 2011.

70. Segura-Egea JJ, Jimenez-Pinzon A, Rios-Santos JV, et al: High prevalence of apical periodontitis amongst type 2 diabetic patients, *Int Endod J* 38:564-569, 2005.

71. Doyle SL, Hodges JS, Pesun IJ, et al: Factors affecting outcomes for single-tooth implants and endodontic restorations, *J Endod* 33:399-402, 2007.

72. Fouad AF, Burleson J: The effect of diabetes mellitus on endodontic treatment outcome: data from an electronic patient record, *J Am Dent Assoc* 134:43-51; quiz, 117-118; 2003.

73. Ng YL, Mann V, Gulabivala K: A prospective study of the factors affecting outcomes of nonsurgical root canal treatment. Part 1. Periapical health, *Int Endod J* 44:583-609, 2011.

74. Fein JE, Caplan DJ, Hicks ML, et al: The relationship between diabetic control and periapical lesion resolution, *J Endod* 38:e37, 2012.

75. Cheraskin E, Ringsdorf WM Jr: The biology of the endodontic patient. Part 3. Variability in periapical

healing and blood glucose, *J Oral Med* 23:87-90, 1968.

76. Fouad AF, Kum KY, Clawson ML, et al: Molecular characterization of the presence of *Eubacterium* spp and *Streptococcus* spp in endodontic infections, *Oral Microbiol Immunol* 18:249-255, 2003.

77. Salvi GE, Beck JD, Offenbacher S: PGE2, IL-1 beta, and TNF-alpha responses in diabetics as modifiers of periodontal disease expression, *Ann Periodontol* 3:40-50, 1998.

78. Lalla E, Lamster IB, Schmidt AM: Enhanced interaction of advanced glycation end products with their cellular receptor RAGE: implications for the pathogenesis of accelerated periodontal disease in diabetes, *Ann Periodontol* 3:13-19, 1998.

79. Mindiola MJ, Mickel AK, Sami C, et al: Endodontic treatment in an American Indian population: a 10-year retrospective study, *J Endod* 32:828-832, 2006.

80. Wang CH, Chueh LH, Chen SC, et al: Impact of diabetes mellitus, hypertension, and coronary artery disease on tooth extraction after nonsurgical endodontic treatment, *J Endod* 37:1-5, 2011.

81. Lilly JP, Cox D, Arcuri M, et al: An evaluation of root canal treatment in patients who have received irradiation to the mandible and maxilla, *Oral Surg Oral Med Oral Pathol Oral Radiol Endod* 86:224-226, 1998.

82. Badros A, Weikel D, Salama A, et al: Osteonecrosis of the jaw in multiple myeloma patients: clinical features and risk factors, *J Clin Oncol* 24:945-952, 2006.

83. Sarathy AP, Bourgeois SL, Goodell GG: Bisphosphonate-associated osteonecrosis of the jaws and endodontic treatment: two case reports, *J Endod* 31:759-763, 2005.

84. Katz H: Endodontic implications of bisphosphonate-associated osteonecrosis of the jaws: a report of three cases, *J Endod* 31:831-834, 2005.

85. Hsiao A, Glickman G, He J: A retrospective clinical and radiographic study on healing of periradicular lesions in patients taking oral bisphosphonates, *J Endod* 35:1525-1528, 2009.

86. Glick M, Abel SN, Muzyka BC, et al: Dental complications after treating patients with AIDS, *J Am Dent Assoc* 125:296-301, 1994.

87. Quesnell BT, Alves M, Hawkinson RW Jr, et al: The effect of human immunodeficiency virus on endodontic treatment outcome, *J Endod* 31:633-636, 2005.

88. Goon WW, Jacobsen PL: Prodromal odontalgia and multiple devitalized teeth caused by a herpes zoster infection of the trigeminal nerve: report of case, *J Am Dent Assoc* 116:500-504, 1988.

89. Gregory WB Jr, Brooks LE, Penick EC: Herpes zoster associated with pulpless teeth, *J Endod* 1:32-35, 1975.

90. Sigurdsson A, Jacoway JR: Herpes zoster infection presenting as an acute pulpitis, *Oral Surg Oral Med Oral Pathol Oral Radiol Endod* 80:92-95, 1995.

91. Sabeti M, Slots J: Herpesviral-bacterial coinfection in periapical pathosis, *J Endod* 30:69-72, 2004.

92. Slots J, Nowzari H, Sabeti M: Cytomegalovirus infection in symptomatic periapical pathosis, *Int Endod J* 37:519-524, 2004.

93. Chen V, Chen Y, Li H, et al: Herpesviruses in abscesses and cellulitis of endodontic origin, *J Endod* 35:182-188, 2009.

94. Li H, Chen V, Chen Y, et al: Herpesviruses in endodontic pathoses: association of Epstein-Barr virus with irreversible pulpitis and apical periodontitis, *J Endod* 35:23-29, 2009.

95. Ferreira DC, Paiva SS, Carmo FL, et al: Identification of herpesviruses types 1 to 8 and human papillomavirus in acute apical abscesses, *J Endod* 37:10-16, 2011.

96. Taylor LB, Nowak AJ, Giller RH, et al: Sickle cell anemia: a review of the dental concerns and a

retrospective study of dental and bony changes, *Spec Care Dentist* 15:38-42, 1995.

97. Andrews CH, England MC Jr, Kemp WB: Sickle cell anemia: an etiological factor in pulpal necrosis, *J Endod* 9:249-252, 1983.

98. Demirbas Kaya A, Aktener BO, Unsal C: Pulpal necrosis with sickle cell anaemia, *Int Endod J* 37:602-606, 2004.

99. Kirkevang LL, Wenzel A: Risk indicators for apical periodontitis, *Community Dent Oral Epidemiol* 31:59-67, 2003.

100. Segura-Egea JJ, Castellanos-Cosano L, Velasco-Ortega E, et al: Relationship between smoking and endodontic variables in hypertensive patients, *J Endod* 37:764-767, 2011.

101. Segura-Egea JJ, Jimenez-Pinzon A, Rios-Santos JV, et al: High prevalence of apical periodontitis amongst smokers in a sample of Spanish adults, *Int Endod J* 41:310-316, 2008.

102. Krall EA, Abreu Sosa C, Garcia C, et al: Cigarette smoking increases the risk of root canal treatment, *J Dent Res* 85:313-317, 2006.

103. Garcia B, Penarrocha M, Marti E, et al: Pain and swelling after periapical surgery related to oral hygiene and smoking, *Oral Surg Oral Med Oral Pathol Oral Radiol Endod* 104:271-276, 2007.

104. Engebretson SP, Lamster IB, Herrera-Abreu M, et al: The influence of interleukin gene polymorphism on expression of interleukin-1 beta and tumor necrosis factor-alpha in periodontal tissue and gingival crevicular fluid, *J Periodontol* 70:567-573, 1999.

105. Morsani JM, Aminoshariae A, Han YW, et al: Genetic predisposition to persistent apical periodontitis, *J Endod* 37:455-459, 2011.

106. Siqueira JF Jr, Rocas IN, Provenzano JC, et al: Relationship between Fcgamma receptor and interleukin-1 gene polymorphisms and post-treatment apical periodontitis, *J Endod* 35:1186-1192, 2009.

107. Aldous JA, Powell GL, Stensaas SS: Brain abscess of odontogenic origin: report of case, *J Am Dent Assoc* 115:861-863, 1987.

108. Li X, Tronstad L, Olsen I: Brain abscesses caused by oral infection, *Endod Dent Traumatol* 15:95-101, 1999.

109. Mylona E, Vadala C, Papastamopoulos V, et al: Brain abscess caused by *Enterococcus faecalis* following a dental procedure in a patient with hereditary hemorrhagic telangiectasia, *J Clin Microbiol* 50:1807-1809, 2012.

110. Saal CJ, Mason JC, Cheuk SL, et al: Brain abscess from chronic odontogenic cause: report of case, *J Am Dent Assoc* 117:453-455, 1988.

111. Bonapart IE, Stevens HP, Kerver AJ, et al: Rare complications of an odontogenic abscess: mediastinitis, thoracic empyema and cardiac tamponade, *J Oral Maxillofac Surg* 53:610-613, 1995.

112. Furst IM, Ersil P, Caminiti M: A rare complication of tooth abscess: Ludwig's angina and mediastinitis, *J Can Dent Assoc* 67:324-327, 2001.

113. Garatea-Crelgo J, Gay-Escoda C: Mediastinitis from odontogenic infection: report of three cases and review of the literature, *Int J Oral Maxillofac Surg* 20:65-68, 1991.

114. Stoykewych AA, Beecroft WA, Cogan AG: Fatal necrotizing fasciitis of dental origin, *J Can Dent Assoc* 58:59-62, 1992.

115. Allareddy V, Lin CY, Shah A, et al: Outcomes in patients hospitalized for periapical abscess in the United States: an analysis involving the use of a nationwide inpatient sample, *J Am Dent Assoc* 141:1107-1116, 2010.

116. Fouad AF, Walton RE, Rittman BR: Induced periapical lesions in ferret canines: histologic and radiographic evaluation, *Endod Dent Traumatol* 8:56-62, 1992.

117. Walton RE, Ardjmand K: Histological evaluation of the presence of bacteria in induced periapical lesions in monkeys, *J Endod* 18:216-227, 1992.

118. Nair P: Light and electron microscopic studies of root canal flora and periapical lesions, *J Endod* 13:29-39, 1987.

119. Ricucci D, Pascon EA, Ford TR, et al: Epithelium and bacteria in periapical lesions, *Oral Surg Oral Med Oral Pathol Oral Radiol Endod* 101:239-249, 2006.

120. Sunde PT, Olsen I, Gobel UB, et al: Fluorescence in situ hybridization (FISH) for direct visualization of bacteria in periapical lesions of asymptomatic root-filled teeth, *Microbiology* 149:1095-1102, 2003.

121. Sunde PT, Olsen I, Debelian GJ, et al: Microbiota of periapical lesions refractory to endodontic therapy, *J Endod* 28:304-310, 2002.

122. Caplan DJ, Chasen JB, Krall EA, et al: Lesions of endodontic origin and risk of coronary heart disease, *J Dent Res* 85:996-1,000, 2006.

123. Willershausen B, Kasaj A, Willershausen I, et al: Association between chronic dental infection and acute myocardial infarction, *J Endod* 35:626-630, 2009.

124. Joshipura KJ, Pitiphat W, Hung HC, et al: Pulpal inflammation and incidence of coronary heart disease, *J Endod* 32:99-103, 2006.

Interaction between the general dentist and the endodontist

Ashraf F. Fouad, Mahmoud Torabinejad

CHAPTER OUTLINE

Specialty Qualifications in the United States
Endodontic Practice Figures in the United States
Communication Between Endodontists and General Dentists
Standards of Endodontic Care and Case Documentation

Identification and Classification of Cases
What Is Expected of a General Practitioner
What Is Expected of an Endodontist

LEARNING OBJECTIVES

After reading this chapter, the student should be able to:
1. Understand the importance of referral.
2. Learn about the educational qualifications that lead to specialty status.
3. Identify the volume of endodontic treatment performed by general dentists and endodontists in the United States.
4. Identify the optimal methods of communication between the general dentist and the endodontist.

5. Define the standards of care for endodontic treatment.
6. Identify the indications for referral to an endodontic specialist.
7. Identify the various sources of information on endodontic materials and procedures.
8. Identify the important elements of record keeping with respect to endodontic treatment.

A patient who seeks root canal treatment to save his or her natural dentition deserves the best quality of care possible. Depending on the experience of the general dentist and the complexity of treatment, the general dentist might be able to deliver that care. However, in more complex cases, an endodontist provides the best care.[1]

Referral to an endodontist is appropriate when the general dentist is not capable of providing treatment that meets the standard of care.[2] By definition, *the standard of care provided to a patient by a general dentist should be similar to that provided by an endodontist.*[3] Studies show that success rates for root canal treatments performed by endodontists are higher than those performed by general dentists.[4,5] One contributing factor might be that general dentists often perform root canal treatments that are beyond their abilities.

This chapter provides information regarding the educational qualification of endodontists, figures related to the number of endodontic procedures performed in the United States by general dentists and endodontists, methods of communication between general dentists and endodontists, and some general guidelines for determining case complexity using the Endodontic Case Difficulty Assessment Form recommended by the American Association of Endodontists. Application of these guidelines should help general practitioners avoid mishaps before, during, and after providing root canal treatment.

SPECIALTY QUALIFICATIONS IN THE UNITED STATES

In the United States, the American Dental Association (ADA) recognizes nine areas of specialization in dentistry. This means that members of these specialty groups can limit their practice to this specialty. These specialties include dental public health, endodontics, oral and maxillofacial radiology, oral and maxillofacial surgery, oral pathology, orthodontics, pediatric dentistry, periodontics, and prosthodontics. The endodontic specialist has had 2 to 3 years of specialty training in an advanced program accredited by the ADA's Commission on Dental Accreditation. Through this training, the endodontics trainee encounters a multitude of cases involving varying degrees of complexity in different types of patients. Advanced endodontics specialty programs also have a mandate to expose the specialist to a vast array of research articles encompassing all aspects of the specialty and its relationship with other dental and medical specialties. Additionally, endodontics trainees have to be involved in a research project, which allows them to understand the fundamental tenets of asking a research question, designing a suitable study, and reporting on the findings using sound scientific principles. After completion of their educational programs, many endodontists pursue the rigorous process of becoming certified by the American Board of Endodontics.

ENDODONTIC PRACTICE FIGURES IN THE UNITED STATES

General dentists perform most of the endodontic procedures in the United States (Fig. 6.1). This is why dental schools must teach endodontics in the predoctoral curriculum to the level of competency required to manage simple endodontic cases. According to the Survey of Dental Procedures Rendered, published by the American Dental Association in 2007 (the latest year for which data are available), 15 million primary endodontic treatment procedures are performed annually.[6] According to this survey, endodontists perform about a quarter of these procedures, almost all retreatments (which number around 600,000 annually), and about two thirds of endodontic surgeries (about 300,000 annually).

The practice of endodontics among general dentists varies significantly and depends on their level of training, their personal interest, and the availability of endodontic specialists in their communities. As the primary provider for most patients, general dentists must be familiar with the principles of endodontic diagnosis and management of emergencies, including those related to traumatic injuries. Even if the general dentist routinely refers endodontic cases to specialists, he or she must have a basic understanding of the pathogenesis of endodontic disease and the accurate interpretation of patients' signs and symptoms, including the ability to perform pulp testing for most routine cases. This level of understanding allows practitioners to make accurate determinations about the need to treat and to refer when indicated; it also helps them establish rapport with patients and specialists with whom they interact.

Generally speaking, large insurance databases show that the retention (also known as *survival*) of teeth treated endodontically ranges from 94% to 97%.[7,8] The survival rate of teeth treated by endodontists tends to be somewhat higher than that of teeth treated by general dentists.[4,5] Similarly, recent information suggests that the survival of cases treated by general dentists is about 81%.[9] As noted before, one contributing factor might be that general dentists often perform root canal treatments that are beyond their abilities. Another possibility may be the compromise of asepsis protocols, such as the failure to use a dental dam seen in some general dentistry offices.[10]

There are many factors involved in the decision on whether the dentist would treat the tooth or refer the patient to an endodontist. Given the large number of endodontic procedures performed by general dentists, it is essential to identify the common practice for how and when cases are referred to endodontists, the specific standards of practice for this treatment, and the optimal methods of communication among the two types of practitioners that would ensure high standards of care for patients.

COMMUNICATION BETWEEN ENDODONTISTS AND GENERAL DENTISTS

Communication between general dentists and specialists takes place in the context of the referral of urgent or complex cases, discussion of optimal treatment plans for the patients, and/or discussion of the latest evidence for a particular procedure or material used in endodontic treatment. Many endodontists also endeavor to speak at local study clubs or regional meetings to promote information on the latest technologies and practices in the field. Most interactions occur by printed forms or letters that are given to the patient (for subsequent delivery) or sent by mail. Phone communication is a common and secure means to efficiently exchange ideas and information about the patient. Electronic forms of communication have become very common. However, many popular methods of electronic communication, such as e-mail, text messages, and online portals, are not inherently secure. Some e-mail programs permit encryption, which must be used for communication related to patients. Some practice management software programs offer online sites where information could be uploaded and viewed in a secure manner. According to the Health Insurance Portability and Accountability Act (HIPAA), there are 19 information items that constitute protected health information (PHI), which can be used to identify a patient. These include the name, birth date, contact information, and health record number, among other items, and they must be kept secure to comply with the law.

STANDARDS OF ENDODONTIC CARE AND CASE DOCUMENTATION

The standards of care in dentistry are difficult to define, and they vary considerably in different communities and

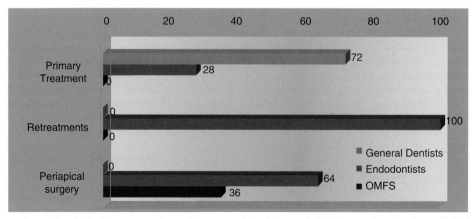

Fig. 6.1 Percentage of endodontic cases performed by general dentists, endodontists, and oral and maxillofacial surgeons. (Data from Molven O: The frequency, technical standard and results of endodontic therapy, *Nor Tannlasg Tidsskr* 86:142, 1976.)

geographic locations. However, it is generally accepted that the legal standard is the degree of skill, knowledge, and care possessed and exercised by prudent dentists under similar circumstances. The question usually asked in cases that are litigated is, "What would a prudent dentist do under similar circumstances?"

In general, endodontics is taught to predoctoral students by endodontists, who write the curriculum of the discipline in dental schools and define the competencies that students have to acquire to graduate. Therefore, endodontists set the standard of care for endodontics, and the general practitioner is expected to meet the same standard. The general dentist learns the principles and applies them to routine cases within his or her level of expertise. It is generally expected that if the general dentist thinks that the same standard cannot be met for a case, due to complexity or lack of training in a certain area, the patient is referred to an endodontist. It is important to emphasize that for training to be adequate, it should be from qualified experts in the area, in the context of approved continuing education courses, and from textbooks and research articles, rather than commercial venues with potential conflicts of interest.

Perhaps it is easier to describe the standard of care in endodontics by recognizing when it is not met. Examples of these negligent situations include the following:

- Failure to refer patients for complicated procedures
- Failure to perform proper pulp tests before diagnosing pulpal disease
- Failure to use the rubber dam for nonsurgical endodontic treatment
- Failure to use aseptic technique and infection control measures

The dentist has an obligation to document the clinical and radiographic findings of the case that led to the diagnosis reached. As noted before, there are many cases that do not fit the recognized patterns and are difficult to diagnose. In these cases, the dentist should still apply the principles, document the findings, and refer as needed. Thus, the correct diagnosis may not be reached in every case, but the clinical evaluation must be performed and documented in every case to satisfy the standard of what a prudent dentist would do. The records are the proof of what took place during the treatment and must describe what was performed in detail. The records must also document cases in which referral to a specialist was offered to the patient and the patient declined to take advantage of this offer. Finally, the records must document the consent of the patient to receive treatment after all available options were discussed and instances when the patient was informed of special risks and potential complications. In endodontic treatment, it is important to remember that the obturation is not the completion of the treatment. Prompt, adequate restoration and follow-up, which can extend up to 2 to 4 years after the obturation, are all necessary to ensure the success of treatment.

IDENTIFICATION AND CLASSIFICATION OF CASES

The decision about what to treat and what to refer depends on different risk factors, including the skills of the dentist and the difficulty of the case.[11]

The AAE Case Selection System

The American Association of Endodontists (AAE) has published guidelines for general dentists to help them classify the degree of difficulty of a case (Fig. 6.2). These guidelines are used in many dental schools to teach predoctoral students how to identify cases that ought to be referred to an endodontist. The guidelines use the classifications minimal difficulty, moderate difficulty, and high difficulty; they assist the practitioner in identifying the parameters of case difficulty and making a judgment as to whether the case is within his or her level of expertise. At first, the process seems cumbersome. However, *repeated* usage and familiarity *reduces risk* for both patients and general dentists. This should allow the dentist to provide optimum quality care. Referral can happen before, during, and after root canal treatment.

I. Referral Before Treatment
Complex Medical and Behavioral Issues
Patients who require significant alterations to the treatment regimen or close interactions with medical specialists due to their fragile health condition or disabilities are best managed by an endodontist. Frequently these patients are unable to stay in the dental chair for a long procedure, may require management under intravenous (IV) sedation or in the operating room, or require premedication and close monitoring during treatment. All these are factors that complicate the treatment, even if the technical aspect of the treatment does not appear to be complicated.

Emotional and Physical Limitations
Anxiety and/or physical limitations may present problems in providing proper treatment. Anxiety usually arises from poor previous dental experiences and can interfere with diagnosis and treatment. Providing assurance and showing patience during consultation and treatment usually result in the cooperation of these patients. Inadequate mouth opening can compromise access to the teeth and root canals. Referral should be considered for patients with significant limitations in mouth opening. Emotional and physical issues should be evaluated carefully; if problems are detected, the patient should be referred. Patients with severe gag reflexes should be treated under IV sedation by an endodontist.

Complex Diagnosis
Appropriate treatment follows accurate diagnosis. Diagnostic difficulties include confusing test results, nonspecific or unusual patterns of pain from periradicular lesions of nonpulpal origin, endodontic or periodontal lesions, and resorption.

As noted in Chapter 5, the practitioner should be able to use the patient's signs and symptoms, the clinical and radiographic findings, and the results of clinical tests to establish a pulpal and periapical diagnosis and make treatment decisions accordingly. Applying these principles should allow the general practitioner to make an accurate diagnosis in most cases (Fig. 6.3). However, there are many cases in which the application of these basic principles is not sufficient, and the practitioner would need the expertise to recognize and manage less common patient presentations or clinical conditions. These complex cases include situations in which diagnostic tests provide conflicting results or results that do not match the radiographic and clinical findings, traumatic injuries to

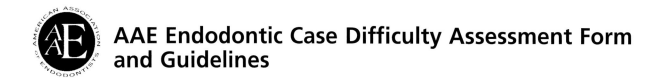

AAE Endodontic Case Difficulty Assessment Form and Guidelines

PATIENT INFORMATION

Name_____

Address_____

City/State/Zip_____

Phone_____

DISPOSITION

Treat in Office: Yes ☐   No ☐

Refer Patient to:

_____

Date:_____

Guidelines for Using the AAE Endodontic Case Difficulty Assessment Form

The AAE designed the Endodontic Case Difficulty Assessment Form for use in endodontic curricula. The Assessment Form makes case selection more efficient, more consistent and easier to document. Dentists may also choose to use the Assessment Form to help with referral decision making and record keeping.

Conditions listed in this form should be considered potential risk factors that may complicate treatment and adversely affect the outcome. Levels of difficulty are sets of conditions that may not be controllable by the dentist. Risk factors can influence the ability to provide care at a consistently predictable level and impact the appropriate provision of care and quality assurance.

The Assessment Form enables a practitioner to assign a level of difficulty to a particular case.

LEVELS OF DIFFICULTY

MINIMAL DIFFICULTY   Preoperative condition indicates routine complexity (uncomplicated). These types of cases would exhibit only those factors listed in the MINIMAL DIFFICULTY category. Achieving a predictable treatment outcome should be attainable by a competent practitioner with limited experience.

MODERATE DIFFICULTY   Preoperative condition is complicated, exhibiting one or more patient or treatment factors listed in the MODERATE DIFFICULTY category. Achieving a predictable treatment outcome will be challenging for a competent, experienced practitioner.

HIGH DIFFICULTY   Preoperative condition is exceptionally complicated, exhibiting several factors listed in the MODERATE DIFFICULTY category or at least one in the HIGH DIFFICULTY category. Achieving a predictable treatment outcome will be challenging for even the most experienced practitioner with an extensive history of favorable outcomes.

Review your assessment of each case to determine the level of difficulty. If the level of difficulty exceeds your experience and comfort, you might consider referral to an endodontist.

The contribution of the Canadian Academy of Endodontics and others to the development of this form is gratefully acknowledged.

Fig. 6.2   Case difficulty classification by the American Association of Endodontists. (Published with permission from the AAE.)

AAE Endodontic Case Difficulty Assessment Form

CRITERIA AND SUBCRITERIA	MINIMAL DIFFICULTY	MODERATE DIFFICULTY	HIGH DIFFICULTY
A. PATIENT CONSIDERATIONS			
MEDICAL HISTORY	☐ No medical problem (ASA Class 1*)	☐ One or more medical problems (ASA Class 2*)	☐ Complex medical history/serious illness/disability (ASA Classes 3-5*)
ANESTHESIA	☐ No history of anesthesia problems	☐ Vasoconstrictor intolerance	☐ Difficulty achieving anesthesia
PATIENT DISPOSITION	☐ Cooperative and compliant	☐ Anxious but cooperative	☐ Uncooperative
ABILITY TO OPEN MOUTH	☐ No limitation	☐ Slight limitation in opening	☐ Significant limitation in opening
GAG REFLEX	☐ None	☐ Gags occasionally with radiographs/treatment	☐ Extreme gag reflex which has compromised past dental care
EMERGENCY CONDITION	☐ Minimum pain or swelling	☐ Moderate pain or swelling	☐ Severe pain or swelling
B. DIAGNOSTIC AND TREATMENT CONSIDERATIONS			
DIAGNOSIS	☐ Signs and symptoms consistent with recognized pulpal and periapical conditions	☐ Extensive differential diagnosis of usual signs and symptoms required	☐ Confusing and complex signs and symptoms: difficult diagnosis ☐ History of chronic oral/facial pain
RADIOGRAPHIC DIFFICULTIES	☐ Minimal difficulty obtaining/interpreting radiographs	☐ Moderate difficulty obtaining/interpreting radiographs (e.g., high floor of mouth, narrow or low palatal vault, presence of tori)	☐ Extreme difficulty obtaining/interpreting radiographs (e.g., superimposed anatomical structures)
POSITION IN THE ARCH	☐ Anterior/premolar ☐ Slight inclination (<10°) ☐ Slight rotation (<10°)	☐ 1st molar ☐ Moderate inclination (10-30°) ☐ Moderate rotation (10-30°)	☐ 2nd or 3rd molar ☐ Extreme inclination (>30°) ☐ Extreme rotation (>30°)
TOOTH ISOLATION	☐ Routine rubber dam placement	☐ Simple pretreatment modification required for rubber dam isolation	☐ Extensive pretreatment modification required for rubber dam isolation
MORPHOLOGIC ABERRATIONS OF CROWN	☐ Normal original crown morphology	☐ Full coverage restoration ☐ Porcelain restoration ☐ Bridge abutment ☐ Moderate deviation from normal tooth/root form (e.g., taurodontism, microdens) ☐ Teeth with extensive coronal destruction	☐ Restoration does not reflect original anatomy/alignment ☐ Significant deviation from normal tooth/root form (e.g., fusion, dens in dente)
CANAL AND ROOT MORPHOLOGY	☐ Slight or no curvature (<10°) ☐ Closed apex (<1 mm in diameter)	☐ Moderate curvature (10-30°) ☐ Crown axis differs moderately from root axis. Apical opening 1-1.5 mm in diameter	☐ Extreme curvature (>30°) or S-shaped curve ☐ Mandibular premolar or anterior with 2 roots ☐ Maxillary premolar with 3 roots ☐ Canal divides in the middle or apical third ☐ Very long tooth (>25 mm) ☐ Open apex (>1.5 mm in diameter)
RADIOGRAPHIC APPEARANCE OF CANAL(S)	☐ Canal(s) visible and not reduced in size	☐ Canal(s) and chamber visible but reduced in size ☐ Pulp stones	☐ Indistinct canal path ☐ Canal(s) not visible
RESORPTION	☐ No resorption evident	☐ Minimal apical resorption	☐ Extensive apical resorption ☐ Internal resorption ☐ External resorption
C. ADDITIONAL CONSIDERATIONS			
TRAUMA HISTORY	☐ Uncomplicated crown fracture of mature or immature teeth	☐ Complicated crown fracture of mature teeth ☐ Subluxation	☐ Complicated crown fracture of immature teeth ☐ Horizontal root fracture ☐ Alveolar fracture ☐ Intrusive, extrusive or lateral luxation ☐ Avulsion
ENDODONTIC TREATMENT HISTORY	☐ No previous treatment	☐ Previous access without complications	☐ Previous access with complications (e.g., perforation, non-negotiated canal, ledge, separated instrument) ☐ Previous surgical or nonsurgical endodontic treatment completed
PERIODONTAL-ENDODONTIC CONDITION	☐ None or mild periodontal disease	☐ Concurrent moderate periodontal disease	☐ Concurrent severe periodontal disease ☐ Cracked teeth with periodontal complications ☐ Combined endodontic/periodontic lesion ☐ Root amputation prior to endodontic treatment

*American Society of Anesthesiologists (ASA) Classification System

Class 1: No systemic illness. Patient healthy.
Class 2: Patient with mild degree of systemic illness, but without functional restrictions, e.g., well-controlled hypertension.
Class 3: Patient with severe degree of systemic illness which limits activities, but does not immobilize the patient.

Class 4: Patient with severe systemic illness that immobilizes and is sometimes life threatening.
Class 5: Patient will not survive more than 24 hours whether or not surgical intervention takes place.

www.asahq.org/clinical/physicalstatus.htm

Fig. 6.2, cont'd

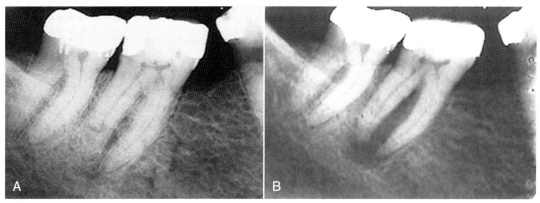

Fig. 6.3 An example of a simple diagnosis. Tooth #30 had caries and was not responsive to pulp testing. **A,** The dentist excavated the restoration and placed a temporary restoration, because "the tooth did not have a pulp exposure." **B,** Three months later, a periapical lesion had developed. Endodontic treatment should have been initiated at the time of diagnosis for pulp necrosis.

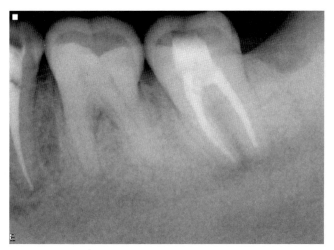

Fig. 6.4 An example of a complex diagnosis. The patient had a chronic, dull ache in the mandibular left quadrant. Endodontic treatment had been completed 2 years earlier by an endodontist, and the lesion appeared to be resolving. The chief complaint could not be reproduced, and the radiographic pattern of the bone suggested a possibility of bone pathosis. The case was diagnosed by an oral and maxillofacial surgeon as chronic sclerosing osteomyelitis.

teeth and their sequelae, diagnosis of symptomatic cases that were previously treated endodontically (Fig. 6.4), and/or orofacial pain or radiolucencies of nonendodontic origin that mimic endodontic pathosis.

Radiographic Difficulties

Radiographs are important tools for proper diagnosis and treatment planning. In cases in which obtaining and interpreting radiographs are difficult, the patient should be referred to an endodontist. This occurs with patients who have muscle trismus, have received radiation therapy to the orofacial musculature, have severe gagging issues, and/or have a small oral cavity.

Position of a Tooth in the Arch

Many dentists perform root canal treatment based on the location of the tooth in the arch. However, there are many other factors, in addition to the location of the tooth in the arch, that make root canal treatment difficult. Depending on these factors, performing a root canal in a second molar in one patient may be easier than performing the procedure on a premolar in another patient.

Local Anesthesia Difficulties

Some patients report an "allergy" to local anesthetics (tachycardia is often confused with an allergy). A patient may report adverse reactions to the epinephrine in a local anesthetic as an allergy. A major dilemma is highly inflamed pulps, particularly in mandibular molars.[12] Difficulty with anesthesia can change a cooperative patient into a phobic and uncooperative patient. When difficulty in obtaining profound anesthesia is encountered, referral should be considered.

Rubber Dam Isolation

Because of severe caries or crown fractures, a tooth may be too difficult to isolate or to restore; extraction may be the best alternative. In some instances, crown lengthening may be necessary to create biologic width before performing root canal treatment. Referral to a periodontist for this type of treatment should be considered if such a problem exists.

Morphologic Difficulties

A number of anatomic factors should be considered in the treatment planning for a tooth intended for root canal therapy.

Pulp Chamber and Root Canal Calcification

As a tooth ages, its pulp chamber and root canals calcify. Pulp chamber and root canal sizes, the presence of pulp stones, and the extent of calcifications in the root canal system must be considered before a decision is made regarding root canal treatment (Fig. 6.5).

Difficult Access and Anatomy of the Tooth Involved

As noted in Fig. 6.2, there are several situations that limit access to the tooth in question, making it difficult to render routine treatment. These cases include limited mouth opening (particularly for the treatment of molars), tooth crowding, severe tilting or rotation, subgingival carious lesions necessitating crown lengthening or other procedures to ensure good isolation, and molars with very long working lengths. In the latter case, although the tooth may be accessible for routine restorative work, the use of long instruments to instrument the canals presents a challenge (Fig. 6.6).

There are a number of anatomic variations that may necessitate referral to an endodontist. These include teeth with an immature apex, teeth with severe canal curvature, or teeth with a very calcified canal space. The general dentist should always be aware of the common anatomic variations of teeth and should rely on consultation or referral if he or she suspects additional canals that cannot be located; if the anatomic variation is unusual; or if the disease process persists despite treatment. Examples of circumstances in which the anatomic variations may render a case difficult to manage by the general dentist include mandibular premolars with more than one canal; maxillary premolars with more than two canals; radix entomolaris (extra roots in the mandibular molars); C-shaped canals; dens invaginatus and evaginatus; fused and geminated teeth; teeth with palatal groove defects; and teeth with lateral or J-shaped lesions (which may have unusual canal branching).

Existing Restorations

Many teeth that require root canal treatment have cast restorations.[13] The restoration anatomy usually does not correspond

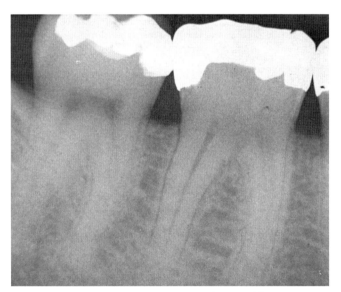

Fig. 6.5 Pulp chamber and root canals show calcific metamorphosis. This situation is rated as an extreme risk.

to the original crown anatomy, and the pulp chamber can be difficult to locate. When the tooth that requires root canal treatment is part of a bridge, the angulation of the restoration to the original crown and its location in the arch must be examined carefully before an access preparation is made. These considerations are particularly important in maxillary first premolars, lateral incisors, and mandibular incisors. These teeth are narrow and prone to crown or root perforations during access cavity preparations. Access through gold is easier than access through nonprecious metals. Porcelain crowns are fragile and can break during access preparation. When the pulp chamber and orifices to the root canals are not visible in the preoperative radiographs, referral to an endodontist should be considered (Fig. 6.7).

Cases with Root Resorption

There are several different types of root resorption (see Chapter 11 for a review of these conditions and their management). However, it is important to note here that root resorption has many different etiologies, pathogeneses, management strategies, and prognoses. The scientific literature that addresses these conditions is covered in advanced educational programs, and because these cases are relatively infrequent, the general dentist is advised to recognize their clinical presentation and refer them to an endodontist. Occasionally, resorption may present in a way that mimics caries. The dentist should realize the differences in clinical presentation between these two conditions (Fig. 6.8).

Endodontic Periodontal Lesion

Another complex diagnostic condition may arise in patients with periodontal pockets that may be related to a tooth with pulpal necrosis. If doubt exists regarding the origin of the periodontal pocket, the patient should be referred to an endodontist or a periodontist. Marginal periodontitis is best evaluated by a periodontist. Both endodontists and periodontists can best differentiate endodontic pathosis from periodontal pathosis. (The differential diagnosis of periodontal and endodontic lesions is discussed in Chapter 7.)

Traumatic Injuries, Retreatments, and Surgeries

Many of the cases that fall into the categories of traumatic injuries, retreatments, and surgeries are further described in the corresponding chapters (Chapters 11, 20, and 21, respectively); a general description of the interaction of the general

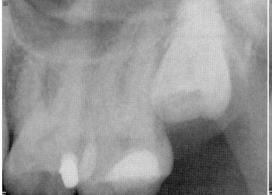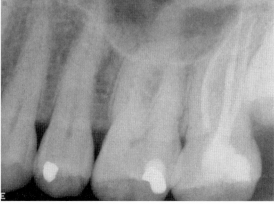

Fig. 6.6   Maxillary left second molar with working lengths that ranged from 26 to 28 mm.

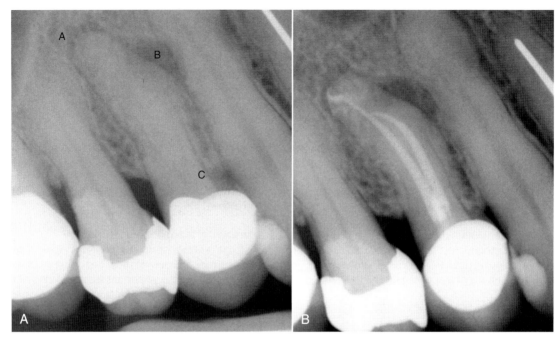

Fig. 6.7 **A,** Periapical radiolucency *(A)* and mesial radiolucency in the apical third *(B)*. The canals are calcified, the root is narrow, and there is a hint of a significant mesial concavity in the coronal third *(C)*. The tooth is also crowned, which increases access complexity. This is considered a high-risk case. **B,** Postoperatively, the mesial radiolucency resulted from the buccal root exiting several millimeters shorter than the palatal root with a significant distal curvature. The practitioner must manage unexpected complications should problems arise during treatment.

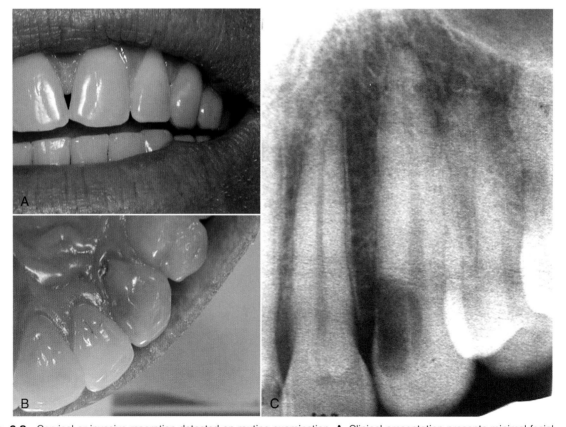

Fig. 6.8 Cervical or invasive resorption detected on routine examination. **A,** Clinical presentation presents minimal facial changes. **B,** Pink discoloration, associated with resorption and the presence of a vital responsive pulp. **C,** Extensive lesion extending below the osseous margin. Management of these cases is within the expertise of a specialist. This condition is different from caries in that it is exclusively subgingival and possibly subosseous, hard when it can be detected clinically (unlike the soft caries), and usually progresses to a large extent without devitalizing the tooth.

dentist and the specialist is given here. Many cases of traumatic injuries are first seen by the patient's general dentist. The general dentist has an obligation to manage the emergency condition and triage the patient appropriately. The latest guidelines for management of traumatic injuries should be posted and frequently reviewed. Diagnosis should include the pulpal and periapical conditions of all the teeth in the line of the trauma after the necessary examination and clinical testing has been performed. Management includes first aid for soft tissue injuries, repositioning of luxated teeth, and/or restoration of fractured teeth. The specialist should be involved in the diagnosis and management of extensive injuries and complications, including luxations, fracture of the alveolar bone and obvious pulpal involvement, root fractures, root resorptions, teeth with immature apices, patients with behavioral or complex medical problems, and late complications of trauma.

The general dentist plays an important role, as the gatekeeper of the patient's oral health, in recognizing and referring cases with failure of previous endodontic treatment. Many of these cases are asymptomatic; therefore, recognizing them requires adequate clinical and radiographic examination of the patient. The general dentist should be aware of the treatment procedures that are within the scope of the endodontic practice and educate the patient accordingly. It is important that the general dentist present the patient with all the available treatment options before recommending that a tooth be extracted and replaced by an implant or prosthesis. There are many cases in which the general dentist recognizes that additional expertise in determining the prognosis and the treatment options is needed and that consultation with an endodontist is warranted. In retrospect, many of the cases that are surgically or nonsurgically retreated by the endodontist should have been referred to the endodontist for primary treatment (Fig. 6.9). The prudent general dentist recognizes a case that is likely to be too complex and refers appropriately, rather than risk the development of treatment problems. There are many cases in which treatment appears to be routine, yet problems are encountered; referral to an endodontist can help ensure a good outcome (Fig. 6.10).

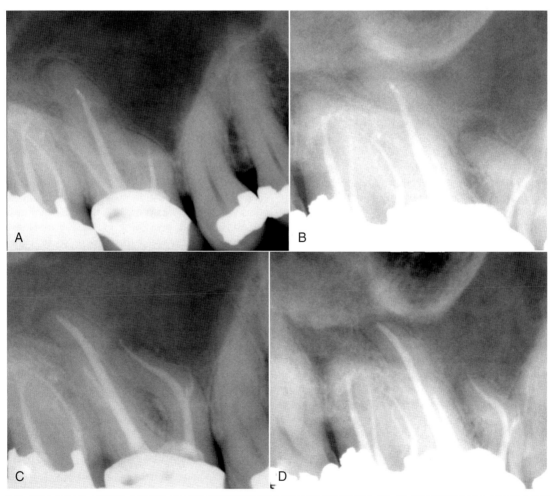

Fig. 6.9 This patient presented to the general dentist for root canal treatment of tooth #3. The tooth had a severe curvature of the mesial buccal (MB) root. The dentist performed root canal treatment and provided a crown for the tooth. **A,** Three months later, the patient was referred to the endodontist with continued pain. The straight radiograph shows that the MB canal could not be negotiated to length and had a possible perforation. There was blockage apically in the palatal and distal buccal canals. The palatal root had a small radiolucency. **B,** Distal shift shows the perforation on the MB canal and the lesion related to this root. The root apex had apical root resorption. **C,** Retreatment was successful in negotiating the MB and palatal canals. The perforation was sealed with mineral trioxide aggregate (MTA). **D,** Six-month follow-up shows healing of the lesions, and signs and symptoms of disease are absent.

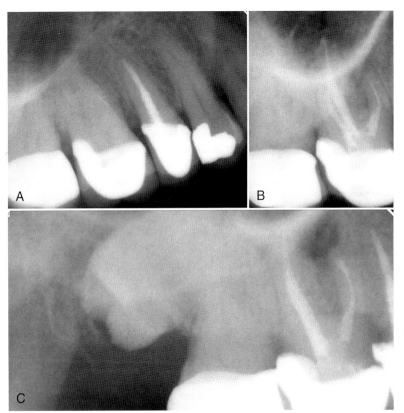

Fig. 6.10 **A,** Rotary instrument was separated in the mesial buccal (MB) canal of the maxillary first molar, which had a periapical lesion. **B,** The instrument was beyond the curvature of the canal and could not be retrieved; therefore, nonsurgical treatment was completed. **C,** Surgical treatment was performed on the MB root, with root-end filling using mineral trioxide aggregate (MTA). This ensured that the portion of the canal that was apical to the instrument was sealed and less likely to cause failure of treatment.

II. Referral During Treatment

The timing and discussion of referral with the patient are important during treatment planning. It is poor practice to initiate treatment with the sense that problems will be encountered and a referral will be made then. An initial referral prevents potential procedural accidents and improves the prognosis of difficult cases. Mid-treatment referral may also result in misunderstanding and loss of confidence by the patient. Another issue is financial problems that may arise during mid-treatment referrals. The endodontist is entitled to a full fee, and the patient should not be responsible for two fees for one tooth.

Despite all precautions and considerations, unanticipated problems may arise during treatments that require referral. A full explanation to the patient and a call to the endodontist are the necessary elements to prevent future problems. Reasons for referral during treatment include flare-ups (pain and/or swelling), procedural accidents, inability to achieve adequate anesthesia, and other factors that hinder completion of root canal therapy.

Flare-ups

Usually most pain or swelling occurs before initial treatment. After emergency treatments, pain usually decreases significantly in most patients within 24 to 48 hours. Flare-ups are not common during root canal treatments.[14] However, some patients develop pain and/or swelling after initial root canal treatment. The general dentist may elect to treat such flare-ups with appropriate local procedures and systemic medications. If these measures prove inadequate, referrals are in order.

Procedural Accidents

Procedural accidents during root canal treatment include ledge formation, creation of an artificial canal, root perforations, separated instruments, hypochlorite accidents, and underfilling and overfilling. (The causes, prevention, and prognosis of these mishaps is discussed in detail in Chapter 19.) Consultation with an endodontist is advisable to handle these accidents nonsurgically or, in some cases, surgically (properly and expediently) with appropriate follow-up. Treatment approaches and long-term assessment of these cases are usually beyond the expertise of a general dentist.

III. Referral After Treatment

Persistent problems, such as pain, pathosis, and sinus tract after root canal treatment, may indicate root canal failure and the need for further evaluation and treatment.

Pain

If pain and/or swelling persist or develop after treatment, the patient should be referred or an endodontist should be consulted. These symptoms may be related to lack of debridement, inadequate obturation, missed canals, root fractures, or other causes. Surgical and/or nonsurgical retreatment procedures or extraction might be in order.

Pathosis

Persistent periapical lesions or the development of new lesions after root canal treatment is indicative of root canal failure. Surgical and/or nonsurgical retreatment procedures are needed to resolve the problem.

Sinus Tract

When a periodontal defect of pulpal origin or a sinus tract does not resolve after treatment, the patient should be referred to an endodontist. The presence of a new defect or sinus tract indicates treatment failure, and the patient must be referred for consultation or treatment by an endodontist.

WHAT IS EXPECTED OF A GENERAL PRACTITIONER

Explicit written instructions, pertinent findings and treatment history, and appropriate radiographs (original or duplicate) are mailed or e-mailed to the endodontist. (Asking the patient to hand-carry these materials is discouraged.) These instructions should include how the tooth fits into the overall treatment plan, including the anticipated restoration.

WHAT IS EXPECTED OF AN ENDODONTIST

Specialists serve both the patient and referring dentist, and their responsibilities are to both. They should deliver appropriate treatment and communicate with the practitioner and the patient. When treatment is complete, the referring dentist should receive written confirmation from the endodontist that includes a radiograph of the obturation. A note is included about how the tooth was treated, anticipated recalls, the prognosis (both short term and long term), and unusual findings or circumstances. A suggestion regarding the definitive restoration is appropriate.

Before and during treatment, the endodontist explains to the patient all of the important aspects of the procedure and the anticipated outcome. After completion of treatment, the patient is informed of the prognosis, appropriate follow-up care, and the need to return to the referring dentist for continued care and any possible additional future procedures.[15]

REFERENCES

1. Molven O: The frequency, technical standard and results of endodontic therapy, *Nor Tannlaeg Tidsskr* 86:142, 1976.
2. Scharwatt BR: The general practitioner and endodontist, *Dent Clin North Am* 23:747, 1974.
3. Cohen S, Schwartz S: Endodontic complications and the law, *J Endod* 13:191, 1987.
4. Ericksen H: Endodontology-epidemiologic consideration, *Endod Dent Trauma* 7:189, 1991.
5. Alley BS, Kitchens GG, Alley LW, et al: A comparison of survival of teeth following endodontic treatment performed by general dentists or by specialists, *Oral Surg Oral Med Oral Pathol Oral Radiol Endod* 98(1):115-118, 2004.
6. American Dental Association: *The 2005-2006 survey of dental services rendered*, Chicago, 2007, The Association.
7. Lazarski MP, Walker WA III, Flores CM, et al: Epidemiological evaluation of the outcomes of nonsurgical root canal treatment in a large cohort of insured dental patients. *J Endod* 27:791-796, 2001.
8. Salehrabi R, Rotstein I: Endodontic treatment outcomes in a large patient population in the USA: an epidemiological studyl, *J Endod* 30:846-850, 2004.
9. Bernstein SD, Horowitz AJ, Man M, et al: Outcomes of endodontic therapy in general practice: a study by the Practitioners Engaged in Applied Research and Learning Network, *J Am Dent Assoc* 143:478-487, 2012.
10. Anabtawi MF, Gilbert GH, Bauer MR, et al: Rubber dam use during root canal treatment: findings from the Dental Practice–Based Research Network, *J Am Dent Assoc* 144:179-186, 2013.
11. Caplan D, Reams G, Weintraub J: Recommendations for endodontic referral among practitioners in a dental HMO, *J Endod* 25:369, 1999.
12. Seltzer S, Bender IB: *The dental pulp: biologic considerations in dental practice*, ed 3, p 127, St Louis, 1990, Ishiyaku Euro-America.
13. Burns R, Herbranson E: Tooth morphology and cavity preparation. In Cohen S, Burns RC, editors: *Pathways of the pulp*, ed 8, St Louis, 2001, Mosby.
14. Walton R, Fouad A: Endodontic interappointment flare-ups: a prospective study of incidence and related factors, *J Endod* 18:172, 1992.
15. Kramer S: Communications regarding referrals, *Risk Manage Rep* I(IV):4, 1989.

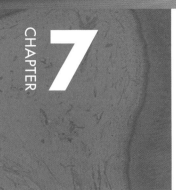

CHAPTER 7

Endodontic-periodontic interrelationship

Mahmoud Torabinejad, Ilan Rotstein

LEARNING OBJECTIVES

After reading this chapter, the student should be able to:

1. Delineate the anatomic pathways of communication between the dental pulp and the periradicular tissues.
2. Describe the effects of pulpal diseases and endodontic procedures on the periodontium.
3. Describe the effects of periodontal disease and procedures on the dental pulp.
4. Identify the clinical and radiographic findings that are important to identify the origin of periodontal pockets.
5. Know the clinical classification of endodontic-periodontal diseases.
6. Identify prognoses and assess which cases should be considered for referral.

A periodontist refers a 46-year-old patient with no contributing medical history to an endodontic office for diagnosis and possible root canal treatment. The patient states that he has been treated for periodontal disease for a few years by a periodontist. His chief complaint is "having a recent localized gumboil in one of his front teeth." Clinical examination shows that the patient has generalized moderate periodontitis and a localized severe periodontitis around the maxillary left lateral incisor. This tooth has no restoration and is sensitive to percussion and palpation. The pulp of the left lateral incisor responds within normal limits compared to the contralateral and adjacent teeth. Periodontal probing of this tooth reveals the presence of pockets with depths ranging from 3 to 9 mm. Radiographic examination of the patient reveals the presence of moderate bone loss around most of the maxillary anterior teeth with localized triangular bone loss around the left lateral incisor. No periapical radiolucency is noted around this tooth.

The endodontist contacts the referring periodontist and informs him that the periodontal pockets around the left lateral incisor are of periodontal origin and root canal treatment would not affect the prognosis of this tooth. The periodontist states that the periodontal condition around this tooth has been stable for some time and that the patient had recently developed deep pockets. The periodontist thinks that the pulp is involved and that root canal treatment will improve the

periodontal condition around this tooth. The endodontist disagrees with his colleague, and the patient is caught in the middle of this discussion. Although it may seem unlikely, this type of scenario is played out daily in dental offices around the world. It demonstrates the clinical importance of the interrelation of endodontic and periodontics lesions.

A number of investigations have shown that the presence of microorganisms is essential for the development of pulpal and/or periradicular pathosis.[1-4] Cultures from infected root canals show the predominant presence of gram-negative anaerobic bacteria.[5,6] These bacteria enter the root canals through direct pulp exposures (caries or traumatic injuries) or by coronal microleakage.[7-11] Egress of bacteria or their byproducts from pathologically involved pulps into the periradicular tissues results in inflammatory and immunologic reactions in this region. The extent of the periradicular lesion depends on the virulence of the bacteria present in the root canal system and the immune response during the disease process. Periradicular changes vary from a confined apical lesion to an extensive lesion communicating with the oral cavity via a sinus tract (Fig. 7.1) along the root surface as a periodontal pocket.[12]

Examination of the pathologic changes in the coronal periodontium during periodontitis shows that the mechanisms involved in periodontal disease are similar to those involved in the pathogenesis of periapical lesions.[13] The main

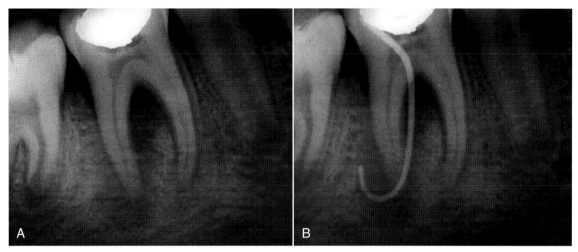

Fig. 7.1 **A,** Pulpal necrosis has caused development of a periradicular lesion extending along the mesial aspect of the distal root and furcation of the first mandibular right molar. **B,** Sinus tract exploration using a gutta-percha cone shows that the lesion communicates with the oral cavity via a narrow pocket on the buccal aspect of this tooth.

differences between the two processes are their original source and the direction of their progression. Periapical lesions extend apically or coronally, whereas periodontal lesions tend to extend only apically. As expected, these lesions can mimic each other at one or another stage of their development and make differential diagnosis difficult (see Fig. 7.1).

The decision on whether a tooth with a periodontal pocket requires endodontic therapy or periodontal treatment (or both) should be based on correct diagnosis. It is critical to examine all systematically obtained data during the patient examination before instituting proper treatment. Careful diagnosis prevents misunderstanding between patients and dentists involved in the treatment of endodontic-periodontic lesions. The purpose of this chapter is to discuss various aspects of this issue, including (1) pathways of communication between pulp and periodontium; (2) effects of periodontal disease and procedures on the pulp; (3) effects of endodontic lesions and procedures on the periodontium; (4) clinical and radiographic diagnostic procedures; and (5) classification of these lesions.

PATHWAYS OF COMMUNICATION BETWEEN THE DENTAL PULP AND THE PERIODONTIUM

Embryonically, the pulp and periodontium have an intimate relationship.[14] The dental papilla, which becomes dental pulp later on in the life of a tooth, is derived from cells that have migrated from the neural crest. Tissues of the periodontium develop from the dental follicle. These ectomesenchymal tissues are separated by Hertwig's epithelial root sheath (Fig. 7.2). After formation of the first layer of dentin in the root, Hertwig's sheath breaks up, allowing cells of the surrounding dental follicle to migrate and contact the newly formed dentin surface. The cells of the dental follicle differentiate into cementoblasts and initiate cementum formation. This acellular cementum ultimately serves as an anchor for the periodontal ligament (PDL) cells. As maturation of the root continues, direct communication between the pulp tissue and the periodontium becomes limited to the apical foramina and lateral canals.[14] Congenital absence of cementum in the coronal portion of roots in some individuals or removal of it during

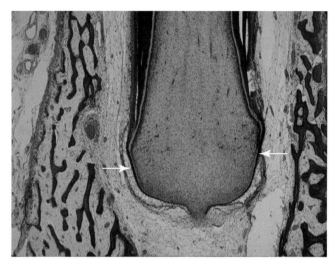

Fig. 7.2 The dental papilla (future pulp) is separated from the dental follicle (future periodontium) by Hertwig's epithelial root sheath *(arrows).*

periodontal treatment can result in communication between the periodontium and the dental pulp through exposed dentinal tubules. The pathways of communication between the pulp tissue and periodontium include the apical foramen, lateral or accessory canals, and dentinal tubules.

Apical Foramen

The apical foramen is the main pathway between the pulp and the PDL (Fig. 7.3). There may be one foramen or multiple foramina at the apex. Multiple foramina occur more often in multirooted teeth. Egress of irritants from pathologically involved root canals via the apical foramen into periapical tissues initiates an inflammatory response and its consequences, such as destruction of the apical PDL and resorption of bone, cementum, and dentin.

Although a clear cause and effect relationship between pulpal diseases and inflammation in the apical periodontium via the apical foramen has been established, there is no substantial evidence that shows that periodontitis affects the viability of the dental pulp.

Lateral Canals

Lateral or accessory canals are formed when a localized area of epithelial root sheath breaks down before the root dentin is laid down.[14] Formation of these canals results in direct communication between the pulp and the PDL. These canals can be single or multiple, small or large, and can be present anywhere along the roots (Fig. 7.4). The incidence of these canals varies not only among different types of teeth, but also at different levels of roots. In general, lateral canals are present more frequently in posterior teeth than in anterior teeth and are found more frequently in the apical portions of roots than in their coronal segments.[15-17] The incidence of lateral canals in the furcation of molars is reported to be as low as 2% to 3% and as high as 76.8%.[18-20] A patent lateral canal can carry

irritants from the pulp to the periodontium or vice versa. A lateral canal can carry enough irritants from a necrotic pulp to the periradicular tissues to induce a lateral lesion (Fig. 7.5, A). However, pulpal pathosis rarely occurs in teeth with periodontal involvement through the lateral canals.[21,22] This phenomenon is attributed to the defense of vital pulp against irritants coming from the periodontium.

Lack of severe changes, such as irreversible pulpitis or pulpal necrosis, has been demonstrated in histologic sections of teeth with severe periodontal disease.[23,24] Despite their frequent presence in the roots, lateral canals are not usually visible on standard radiographs.[25] They are usually revealed only when filled with radiopaque materials such as endodontic sealers, after obturation of the root canal system (Fig. 7.5, B). The main radiographic indicators of the presence of lateral canals before obturation are (1) a notch on the lateral root surface, (2) localized thickening of the PDL on the lateral surface of the root, and (3) a frank lateral lesion in periradicular tissues (Fig. 7.6). The location and size of lateral canals are usually revealed when they are filled with root canal filling materials (Fig. 7.7). The presence of infected lateral canals can be the cause of persistent narrow periodontal pockets that do not extend into the apical foramen after adequate root canal therapy.

Dentinal Tubules

In the root, the dentinal tubules extend from the pulp to the cementodentinal junction (CDJ). These tubules run a relatively straight course between the pulp and the cementum on the root surfaces. Their diameter ranges from about 1 to 3 μm.[26,27] The tubules in the coronal root are larger than those in the apical root (Fig. 7.8). The number of dentinal tubules per square millimeter has been reported to range from 4,900 to 90,000.[26] The size and number of dentinal tubules decreases in the coronal-apical direction (Fig. 7.8). At the cemento-enamel junction (CEJ), the number of dentinal tubules has been estimated to be approximately 15,000 per square millimeter. The dentinal tubules contain odontoblastic processes, nerve fibers, and tissue fluid. As the tooth ages or becomes irritated, the tubules calcify and decrease in number.

Studies have shown that bacteria present in infected root canals invade the dentinal tubules (Fig. 7.9).[28-37] The presence of a continuous layer of cementum is an effective barrier

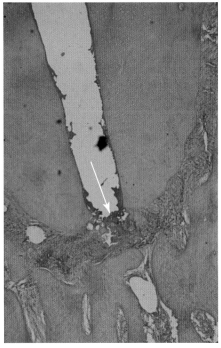

Fig. 7.3 The apical foramen *(arrow)* is the main pathway of communication between the pulp and the periodontal ligament (PDL).

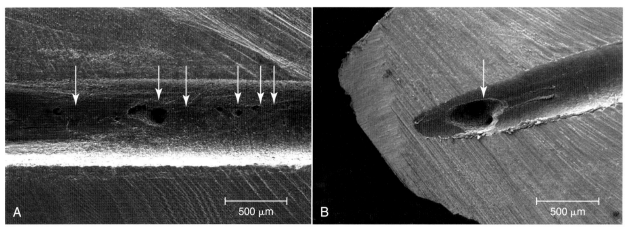

Fig. 7.4 A scanning electron micrograph reveals the presence of multiple lateral canals of various size in the middle **(A)** and apical **(B)** surfaces of the root canal of a lateral incisor after removal of the smear layer using MTAD. (Original magnification, ×100.)

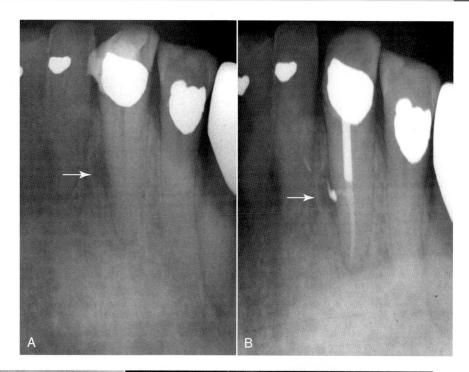

Fig. 7.5 **A,** A periapical radiograph reveals the presence of a lateral canal *(arrow)* in a mandibular cuspid with necrotic pulp. **B,** The location of this canal is revealed only after obturation of the root canal and placement of a post.

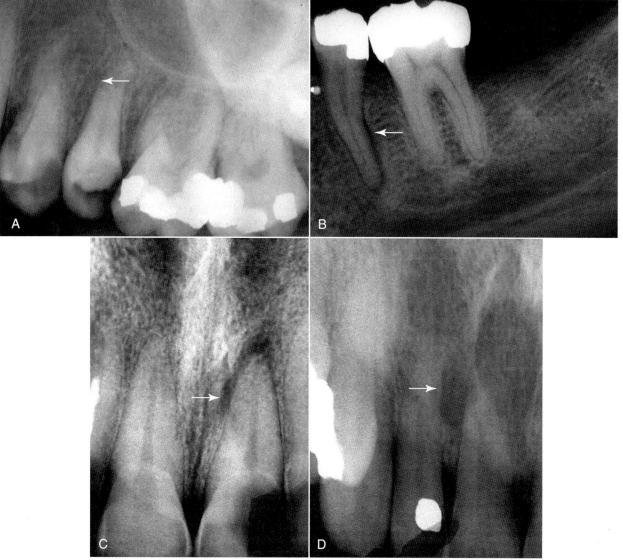

Fig. 7.6 Presence of a lateral canal is suspected when a notch is observed on the surface of roots **(A),** or there is a localized thickening of the PDL on the lateral surface of the root **(B),** or there is a small **(C)** or a large **(D)** lateral lesion in periradicular tissues.

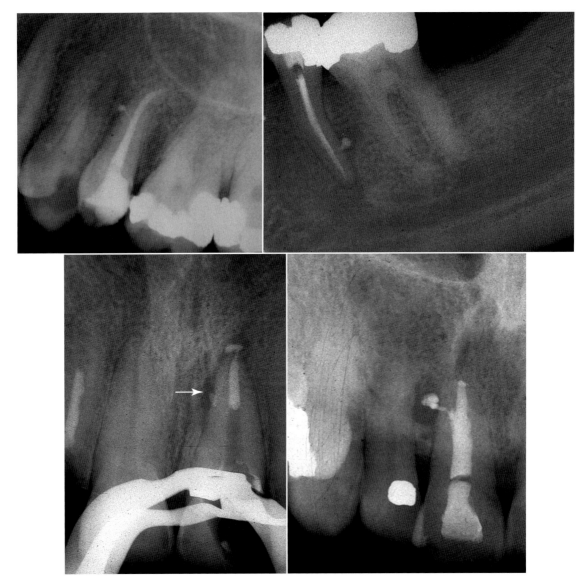

Fig. 7.7 The location of lateral canals is revealed after obturation of the root canal system and extrusion of root canal filling materials into pathways of communication between the pulp and periodontium.

against the penetration of bacteria and their byproducts from the pathologically involved root canals into the periodontium and vice versa. Congenital absence of cementum over root dentin at the CEJ,[38] caries, or removal of the cementum during periodontal treatment can result in the opening of numerous channels of communication between the pulp and the periradicular tissues. Theoretically, these channels can carry toxic metabolites present in infected root canals or infected periodontium in both directions. However, it has been shown that root surfaces denuded of cementum and exposed to the oral cavity do not cause significant changes in the pulp.[39,40]

Outward movement of dentinal tissue fluid and the tubular contents of vital pulps can delay intratubular invasion by bacteria. Accumulated host defense cells and inflammatory mediators at the site of exposure, dentinal sclerosis, and reparative dentin also limit or even prevent bacterial invasion of the pulp via dentinal tubules.[41] These protective factors become less effective when dentin thickness is considerably reduced and dentin permeability, therefore, is significantly

increased. On the other hand, if the pulp is necrotic, exposed dentinal tubules can become true avenues for bacteria to reach and colonize the pulp. Nagaoka and associates have shown that bacterial invasion of dentinal tubules occurs more rapidly in teeth with necrotic pulps than in those with vital pulps.[42]

EFFECT OF PULPAL DISEASES AND ENDODONTIC PROCEDURES ON THE PERIODONTIUM

Pulpal diseases may induce pathologic alterations in the periodontium.

Etiology
Irritants present in pathologically involved root canal systems or those induced by root canal procedures can be divided into living and nonliving.[12] Living irritants are various microorganisms and viruses. Nonliving irritants can be mechanical,

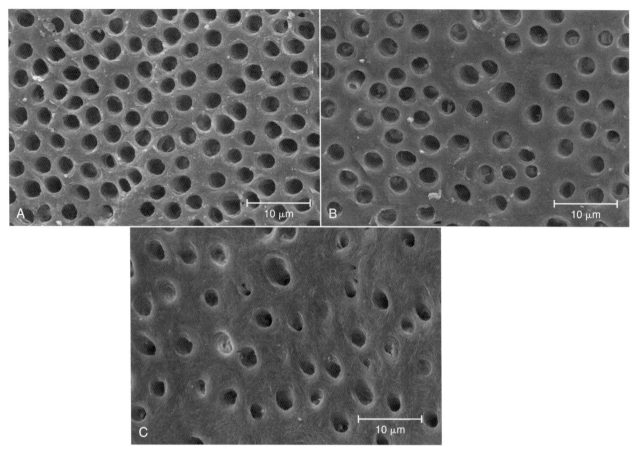

Fig. 7.8 A scanning electron micrograph reveals the presence of dentinal tubules in the coronal **(A)**, middle **(B)**, and apical **(C)** third of a single-rooted tooth after removal of the smear layer using MTAD. The size and number of dentinal tubules decrease in a coronal-apical direction. (Original magnification, ×5,000.)

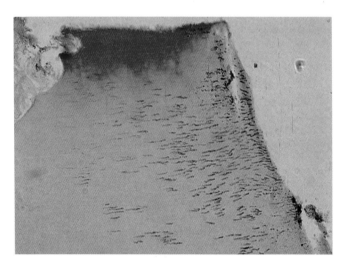

Fig. 7.9 A histologic section of a root shows the invasion of dentinal tubules by bacteria present in an infected root canal of dog premolar. (Brown and Brenn staining; original magnification, ×60.)

thermal, or chemical in nature. The inflammatory effect of mechanical, thermal, and chemical irritants is usually transient and nonlingering for the patient. Bacteria are the major cause of pathologic changes in periradicular tissues.[1] Anaerobic gram-negative bacteria appear to be the most common microorganisms found in infected root canals.[43] In addition to bacteria,[44] several other pathogens, such as spirochetes,[45-49] fungi,[50-53] and viruses,[54-56] have been identified in infected root canals. Nonliving irritants include foreign bodies such as dentin and cementum chips, root canal filling materials, and food debris.

Pathogenesis

Pathologic changes can occur in the periradicular tissues as a consequence of pulpal inflammation and necrosis. Irreversible pulpitis can cause inflammatory reactions in periradicular tissues and can increase the sensitivity of teeth to pressure. Subsequent to pulpal necrosis, interaction between irritants emanating from infected root canals and the host defense system results in the activation of an extensive array of reactions in periradicular tissues attempting to localize the infection and protect the host from osteomyelitis.[12] The reactions involved are highly complex and usually mediated by nonspecific mediators of inflammation and specific immune reactions (Fig. 7.10). Depending on the nature of irritation, duration, and host response, periradicular reactions can range from slight inflammation to extensive tissue destruction.

Effect

As expected, periradicular changes after pulpal necrosis are not always confined to the apical tissues. They can also be found anywhere adjacent to the root surfaces and drain **111**

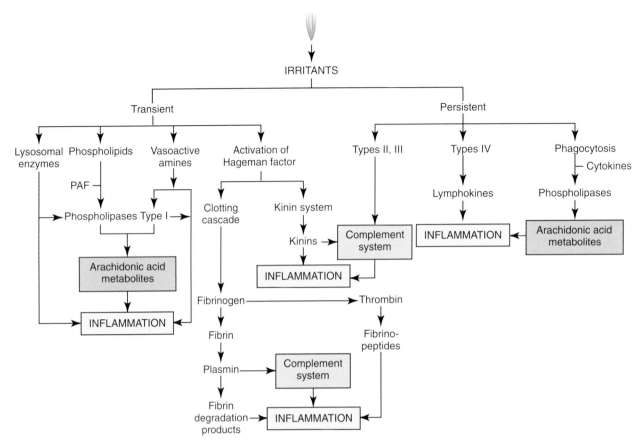

Fig. 7.10 Pathways of nonspecific and specific inflammatory reactions for pathogenesis of periapical lesions.

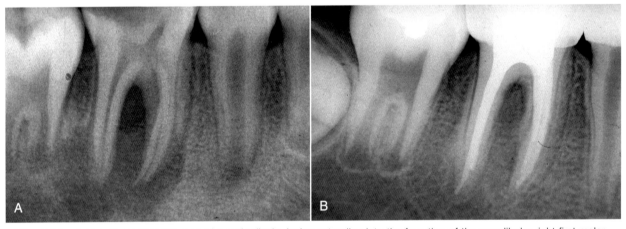

Fig. 7.11 A, Pulpal necrosis has caused a periradicular lesion extending into the furcation of the mandibular right first molar. **B,** Complete cleaning, shaping, and obturation of the root canal system in this tooth resulted in resolution of this lesion.

through a sulcus, simulating a periodontal pocket (Fig. 7.11, *A*). As a result of such a lesion, the periradicular tissues are replaced by an inflammatory connective tissue. This phenomenon is in contrast to the periodontal detachment caused by periodontal diseases. After complete cleaning and obturation of the root canal system in three dimensions, the pathologic changes in the periradicular tissues usually disappear and the periodontium returns to normalcy (Fig. 7.11, *B*, and Fig. 7.12). It has been speculated that root canal materials, such as sealers or medicaments, may penetrate through dentinal tubules, cause cementum necrosis, and delay or prevent tissue

healing after periodontal therapy. However, there is not enough evidence to support the idea that root canal treatment has adverse long-term effects on periodontal treatment.[57]

Procedural accidents, such as furcation perforation of the floor of the pulp chamber in multirooted teeth during access preparation, strip root perforations during cleaning and shaping, and root perforation during post space preparation, damage the periodontium (Fig. 7.13, *A*). Sealing of these perforations with biocompatible repair material eliminates the infection and periodontal pocket of endodontic origin (Fig. 7.13, *B* to *D*). Vertical root fracture after root canal treatment

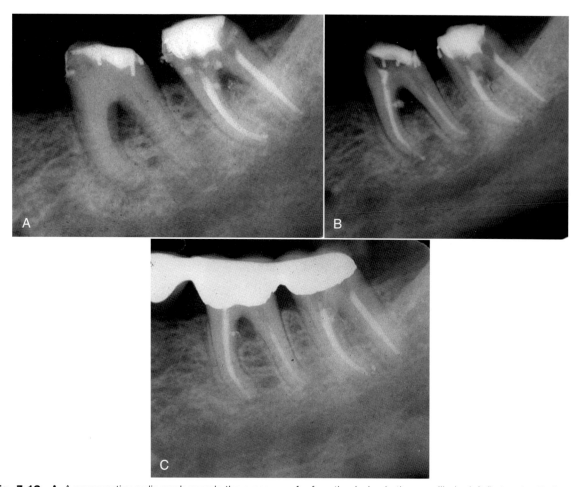

Fig. 7.12 **A,** A preoperative radiograph reveals the presence of a furcation lesion in the mandibular left first molar. **B,** A postoperative radiograph after root canal treatment shows the presence of a lateral canal. **C,** Another postoperative radiograph (18 months later) reveals the resolution of most of the furcation lesion.

can often produce narrow probing defects that simulate periodontal disease (Fig. 7.14).

EFFECT OF PERIODONTAL DISEASE AND PROCEDURES ON THE PULP

As discussed earlier, irritants from the root canal system can enter the periodontium through the apical foramen or lateral canals and cause pathologic changes in surrounding tissues.[12] However, the effect of periodontal disease on the pulp via the same channels is the subject of debate.[17,23,24,58] Differences in etiologic factors, pathogenesis, and progression of the two diseases may explain why the reactions differ in each tissue.

Etiology

Like pulpal and periapical pathosis, periodontitis is an infectious disease. Examination of plaque samples from human subgingival specimens shows the presence of 300 to 400 bacterial species.[59] Of these, 10 to 20 species may play a role in the pathogenesis of destructive periodontal disease.[60] The microorganisms involved in periodontal disease are largely gram-negative anaerobic bacilli with some anaerobic cocci and a large number of anaerobic spirochetes.[59] The main organisms associated with destructive periodontal lesions are

Porphyromonas gingivalis, Prevotella intermedia, Bacteroides forsythus, Actinobacillus actinomycetemcomitans, and *Treponema denticola.*[61] Page and associates propose that the subgingival microbial flora are highly organized as biofilms and bacteria present in this complex environment are protected from the host defenses and are highly resistant to chemotherapeutic agents.[62] In addition to microbial biofilms present during periodontitis, periodontal procedures, such as scaling and root planing, can also affect the dental pulp.

Pathogenesis

As mentioned, interaction between pathogens present in the periodontal pocket and host defense mechanisms can lead to highly complex reactions mediated by specific and nonspecific reactions. Several reviews focusing on the pathogenesis of chronic marginal periodontitis have been published.[59,61-65] These reviews show major advances in our understanding of cellular and molecular pathways of interaction between biofilms and host responses that destroy the gingivae, PDL, and alveolar bone. Although the presence of bacteria is essential for periodontal disease to occur, bacteria alone are insufficient to sustain the process over time.[62] Host susceptibility and acquired and environmental risk factors, such as tobacco smoking and the genetic makeup of the host, also determine the onset, progression, and outcome of this interaction.[62]

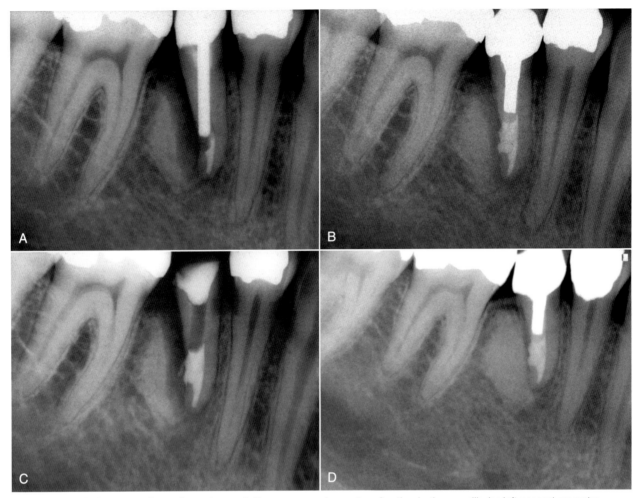

Fig. 7.13 **A,** A preoperative radiograph reveals the presence of a post perforation in the mandibular left second premolar. There is a periodontal pocket on the distal aspect of this tooth. **B,** A postoperative radiograph after removal of the post and repair of the perforation with mineral trioxide aggregate (MTA). **C,** A postoperative radiograph (14 months later) reveals the advanced resolution of the lesion. **D,** Another postoperative radiograph (5 years later) reveals the complete resolution of the lesion. (Courtesy Dr. N. Chivian.)

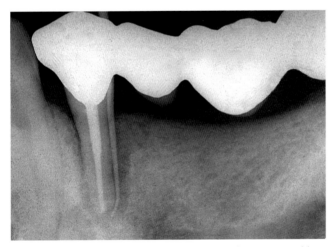

Fig. 7.14 A vertical root fracture has produced a narrow probing defect in the mandibular left first premolar. A gutta-percha cone shows the presence and extent of the lesion.

Depending on these factors, periodontal reactions can range from slight inflammation to extensive destruction of periodontal tissue.

Effect

Severe periodontitis is associated with the formation of a granulomatous tissue that is infiltrated with defensive cells and that normally contains little or no bacteria. This is in contrast to a necrotic pulp, which contains potent irritants, particularly bacteria and their byproducts, that cause pathologic changes in the periodontium. Although it has been stated in textbooks and articles that periodontal lesions can cause inflammation or even necrosis of the pulp,[17] such a reaction has not been fully substantiated (Fig. 7.15).[23,24] Seltzer and associates[17] stated that lateral canals open to oral flora can transmit toxic products into the pulp, causing atrophic, degenerative, inflammatory, and resorptive alterations. In contrast, other investigators have found little or no cause and effect relationship between periodontal disease and inflammatory changes in the pulp.[23,39,66] There is some evidence that severe periodontal involvement that includes plaque on the root close to or at the apex causes necrosis and inflammation in the pulp.[21]

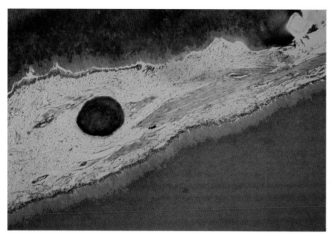

Fig. 7.15 No significant atrophic, degenerative, inflammatory, or resorptive alterations are found in the pulp of a tooth with severe periodontitis.[24]

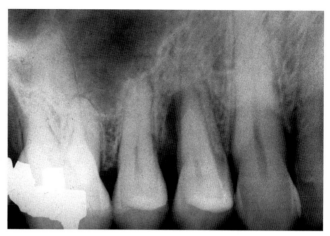

Fig. 7.16 Periapical radiograph of the right maxillary region reveals the presence of generalized periodontal lesions in this area, with angular bone loss and also the absence of buccal and lingual plates around the premolars and cuspid.

In a 3-year, retrospective radiographic study, Jansson and associates reported an approximately threefold increase in marginal bone loss in patients with infected root canals compared to those without endodontic infection.[67] In another report, Jansson and Ehnevid examined the effect of endodontic infection on periodontal probing depth and the presence of furcation involvement in mandibular molars.[68] They reported that endodontic infection in mandibular molars is associated with more attachment loss in the furcation of mandibular molars. These authors attributed the results to penetration of pathogens from infected canals into the furcation of mandibular molars through accessory canals and dentinal tubules. In contrast to these findings, other investigators failed to observe a correlation between reduced marginal bone support and endodontic infection.[69]

Deep scaling and planing of the root surfaces remove cementum and result in opening of the dentinal tubules and, possibly, lateral canals. Invasive periodontal treatment, such as deep curettage that severs apical vessels, can cause necrosis of the dental pulp.

CLINICAL AND RADIOGRAPHIC TESTS FOR DIAGNOSIS OF ENDODONTIC-PERIODONTIC LESIONS

To come up with the correct diagnosis and administer proper treatment, the clinician must take a systematic approach to subjective and objective tests required. Reliance on one test is a prelude to misdiagnosis and improper treatment. Diagnostic tests include subjective signs and symptoms, visual and radiographic examinations, and clinical tests.

Subjective Signs and Symptoms
A complete history of the location, duration, intensity, and frequency of pain and of medications used for pain relief can provide valuable information to help determine the nature of a patient's complaint. In general, periodontal disease is a chronic and generalized process that is associated with little or no significant pain. In contrast, pulpal and periapical lesions are localized conditions and are more likely to be associated with acute symptoms that require analgesics.

Visual Examination
Visual examination of the teeth and gingival tissues provides valuable initial information for diagnosis. The presence of caries, extensive restorations, and discolored crowns is usually associated with endodontic lesions. The absence of obvious coronal defects in conjunction with plaque, calculus, and a generalized gingivitis or periodontitis indicates the presence of periodontal disease.

Radiographic Examination
Periodontal lesions are usually associated with angular bone loss extending from the cervical region toward the apex (Fig. 7.16). In contrast, periapical lesions cause destruction of apical periodontium that occasionally extends coronally toward the CEJ (Fig. 7.17, *A*). In addition to angular bone loss, which is usually pathognomonic for periodontal disease, the absence of the buccal or lingual plate (or both) may result in a clear definition of the tooth and the root canal or canals to the level of the bone loss.[39] Localized or generalized bone loss is an important radiographic finding for differentiation between a lesion of pulpal origin and one of periodontal origin. Usually, periodontal lesions are found around multiple teeth (Fig. 7.16), although this may not always be the case. In contrast, periapical lesions are usually isolated to a single tooth and heal after complete cleaning, shaping, and obturation of root canals (Fig. 7.17, *B*).

Clinical Tests
Clinical tests include vitality tests, percussion and palpation tests, and periodontal probing.

Vitality Tests
The results of vitality tests are generally, but not totally, reliable. Irreversible pulpitis is invariably associated with exaggerated pulpal reaction to cold or heat. Teeth with necrotic pulps have usually no response to thermal or electric stimuli. In contrast, teeth with periodontal lesions often have vital and responsive pulps.

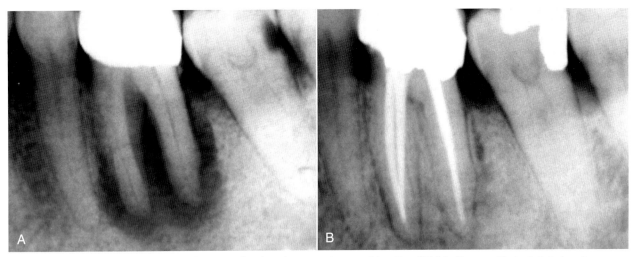

Fig. 7.17 **A,** Large periradicular lesion extending into the cementoenamel junction (CEJ) in the mandibular left first molar. **B,** Complete cleaning, shaping, and obturation of the root canal system resulted in resolution of this lesion.

Palpation and Percussion

Palpation sensitivity of coronal soft tissues is indicative of gingivitis or periodontitis. Palpation sensitivity over the root apex of a tooth with pulpal necrosis indicates the presence of periapical lesions. Percussion, when positive, to some degree shows the presence of an inflammatory response in the periodontal ligament. (The inflammation can be from a pulp or a periodontal lesion.) However, the percussion test is not reliable for differentiating between the two diseases.

Probing

Probing defects originating from a periodontal lesion are usually wide and usually do not extend to the apices of the involved teeth. In contrast, probing defects of pulpal origin are usually narrow and extend either to the openings of lateral canals or to the apical foramen. Developmental grooves (Fig. 7.18), vertical root fractures (see Fig. 7.14), and enamel spurs (Fig. 7.19) may create a narrow pocket simulating a lesion of pulpal origin.[70]

CLASSIFICATION AND DIFFERENTIAL DIAGNOSIS OF ENDODONTIC-PERIODONTIC LESIONS

Periodontal defects such as osseous lesions, periodontal pockets, and pathologic changes in the soft tissues manifested by swelling, presence of sinus tract stoma, and discomfort can be produced by periodontal disease and periradicular lesions of pulpal origin.[57] Based on their genesis, several authors have classified these lesions into several categories.[70-72] Periodontal defects can be classified into three primary types:

- Pulpal (endodontic) origin
- Periodontal (periodontic) origin
- Endodontic-periodontic origin (true combined lesions)

This classification is based on the way these lesions develop, and it provides an understanding of their pathogenesis, clinical signs and symptoms, treatment, and prognosis. In rare instances, long-standing primary defects of pulpal or periodontic origin can be converted into secondary combined lesions.

Primary Periodontal Defects of Pulpal (Endodontic) Origin

A periodontal defect of pulpal/periapical origin is usually associated with a single-rooted tooth (Fig. 7.20, A) with necrotic pulp or a multirooted tooth with a partially necrotic pulp (see Figs. 7.11, A; 7.12, A; and 7.17, A). The patient may or may not have any discomfort. Occasionally, there is evidence of a localized abscess with some swelling.

Visual examination of the involved tooth reveals the presence of caries and/or extensive restoration, which can cause pulp necrosis. Radiographic examination reveals the presence of periapical lesions isolated to a single tooth. Vitality tests show the absence of a response to thermal or electric stimuli. The involved tooth may or may not test positive on palpation or percussion sensitivity tests. Periodontal probing usually shows normal sulci around the tooth except in one area with a narrow defect (video). Placement of a gutta-percha cone or a periodontal probe into this sinus tract shows that the defect is deep, usually to the apex or possibly to the opening of a lateral canal.

Treatment and Prognosis

A periodontal defect of pulpal (endodontic) origin should be considered a coronally extended periradicular lesion, which is initiated and perpetuated by the toxic materials within the root canal system (see Fig. 7.20, A). This defect is not a true periodontal pocket, and adequate cleaning and shaping, in addition to obturation of the root canal system, usually result in complete resolution (see Figs. 7.11, B; 7.12, B; 7.17, B; and 7.20, B). The defect does not require any adjunctive periodontal treatment, disappears quickly, and has an excellent prognosis.

Primary Periodontal Defects of Periodontic Origin

A periodontal defect of periodontic origin is usually associated with generalized gingivitis and/or periodontitis resulting from the accumulation of plaque and/or calculus formation. Except in cases of acute periodontal abscesses, patients usually have no significant symptoms. The affected tooth may or may not have undergone extensive restorative procedures

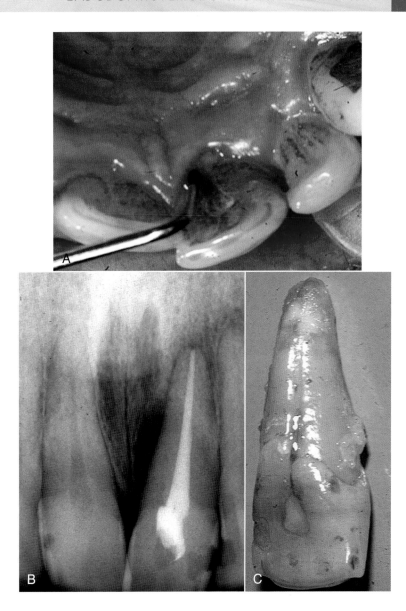

Fig. 7.18 A, A lingual groove in the left central incisor has resulted in the development of a narrow pocket. **B,** This groove caused a visible radiolucency and a nonmanageable periodontal defect that eventually resulted in extraction **(C)** of this tooth.

and is often associated with various degrees of mobility. Radiographic examination of the involved tooth and its adjacent teeth shows the presence of generalized vertical and horizontal bone loss along the root surfaces (Fig. 7.21). Teeth with these defects respond within normal limits to pulp testing procedures. Unlike lesions of pulpal origin, defects of periodontal disease origin are wide and V-shaped.[57] On probing, the crest is within normal limits. Then, in a "step-down" fashion, the probe reaches deeper. The pocket depth decreases in a "step-up" manner and reaches the normal depth on the other side of the pocket.[70]

Treatment and Prognosis

Because primary periodontal defects of periodontic origin are not of pulpal/periapical origin, root canal treatment does not result in resolution. Only periodontal treatment is indicated. The prognosis for these defects is totally dependent on the periodontal treatment. Occasionally, in multirooted teeth that require root amputation or hemisection to remove an unsalvageable root, root canal treatment is necessary as an adjunct to periodontal treatment.

Primary Periodontal Defects of Endodontic-Periodontic Origin (True Combined Lesions)

Primary periodontal defects of endodontic-periodontic origin, or true combined lesions, have two concurrent components and occur less often than the previous two types. One component is an independent periapical lesion originating from a necrotic pulp. The other is an independent periodontal lesion that has progressed apically toward the periapical lesion (Fig. 7.22, *A*) Missing. Depending on their stage of development, the lesions may or may not communicate with one another. A true combined defect is usually associated with clinical signs and symptoms of generalized gingivitis and/or periodontitis with little or no discomfort. The affected tooth may or may not have undergone extensive operative procedures and is often mobile. Radiographically, the involved tooth and its adjacent teeth may show the presence of generalized vertical and horizontal bone loss along the root surfaces and periapical lesions isolated to that tooth. A tooth with true combined lesions is unresponsive to cold, heat, electricity, or cavity tests. Unlike a lesion of pulpal origin, a defect of this type is wide and V-shaped.[57] Periodontal examinations and probing of a tooth with a combined lesion reveal the presence of plaque, calculus, periodontitis, and wide and conical periodontal pockets characteristic of periodontal defects of periodontal disease origin.

Treatment and Prognosis

Treatment of true combined lesions consists of endodontic and periodontal treatments (see Fig. 7.22, *B*). The overall prognosis for the affected tooth depends on the prognosis for each individual lesion. If the periapical and periodontal lesions communicate, successful root canal treatment eliminates perpetuation of the lesion of pulpal origin and converts the combined lesion into a defect of periodontal origin. Therefore, the prognosis for the affected tooth depends primarily on the outcome of periodontal therapy. Generally, however, the prognosis of such conditions is guarded.

Secondary Endodontic-Periodontic Defects

Theoretically, long-standing defects of pulpal or periodontic origin can be converted into combined lesions.[71,72] Hiatt has speculated that a long-standing defect of pulpal origin can become a self-sustaining true periodontal defect.[73] This then becomes a true combined lesion, which requires adjunctive periodontal treatment in addition to root canal treatment. However, there is no evidence that this occurs. Clinical observations show that "old" defects of pulpal origin resolve successfully with root canal treatment without adjunctive periodontal treatment. Long-standing periodontal defects of periodontal origin may also cause pulpal necrosis, although this is a rare phenomenon. If this happens, the periodontal defect becomes a true combined lesion that requires root canal and periodontic treatments.

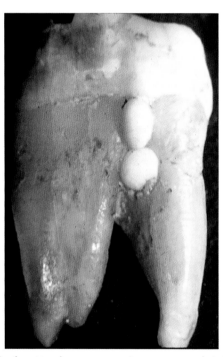

Fig. 7.19 An enamel spur can create a narrow pocket simulating a lesion of pulpal origin in multirooted teeth.

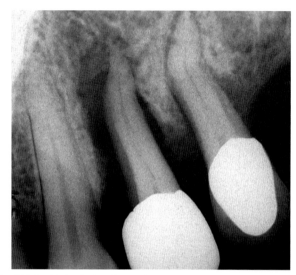

Fig. 7.21 Periapical radiograph of left maxillary premolar region reveals the presence of severe periodontal lesions in this area with generalized vertical and horizontal bone loss along the root surfaces.

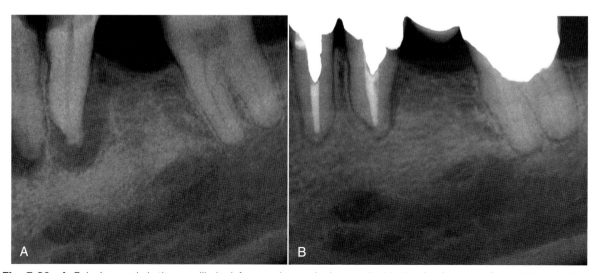

Fig. 7.20 **A,** Pulpal necrosis in the mandibular left second premolar has resulted in the development of a periodontal defect on the distal aspect of this tooth. **B,** Complete cleaning, shaping, and obturation of the root canal system in this tooth resulted in resolution of the lesion a year later.

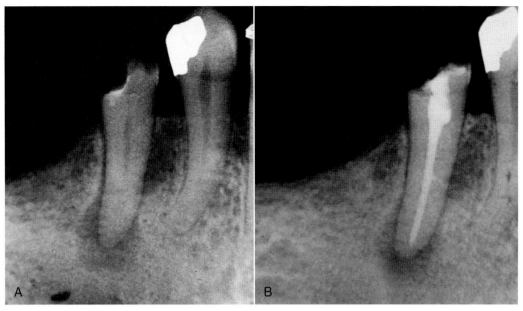

Fig. 7.22 **A,** A true combined endodontic-periodontic lesion is observed in the second mandibular premolar. **B,** Endodontic and periodontal treatments of this tooth resulted in the decrease of these lesions in 6 months.

REFERENCES

1. Kakehashi S, Stanley HR, Fitzgerald RJ: The effects of surgical exposures of dental pulps in germ-free and conventional laboratory rats, *Oral Surg Oral Med Oral Pathol* 20:340, 1965.
2. Bergenholtz G: Micro-organisms from necrotic pulp of traumatized teeth, *Odontol Revy* 25:347, 1974.
3. Sundqvist G: Bacteriological studies of necrotic dental pulps, odontol doctoral dissertation no 7, Umeå, Sweden, 1976, University of Umeå.
4. Möller ÅJR, Fabricius L, Dahlén G, et al: Influence on periapical tissues of indigenous oral bacteria and necrotic pulp tissue in monkeys, *Scand J Dent Res* 89:475, 1981.
5. Fabricius L, Dahlén G, Öhman AE, et al: Predominant indigenous oral bacteria isolated from infected root canals after varied times of closure, *Scand J Dent Res* 90:134, 1982.
6. Kantz WE, Henry CA: Isolation and classification of anaerobic bacteria from intact pulp chambers of non-vital teeth in man, *Arch Oral Biol* 19:91, 1974.
7. Swanson K, Madison S: An evaluation of coronal microleakage in endodontically treated teeth. I. Time periods, *J Endod* 13:56, 1987.
8. Madison S, Swanson K, Chiles S: An evaluation of coronal microleakage in endodontically treated teeth. II. Sealer types, *J Endod* 13:109, 1987.
9. Madison S, Wilcox LR: An evaluation of coronal microleakage in endodontically treated teeth. III. In vivo study, *J Endod* 14:455, 1988.
10. Torabinejad M, Ung B, Kettering JD: In vitro bacterial penetration of coronally unsealed endodontically treated teeth, *J Endod* 16:566, 1990.
11. Magura ME, Kafrawy AH, Brown CE Jr, et al: Human saliva coronal microleakage in obturated root canals: an in vitro study, *J Endod* 17:324, 1991.
12. Torabinejad M, Shabahang S: Pulp and periapical pathosis. In Torabinejad M, Walton RE, editors: *Endodontics: principles and practice*, ed 4, St Louis, 2009, Saunders/Elsevier.
13. Seymour GJ: Possible mechanisms involved in the immunoregulation of chronic inflammatory periodontal disease, *J Dent Res* 66:2, 1987.
14. Holland GR, Torabinejad M: The dental pulp and periradicular tissues. In Torabinejad M, Walton RE, editors: *Endodontics: principles and practice*, ed 4, St Louis, 2009, Saunders/Elsevier.

15. Hess W: *The anatomy of the root canals of the teeth of the permanent dentition*, London, 1925, John Bale Sons, Danielsson.
16. Green D: Morphology of the pulp cavity of the permanent teeth, *Oral Surg Oral Med Oral Pathol* 8:743, 1955.
17. Seltzer S, Bender IB, Ziontz M: The interrelationship of pulp and periodontal disease, *Oral Surg Oral Med Oral Pathol* 16:1474, 1963.
18. DeDeus DD: Frequency, location, and direction of the labial secondary and accessory canals, *J Endod* 1:361, 1975.
19. Burch JG, Hulen S: A study of the presence of accessory foramina and the topography of molar furcations, *Oral Surg Oral Med Oral Pathol* 38:451, 1974.
20. Vertucci FJ, Anthony RL: A scanning electron microscopic investigation of accessory foramina in the furcation and pulp chamber floor of molar teeth, *Oral Surg Oral Med Oral Pathol* 62:312, 1986.
21. Langeland K, Rodrigues H, Dowden W: Periodontal disease, bacteria and pulpal histopathology, *Oral Surg Oral Med Oral Pathol* 37:257, 1974.
22. Nicholls E: Lateral radicular disease due to labial branching of the root canal, *Oral Surg Oral Med Oral Pathol* 16:837, 1963.
23. Czarnecki R, Schilder H: A histological evaluation of the human pulp in teeth with varying degrees of periodontal disease, *J Endod* 5:242, 1979.
24. Torabinejad M, Kiger RD: A histologic evaluation of dental pulp tissue of a patient with periodontal disease, *Oral Surg Oral Med Oral Pathol* 59:198, 1985.
25. Pineda F, Kuttler Y: Mesiodistal and buccolingual roentgenographic investigation of 7,275 root canals, *Oral Surg Oral Med Oral Pathol* 33:101, 1972.
26. Mjör IA, Nordahl I: The density and branching of dentinal tubules in human teeth, *Arch Oral Biol* 41:401, 1996.
27. Garberoglio R, Brännström M: Scanning electron microscopic investigation of human dentinal tubules, *Arch Oral Biol* 21:355, 1976.
28. Ando N, Hoshino E: Predominant obligate anaerobes invading the deep layers of root canal dentine, *Int Endod J* 23:20, 1990.
29. Armitage GC, Ryder MI, Wilcox SE: Cemental changes in teeth with heavily infected root canals, *J Endod* 9:127, 1983.

30. Sen BH, Piskin B, Demirci T: Observation of bacteria and fungi in infected root canals and dentinal tubules by SEM, *Endod Dent Traumatol* 11:6, 1995.
31. Horiba N, Maekawa Y, Matsumoto T, et al: A study of the distribution of endotoxin in the dentinal wall of infected root canals, *J Endod* 16:331, 1990.
32. Akpata ES, Blechman H: Bacterial invasion of pulpal dentin wall in vitro, *J Dent Res* 61:435, 1982.
33. Haapasalo M, Ørstavik D: In vitro infection and disinfection of dentinal tubules, *J Dent Res* 66:1375, 1987.
34. Ørstavik D, Haapasalo M: Disinfection by endodontic irrigants and dressings of experimentally infected dentinal tubules, *Endod Dent Traumatol* 6:142, 1990.
35. Siqueira JF Jr, de Uzeda M, Fonseca MEF: A scanning electron microscopic evaluation of in vitro dentinal tubule penetration by selected anaerobic bacteria, *J Endod* 22:308, 1996.
36. Perez F, Rochd T, Lodter J-P, et al: In vitro study of the penetration of three bacterial strains into root dentine, *Oral Surg Oral Med Oral Pathol* 76:97, 1993.
37. Peters LB, Wesselink PR, Buijs JF, et al: Viable bacteria in root dentinal tubules of teeth with apical periodontitis, *J Endod* 27:76, 2001.
38. Muller CJ, Van Wyk CW: The amelo-cemental junction, *J Dent Assoc S Afr* 39:799, 1984.
39. Bergenholtz G, Lindhe J: Effect of experimentally induced marginal periodontitis and periodontal scaling on the dental pulp, *J Clin Periodontol* 5:59, 1978.
40. Walton RE, Leonard L, Sharawy M, et al: Effects on pulp and dentin of iontophoresis of sodium fluoride on exposed roots in dogs, *Oral Surg Oral Med Oral Pathol* 48:454, 1979.
41. Pashley DH: Dynamics of the pulpo-dentin complex, *Crit Rev Oral Biol Med* 7:104, 1996.
42. Nagaoka S, Miyazaki Y, Liu HJ, et al: Bacterial invasion into dentinal tubules of human vital and nonvital teeth, *J Endod* 21:70, 1995.
43. Siqueira JF, Rocas I: Endodontic microbiology. In Torabinejad M, Walton RE, editors: *Endodontics: principles and practice*, ed 4, St Louis, 2009, Saunders/Elsevier.

44. Baumgartner JC: Microbiologic aspects of endodontic infections, *J Calif Dent Assoc* 32:459, 2004.
45. Molven O, Olsen I, Kerekes K: Scanning electron microscopy of bacteria in the apical part of root canals in permanent teeth with periapical lesions, *Endod Dent Traumatol* 7:226, 1991.
46. Dahle UR, Tronstad L, Olsen I: Observation of an unusually large spirochete in endodontic infection, *Oral Microbiol Immunol* 8:251, 1993.
47. Siqueira JF Jr, Rocas IN, Souto R, et al: Checkerboard DNA-DNA hybridization analysis of endodontic infections, *Oral Surg Oral Med Oral Pathol Oral Radiol Endod* 89:744, 2000.
48. Rocas IN, Siqueira JF Jr, Santos KR, et al: "Red complex" (*Bacteroides forsythus, Porphyromonas gingivalis,* and *Treponema denticola*) in endodontic infections: a molecular approach, *Oral Surg Oral Med Oral Pathol Oral Radiol Endod* 91:468, 2001.
49. Jung IY, Choi BK, Kum KY, et al: Identification of oral spirochetes at the species level and their association with other bacteria in endodontic infections, *Oral Surg Oral Med Oral Pathol Oral Radiol Endod* 92:329, 2001.
50. Siqueira JF, Sen BH: Fungi in endodontic infections, *Oral Surg Oral Med Oral Pathol Oral Radiol Endod* 97:632, 2004.
51. Sen BH, Piskin B, Demirci T: Observations of bacteria and fungi in infected root canals and dentinal tubules by SEM, *Endod Dent Traumatol* 11:6, 1995.
52. Nair PNR, Sjogren U, Krey G, et al: Intraradicular bacteria and fungi in root-filled, asymptomatic human teeth with therapy resistant periapical lesions: a long term light and electron microscopic follow-up study, *J Endod* 16:580, 1990.
53. Waltimo TM, Siren EK, Torkko HL, et al: Fungi in therapy-resistant apical periodontitis, *Int Endod J* 30:96, 1997.
54. Contreras A, Nowzari H, Slots J: Herpes viruses in periodontal pocket and gingival tissue specimens, *Oral Microbiol Immunol* 15:15, 2000.
55. Sabeti M, Simon JH, Nowzari H, et al: Cytomegalovirus and Epstein-Barr virus active infection in periapical lesions of teeth with intact crowns, *J Endod* 29:321, 2003.
56. Contreras A, Slots J: Herpesvirus in human periodontal disease, *J Periodont Res* 35:3, 2000.
57. Bergenholtz G: Interrelationship between periodontics and endodontics. In Lindhe J, editor: *Textbook of clinical periodontology*, Copenhagen, 1983, Munksgaard.
58. Bender IB, Seltzer S: The effect of periodontal disease on the pulp, *Oral Surg Oral Med Oral Pathol* 33:458, 1972.
59. Kinane DF: Causation and pathogenesis of periodontal disease, *Periodontol 2000* 25:8, 2001.
60. Socransky S, Haffajee A: Evidence of bacterial aetiology: a historical perspective, *Periodontol 2000* 5:7, 1994.
61. Zambon JJ: Periodontal diseases: microbial factors, *Ann Periodontol* 1:879, 1996.
62. Page RC, Offenbacher S, Schroeder HE, et al: Advances in the pathogenesis of periodontitis: summary of developments, clinical implications and future directions, *Periodontol 2000* 14:216, 1997.
63. Page RC, Kornman KS: The pathogenesis of human periodontitis: an introduction, *Periodontol 2000* 14:9, 1997.
64. Hart TC, Kornman KS: Genetic factors in the pathogenesis of periodontitis, *Periodontol 2000* 14:202, 1997.
65. Schenkein HA, Van Dyke TE: Early-onset periodontitis: systemic aspects of etiology and pathogenesis, *Periodontol 2000* 6:7, 1994.
66. Mazur B, Massler M: Influence of periodontal disease on the dental pulp, *Oral Surg Oral Med Oral Pathol* 17:592, 1964.
67. Jansson L, Ehnevid H, Lindskog S, et al: The influence of endodontic infection on progression of marginal bone loss in periodontitis, *J Clin Periodontol* 22:729, 1995.
68. Jansson L, Ehnevid H: The influence of endodontic infection on periodontal status in mandibular molars, *J Clin Periodontol* 69:1392, 1998.
69. Miyashita H, Bergenholtz G, Gröndahl K: Impact of endodontic conditions on marginal bone loss, *J Clin Periodontol* 69:158, 1998.
70. Harrington GW: The perio-endo question: differential diagnosis, *Dent Clin North Am* 23:673, 1979.
71. Simon JHS, Glick DH, Frank AL: The relationship of endodontic-periodontic lesions, *J Clin Periodontol* 43:202, 1972.
72. Rotstein I, Simon JHS: Diagnosis, prognosis and decision-making in the treatment of combined periodontal-endodontic lesions, *Periodontol 2000* 34:165, 2004.
73. Hiatt W: Pulpal periodontal disease, *J Clin Periodontol* 48:598, 1977.

Longitudinal tooth fractures

Eric M. Rivera, Richard E. Walton

CHAPTER OUTLINE

Incidence

Categories

Craze Lines

Fractured Cusp

Cracked Tooth

Split Tooth

Vertical Root Fracture

LEARNING OBJECTIVES

After reading this chapter, the student should be able to:

1. Define and differentiate craze line, cusp fracture, cracked tooth, split tooth, and vertical root fracture.
2. Describe the causes of these fractures of tooth structure.
3. List and describe the five considerations (characteristics) of fractures in dentin.

4. Describe in general each of the five categories of fracture regarding incidence, pathogenesis, clinical features, etiologies, diagnosis, treatment, prognosis, and prevention.
5. Identify patients with difficult tooth fracture situations who should be considered for referral.

Cracked teeth and their related entities, in addition to vertical root fractures, are longitudinal fractures of the crown and/or root that grow over time. These contrast with horizontal fractures, which predominate in anterior teeth and result from impact trauma. Longitudinal (vertical) fractures occur in all tooth groups and are caused by occlusal forces and dental procedures. *Longitudinal* implies a vertical direction and a time component.[1]

There remains relatively little research on longitudinal tooth fractures, particularly on clinical outcomes related to diagnosis and treatment. Most treatment modalities are based on opinion and anecdotal information.[2,3] Therefore, many recommendations have not been substantiated in controlled clinical trials but are based on experience. This chapter deals with longitudinal fractures in the vertical plane, or long axis of the crown or root, that propagate over time.[1,4]

Treating longitudinal fractures is usually challenging. Sometimes these fractures are not difficult to diagnose or manage, whereas at other times they are so devastating that the involved tooth must be extracted. Notwithstanding, many situations present with significant problems in both diagnosis and treatment; these patients should be considered for referral.

INCIDENCE

The incidence of longitudinal fractures is increasing. There are several reasons for this unfortunate occurrence. One is the increasing age of patients with decreased numbers of tooth extractions. Therefore, more teeth undergo complex procedures and are present for a longer time. These procedures include restorative and endodontic treatments that remove dentin, thereby compromising internal strength. Excessive uses of ethylenediaminetetraacetic acid (EDTA), bleaching materials, and calcium hydroxide have also been recently implicated,[5-7] although a recent systematic review was inconclusive whether calcium hydroxide exposure for 1 month or less had a negative effect.[8] Also, the teeth absorb external forces, usually occlusal, that exceed the strength of dentin and gradually alter tooth structure. When the destructive force is beyond the elastic limit of dentin or enamel, a fracture occurs.[9] Therefore, the longer a tooth is present and the more forces it undergoes, the greater the chances of an eventual fracture. Another reason for the increased incidence is clinicians' greater awareness and better diagnosis and identification of the problem. Such fractures are not confined to elderly patients and do not occur only in restored or endodontically treated teeth.[10-13]

CATEGORIES

There are five categories of longitudinal fractures. From least to most severe, they are (1) craze lines, (2) fractured cusp, (3) cracked tooth, (4) split tooth, and (5) vertical root fracture. Although these fractures differ, they are often confused or combined in clinical articles.[14-18] This leads to misunderstanding, with incorrect diagnosis and inappropriate treatment. All of these could be referred to as vertical cracks or fractures, but each category is distinct with regard to incidence, pathogenesis, clinical features, etiologies, diagnosis, treatment, prognosis, and prevention. Epidemiologic research in the future to establish better ways to prevent these longitudinal fractures can benefit from an analysis of these distinctions. Table 8.1 identifies the five entities by findings, diagnostic methods, and treatment. The reader is referred to this table throughout the chapter.

Fractures occur primarily in two areas, the crown and the root. Either area may be the site of initiation and the region of principal damage. In the crown (usually extending to the root), these lesions take the form of a craze line, fractured cusp, cracked tooth, or split tooth (Fig. 8.1); the latter three usually extend to the root. Roots show vertical root fracture

(Fig. 8.2). Clinical determination and treatment of longitudinal cracks and fractures are based on location and separable segments.[4]

CRAZE LINES

Craze lines are common, particularly in permanent teeth in adults (Box 8.1). They usually extend over marginal ridges and along buccal and lingual surfaces in posterior teeth, but also appear as long vertical defects from the incisal to the cervical aspect on anterior teeth (Fig. 8.3). Craze lines are confined to enamel.[2,3,14]

Craze lines occur naturally, but their incidence increases in patients who have had restorations or impact injuries. It is

Table 8.1 Categories of longitudinal tooth fractures

	Craze line	Fractured cusp	Cracked tooth	Split tooth	Vertical root fracture
Location	Enamel only Common on marginal ridges	Crown and cervical margin of root	Crown only or crown to root extension (depth varies)	Crown and root; extension to proximal surfaces	Root only
Direction	Occlusogingival	Mesiodistal and faciolingual	Mesiodistal	Mesiodistal	Faciolingual
Origination	Occlusal surface	Occlusal surface	Occlusal surface	Occlusal surface	Root (any level)
Etiologies	Occlusal forces, thermocycling	Undermined cusp, damaging habits	Damaging habits, weakened tooth structure	Damaging habits, weakened tooth structure	Wedging posts, obturation forces, excessive root-dentin removal
Symptoms	Asymptomatic	Sharp pain with mastication and with cold	Highly variable	Pain with mastication	None to slight
Signs	None	None of significance	Variable	Separable segments, periodontal abscess	Variable
Identification	Direct visualization, transillumination	Visualize, remove restoration	Biting, remove restoration	Remove restoration	Reflect flap and transilluminate
Diagnostic tests	None	Visible fractures of cusps, biting test, transillumination	Transillumination, staining, wedge segments (inseparable), isolated/narrow perio probing, biting test, magnification	Wedge segments (separable)	Reflect flap and transilluminate
Treatment	No treatment needed, esthetic	Remove cusp and/or restore	Root canal treatment depends on pulpal and periradicular diagnosis; restore with full cuspal coverage	Variable, must remove one segment, restore, or extract	Remove tooth or fractured root; consider fixed and/or removable bridge or implant
Prognosis	Very good	Very good	Always questionable to poor	Maintain intact (hopeless) Remove segment (variable)	Hopeless for fractured root
Prevention	None needed	Place conservative Class II restorations, coronal protection (onlay undermined cusps)	Eliminate damaging habits (e.g., ice chewing), coronal protection (onlay undermined cusps)	Eliminate damaging habits, coronal protection (onlay cusps)	Minimize root-dentin removal, avoid wedging posts, reduce condensation forces

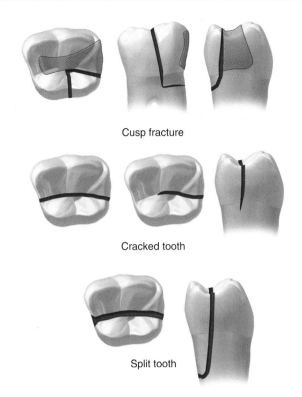

Cusp fracture

Cracked tooth

Split tooth

Fig. 8.1 The three fracture types that originate occlusally and then extend toward the root.

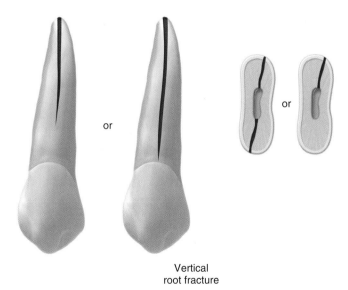

or

or

Vertical
root fracture

Fig. 8.2 This fracture begins and ends on the root. Usually the fracture extends facially and lingually but may not extend to both surfaces or from apical to cervical.

unknown whether they are precursors to dentin fractures (but this is unlikely). Craze lines are unimportant other than as a common source of misidentification and confusion with cracked teeth.

FRACTURED CUSP

Fractured cusps are usually relatively easy to diagnose and treat and generally have a good prognosis (see Table 8.1).

Box 8.1   Considerations for Longitudinal Fractures

Patients must be informed of the following facts.
1. Longitudinal fractures are not diagnoses, they are findings. Pulpal and periradicular diagnoses are usually not affected by longitudinal fractures that do not communicate with the pulp. Longitudinal fractures with pulpal communication allow bacterial contamination, which affects pulpal and periapical diagnoses.
2. Longitudinal fractures result from excessive forces that are usually (but not always) long-term forces.
3. The presence or extent of the fracture may be difficult to identify clinically, because these fractures are often tiny and are not demonstrable until growth or expansion occurs. Also, they may be hidden under restorations or bone and gingiva and thus are not visible even after flap reflection.
4. With time, fracture spaces tend to acquire stains and become more visible.
5. Fractures have a tendency to grow, although initially they are very small. This propagation may be very slow. An analogy is a small crack in a windshield that may lengthen over months or years.
6. Signs and symptoms often are not present early but become manifest months, years, or decades after fracture initiation.

Incidence

Fractured cusps are more common than the other major entities discussed in this chapter, which is fortunate, because these are the least devastating and the most manageable.[2,3] This fracture occurs often in teeth with extensive caries or large restorations that do not protect undermined cusps.[19]

Pathogenesis

Cusp fractures are related to lack of cusp support, especially when restorations are placed after loss of tooth structure because of extensive caries. A confusing entity is the type of cusp fracture that occurs as the result of a traumatic injury, usually an upward blow to the mandible that results in a sharp impact between the maxillary and mandibular teeth. These fractures occur immediately (i.e., not over time), so they are technically not classified as longitudinal fractures, even though the end result is the loss of one or more cusps. As mentioned, the term *longitudinal* implies both a vertical direction and a time component. Fortunately, this mishap does not occur often. A single injury may cause fracture or loss of several cusps, particularly of the maxillary premolars.

Clinical Features

Cusp fractures are usually associated with a weakened marginal ridge in conjunction with an undermined cusp. These conditions compromise dentin support for the cusp, which is supplied primarily by the marginal ridge.[20] Either a single cusp or two cusps (in molars) are involved. The single-cusp fracture includes a mesiodistal and a faciolingual component (Fig. 8.4). Therefore, the crack lines (see Fig. 8.1) cross the marginal ridge and then extend down a facial or lingual groove and often into the cervical region parallel to the gingival margin (or somewhat subgingivally, which is more common). If two cusps are involved, the fracture lines are mesial and **123**

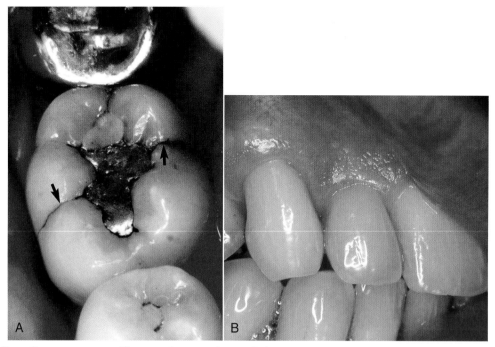

Fig. 8.3 Craze lines are common. These are fractures that are limited to the enamel and do not extend to dentin. **A,** This molar shows craze lines over marginal ridges and through buccal and lingual grooves *(arrows).* **B,** Vertical craze lines are common in anterior teeth, particularly in older patients.

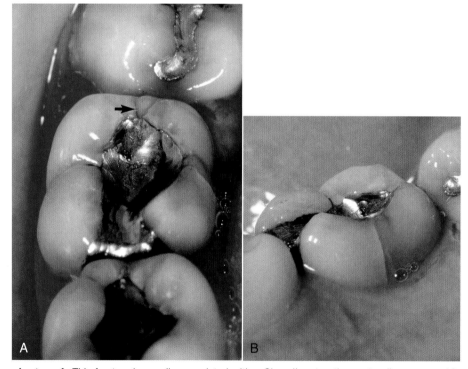

Fig. 8.4 Cusp fracture. **A,** This fracture is usually associated with a Class II restoration, extending across at least one marginal ridge *(arrow)* and often down a lingual or buccal surface **(B).** These fractures tend to acquire stain with time, are usually symptomatic, and stop light with transillumination.

distal, without a facial or lingual component. Two mesial or two distal cusps are seldom fractured together.

Cusp fractures are oblique shearing fractures that extend from the occlusal surface, often from a line angle at the base of a cavity (Fig. 8.5). The defect often includes the region of epithelial attachment and usually does not extend beyond the cervical third of the root.[21] Usually, there is no pulp exposure, particularly in older teeth with smaller pulp chambers.

Etiologies

Typically, there is a history of extensive deep interproximal caries or a subsequent Class II restoration. Occasionally, these

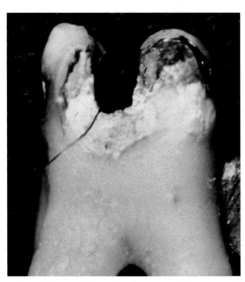

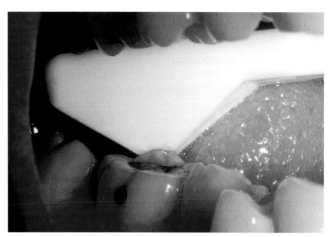

Fig. 8.6 Special diagnostic biting instruments, such as a Tooth Slooth, are placed on one cusp at a time while the patient grinds with the opposing teeth. Sharp pain on pressure or release may indicate a cusp fracture or cracked tooth.

Fig. 8.5 Cusp fracture. Typically, the separation occurs from the line angle of the cavity to the cervical surface.

cusp fractures occur in nonrestored teeth with extensive undermining caries.

Diagnosis
Subjective Findings
Frequently, the patient reports brief, sharp pain on mastication. There may be sensitivity to temperature changes, particularly cold. Often the pain is more distinct with masticatory release (not with closure, but with separation of the teeth after biting). Pain is neither severe nor spontaneous and occurs only on stimulus. Interestingly, the symptoms are often relieved when the cusp finally breaks off.

Objective Tests
The most indicative test is biting.[13] The patient may close onto a cotton swab applicator, a rubber polishing (Burlew) wheel, or a specially designed bite-testing instrument (Tooth Slooth or Frac Finder) (Fig. 8.6). An occlusal, gnashing force on the involved cusp or upon quickly opening the mouth elicits pain.[22] Patients ordinarily respond to pulp testing, unless the pulp has been exposed to bacteria for prolonged periods, which may result in pulp necrosis.

Radiographic Findings
Radiographs are not useful, because cusp fractures are usually not visible radiographically.

Other Findings
The restoration often has to be removed to observe the underlying dentin. The fracture may then be readily visible, or it may be disclosed by either staining or transillumination.[23,24] Older fractures may have already acquired stain (see Fig. 8.4). The cusp fracture line usually originates at the cavity floor at a line angle. A surgical microscope is very useful for identification.

Treatment
Retaining the fractured cusp is often not indicated. The cusp is removed, and the tooth is restored as appropriate. The restoration will probably be a three-fourths or full crown extending apical or to the fracture margin. Root canal treatment is often not required, because the pulp is usually not exposed. Occasionally, restoration is unnecessary, and the tooth functions minus a cusp.

If the cusp is not mobile, the fracture line probably does not extend to a root surface subgingivally. In these cases, the cusp need not be removed, and a cuspally reinforced restoration should be placed to hold the segments.

Prognosis
Long-term success with cusp fractures is good, because these fractures tend to be shallow. They occasionally extend deeper, below the gingival attachment, and treatment of these fractures is more challenging. An approach to restoring deep-extending cusp fractures is described later in this chapter.

Prevention
Extensive removal of dentin support should be avoided. The width and particularly the depth of restorations should be minimized.[25] Restorations that wedge, such as inlays, require adequate dentin support. Cusps should be reduced and onlayed if undermined; both amalgam and gold onlays provide fracture resistance.[26-28] Composite resins that are bonded to enamel or dentin and improperly placed may shrink excessively on polymerization. This contraction may displace and weaken cusps, rendering them susceptible to occlusal forces and fracture.

Construction of a crown with a 1 to 2 mm ferrule appears to be the most important factor with respect to restoration.[29-32]

In terms of bonding, adhesive resins, if placed with special techniques, may reinforce weakened cusps.[33-35] However, resin-based composites are equivalent to amalgams with regard to the occurrence of cusp fractures.[36-39] Therefore, bonded restorations may provide only temporary reinforcement.[40]

CRACKED TOOTH

Cracked teeth are defined as an incomplete fracture initiated from the crown and extending subgingivally, usually directed **125** mesiodistally.[12] The fracture may extend through either or both of the marginal ridges and through the proximal surfaces. The fracture is located in the crown portion of the tooth only or may extend from the crown to the proximal root (see Table 8.1). Cracked teeth are also described as incomplete (greenstick) fractures, which indicates their form.[14,23,41] Cracked tooth is a variation of the cusp fracture, but the associated fracture is centered more occlusally (see Fig. 8.1). The effects of cracked teeth tend to be more devastating, because the extent and direction of these fractures are more centered and more apical (see Table 8.1).

Incidence

The occurrence of cracked tooth is unknown but is apparently increasing.[14,42,43] Ten percent of teeth referred to endodontists in one study were determined to have a crack involving one or both marginal ridges.[43] Cracked teeth are predominantly seen in older patients, although they may occur at any age in adults.[10,12] The longevity and complexity of restorations are related factors, although cracked teeth often are minimally restored or not restored at all.[12,14] Mastication for many years, particularly of hard objects, is also a factor. Continued and repeated forces finally cause fatigue of the tooth structure, resulting in a small fracture that is followed by continued growth of the fracture.[44]

The teeth usually involved are the mandibular second molars (both restored and nonrestored), followed closely by the mandibular first molars and then by either the maxillary second molars or the maxillary premolars, depending on the study.[12,13,43,45] Anterior teeth occasionally develop true cracks, usually as a result of weakened tooth structure from a traumatic impact or from restorations. Cracks rarely occur on mandibular premolars. Furthermore, Class I restored teeth fracture as often as do Class II restored teeth, particularly molars. Therefore, the phenomenon is not always dependent on violation of tooth structure by access preparations, caries, or restorations.[22,46] There has been speculation that teeth treated by root canals are more brittle and weakened and therefore are more susceptible to fracture. However, the evidence does not support this assumption.[20,47-51]

Pathogenesis

As stated previously, cracks in teeth tend to depend on time and the patient's habits. Obviously, forces in excess of dentin strength are responsible. These forces are greater in the posterior region (i.e., close to the fulcrum of the mandible), invoking the "nutcracker" effect.[12,52]

Although occlusal anatomy (deep fissures or prominent or functional cusps) and occlusal dysfunction might render a tooth more susceptible to cracking, these factors are only speculative, because no relationship to cracked teeth has been demonstrated.

Clinical Features

Cracks in teeth are almost invariably mesiodistal fractures[12] (Fig. 8.7), although mandibular molars occasionally (rarely) fracture toward the faciolingual surface. The diagnosis of a faciolingual cracked molar is a common misinterpretation because of visualization of facial and lingual fractures (see Fig. 8.3, A). These are actually craze lines, which follow the buccal and lingual grooves.

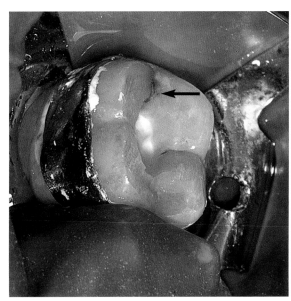

Fig. 8.7 Cracked tooth. The fracture extends along the cavity floor and across both marginal ridges but is most evident on the distal side *(arrow)*. Fractures in the mesiodistal direction are by far the most common.

Cracks cross one or both marginal ridges. They generally shear toward the facial or lingual side toward a root surface, usually lingual. Because the fracture begins on the occlusal surface, it grows from this surface toward the cervical surface and down the root. The more centered the fracture (initiated on the midocclusal surface), the more it has a tendency to extend deeper before it shears toward the root surface. The fracture is considered greenstick because it is incomplete (either to the mesial or distal surface) or does not extend to the facial or lingual root surface.[14] Wedging forces produce no separable segments that would indicate a complete fracture, as with split teeth (see the section on split tooth later in the chapter). The direct midocclusal fracture may be very deep. On maxillary molars, it may extend toward the furcation (Fig. 8.8) or occasionally toward the apex on mandibular molars (Fig. 8.9).

The fracture may or may not include the pulp. The more centered the fracture, the greater the chance of pulp exposure now or later. Occasionally, fractures oriented toward the faciolingual surface shear away from the pulp, although this is not likely and difficult to determine clinically. Therefore many cracked teeth require root canal treatment, preferably before restoration for coronal protection. Wedging forces must be minimized during both root canal treatment and restoration to avoid aggravating the fracture.

Etiologies

Cracked teeth are often found in patients who chew hard, brittle substances (ice, unpopped popcorn kernels, hard candy, and so on). These patients may have prominent masticatory muscles and show excessive occlusal wear as a result of heavy occlusal forces.[52]

However, cracked teeth may occur in patients who do not have these damaging parafunctional habits and who do not display heavy musculature. If these teeth are restored, the

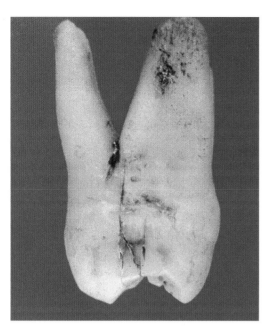

Fig. 8.8 Cracked tooth. The fracture extends mesiodistally across the marginal ridge and down the proximal close to the furcation (greenstick fracture). The extent of the crack is usually difficult to determine due to the position of the crack below the periodontium and the close approximation of adjacent teeth.

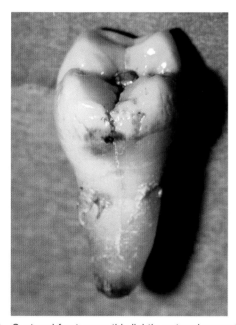

Fig. 8.9 Centered fracture on this lightly restored second molar extends toward the apex. Treatment of these fractures is hopeless.

restorations may be Class I or a deep Class II. Interestingly, cracks associated with wide Class II restorations are more likely to be cusp fractures, and their effects are not as devastating.[53]

Thermal stresses are also thought to be a cause of fractures, although the evidence on this is inconclusive. Supposedly, differences in expansion and contraction of restorations versus tooth structure may weaken and crack dentin.[54]

Diagnosis

Cracked teeth show a variety of test results, radiographic findings, and signs and symptoms, depending on many factors. This variety and unpredictability often make the cracked tooth a perplexing diagnostic and treatment entity. Again, cracks are findings only, and the pulpal/periradicular diagnosis is determined as in other clinical situations.

Subjective Findings

Often cracked teeth manifest as the so-called cracked tooth syndrome.[52] This syndrome is characterized by acute pain on mastication (pressure or release) of grainy, tough foods and sharp, brief pain with cold.[53,55,56] These findings are also related to cusp fracture. However, cracked teeth may present with a variety of symptoms, ranging from slight to very severe spontaneous pain consistent with irreversible pulpitis, pulp necrosis, or apical periodontitis.[24] Even an acute apical abscess, with or without swelling or a draining sinus tract, may be present if the pulp has undergone necrosis. In other words, once the fracture has extended to and exposed the pulp, severe pulp and/or periapical pathosis will be present. This explains the variation in signs and symptoms, which can be confusing and misleading in determining the diagnosis; it also prevents these signs and symptoms, and therefore are not to be termed a syndrome.[57]

Objective Tests

Pulp and periapical tests have variable results. The pulp is usually responsive (vital)[52] but may be nonresponsive (necrosis). Periapical tests also vary, but usually pain is not elicited with percussion or palpation if the pulp is vital. Directional percussion is also advocated. Percussion that separates the crack may cause pain. Opposite-direction percussion usually is asymptomatic. This pain is probably related to stimulation of the periodontal ligament proprioceptors.

Radiographic Findings

Because of the mesiodistal direction of the fracture, it is not visible radiographically. Radiographs are made to help determine the pulp/periapical status. Usually there are no significant findings, although occasionally different entities occur. At times, loss of proximal bone (horizontal, vertical, or furcal) is related to the fracture; bone loss increases as the severity of the crack increases.

Newer methods of analysis are currently being studied, such as cone beam computed tomography (CBCT), ultrasound, and infrared thermography, to help identify longitudinal fractures in a nondestructive fashion.[58-71]

Other Findings

Craze lines in posterior teeth that cross marginal ridges or buccal and lingual surfaces must be differentiated with transillumination. With craze lines, transilluminated light from the facial or lingual surface is not blocked or reflected, and the entire tooth in a faciolingual orientation is illuminated.

When a crack is suspected, it is important to try to visualize the length and location of the fracture. Direct inspection (again, a microscope is helpful), staining, and transillumination are usually effective.[24,72,73] Occlusal and proximal restorations are first removed.[74] Then transillumination (Fig. 8.10), which often shows a characteristic abrupt blockage of

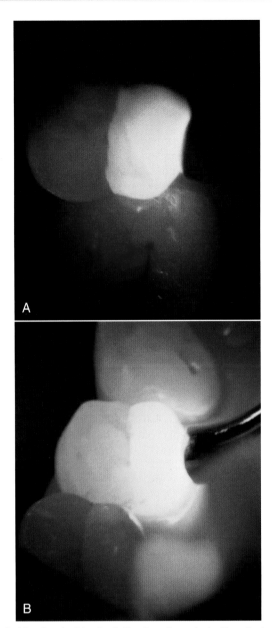

Fig. 8.10 Cracked tooth. **A,** Fracture through dentin reflects transilluminated light, showing abrupt change in brightness. **B,** For comparison, an adjacent noncracked premolar with a craze line transmits light readily.

transmitted light, is performed. With transillumination the portion of the tooth where the light originates illuminates to the fracture. A fracture contains a thin air space, which does not readily transmit light. Therefore, the crack (or fracture) blocks or reflects the light, causing the other portion to appear dark.

Staining with methylene blue, iodine, or caries detection dyes may also disclose the fracture, although not predictably. A cotton pledget soaked with methylene blue or other dye is placed against the cavity floor. The dye may be washed away immediately to reveal the crack, or it may be held in by a temporary sealing, such as intermediate restorative material (IRM). The temporary restoration and pledget are removed after a few days. The dye may have been in contact with the

crack long enough to disclose it clearly (Fig. 8.11). Patients should be advised that the tooth may temporarily turn blue (Fig. 8.11); they may wish to forego this test.

Viewing with a surgical microscope is particularly useful for identifying both the presence and the extent of the fracture (Fig. 8.12).

Occasionally (particularly if the crack is centered), an access preparation is necessary to disclose the extent of the crack (see Fig. 8.12). After the chamber roof and coronal pulp have been removed, the floor is transilluminated as for a fracture (not to be confused with anatomic grooves). Sealing in a disclosing dye for a few days may be helpful. Again, visualization with the microscope allows for more definitive identification.

Removal of the fracture line in the area of the cavity floor that would include an ideal endodontic access opening is helpful in removing and/or determining the apical extent of the crack and assessing whether the pulp is involved (Fig. 8.13). However, the fracture is small and invisible at the furthest extent (even after staining). Therefore, the crack probably continues deeper into dentin than can be visualized. Removal of the fracture line in the proximal portion of the tooth may provide information on the extent but also may cause the tooth to become nonrestorable. Both of these procedures, particularly removal of proximal marginal ridge and tooth structure, remove sound tooth structure, thereby decreasing tooth strength and resistance to fracture.[75,76]

Wedging forces are used to determine whether the tooth segments are separable (see Fig. 8.13). If a fracture is detected, any restorations are removed and an instrument is placed in the cavity with moderate pressure exerted on opposing walls to try to separate the segments. If no movement is detected, the classification is a *cracked tooth;* if the segments separate, it is a *split tooth* (discussed later). The patient must be informed of possible sequelae (i.e., hearing a cracking sound and/or feeling pain) before this test is performed. Clinicians and patients may be hesitant to perform wedging of the segments for fear of splitting the tooth iatrogenically or causing pain. However, if controlled force exacerbates the crack, the tooth is predisposed to a later split anyway, and the patient is best served to know this expeditiously.

Periodontal probing is important and may disclose the approximate depth and severity of the fracture. Removal of interproximal restorations is helpful, because it allows improved access for placement of the periodontal probe. However, subgingival fractures often do not create a probing defect. Therefore, the absence of deep probing does not preclude a cracked tooth. The presence of deep probing is serious and indicates a poorer prognosis.[77] Recording of probing depths on the mesial and distal portions of the tooth for a total of eight points of probing must be included with the other, normal six points of probing.

Selective biting on objects is helpful (see the earlier section on cusp fractures; also see Fig. 8.6), particularly when pain is reported on mastication.[13]

Treatment

Six important considerations for longitudinal fractures are listed in Box 8.1. When both clinician and patient are aware of the complications and questionable outcomes, a treatment plan is formulated. Extraction is a reasonable solution in many situations. Much depends on the nature (depth and location)

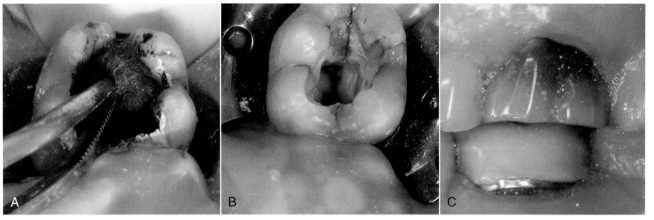

Fig. 8.11 **A,** Disclosing solution on a cotton pellet (in this case, methylene blue) is placed in the cavity for a few minutes or sealed in for a week. **B,** This technique may clearly disclose the fracture and its extent. **C,** Staining solutions may discolor the tooth.

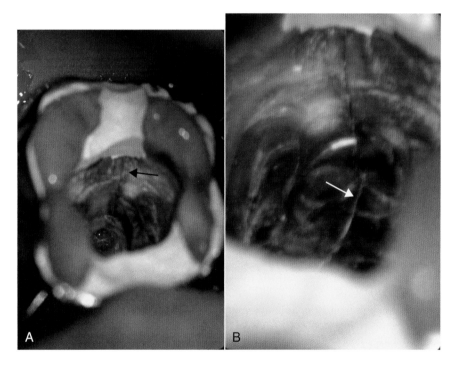

Fig. 8.12 Evaluation with magnification and illumination. **A,** To minimize movement of segments, an orthodontic band has been placed. The access is now completed to determine the depth of the fracture *(arrow)*. **B,** The fracture *(arrow)* extends across the pulpal floor. The prognosis is poor.

of the fracture (Box 8.2). Again, the segments must not separate on wedging. If they do not separate, there are many treatment alternatives for retaining the tooth intact. If the occlusal-proximal fracture is centered in the faciolingual aspect and involves the floor of the cavity preparation, there are treatment options. If there are no symptoms of irreversible pulpitis or pulpal necrosis, a crown may be placed, although some of these teeth eventually manifest irreversible pulpitis or pulp necrosis,[43,78] and they then require endodontic treatment through the crown.

Further Examination

After endodontic access, the pulp chamber floor is examined. If the fracture extends through the chamber floor, generally further treatment is hopeless and extraction is preferred (see Fig. 8.12).[79] An exception is the maxillary molar, which may be hemisected along the fracture, saving half (or both halves) of the crown and supporting roots. Many of these treatments

are complex, and the patient should be considered for referral to an endodontist. If a partial fracture of the chamber floor is detected, the crown may be bound with a stainless steel or an orthodontic band (see Fig. 8.12) or a temporary crown to protect the cusps until final restoration is performed.[23,80] This also helps to determine whether symptoms decrease during root canal treatment. The rationale (unsupported) is that if pain symptoms are not relieved, the prognosis is significantly poorer and extraction may be necessary.

Restoration

If the fracture appears to be incomplete (not terminating on a root surface), the tooth is restored to bind the fractured segments (barrel stave effect) and also to protect the cusps. For a permanent restoration, a full crown is preferred, although an onlay with bevels may suffice. Posts and internally wedging foundations are to be avoided. Acid-etch dentin bonding resins may help to provide a foundation for the crown to

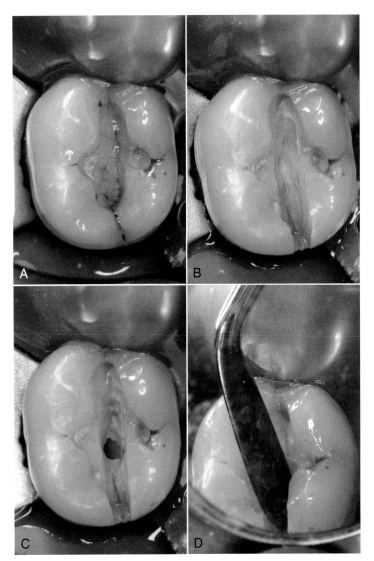

Fig. 8.13 **A,** Removal of amalgam restoration reveals cracked tooth in mesiodistal direction on the cavity floor. **B,** Removal of fracture line distally and also apically only in the area of the cavity floor that would include an ideal endodontic access opening. **C,** Further removal reveals fracture extending into pulp chamber. **D,** Wedging forces used to determine whether segments are mobile.

prevent crack propagation, although more research is necessary to support this concept.[81-83] Amalgam, which tends to expand and which requires a wedging effect with condensation, is not a good choice.

Prognosis

The overall prognosis depends on the situation but is always questionable at best. The patient is informed of the possible outcomes and the unpredictability of the duration of treatment. The fracture may continue to grow to become a split tooth, with devastating consequences, requiring tooth extraction or additional treatments (Fig. 8.14). Furthermore, the patient should be informed that cracks also may be present in other teeth and could manifest in the future.

In general, the more centered the origin of the fracture is on the occlusal surface, the poorer the long-term prognosis. These fractures tend to *remain* centered and grow deeper. The result is major damage to the tooth and periodontium. In other words, the cracked tooth may ultimately evolve to a split tooth or develop severe periodontal defects.

In one study, 20% of teeth with a cracked tooth and a pulpal diagnosis of reversible pulpitis referred back to the general dentist for crown placement resulted in progression to irreversible pulpitis or necrosis, with a subsequent need for endodontic therapy or extraction.[43] Similarly, another study found that teeth with reversible pulpitis due to cracks can be treated conservatively without endodontic treatment in about 80% of cases.[84]

Prevention

Generally, patients are encouraged to forego destructive habits such as ice chewing. In addition, most suggestions made earlier for prevention of cusp fractures apply here. The use of deep Class I or Class II restorations should be minimized, particularly on maxillary premolars (cusp protection may be helpful).[85] Altering the occlusal anatomy or changing occlusal relationships is not useful.

SPLIT TOOTH

A split tooth is the evolution of a cracked tooth. The fracture is now complete and extends to a surface in all areas.[11] The root surface involved is in the middle or apical third. There are no dentin connections; tooth segments are entirely separate (see Fig. 8.14, *C*). The split may occur suddenly, but it

Box 8.2 Prognosis and Treatment Suggestions for Cracked Teeth

1. Pulpal and periapical diagnoses are established. The diagnosis determines the treatment. Included in this assessment is a determination of how the finding of a cracked tooth relates to the diagnosis, prognosis, and treatment (see Box 8.1, number 1).
2. Treatment alternatives are provided to the patient.
3. The patient's questions are answered, and the patient chooses the treatment to be performed.
4. Prognosis is more variable with cracks than with other longitudinal fractures. Determining the position and extent of cracks may be helpful in arriving at a prognosis and deciding when to recommend extraction. Techniques that provide more information related to the extent of cracks internally and on the proximal surfaces below the cementoenamel junction are needed. It is hypothesized that the prognosis declines from questionable to poor when cracks involve the following (in order):
   - One marginal ridge limited to the crown
   - Two marginal ridges limited to the crown
   - One or more marginal ridges and an internal proximal cavity wall only
   - One or more marginal ridges and a floor of the cavity preparation (may involve restoration removal)
   - One marginal ridge extending from the crown to the root surface (difficult to visualize)
   - Two marginal ridges extending from the crown to the root surface (difficult to visualize)
   - One or more marginal ridges extending into a canal orifice (or orifices)
   - One or more marginal ridges and the pulpal floor
   - Furcation involvement (can be confirmed only after exploratory surgery or extraction)

more likely results from long-term growth of an incomplete fracture (see Table 8.1).

Incidence

As with cracked tooth, the occurrence of split tooth is apparently increasing.[86] Obviously, many factors related to cracked tooth are endemic to split tooth. An assumption is that root canal treatment weakens dentin and renders teeth more susceptible to severe fractures, but this is unlikely.[20,48-50]

Pathogenesis

Causative factors related to cracked tooth also apply to split tooth. Why some cracked tooth fractures continue to grow to a complete split is unknown. Two major causes are probably (1) persistent destructive wedging or displacing forces on existing restorations and (2) new traumatic forces that exceed the elastic limits of the remaining intact dentin.

Clinical Features

Split tooth fractures are primarily mesiodistal fractures that cross both marginal ridges and extend deep to shear onto the root surfaces. The more centered the fracture is occlusally, the greater the tendency to extend apically. These fractures are more devastating. Mobility (or separation) of one or both segments is present. These fractures usually include the pulp. The more centered the fracture, the greater the probability of exposure.

Etiologies

Split tooth has the same causes as cracked tooth. Split tooth may be more common in root canal–treated teeth. However, this is not because the treatment per se weakens the tooth by dehydrating or altering dentin.[87] Rather, the strength of these teeth has already been compromised by caries, restorations, or overextended access preparations.[10]

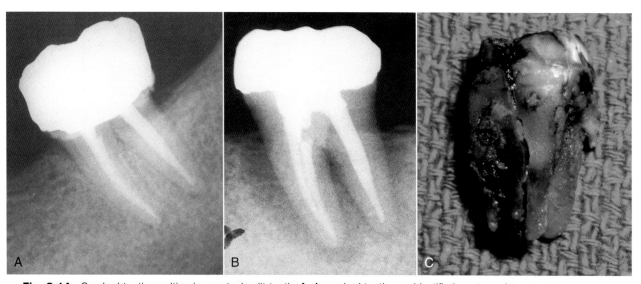

Fig. 8.14 Cracked tooth resulting in eventual split tooth. **A,** A cracked tooth was identified, root canal treatment was completed, and a full crown was placed. **B,** After 3½ years the fracture became manifest with extensive bony destruction. **C,** The fracture had grown over time to become a split tooth. Note the mesiodistal orientation of the fracture and the involvement of both the coronal and root segments of the tooth.

Diagnosis

Split tooth does not have the same variety of confusing signs, symptoms, and test results as cracked tooth. In general, split teeth are easier to identify. Damage to the periodontium is usually significant and is detected by both the patient and the dentist.

Subjective Findings

Commonly, the patient reports marked pain on mastication. These teeth tend to be less painful with occlusal centric contacts than with mastication. A periodontal abscess may be present, often resulting in mistaken diagnosis.

Objective Findings

Objective findings are not particularly helpful but should include both pulp and periapical tests.

Radiographic Findings

Findings on radiographs depend partially on the pulp's status but are more likely to reflect damage to the periodontium. Often there is marked horizontal loss of interproximal or interradicular bone (see Fig. 8.14, B; also Fig. 8.15, A). The fracture line, which is usually mesiodistal, is not visible. Fractures of this type, if visualized with the aid of CBCT, are more significant and likely deleterious, indicating the probable need for extraction.

Other Findings

The most important consideration is to identify the extent and severity of the fracture, which often requires removal of a restoration. With split tooth, the fracture line is usually readily visible under or adjacent to the restoration; it includes the occlusal surface and both marginal ridges.

Wedging to determine separability of the segments is also important. As with cracked tooth, an instrument is placed in the cavity after the patient has been informed of possible sequelae. Wedging against the walls is done with moderate pressure; the walls are then visualized for separation (Fig. 8.15, B).

The surgical microscope is a very useful aid. A separating movement indicates a through-and-through fracture.

Periodontal probing generally shows deep defects; probings tend to be adjacent to the fracture. Here again, removal of existing restorations is helpful in visualizing interproximal areas.

Treatment

Maintaining an intact tooth is impossible. If the fracture is severe (i.e., deep apically), the tooth must be extracted. If the fracture shears to a root surface that is not too far apical (middle to cervical third of the root), the smaller segment will be very mobile; then there is a good possibility that the small segment can be removed and the remainder of the tooth salvaged.

Different approaches to maintenance are used, depending on conditions. Some of the practitioner's options are as follows.

- *Remove the fractured segment.* The type of treatment and restoration are then determined. However, the following choice (temporary retention of the fractured segment) is preferred and is generally less complicated.
- *Retain the fractured segment temporarily* (Fig. 8.16). First, a rubber dam is applied with a strong rubber dam clamp to isolate and hold the segments together. Root canal treatment is completed (if not already performed), and restoration with a retentive amalcore (onlaying the undermined cusps) or bonded restoration is performed. The fractured segment then is removed. Granulation tissue proliferates to occupy the space and reattach the periodontium to the root dentin surface. The final restoration usually is the amalcore but may be a full crown with a margin related to the new attachment.
- *Remove the fractured segment and perform crown lengthening or orthodontic extrusion.* The mobile segment is removed first; root canal treatment is then performed, followed by crown lengthening or orthodontic extrusion and placement of an appropriate

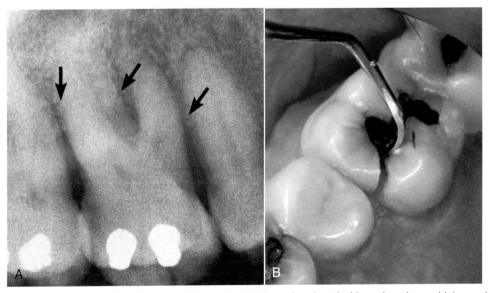

Fig. 8.15 Split tooth. **A,** Often split teeth demonstrate marked horizontal and vertical bone loss *(arrows)* interproximally and in the furcation. **B,** This molar shows the definitive sign: separation of the segments on wedging.

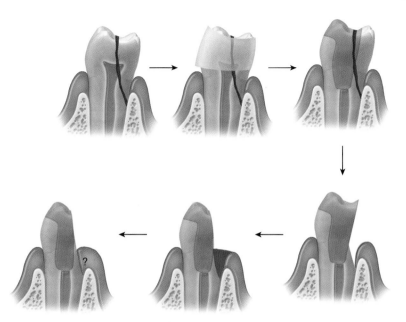

Fig. 8.16 A technique for managing certain split teeth and cusp fractures. *Upper left to lower left:* Separable segment is held with a matrix or band. Root canal treatment is followed by an amalcore onlay. The fractured segment is removed, and the amalgam is contoured. The tissue will heal and usually reattaches. The nature of the attachment (connective or epithelial tissue) is unknown. Usually, normal sulcus depth is reestablished.

restoration. This is not feasible in most situations because the fracture is too deep on the root surface.

- *Remove the fractured segment and perform no further treatment.* This choice is appropriate when root canal treatment has been completed previously and the tooth already restored. All pulp space areas *must* be filled to the margins with permanent restorative material (e.g., amalgam) with no root canal filling material exposed (Fig. 8.17). The defect often granulates in, and reattachment to the fractured dentin surface occurs.

If the fracture does not extend to the pulp, the segment is removed; the epithelial and periodontal tissues usually reattach to the fresh, raw dentin surface (see Fig. 8.17).

In summary, treatment may be complex or relatively simple, depending on the situation. Because of the possible complexity of these cases, these patients should be considered for referral to an endodontist for diagnosis and treatment.

Prognosis

As expected, the prognosis is variable. Some treatments of split tooth are successful, whereas others are doomed to failure if attempted. When the fracture extends to and surfaces in the middle to cervical third of the root, there is a reasonable chance of successful treatment and restoration. If the fracture surfaces in the middle to apical third, the prognosis is poor. With these deep fractures, usually too much of the pulp space is exposed to the periodontium. Root canal treatment with restoration of this space would result in deep periodontal defects.

Sometimes a prediction of success or failure cannot be determined before treatment is completed if the more conservative approach is taken (i.e., if the segment is temporarily held in place during root canal treatment and restoration). After root canal treatment has been completed and the segment has been removed, the dentist may discover that unfortunately the fracture is indeed very deep and the tooth cannot be salvaged. The patient must be informed of all these possibilities before treatment is begun.

Prevention

In general, preventive measures are similar to those recommended for cracked tooth: eliminating oral habits that damage tooth structure and impose wedging forces. Teeth requiring large, deep access preparations should be protected by an onlay or full crown. Large access preparations also require appropriate cusp protection.[20] Of course, teeth with cracks generally require a cuspally reinforced restoration to help prevent propagation and the development of a split tooth.

VERTICAL ROOT FRACTURE

Vertical root fracture (VRF) differs from the entities previously described (see Table 8.1) because the treatment plan is easy; however, diagnosis often is tricky and elusive, because the VRF mimics other conditions.[28,88-91] Because treatment invariably consists of either tooth extraction or removal of the fractured root, an error in diagnosis has serious consequences.

Incidence

The overall occurrence is unknown, but VRF is not uncommon.[28,92] These defects occur more often in teeth that have undergone complex restorative procedures, such as root canal treatment and intraradicular post retention.

Pathogenesis

VRFs result from wedging forces within the canal. These excessive forces exceed the binding strength of root dentin, causing fatigue and fracture. Irritants that induce severe inflammation in the adjacent periodontium result from the fracture.[93] In general, this periodontal destruction and the accompanying findings, signs, and symptoms bring the fracture to the attention of the patient or dentist.

Clinical Features

VRFs occur primarily in the faciolingual plane (see Fig. 8.2).[88,92,94-100] They are longitudinal and may either be short or **133**

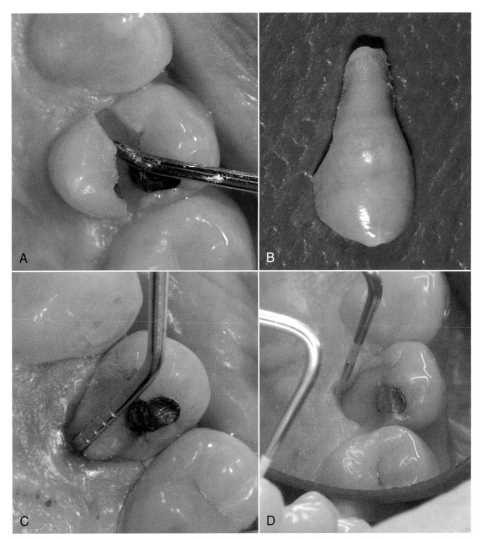

Fig. 8.17 A technique for managing fractures: "cuspidization" of a premolar. **A,** Fractured lingual cusp. **B,** Fracture extends to deep subgingival tissue. **C,** Deep probing defect. **D,** After a brief healing period, the tissue has reattached to form a normal sulcus depth.

extend the length of the root from apical to cervical (Fig. 8.18). The fracture probably begins internally (canal wall) and grows outward to the root surface. In addition, the fracture may begin at the apex or at midroot.[101] Therefore, it may be incomplete (see Fig. 8.2), extending neither to both facial and lingual root surfaces nor from apical to cervical root surfaces.

Although VRFs usually show only mild clinical signs and symptoms, the effects on the periodontium are eventually devastating and irresolvable.

Etiologies

There are two major causes (the only demonstrated ones) of VRFs: (1) post placement (cementation) and (2) condensation during root canal filling.[102-105] The only reported cases of VRF occurring in nonendodontically treated teeth were in Chinese patients.[106,107] Other causes, such as occlusal forces, wedging of restorations, corrosion and expansion of metallic posts, and expansion of postsurgical retrograde restorations, have been mentioned but not convincingly shown to cause VRF.

Condensation during root canal filling procedures, both lateral and vertical, may cause excessive wedging forces,

creating a VRF.* Intraradicular retentive posts have also been implicated[102,103,114-116]; however, endodontically treated and crowned teeth without root canal posts can develop VRF.[117] Two aspects of posts cause wedging forces. Wedging occurs during cementation of posts and also during the seating of tapered posts or with posts that depend on frictional retention.[102,109] Occlusal forces exerted on the post after cementation and restoration may also be a factor but probably a minor one. Post placement (cementation) has been shown to exert a greater wedging force than lateral condensation.[109]

Certain root shapes and sizes are more susceptible to VRF. Roots that are curved and deep facially and lingually but narrow mesially and distally are particularly prone to fracture.[98,101,113] Examples are mandibular incisors and premolars, maxillary second premolars, mesiobuccal roots of maxillary molars, and mesial and distal roots of mandibular molars. Round, oval, or bulky roots (e.g., maxillary central incisors, lingual roots of maxillary molars, and maxillary canines) are resistant to fracture.

---

*References 92, 96, 100, 101, 103, and 108 to 113.

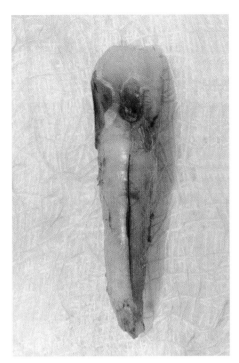

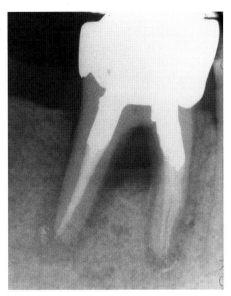

Fig. 8.19 Vertical root fracture of the distal root. A common radiographic pattern of bone resorption is seen. The defect extends along the fractured root and into the furcation.

Fig. 8.18 Vertical root fracture in this anterior tooth extends facially and lingually and also in an apical to cervical direction.

Susceptibility of any root to fracture is markedly increased by excessive dentin removal during canal instrumentation or post preparation.[96,114,118] An additional factor during condensation is the placement of excessive numbers of accessory cones, requiring multiple spreader insertions.[101,108] Also, the insertion of tapered, inflexible condensing instruments into curved canals creates root distortion and the potential for fracture.[110] The root canal filling material used is apparently unable to increase fracture resistance in canals submitted to chemomechanical preparation.[116] Glass ionomer and composite, but not mineral trioxide aggregate (MTA), have been shown to improve fracture resistance when used as intraorifice barriers.[119] Retrospective surveys of success and failure of restored endodontically treated teeth have shown that 3% to 13% of failures are due to cracks or fractures.[92,120-122]

Diagnosis

Vertical root fractures become manifest by a variety of signs, symptoms, and other clinical findings. They may mimic other entities, such as periodontal disease or failed root canal treatment. This variety of findings often makes VRF a perplexing diagnosis.[94] Interestingly, because VRFs are often mistaken for periodontal lesions or for failed root canal treatment, the dentist may refer these cases of difficult diagnosis to the periodontist or endodontist, presumably for periodontal therapy or endodontic retreatment.

Diagnostic findings of VRF were reported in a series of 42 clinical cases in a study performed by Michelich et al.[28] Much of the information that follows is derived from the findings in that study, in conjunction with other reports. Evidence-based data concerning the diagnostic accuracy and clinical effectiveness of clinical and radiographic dental evaluation for the diagnosis of VRF in endodontically treated teeth are lacking.[123]

Subjective Findings

Symptoms tend to be minimal. Seldom is the VRF painful; it is often asymptomatic or shows mild, insignificant signs and symptoms. Often some mobility is detectable, but many teeth are stable. Periradicular symptoms (pain on pressure or mastication) are common but mild.

Because many VRFs resemble periodontal lesions, a periodontal-type abscess (either as a presenting sign or in the history) is a common occurrence.[93,103] In fact, this localized swelling is often what brings the patient to the dentist's office.

Objective Tests

Periradicular tests of palpation and percussion are not particularly helpful. Periodontal probing patterns are more diagnostic. Significantly, some teeth with VRFs have normal probing patterns.[28,92,100] Most show significant probing depths with narrow or rectangular patterns, which are more typical of endodontic-type lesions.[94,97,103,124] These deep probing depths are not necessarily evident on both the facial and lingual aspects. Overall, probing patterns are not in themselves totally diagnostic, but they are helpful.

Radiographic Findings

Radiographs also show a variety of patterns. At times there are no significant changes.[28,125] However, when such changes are present, bone resorptive patterns tend to be marked, extending from the apex along the lateral surface of the root, and often include angular resorption at the cervical root (Fig. 8.19).[92,100,125,126] Many of the resorptive patterns related to VRF mimic other entities. The resorptive pattern may extend over the apex and along one root surface, described as a "J-shaped" or "halo" pattern.[92,100,125,126] Lesions may resemble failed root canal treatment because they have an apical "hanging drop" appearance.[92,100,125,126] Only a small percentage of teeth have a visible separation of fractured root segments (Fig. 8.20).[28] Interestingly, VRFs may be more readily identified using CT rather than conventional radiography.[58-68] It is more often the **135**

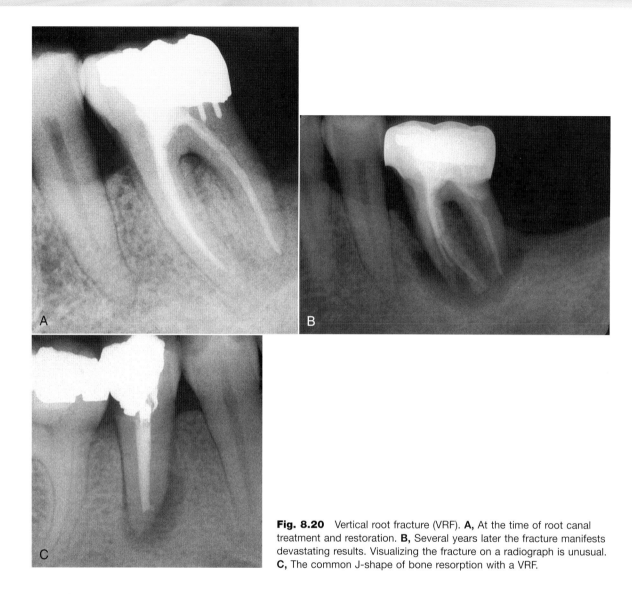

Fig. 8.20 Vertical root fracture (VRF). **A,** At the time of root canal treatment and restoration. **B,** Several years later the fracture manifests devastating results. Visualizing the fracture on a radiograph is unusual. **C,** The common J-shape of bone resorption with a VRF.

pattern of bone loss, rather than visualizing an actual fracture, that is helpful when using CBCT.

The idea that a radiolucent line separating the root canal filling material from the canal wall is diagnostic has been advocated. However, this radiolucent line may be a radiographic artifact, incomplete root canal filling, an overlying bony pattern, or other radiographic structure that is confused with a fracture. Therefore, radiographs are helpful but are not solely diagnostic except in those few instances in which the fracture is obvious.

Dental History

Virtually all teeth with a VRF have had root canal treatment,[16] and many have been restored with cast or prefabricated posts. Conventional tapered wedging posts and cores have higher failure thresholds but potentially result in greater destructive forces involving tooth fracture.[127,128] The newer fiber post and core systems have lower failure thresholds and are more likely to fail by core fracture rather than by tooth fracture.[82,128-132] Posts that are poorly designed (too long or too wide) are a frequent culprit.[15]

Endodontic and restorative treatment may have been done months or years before the fracture. Forces (without fracture) are established at the time of treatment or restoration.[96,103,107,109] These forces are stored in root dentin but may not result in an actual fracture until later. Neither patient nor dentist may relate the fracture to earlier procedures.

Other Findings

Signs, symptoms, and radiographs all give variable findings. However, the presence of a sinus tract, especially on attached gingiva, and a narrow, isolated periodontal probing defect in association with a tooth that has had root canal treatment, with or without post placement, are considered pathognomonic for a vertical root fracture.[92,94,100,133]

Conventional radiographs using multiple angles and/or CBCT may be helpful; however, flap reflection remains the only reliable diagnostic approach for fracture confirmation. Surgical exposure of soft tissue and bone overlying the root surface is the best method of identification.[28,88] VRFs have consistent patterns (Fig. 8.21). There is typically a "punched out" bony defect that tends to be oblong and overlies the root

Patterns of Bone Resorption

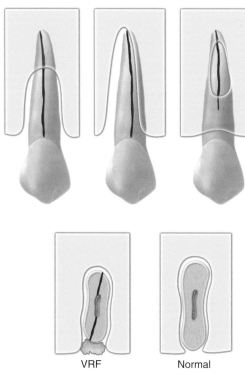

VRF   Normal

Fig. 8.21 Vertical root fracture after flap reflection and visualization. The pattern of bony changes tends to be consistent with oval or oblong "punched-out" defects filled with granulomatous tissue (VRF). This is differentiated from the normal bony fenestration.

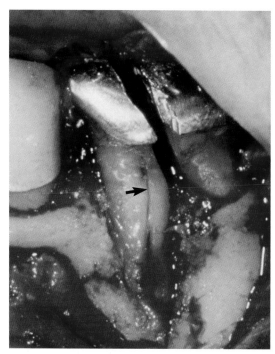

Fig. 8.22 Vertical root fracture is usually but not always identified *(arrow)* after flap reflection. Usually (as in this case), the bone has been resorbed, showing a long defect. This molar has been hemisected, and the fractured mesial segment must now be removed.

surface. This defect may take the form of a dehiscence or fenestration at various root levels. The defect is filled with granulomatous tissue.

After inflammatory tissue has been removed, the fracture is usually (but not always) visible on the root (Fig. 8.22). The operating microscope is useful. If not obvious, the fracture line may be hidden or very small and undeveloped. However, the characteristic punched-out, granulomatous tissue–filled defect is diagnostic of VRF, which should be strongly suspected.[28] Transillumination or staining with dyes is helpful. Also, the root end could be resected and examined under magnification to detect the fracture.

Fracture Characteristics

Histologic fracture characteristics have been described with VRF after removal.[93] All fractures extended from the canal to at least one root surface but not necessarily to both (Fig. 8.23). Usually fractures extend to facial and lingual surfaces (Fig. 8.23). Similarly, fractures often extend only the partial length of the root, usually to the apex but not always to the cervix.

Walton and colleagues found that many irritants occupy the fracture space and adjacent canal, resulting in inflammation at the surface.[93] Fractures harbor bacteria, sealer particles, and amorphous material. Canals adjacent to the fracture often contain necrotic tissue, in addition to concentrations of bacteria. Periodontal tissues adjacent to the fracture are chronically inflamed. Occasionally, connective tissue grows into the fracture toward the canal; this is often associated with

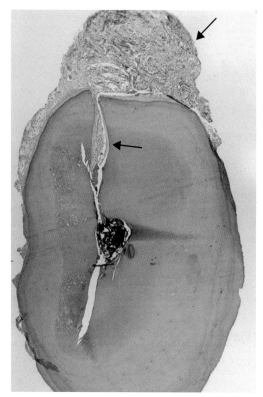

Fig. 8.23 Vertical root fracture. This histologic cross section shows a fracture extending to only one surface and to the canal. The fracture space and root surface show inflammatory tissue *(arrows)*.

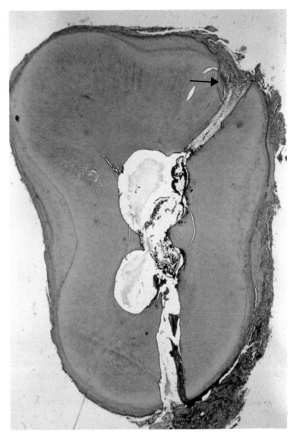

Fig. 8.24 Vertical root fracture extends to both surfaces (facial and lingual). The facial surface shows resorption *(arrow)* and ingrowth of connective tissue. The lingual component contains necrotic debris and bacteria.

resorption at the root surface (Fig. 8.24). VRFs resemble a very long apical foramen that communicates with necrotic pulp containing bacteria—thus the hopeless prognosis.

Treatment

As stated earlier, the only predictable treatment is removal of the fractured root. In multirooted teeth, this could be done by root resection (amputation) or hemisection (see Fig. 8.22).[134]

Other surgical and nonsurgical modalities have been suggested in attempts to reduce the fracture or retain the root: placement of calcium hydroxide, ligation of the fractured segments, or cementation of the fractured segments, trying to bind them with adhesive resins, epoxies, glass ionomer, or MTA.[7,135-137] A unique approach is to extract the tooth, repair the fracture with a laser, cement, or bonding agent, and then replant the tooth.[138-141] Another unusual approach is to perform intentional replantation of a vertically fractured root with intentional rotation 180 degrees so that the surface with the fracture and breakdown of bone with granulomatous tissue is positioned against healthy bone on the opposite side, and healthy periodontal ligament fibers are positioned along the surface with previous bony breakdown; with this arrangement, it is hoped, both surfaces are better able to heal effectively.[142,143] Many of these suggested methods are impractical and have not been shown to have long-term effectiveness. Surgical repairs, such as removal of one of the fractured segments or repair with amalgam or resin after surgical exposure and preparation, have also been suggested, but successful results have limited documentation.

Prognosis

At present, the prognosis is virtually hopeless for a tooth with a vertically fractured root.

Prevention

Because the causes of VRF are well known, prevention is not difficult. The cardinal rules for safety are to (1) *avoid excessive removal of intraradicular dentin* and (2) *minimize internal wedging forces*. The binding strength of root dentin is considerable but is easily compromised. Treatment and restorative procedures that require minimal dentin preparation should be selected. Canal preparation techniques that overenlarge the canal and overly aggressive instruments, such as nickel titanium files that are more tapered, must be continually evaluated with respect to their effect on changing the fracture resistance of teeth.[99,112,144-146]

Condensation of obturating materials should be carefully controlled. More flexible and less tapered finger pluggers or spreaders are preferred, because they are safer than stiff, conventional hand-type spreaders.[108,110,147,148] Posts weaken roots and should not be used unless they are necessary to retain a foundation (see Chapter 17).[149] The post design least likely to cause stress and to fracture dentin is the flexible (including carbon fiber) or cylindrical (parallel-sided) preformed post,[102,128,150] although these designs are not suitable in all restorative situations. Cast posts or some of the tapered preformed posts may be necessary. Their shape may exert wedging forces that readily split roots or cause dentin strain, particularly if they lack a stop or ferrule on the root seat.[29-32,151-153] Any post used should be as small as possible, have a passive fit, and not lock or grip the root internally with threads.[102] Cementation should be done carefully and slowly; an escape vent for the cement is probably helpful. Choosing a post design in which the post is more likely to fracture rather than the tooth (lending itself to multiple repair procedures) is certainly more beneficial for maintaining the natural tooth in the mouth.

REFERENCES

1. Rivera EM, Williamson A: Diagnosis and treatment planning: cracked tooth, *Tex Dent J* 120(3):278-283, 2003.
2. American Association of Endodontists: Cracking the cracked tooth code, *Endodontics: Colleagues for Excellence* [newsletter], fall/winter 1997, Chicago, 1997, The Association.
3. Rivera EM, Walton RE: Cracking the cracked tooth code: detection and treatment of various longitudinal tooth fractures, *Endodontics: Colleagues for Excellence* [newsletter], summer 2008, Chicago, 2008, American Association of Endodontists.
4. Rivera EM, Walton RE: Longitudinal tooth fractures: findings that contribute to complex endodontic diagnoses, *Endod Topics* 16(1):82-111, 2009.
5. Woo JM, Ho S, Tam LE: The effect of bleaching time on dentin fracture toughness in vitro, *J Esthet Restor Dent* 22(3):179-184, 2010.
6. Mai S, Kim YK, Arola DD, et al: Differential aggressiveness of ethylenediamine tetraacetic acid in causing canal wall erosion in the presence of sodium hypochlorite, *J Dent* 38(3):201-206, 2010.
7. Andreasen JO, Munksgaard EC, Bakland LK: Comparison of fracture resistance in root canals of immature sheep teeth after filling with calcium hydroxide or MTA, *Dent Traumatol* 22(3):154-156, 2006.
8. Yassen GH, Platt JA: The effect of nonsetting calcium hydroxide on root fracture and mechanical properties of radicular dentine: a systematic review, *Int Endod J* 46(2):112-118 2013.

9. Carter JM, Sorenson SE, Johnson RR, et al: Punch shear testing of extracted vital and endodontically treated teeth, *J Dent Biomech* 16(10):841-848, 1983.

10. Eakle WS, Maxwell EH, Braly BV: Fractures of posterior teeth in adults, *J Am Dent Assoc* 112(2):215-218, 1986.

11. Ehrmann EH, Tyas MJ: Cracked tooth syndrome: diagnosis, treatment and correlation between symptoms and post-extraction findings, *Aust Dent J* 35(2):105-112, 1990.

12. Hiatt WH: Incomplete crown-root fracture in pulpal-periodontal disease, *J Periodontol* 44(6):369-379, 1973.

13. Seo DG, Yi YA, Shin SJ, et al: Analysis of factors associated with cracked teeth, *J Endod* 38(3):288-292, 2012.

14. Abou-Rass M: Crack lines: the precursors of tooth fractures—their diagnosis and treatment, *Quintessence Int* 14(4):437-447, 1983.

15. Cohen S, Blanco L, Berman L: Vertical root fractures: clinical and radiographic diagnosis, *J Am Dent Assoc* 134(4):434-441, 2003.

16. Gher ME Jr, Dunlap RM, Anderson MH, et al: Clinical survey of fractured teeth [published erratum appears in *J Am Dent Assoc* 114(5):584, 1987], *J Am Dent Assoc* 114(2):174-177, 1987.

17. Opdam NJ, Roeters JM: The effectiveness of bonded composite restorations in the treatment of painful, cracked teeth: six-month clinical evaluation, *Oper Dent* 28(4):327-333, 2003.

18. Cohen S, Berman LH, Blanco L, et al: A demographic analysis of vertical root fractures, *J Endod* 32(12):1160-1163, 2006.

19. Fennis WM, Kuijs RH, Kreulen CM, et al: A survey of cusp fractures in a population of general dental practices, *Int J Prosthodont* 15(6):559-563, 2002.

20. Reeh ES, Messer HH, Douglas WH: Reduction in tooth stiffness as a result of endodontic and restorative procedures, *J Endod* 15(11):512-516, 1989.

21. Cavel WT, Kelsey WP, Blankenau RJ: An in vivo study of cuspal fracture, *J Prosthet Dent* 53(1):38-42, 1985.

22. Kahler B, Moule A, Stenzel D: Bacterial contamination of cracks in symptomatic vital teeth, *Aust Endod J* 26(3):115-118, 2000.

23. Ailor JE Jr: Managing incomplete tooth fractures, *J Am Dent Assoc* 131(8):1168-1174, 2000.

24. Brynjulfsen A, Fristad I, Grevstad T, et al: Incompletely fractured teeth associated with diffuse longstanding orofacial pain: diagnosis and treatment outcome, *Int Endod J* 35(5):461-466, 2002.

25. Re GJ, Norling BK, Draheim RN: Fracture resistance of lower molars with varying faciocclusolingual amalgam restorations, *J Prosthet Dent* 47(5):518-521, 1982.

26. Salis SG, Hood JA, Kirk EE, et al: Impact-fracture energy of human premolar teeth, *J Prosthet Dent* 58(1):43-48, 1987.

27. El Ayouti A, Serry MI, Geis-Gerstorfer J, et al: Influence of cusp coverage on the fracture resistance of premolars with endodontic access cavities, *Int Endod J* 44(6):543-549, 2011.

28. Michelich RJ, Smith GN, Walton RE: Vertical root fractures: clinical features, Unpublished data, 2012.

29. Sorensen JA, Engelman MJ: Ferrule design and fracture resistance of endodontically treated teeth, *J Prosthet Dent* 63(5):529-536, 1990.

30. Ng CC, Dumbrigue HB, Al-Bayat MI, et al: Influence of remaining coronal tooth structure location on the fracture resistance of restored endodontically treated anterior teeth, *J Prosthet Dent* 95(4):290-296, 2006.

31. Tan PL, Aquilino SA, Gratton DG, et al: In vitro fracture resistance of endodontically treated central incisors with varying ferrule heights and configurations, *J Prosthet Dent* 93(4):331-336, 2005.

32. Juloski J, Radovic I, Goracci C, et al: Ferrule effect: a literature review, *J Endod* 38(1):11-19, 2012.

33. Reeh ES, Douglas WH, Messer HH: Stiffness of endodontically treated teeth related to restoration technique, *J Dent Res* 68(11):1540-1544, 1989.

34. Rasheed AA: Effect of bonding amalgam on the reinforcement of teeth, *J Prosthet Dent* 93(1):51-55, 2005.

35. Santos MJ, Bezerra RB: Fracture resistance of maxillary premolars restored with direct and indirect adhesive techniques, *J Can Dent Assoc* 71(8):585, 2005.

36. Allara FW Jr, Diefenderfer KE, Molinaro JD: Effect of three direct restorative materials on molar cuspal fracture resistance, *Am J Dent* 17(4):228-232, 2004.

37. Hurmuzlu F, Serper A, Siso SH, et al: In vitro fracture resistance of root-filled teeth using new-generation dentine bonding adhesives, *Int Endod J* 36(11):770-773, 2003.

38. Zidan O, Abdel-Keriem U: The effect of amalgam bonding on the stiffness of teeth weakened by cavity preparation, *Dent Mater* 19(7):680-685, 2003.

39. Wahl MJ, Schmitt MM, Overton DA, et al: Prevalence of cusp fractures in teeth restored with amalgam and with resin-based composite, *J Am Dent Assoc* 135(8):1127-1132; quiz, 64-65; 2004.

40. Setcos JC, Staninec M, Wilson NH: Bonding of amalgam restorations: existing knowledge and future prospects, *Oper Dent* 25(2):121-129, 2000.

41. Bakland LK: Tooth infractions. In Ingle JI, Bakland LK, Baumgartner JC, editors: Ingle's endodontics 6, ed 6, pp 660-675, Hamilton, Ontario, 2008, BC Decker.

42. Ehrmann EH: Endodontics or root canal therapy, *Aust Fam Physician* 6(10):1227-1241, 1977.

43. Krell KV, Rivera EM: A six year evaluation of cracked teeth diagnosed with reversible pulpitis: treatment and prognosis, *J Endod* 33(12):1405-1407, 2007.

44. Ivancik J, Neerchal NK, Romberg E, et al: The reduction in fatigue crack growth resistance of dentin with depth, *J Dent Res* 90(8):1031-1036, 2011.

45. Weine FS: Initiating endodontic therapy in posterior teeth. III. Mandibular molars, *Compend Contin Educ Dent* 4(2):153-161, 1983.

46. Berman LH, Kuttler S: Fracture necrosis: diagnosis, prognosis assessment, and treatment recommendations, *J Endod* 36(3):442-446, 2010.

47. Howe CA, McKendry DJ: Effect of endodontic access preparation on resistance to crown-root fracture, *J Am Dent Assoc* 121(6):712-715, 1990.

48. Rivera EM, Yamauchi M: Site comparisons of dentine collagen cross-links from extracted human teeth, *Arch Oral Biol* 38(7):541-546, 1993.

49. Rivera EM, Yamauchi M: Collagen cross-links of root-filled and normal dentin, *J Dent Res* Special Issue, Abstract #98(69):121, 1990.

50. Sedgley CM, Messer HH: Are endodontically treated teeth more brittle? *J Endod* 18(7):332-335, 1992.

51. Cheron RA, Marshall SJ, Goodis HE, et al: Nanomechanical properties of endodontically treated teeth, *J Endod* 37(11):1562-1565, 2011.

52. Cameron CE: The cracked tooth syndrome: additional findings, *J Am Dent Assoc* 93(5):971-975, 1976.

53. Homewood CI: Cracked tooth syndrome: incidence, clinical findings and treatment, *Aust Dent J* 43(4):217-222, 1998.

54. Brown WS, Jacobs HR, Thompson RE: Thermal fatigue in teeth, *J Dent Res* 51(2):461-467, 1972.

55. Nguyen V, Palmer G: A review of the diagnosis and management of the cracked tooth, *Dent Update* 36(6):338-340; 42, 45-46 passim; 2009.

56. Banerji S, Mehta SB, Millar BJ: Cracked tooth syndrome. Part 1. Aetiology and diagnosis, *Br Dent J* 208(10):459-463, 2010.

57. Kahler W: The cracked tooth conundrum: terminology, classification, diagnosis, and management, *Am J Dent* 21(5):275-282, 2008.

58. Youssefzadeh S, Gahleitner A, Dorffner R, et al: Dental vertical root fractures: value of CT in detection, *Radiology* 210(2):545-549, 1999.

59. Hannig C, Dullin C, Hulsmann M, et al: Three-dimensional, non-destructive visualization of vertical root fractures using flat panel volume detector computer tomography: an ex vivo in vitro case report, *Int Endod J* 38(12):904-913, 2005.

60. Mora MA, Mol A, Tyndall DA, et al: Effect of the number of basis images on the detection of longitudinal tooth fractures using local computed tomography, *Dentomaxillofac Radiol* 36(7):382-386, 2007.

61. Mora MA, Mol A, Tyndall DA, et al: In vitro assessment of local computed tomography for the detection of longitudinal tooth fractures, *Oral Surg Oral Med Oral Pathol Oral Radiol Endod* 103(6):825-829, 2007.

62. Hassan B, Metska ME, Ozok AR, et al: Detection of vertical root fractures in endodontically treated teeth by a cone beam computed tomography scan, *J Endod* 35(5):719-722, 2009.

63. Kamburoglu K, Murat S, Yuksel SP, et al: Detection of vertical root fracture using cone-beam computerized tomography: an in vitro assessment, *Oral Surg Oral Med Oral Pathol Oral Radiol Endod* 109(2):e74-e81, 2010.

64. Ozer SY: Detection of vertical root fractures by using cone beam computed tomography with variable voxel sizes in an in vitro model, *J Endod* 37(1):75-79, 2011.

65. Tang L, Zhou XD, Wang Y, et al: Detection of vertical root fracture using cone beam computed tomography: report of two cases, *Dent Traumatol* 27(6):484-488, 2011.

66. Wang P, Yan XB, Lui DG, et al: Detection of dental root fractures by using cone-beam computed tomography, *Dentomaxillofac Radiol* 40(5):290-298, 2011.

67. Kajan ZD, Taromsari M: Value of cone beam CT in detection of dental root fractures, *Dentomaxillofac Radiol* 41(1):3-10, 2012.

68. Metska ME, Aartman IH, Wesselink PR, et al: Detection of vertical root fractures in vivo in endodontically treated teeth by cone-beam computed tomography scans, *J Endod* 38(10):1344-1347, 2012.

69. Kambungton J, Janhom A, Prapayasatok S, et al: Assessment of vertical root fractures using three imaging modalities: cone beam CT, intraoral digital radiography and film, *Dentomaxillofac Radiol* 41(2):91-95, 2012.

70. Culjat MO, Singh RS, Brown ER, et al: Ultrasound crack detection in a simulated human tooth, *Dentomaxillofac Radiol* 34(2):80-85, 2005.

71. Matsushita-Tokugawa M, Miura J, Iwami Y, et al: Detection of dentinal microcracks using infrared thermography, *J Endod* 39(1):88-91, 2013.

72. Wright HM Jr, Loushine RJ, Weller RN, et al: Identification of resected root-end dentinal cracks: a comparative study of transillumination and dyes, *J Endod* 30(10):712-715, 2004.

73. Alassaad SS: Incomplete cusp fractures: early diagnosis and communication with patients using fiber-optic transillumination and intraoral photography, *Gen Dent* 59(2):132-135, 2011.

74. Abbott PV: Assessing restored teeth with pulp and periapical diseases for the presence of cracks, caries and marginal breakdown, *Aust Dent J* 49(1):33-39; quiz, 45; 2004.

75. Gorucu J, Ozgunaltay G: Fracture resistance of teeth with Class II bonded amalgam and new tooth-colored restorations, *Oper Dent* 28(5):501-507, 2003.

76. Seow LL, Toh CG, Wilson NH: Remaining tooth structure associated with various preparation designs for the endodontically treated maxillary second premolar, *Eur J Prosthodont Restor Dent* 13(2):57-64, 2005.

77. Tan L, Chen NN, Poon CY, et al: Survival of root filled cracked teeth in a tertiary institution, *Int Endod J* 39(11):886-889, 2006.

78. Paul RA, Tamse A, Rosenberg E: Cracked and broken teeth: definitions, differential diagnosis and treatment, *Refuat Hapeh Vehashinayim* 24(2):7-12; 68; 2007.

79. Turp JC, Gobetti JP: The cracked tooth syndrome: an elusive diagnosis, *J Am Dent Assoc* 127(10):1502-1507, 1996.

80. Pane ES, Palamara JE, Messer HH: Stainless steel bands in endodontics: effects on cuspal flexure and fracture resistance, *Int Endod J* 35(5):467-471, 2002.

81. Franchi M, Breschi L, Ruggeri O: Cusp fracture resistance in composite-amalgam combined restorations, *J Dent* 27(1):47-52, 1999.

82. Fennis WM, Tezvergil A, Kuijs RH, et al: In vitro fracture resistance of fiber reinforced cusp-replacing composite restorations, *Dent Mater* 21(6):565-572, 2005.

83. Kruzic JJ, Nalla RK, Kinney JH, et al: Mechanistic aspects of in vitro fatigue-crack growth in dentin, *Biomaterials* 26(10):1195-1204, 2005.

84. Abbott P, Leow N: Predictable management of cracked teeth with reversible pulpitis, *Aust Dent J* 54(4):306-315, 2009.

85. Blaser PK, Lund MR, Cochran MA, et al: Effect of designs of Class II preparations on resistance of teeth to fracture, *Oper Dent* 8(1):6-10, 1983.

86. Geurtsen W, Schwarze T, Gunay H: Diagnosis, therapy, and prevention of the cracked tooth syndrome, *Quintessence Int* 34(6):409-417, 2003.

87. Huang T-JG, Schilder H, Nathanson D: Effect of moisture content and endodontic treatment on some mechanical properties of human dentin, *J Endod* 18(5):209-215, 1992.

88. Pitts DL, Natkin E: Diagnosis and treatment of vertical root fractures, *J Endod* 9(8):338-346, 1983.

89. Bhaskar U, Logani A, Shah N: True vertical tooth root fracture: case report and review, *Contemp Clin Dent* 2(3):265-268, 2011.

90. Tamse A: Iatrogenic vertical root fractures in endodontically treated teeth, *Endod Dent Traumatol* 4(5):190-196, 1988.

91. Moule AJ, Kahler B: Diagnosis and management of teeth with vertical root fractures, *Aust Dent J* 44(2):75-87, 1999.

92. Tamse A: Vertical root fractures in endodontically treated teeth. In Ingle JI, Bakland LK, Baumgartner JC, editors: Ingle's endodontics 6, ed 6, pp 676-689, Hamilton, Ontario, 2008, BC Decker.

93. Walton RE, Michelich RJ, Smith GN: The histopathogenesis of vertical root fractures, *J Endod* 10(2):48-56, 1984.

94. Tamse A, Fuss Z, Lustig J, et al: An evaluation of endodontically treated vertically fractured teeth, *J Endod* 25(7):506-508, 1999.

95. Pitts DL, Matheny HE, Nicholls JI: An in vitro study of spreader loads required to cause vertical root fracture during lateral condensation, *J Endod* 9(12):544-550, 1983.

96. Ricks-Williamson LJ, Fotos PG, Goel VK, et al: A three-dimensional finite-element stress analysis of an endodontically prepared maxillary central incisor, *J Endod* 21(7):362-367, 1995.

97. Lustig JP, Tamse A, Fuss Z: Pattern of bone resorption in vertically fractured, endodontically treated teeth, *Oral Surg Oral Med Oral Pathol Oral Radiol Endod* 90(2):224-227, 2000.

98. Lertchirakarn V, Palamara JE, Messer HH: Patterns of vertical root fracture: factors affecting stress distribution in the root canal, *J Endod* 29(8):523-528, 2003.

99. Lam PP, Palamara JE, Messer HH: Fracture strength of tooth roots following canal preparation by hand and rotary instrumentation, *J Endod* 31(7):529-532, 2005.

100. Tamse A: Vertical root fractures in endodontically treated teeth: diagnostic signs and clinical management, *Endod Topics* 13:84-94, 2006.

101. Holcomb JQ, Pitts DL, Nicholls JI: Further investigation of spreader loads required to cause vertical root fracture during lateral condensation, *J Endod* 13(6):277-284, 1987.

102. Ross R, Nicholls J, Harrington G: A comparison of strains generated during placement of five endodontic posts, *J Endod* 17(9):450-456, 1991.

103. Meister F Jr, Lommel TJ, Gerstein H: Diagnosis and possible causes of vertical root fractures, *Oral Surg Oral Med Oral Pathol* 49(3):243-253, 1980.

104. Fuss Z, Lustig J, Tamse A: Prevalence of vertical root fractures in extracted endodontically treated teeth, *Int Endod J* 32(4):283-286, 1999.

105. Testori T, Badino M, Castagnola M: Vertical root fractures in endodontically treated teeth: a clinical survey of 36 cases, *J Endod* 19(2):87-91, 1993.

106. Yang SF, Rivera EM, Walton RE: Vertical root fracture in nonendodontically treated teeth, *J Endod* 21(6):337-339, 1995.

107. Chan CP, Lin CP, Tseng SC, et al: Vertical root fracture in endodontically versus nonendodontically treated teeth: a survey of 315 cases in Chinese patients, *Oral Surg Oral Med Oral Pathol Oral Radiol Endod* 87(4):504-507, 1999.

108. Dang DA, Walton RE: Vertical root fracture and root distortion: effect of spreader design, *J Endod* 15(7):294-301, 1989.

109. Obermayr G, Walton RE, Leary JM, et al: Vertical root fracture and relative deformation during obturation and post cementation, *J Prosthet Dent* 66(2):181-187, 1991.

110. Murgel CA, Walton RE: Vertical root fracture and dentin deformation in curved roots: the influence of spreader design, *Endod Dent Traumatol* 6(6):273-278, 1990.

111. Okitsu M, Takahashi H, Yoshioka T, et al: Effective factors including periodontal ligament on vertical root fractures, *Dent Mater J* 24(1):66-69, 2005.

112. Sathorn C, Palamara JE, Messer HH: A comparison of the effects of two canal preparation techniques on root fracture susceptibility and fracture pattern, *J Endod* 31(4):283-287, 2005.

113. Sathorn C, Palamara JE, Palamara D, et al: Effect of root canal size and external root surface morphology on fracture susceptibility and pattern: a finite element analysis, *J Endod* 31(4):288-292, 2005.

114. Kishen A: Mechanisms and risk factors for fracture predilection in endodontically treated teeth, *Endod Topics* 13:57-83, 2006.

115. Kishen A, Kumar GV, Chen NN: Stress-strain response in human dentine: rethinking fracture predilection in postcore restored teeth, *Dent Traumatol* 20(2):90-100, 2004.

116. Al-Omiri MK, Rayyan MR, Abu-Hammad O: Stress analysis of endodontically treated teeth restored with post-retained crowns: a finite element analysis study, *J Am Dent Assoc* 142(3):289-300, 2011.

117. Schwarz S, Lohbauer U, Petschelt A, et al: Vertical root fractures in crowned teeth: a report of 32 cases, *Quintessence Int* 43(1):37-43, 2012.

118. Trope M, Ray HL Jr: Resistance to fracture of endodontically treated roots, *Oral Surg Oral Med Oral Pathol* 73(1):99-102, 1992.

119. Nagas E, Uyanik O, Altundasar E, et al: Effect of different intraorifice barriers on the fracture resistance of roots obturated with Resilon or gutta-percha, *J Endod* 36(6):1061-1063, 2010.

120. Spielman H, Schaffer SB, Cohen MG, et al: Restorative outcomes for endodontically treated teeth in the Practitioners Engaged in Applied Research and Learning network, *J Am Dent Assoc* 143(7):746-755, 2012.

121. Toure B, Faye B, Kane AW, et al: Analysis of reasons for extraction of endodontically treated teeth: a prospective study, *J Endod* 37(11):1512-1515, 2011.

122. Goodacre CJ, Spolnik KJ: The prosthodontic management of endodontically treated teeth: a literature review. I. Success and failure data, treatment concepts, *J Prosthodont* 3(4):243-250, 1994.

123. Tsesis I, Rosen E, Tamse A, et al: Diagnosis of vertical root fractures in endodontically treated teeth based on clinical and radiographic indices: a systematic review, *J Endod* 36(9):1455-1458, 2010.

124. Harrington GW: The perio-endo question: differential diagnosis. *Dent Clin North Am* 23(4):673-690, 1979.

125. Tamse A, Kaffe I, Lustig J, et al: Radiographic features of vertically fractured endodontically treated mesial roots of mandibular molars, *Oral Surg Oral Med Oral Pathol Oral Radiol Endod* 101(6):797-802, 2006.

126. Tamse A, Fuss Z, Lustig J, et al: Radiographic features of vertically fractured, endodontically treated maxillary premolars, *Oral Surg Oral Med Oral Pathol Oral Radiol Endod* 88(3):348-352, 1999.

127. Standlee JP, Caputo AA, Collard EW, et al: Analysis of stress distribution by endodontic posts, *Oral Surg Oral Med Oral Pathol* 33(6):952-960, 1972.

128. Sirimai S, Riis DN, Morgano SM: An in vitro study of the fracture resistance and the incidence of vertical root fracture of pulpless teeth restored with six post-and-core systems, *J Prosthet Dent* 81(3):262-269, 1999.

129. Hayashi M, Takahashi Y, Imazato S, et al: Fracture resistance of pulpless teeth restored with post-cores and crowns, *Dent Mater* 22(5):477-485, 2006.

130. Fernandes AS, Shetty S, Coutinho I: Factors determining post selection: a literature review, *J Prosthet Dent* 90(6):556-562, 2003.

131. Maccari PC, Conceicao EN, Nunes MF: Fracture resistance of endodontically treated teeth restored with three different prefabricated esthetic posts, *J Esthet Restor Dent* 15(1):25-30; discussion, 31; 2003.

132. Newman MP, Yaman P, Dennison J, et al: Fracture resistance of endodontically treated teeth restored with composite posts, *J Prosthet Dent* 89(4):360-367, 2003.

133. Nicopoulou-Karayianni K, Bragger U, Lang NP: Patterns of periodontal destruction associated with incomplete root fractures, *Dentomaxillofac Radiol* 26(6):321-326, 1997.

134. Kurtzman GM, Silverstein LH, Shatz PC: Hemisection as an alternative treatment for vertically fractured mandibular molars, *Compend Contin Educ Dent* 27(2):126-129, 2006.

135. Doyon GE, Dumsha T, von Fraunhofer JA: Fracture resistance of human root dentin exposed to intracanal calcium hydroxide, *J Endod* 31(12):895-897, 2005.

136. Taschieri S, Tamse A, Del Fabbro M, et al: A new surgical technique for preservation of endodontically treated teeth with coronally located vertical root fractures: a prospective case series, *Oral Surg Oral Med Oral Pathol Oral Radiol Endod* 110(6):e45-e52, 2010.

137. Floratos SG, Kratchman SI: Surgical management of vertical root fractures for posterior teeth: report of four cases, *J Endod* 38(4):550-555, 2012.

138. Arikan F, Franko M, Gurkan A: Replantation of a vertically fractured maxillary central incisor after repair with adhesive resin, *Int Endod J* 41(2):173-179, 2008.

139. Ozturk M, Unal GC: A successful treatment of vertical root fracture: a case report and 4-year follow-up, *Dent Traumatol* 24(5):e56-e60, 2008.

140. Unver S, Onay EO, Ungor M: Intentional re-plantation of a vertically fractured tooth repaired with an adhesive resin, *Int Endod J* 44(11):1069-1078, 2011.

141. Ozer SY, Unlu G, Deger Y: Diagnosis and treatment of endodontically treated teeth with vertical root fracture: three case reports with two-year follow-up, *J Endod* 37(1):97-102, 2011.

142. Kudou Y, Kubota M: Replantation with intentional rotation of a complete vertically fractured root using adhesive resin cement, *Dent Traumatol* 19(2):115-117, 2003.

143. Kawai K, Masaka N: Vertical root fracture treated by bonding fragments and rotational replantation, *Dent Traumatol* 18(1):42-45, 2002.

144. Milani AS, Froughreyhani M, Rahimi S, et al: The effect of root canal preparation on the development of dentin cracks, *Iran Endod J* 7(4):177-182, 2012.

145. Zandbiglari T, Davids H, Schafer E: Influence of instrument taper on the resistance to fracture of endodontically treated roots, *Oral Surg Oral Med Oral Pathol Oral Radiol Endod* 101(1):126-131, 2006.

146. Wilcox LR, Roskelley C, Sutton T: The relationship of root canal enlargement to finger-spreader induced vertical root fracture [in process citation], *J Endod* 23(8):533-534, 1997.

147. Lindauer PA, Campbell AD, Hicks ML, et al: Vertical root fractures in curved roots under simulated clinical conditions, *J Endod* 15(8):345-349, 1989.

148. Piskin B, Aydin B, Sarikanat M: The effect of spreader size on fracture resistance of maxillary incisor roots, *Int Endod J* 41(1):54-59, 2008.

149. Rosen E, Tsesis I, Tamse A, et al: Medico-legal aspects of vertical root fractures in root filled teeth, *Int Endod J* 45(1):7-11, 2012.

150. Goodacre CJ: Carbon fiber posts may have fewer failures than metal posts, *J Evid Based Dent Pract* 10(1):32-34, 2010.

151. Mezzomo E, Massa F, Libera SD: Fracture resistance of teeth restored with two different post-and-core designs cemented with two different cements: an in vitro study. I, *Quintessence Int* 34(4):301-306, 2003.

152. Naumann M, Preuss A, Rosentritt M: Effect of incomplete crown ferrules on load capacity of endodontically treated maxillary incisors restored with fiber posts, composite build-ups, and all-ceramic crowns: an in vitro evaluation after chewing simulation, *Acta Odontol Scand* 64(1):31-36, 2006.

153. Peroz I, Blankenstein F, Lange KP, et al: Restoring endodontically treated teeth with posts and cores: a review, *Quintessence Int* 36(9):737-746, 2005.

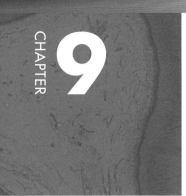

9

Local anesthesia

Al Reader, John M. Nusstein, Richard E. Walton

CHAPTER OUTLINE

Factors Affecting Endodontic Anesthesia
Initial Management
Conventional Pulpal Anesthesia for Restorative Dentistry
Mandibular Anesthesia for Restorative Dentistry
Maxillary Anesthesia for Restorative Dentistry
Supplemental Anesthesia for Restorative Dentistry in the Mandible

and Maxilla
Anesthesia Difficulties in Endodontics
Supplemental Techniques for Mandibular Teeth in Endodontics
Anesthetic Management of Pulpal or Periapical Pathoses
Anesthesia for Surgical Procedures

LEARNING OBJECTIVES

After reading this chapter, the student should be able to:

1. Explain why apprehension and anxiety, fatigue, and tissue inflammation create difficulties in obtaining profound anesthesia.
2. Define the pain threshold and the factors affecting it.
3. Describe patient management techniques that facilitate obtaining adequate anesthesia.
4. List techniques that are helpful in reducing the pain of injections.
5. Describe the "routine" approach to conventional local anesthesia: when and how to anesthetize.

6. Describe circumstances that create difficulties in obtaining profound anesthesia using conventional techniques.
7. Describe when to use supplemental methods of obtaining pulpal anesthesia if standard block or infiltration methods fail.
8. Review techniques of infiltration intraosseous, periodontal ligament, and intrapulpal injections.
9. Discuss how to obtain anesthesia for specific pulpal and periapical pathoses: symptomatic irreversible pulpitis, symptomatic teeth with pulpal necrosis, asymptomatic teeth with pulpal necrosis, and surgical procedures.

When a tooth which is loose or painful is to be extracted, the nose of the patient should be rubbed with brown sugar, ivy and green oil; he is advised to hold his breath, a stone is then placed between his teeth, and he is made to close his mouth. The fluid which causes the pain is then seen to flow from the mouth in such quantity as frequently to fill three pots; after having cleansed the nose with pure oil, rinsed the mouth with wine, the tooth is no longer painful, and may easily be extracted.

Scribonius, AD 47

This quotation sets forth Scribonius' method of obtaining "anesthesia" almost 2,000 years ago. He was convinced that he could perform painless extractions using what was apparently a rather crude technique of pressure anesthesia. Even in modern times, this concern remains for dentists—how can they attain adequate levels of anesthesia to keep their patients relatively comfortable during endodontic procedures? Obtaining profound anesthesia for the endodontic patient is difficult and challenging. Many patients recount vivid (and often valid) accounts of painful experiences. Although routine

anesthetic techniques are usually effective for restorative dentistry, endodontic procedures present special situations that require additional techniques and special approaches.

FACTORS AFFECTING ENDODONTIC ANESTHESIA

Emotional considerations, in addition to tissue changes, impair the effectiveness of local anesthesia.[1] A patient who is psychologically distraught and has an inflamed pulp or periapex has a lower pain threshold (i.e., less stimulus is required to produce pain).[2] In addition, the trigeminal nerve, which supplies primary sensory innervation to oral structures, is a complex entity. Knowledge of its more common anatomic features aids the clinician in successfully obtaining anesthesia.

Apprehension and Anxiety

Many endodontic patients have heard horror stories about root canal treatment. The cause may not be the treatment but the experience of a painful or "infected" tooth. They vividly recall the pain, swelling, and sleepless nights associated with the tooth before treatment. The procedure itself is generally less threatening; a survey of endodontic patients completing therapy indicated that 96% would agree to have future root canal treatment.[3] Therefore, because they fear the unknown and have heard unfavorable stories, patients are apprehensive or anxious. This emotion plays a role in their perceptions and also affects how they react to pain. Many patients can effectively mask this apprehension!

Fatigue

Over a course of days, many patients with a toothache have not slept well, not eaten properly, or otherwise have not functioned normally. In addition, many are apprehensive or anxious about the appointment. The end result is a patient with a decreased ability to manage stress and less tolerance for pain.

Tissue Inflammation

Inflamed tissues have a lower threshold of pain perception[4]; this is called the *allodynia phenomenon*. In other words, a tissue that is inflamed is much more sensitive and reactive to a mild stimulus.[4] Therefore, an inflamed tissue responds painfully to a stimulus that otherwise would be unnoticed or perceived only mildly. Because root canal treatment procedures generally involve inflamed pulpal or periradicular tissues, this phenomenon has obvious importance. A related complication is that inflamed tissues are more difficult to anesthetize.[5]

A good example of the phenomenon of increased sensitivity is sunburn. Exposed tissues that have been sunburned are irritated and inflamed. The skin has now become quite sensitive (lower pain threshold) to contact and is painful. This same principle applies to inflamed pulpal and periapical tissues.[6]

Previous Unsuccessful Anesthesia

Unfortunately, profound pulpal anesthesia is not always obtained with conventional techniques. Previous difficulty with teeth becoming anesthetized is associated with a likelihood of subsequent unsuccessful anesthesia.[7] These patients are likely to be apprehensive (lower pain threshold) and generally identify themselves by comments such as, "Novocain never seems to work very well on me" or "A lot of shots are always necessary to deaden my teeth." The practitioner should anticipate difficulties in obtaining anesthesia in such patients. Often, psychological management and supplemental local anesthesia techniques are required.

INITIAL MANAGEMENT

The early phase of treatment is most important. If the patient is managed properly and anesthetic techniques are performed smoothly, the pain threshold elevates. The result is more predictable anesthesia and a less apprehensive, more cooperative patient.

Psychological Approach

The psychological approach involves the four Cs: control, communication, concern, and confidence. *Control* is important and is achieved by obtaining and maintaining the upper hand. *Communication* is accomplished by listening to the patient and explaining what is to be done and what the patient should expect. *Concern* is shown by verbalizing awareness of the patient's apprehensions. *Confidence* is expressed in body language and in a professional approach and communication style, giving the patient confidence in the management, diagnostic, and treatment skills of the dentist. Management of the four Cs effectively calms and reassures the patient, thereby raising the pain threshold.

Topics Related to Injection Pain
Obtaining the Patient's Confidence

Obtaining the patient's confidence is critical. Before any injection is given, establishing communication, exhibiting empathy, and informing patients of an awareness of their apprehension, in addition to their dental problem, markedly increases the patient's confidence levels.[8] Most important, having the patient's confidence gives control of the situation to the dentist; this is a requisite!

Topical Anesthetic

Use of a topical anesthetic is popular as an adjunct to painless injections. Some investigators have shown topical anesthetics to be effective,[9-11] whereas others have not.[12,13] The most important aspect of using topical anesthesia is not primarily the actual decrease in mucosal sensitivity, but rather the demonstrated concern that everything possible is being done to prevent pain. Another aspect is the power of suggestion that the topical anesthetic will reduce the pain of injection.[13] When a topical anesthetic gel is used, a small amount on a cotton-tipped applicator is placed on the dried mucosa for 1 to 2 minutes before the injection.[14]

Solution Warming

A common belief is that an anesthetic solution warmed to or above body temperature is better tolerated and results in less pain during injection. Although some studies have shown that warming anesthetic solutions did not reduce the pain of injection,[15-17] other studies have found that warming did reduce this pain.[18-20] Further research is needed to determine whether warming anesthetic solutions is beneficial.

Needle Insertion

Initially, the needle is inserted *gently* into the mucosal tissue.

Small-Gauge Needles

A common misconception is that smaller needles cause less pain; this is not true for dental needles. Patients cannot differentiate between 25-, 27-, and 30-gauge needles during injections.[21] These sizes have similar deflection patterns and resistance to breakage.[22,23] However, to prevent broken needles when administering inferior alveolar nerve blocks, do not use 30-gauge needles, bury the needle to the hub, or bend needles at the hub.[24] As a recommendation, a 27-gauge needle is suitable for most conventional dental injections.

Slow Injection

A slow injection decreases both pressure and the patient's discomfort.[25] A slow inferior alveolar nerve block is more comfortable than a rapid injection.[25,26] A technique for slow injection is to use a computer-controlled anesthetic delivery system (CCLAD)(Fig. 9.1). Most studies on CCLADs **143**

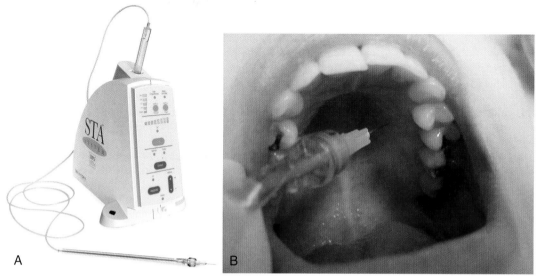

Fig. 9.1 **A,** Computer-controlled injection device. Note the handpiece assembly and microtubing. **B,** The specialized handpiece and needle may be used in most situations. (A courtesy of Milestone Scientific, Inc., Livingston, N.J.)

compared the pain of injection with the delivery system to that with standard syringe injections,[27-33] generally with favorable results.[29-33] Therefore, although the CCLAD reduces the pain of the injection, the system does not produce a painless injection.[27-33]

Two-Stage Injection

A two-stage injection consists of initial very slow administration of approximately a quarter-cartridge of anesthetic just under the mucosal surface. After regional numbness has been obtained, the remainder of the cartridge is deposited to the full depth at the target site. The two-stage injection decreases the pain of needle placement for females in the inferior alveolar nerve block.[34] This injection technique is indicated for apprehensive and anxious patients or pediatric patients, but it may be used on anyone. It is also effective for any injection, including the inferior alveolar nerve block.

Gender Differences in Pain

Women try to avoid pain more than men, accept it less, and fear it more.[35,36] Anxiety may also modulate differences in pain responses between males and females.[36] Apparently, women react differently to pain than men do and are more likely to present anesthesia challenges.

When to Anesthetize

Preferably, anesthesia should be given at each appointment. There is a common belief that instruments may be used in canals with necrotic pulps and periapical lesions painlessly without anesthesia. Occasionally there may be vital tissue in the apical few millimeters of the canal.[37] This inflamed tissue contains nerves and is sensitive. Not only is this vital tissue contacted during instrumentation, but also pressure is created. These factors may cause discomfort if the patient is not anesthetized.

There is an antiquated notion that canal length can be determined in a nonanesthetized patient by passing an instrument into a necrotic canal until the patient shows an "eye-blink response." Unfortunately, patient perceptions and responses are too variable for accuracy. Pain may be felt when the instrument is far short of the apex, or some patients may have no sensation even when the instrument is several millimeters beyond the apex. Not using anesthesia to aid in length determination cannot replace radiographs or an electronic apex locator for accuracy. Another misconception is that after the canals have been cleaned and shaped, it is not necessary to anesthetize the patient at the obturation appointment. Unfortunately, during obturation, pressure is created and small amounts of sealer may be extruded beyond the apex. This may be quite uncomfortable for the patient. Many patients (and the dentist) are more at ease if regional hard and soft tissue anesthesia is present.

Adjunctive Pharmacologic Therapy

Anxious patients may benefit from sedation (oral, inhalation, intravenous). However, even with conscious sedation, profound local anesthesia is required to eliminate pain during dental treatment.[38-40] Nitrous oxide administration helps reduce pain during treatment in patients presenting with symptomatic irreversible pulpitis.[39] A discussion on agents that control anxiety is included in Chapter 10.

CONVENTIONAL PULPAL ANESTHESIA FOR RESTORATIVE DENTISTRY

Success of local anesthesia is variable. Two surveys of patients and dentists indicated that inadequate anesthesia was common during restorative treatment.[7,41] Several factors affect anesthesia, such as the type of procedure (endodontic, extraction, restorative, periodontal, and so on), arch location (maxillary or mandibular), the patient's anxiety level, and the presence of inflamed tissue. This chapter emphasizes the evidence-based requirements for pulpal anesthesia, which differ from

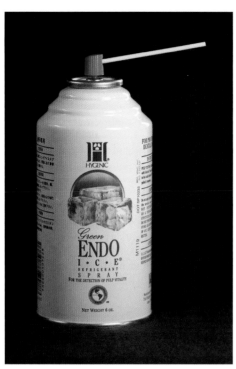

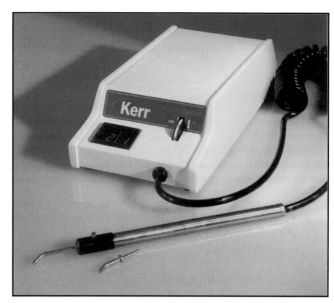

Fig. 9.3 An electrical pulp tester (EPT) also may be used to test for pulpal anesthesia before a clinical procedure is started. (Courtesy SybronEndo, Glendora, Calif.)

Fig. 9.2 A cold refrigerant may be used to test for pulpal anesthesia before the start of a clinical procedure. (Courtesy Coltene/Whaledent, Cuyahoga Falls, Ohio.)

those for oral surgery, implant dentistry, periodontics, and pediatric dentistry.

Many clinical studies have objectively evaluated local anesthetic agents and techniques. A measurement of pulpal anesthesia before beginning a clinical procedure is obtained with a cold spray refrigerant (Fig. 9.2) or electric pulp tester (Fig. 9.3). The cold spray refrigerant is the easiest to use clinically. The cold refrigerant is sprayed on a large cotton pellet held with cotton tweezers. The cold pellet is then placed on the tooth (Fig. 9.4). No pulpal response to the stimuli after administration of anesthetic means probable profound pulpal anesthesia in asymptomatic teeth with vital pulps.[42,43] Experimental studies that have investigated the use of local anesthesia are discussed in the following sections. Conventional injection techniques are detailed in other textbooks.

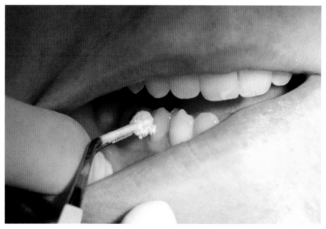

Fig. 9.4 The pellet with the cold refrigerant is applied to the surface of the tooth.

MANDIBULAR ANESTHESIA FOR RESTORATIVE DENTISTRY

Lidocaine with Epinephrine and Vasoconstrictors

The most commonly used local anesthetic agent is 2% lidocaine with 1:100,000 epinephrine, which is a safe and effective drug.[14,44] This agent is indicated for procedures in this chapter unless specified otherwise.

Vasoconstrictors are also generally safe. It has been stated that vasoconstrictors should be avoided in patients who have high blood pressure (higher than 200 mmHg systolic or 115 mmHg diastolic), cardiac dysrhythmias, severe cardio-

vascular disease, or unstable angina or who are less than 6 months past a myocardial infarction or cerebrovascular accident.[14] These conditions are contraindications to routine dental treatment. Patients taking antidepressants, nonselective beta-blocking agents, medicine for Parkinson disease, and cocaine are at risk for problems.[14,44] In patients taking these medications, plain mepivacaine (3% Carbocaine) can be used for the inferior alveolar nerve block.

Anesthetic Factors Associated with the Inferior Alveolar Nerve Block

Although the most common method of mandibular anesthesia is the inferior alveolar nerve block, this injection also has the greatest number of failures.[44] The following sections discuss the expected signs of successful (and unsuccessful) anesthesia after administration of one cartridge of 2% lidocaine with 1:100,000 epinephrine.

Lip Numbness

Lip numbness usually occurs in 4 to 6 minutes after injection.[44-51] Lip numbness indicates only that the injection blocked the nerves to the soft tissues of the lip, not necessarily that pulpal anesthesia has been obtained.[44-54] If lip numbness is not obtained, the block has been "missed." If this occurs frequently, the injection technique should be reviewed.

Soft Tissue Anesthesia

Lack of mucosal or gingival response to a sharp explorer does not indicate pulpal anesthesia.[44-54]

Onset of Pulpal Anesthesia

Pulpal anesthesia usually occurs in 5 to 9 minutes in the molars and premolars and 14 to 19 minutes in the anterior teeth.[44-54] In some patients, onset occurs sooner, and in others it is delayed.[44-54]

Duration

The duration of pulpal anesthesia in the mandible is very good.[44-54] Therefore, if successful, anesthesia usually (but not always) persists for approximately $2\frac{1}{2}$ hours.[52]

Success

The incidence of successful mandibular pulpal anesthesia tends to be higher in molars and premolars and lower in anterior teeth.[44-54] Pulpal anesthesia is not achieved in all patients after what appears to be a clinically successful inferior alveolar nerve block (i.e., numb lip and chin). In such cases other approaches are required.

Alternative Attempts to Increase Anesthetic Success
Increasing the Volume

Increasing the volume of anesthetic from one to two cartridges does not increase the success rate for obtaining pulpal anesthesia with the inferior alveolar nerve block.[44,45,53,54]

Increasing the Epinephrine Concentration

There is no improvement in pulpal anesthesia with a higher concentration (1:50,000) of epinephrine in an inferior alveolar nerve block.[54,55]

Alternative Solutions
2% Mepivacaine with 1:20,000 Levonordefrin, 4% Prilocaine with 1:200,000 Epinephrine, and Plain Solutions (3% Mepivacaine and 4% Prilocaine)

As alternative solutions, 2% mepivacaine with 1:20,000 levonordefrin; 4% prilocaine with 1:200,000 epinephrine; and plain solutions (3% mepivacaine and 4% prilocaine) are equivalent to 2% lidocaine with 1:100,000 epinephrine in providing pulpal anesthesia for at approximately 1 hour after an inferior alveolar nerve block.[48,51]

4% Articaine with Epinephrine for Inferior Alveolar Nerve Blocks

Articaine is a safe and effective local anesthetic agent.[56-65] Articaine has a reputation for providing an improved local anesthetic effect.[66] However, clinical trials have failed to detect any superiority of articaine over lidocaine in inferior alveolar nerve block anesthesia.[61,64]

Articaine, like prilocaine, has the potential to cause neuropathies.[67] Some authors have found the incidence of paresthesia (involving the lip and/or tongue) associated with articaine and prilocaine to be higher than that found with either lidocaine or mepivacaine.[67-69] Other authors have not found a higher incidence when using articaine.[70] However, because there is no difference in success of pulpal anesthesia between articaine and lidocaine for inferior alveolar nerve blocks, and some attorneys are aware of the proposed association of articaine to paresthesia, it seems reasonable to use articaine for infiltrations but not for nerve blocks.

Long-Acting Agents

Clinical trials of bupivacaine and etidocaine have been conducted in oral surgery, endodontics, and periodontics.[71-74] These agents provide a prolonged analgesic period and are indicated when postoperative pain is anticipated. However, not all patients want prolonged lip numbness.[72] For those patients, analgesics may be prescribed. Compared with lidocaine, bupivacaine has a somewhat slower onset but almost double the duration of pulpal anesthesia in the mandible (approximately 4 hours).[52]

Buffered Lidocaine

Buffering lidocaine with sodium bicarbonate raises the pH of the anesthetic solution. In medicine there is evidence that buffering lidocaine results in less pain during the injection.[75,76] In dentistry, some studies[77-80] found that buffered lidocaine produced less pain on injection and a faster onset of anesthesia. However, other dental studies[81,82] did not find less pain on injection or a faster onset with buffered lidocaine for inferior alveolar nerve block. There is a commercial buffering system available (OnPharma, Los Gatos, California), but there are no peer-reviewed studies on this system. Further studies are needed.

Alternative Injections and Locations
Gow-Gates and Vizarani-Akinosi Techniques

Neither the Gow-Gates[83] nor the Vizarani-Akinosi[84] technique is superior to the standard inferior alveolar nerve block injection.[85-90] These techniques are not replacements for the inferior alveolar nerve block, but rather are useful when standard approaches cannot be used; for example, with trismus the Vizarani-Akinosi closed mouth technique can be used.

Incisive Nerve Block/Infiltration at the Mental Foramen

The incisive nerve block is successful 80% to 83% of the time in anesthetizing the premolar teeth for about 20 to 30 minutes.[50,91-93] It is not effective for the central and lateral incisors.[50]

Lidocaine Infiltration Injections

Labial or lingual infiltration injections of a lidocaine solution alone are not effective for pulpal anesthesia in the mandible.[94-96]

Articaine Infiltration Injections

Articaine is significantly better than lidocaine for buccal infiltration of the mandibular first molar.[97-100] However, articaine alone does not predictably provide pulpal anesthesia of the first molar. There is no difference between 4% articaine with 1:100,000 and 1:200,000 epinephrine for buccal infiltration.[101]

In anterior teeth, buccal and lingual infiltrations of articaine provide initial pulpal anesthesia, but anesthesia declines over 60 minutes.[102,103]

Evaluating Mechanisms of Failure with the Inferior Alveolar Nerve Block
Accuracy of Needle Placement

Accurate anatomic positioning of the needle is no guarantee of a successful block.[104,105] Interestingly, even locating the inferior alveolar nerve with ultrasound or with a peripheral nerve stimulator before the injection did not improve success.[106,107] The anesthetic solution may not completely diffuse into the nerve trunk (Fig. 9.5) to reach and block all nerves, even if deposited at the correct site, thus resulting in failure.[108]

Needle Deflection and Needle Bevel

Needle deflection has been theorized to be a cause of failure of the inferior alveolar nerve block.[23,109-112] However, two studies have shown that needle bevel orientation (away or toward the mandibular foramen or ramus) does not affect the success of the inferior alveolar nerve block.[113,114]

Accessory Innervation

Anatomic evidence suggests that accessory innervation exists from branches of the mylohyoid nerve.[115] A study using a mylohyoid injection lingual and inferior to the retromolar fossa, in addition to an inferior alveolar nerve block, showed no enhancement of pulpal anesthesia.[116] Therefore, the mylohyoid nerve is not a major factor in failure of the inferior alveolar nerve block.

Cross-Innervation

Cross-innervation from the contralateral inferior alveolar nerve has been implicated in failure to achieve anesthesia in anterior teeth after an inferior alveolar nerve block injection. Cross-innervation does occur in incisors but is not the major reason for failure in incisor teeth with the inferior alveolar nerve block.[117]

Red Hair

In medicine, red-haired females have shown reduced subcutaneous efficacy of lidocaine and increased requirements for desflurane.[118] However, in dentistry, red hair was unrelated to success rates for the inferior alveolar nerve block. Red hair was associated with higher levels of dental anxiety.[118]

Methods to Increase Success of the Inferior Alveolar Nerve Block
Infiltrations of Articaine After an Inferior Alveolar Nerve Block

An important clinical finding is that an articaine infiltration of the first molar, premolars, and anterior teeth after an inferior alveolar nerve block should provide pulpal anesthesia for approximately 1 hour.[102,119,120] The second molar may require a supplemental intraosseous or periodontal ligament injection to achieve success.

Intraosseous Anesthesia After an Inferior Alveolar Nerve Block

Supplemental intraosseous injections of lidocaine and mepivacaine with vasoconstrictors allow quick onset and increase the success of the inferior alveolar nerve block for approximately 60 minutes.[121,122] Using 3% mepivacaine plain results in pulpal anesthesia for approximately 30 minutes.[123]

Periodontal Ligament Anesthesia After an Inferior Alveolar Nerve Block

Supplemental periodontal ligament injections of 2% lidocaine with 1:100,000 epinephrine increase the success of the inferior alveolar nerve block, but the duration is approximately 23 minutes.[124]

Injection Speed and Success

A slow inferior alveolar nerve block increases success over a fast injection[25] but not for patients diagnosed with irreversible pulpitis.[26]

Pain and Inflammation

Most studies have evaluated anesthesia in the absence of symptoms and inflammation; results differ if these conditions are present.[5,125] As discussed later, patients who have symptomatic pulpal or periapical pathosis (and/or who are anxious) present significant anesthesia problems.

MAXILLARY ANESTHESIA FOR RESTORATIVE DENTISTRY

Unless otherwise specified, the conventional solution used is 2% lidocaine with 1:100,000 epinephrine.

Anesthesia-Related Factors

Anesthesia is more successful in the maxilla than in the mandible. The most common injection for the maxillary teeth is

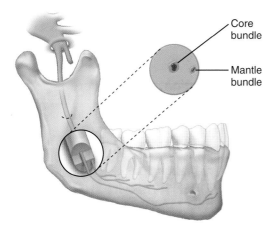

Fig. 9.5 Central core theory. The large diameter and density of the bundle may inhibit diffusion of a sufficient quantity of anesthetic to provide profound pulpal anesthesia.

Core bundle

Mantle bundle

infiltration. Several events can be expected with this technique when one cartridge of anesthetic is used.

Lip/Cheek Numbness or Dead Feeling of the Teeth

Lip/cheek numbness usually occurs within a few minutes. Lip or cheek numbness or a dead feeling when tapping the teeth together does not always indicate pulpal anesthesia. Additionally, lip or cheek numbness does not correspond to the duration of pulpal anesthesia, because the pulp does not remain anesthetized as long as the soft tissues.[44,126-134]

Success

Infiltration results in a fairly high incidence of successful pulpal anesthesia (around 87% to 92%).[11,44,126-134] However, some patients may not be anesthetized due to individual variations in response to the drug administered, operator differences, and variations of anatomy, in addition to tooth position.

Onset of Pulpal Anesthesia

Pulpal anesthesia usually occurs in 3 to 5 minutes.[44,126-134]

Duration of Pulpal Anesthesia

A problem with maxillary infiltration is the duration of pulpal anesthesia.[44,126-134] Pulpal anesthesia of the anterior teeth declines after about 30 minutes, with most losing anesthesia by 60 minutes.[44,126-134] In premolars and first molars, pulpal anesthesia is good until about 40 to 45 minutes and then it starts to decline.[44,126-134] Additional local anesthetic must be administered, depending on the duration of the procedure and the tooth group affected.

Alternative Anesthetic Solutions
Plain Solutions of Mepivacaine and Prilocaine

Anesthesia duration is shorter with plain solutions of mepivacaine and prilocaine.[132,133] Therefore, these anesthetics are used for procedures of short duration (10 to 15 minutes).

4% Prilocaine with 1:200,000 Epinephrine, 2% Mepivacaine with 1:20,000 Levonordefrin, and 4% Articaine with 1:100,000 Epinephrine

The duration of anesthesia with 4% prilocaine with 1:200,000 epinephrine; 2% mepivacaine with 1:20,000 levonordefrin; and 4% articaine with 1:100,000 epinephrine is similar to that for 2% lidocaine with 1:100,000 epinephrine.[129,133,134]

Bupivacaine with Epinephrine

Bupivacaine has a lower success rate than a lidocaine formulation in anterior teeth.[127,135] There is no difference in the first molar between the two formulations.[127] Neither agent provides pulpal anesthesia for an hour.[127,135]

Increasing the Duration of Pulpal Anesthesia
Increasing the Volume of Solution

A two-cartridge volume of 2% lidocaine with epinephrine extends the duration of pulpal anesthesia but not for 60 minutes.[128]

Increasing the Epinephrine Concentration

Increasing the epinephrine concentration to 1:50,000 epinephrine increases duration for the lateral incisor but not for the first molar.[132] Neither tooth achieved a duration of 60 minutes.[132]

Repeating an Infiltration after 30 Minutes

Adding a cartridge of 2% lidocaine with epinephrine at 30 minutes in anterior teeth and 45 minutes in posterior teeth significantly improves the duration of pulpal anesthesia and may be the best way to extend the duration of pulpal anesthesia.[131]

Alternative Injection Techniques

The *posterior superior alveolar (PSA) nerve block* anesthetizes the second molars and about 80% of first molars.[136,137] An additional mesial infiltration injection may be necessary to anesthetize the first molar. Generally, the PSA block injection is not advocated for routine restorative procedures. An infiltration of the molars is preferred.

The *infraorbital block* results in lip numbness but does not predictably anesthetize incisor pulps.[138,139] It usually anesthetizes the canines and premolars, but duration is less than 1 hour.[138,139] Generally, the infraorbital injection is not advocated for routine restorative procedures. An infiltration of the individual teeth is preferred.

The *second division block* usually anesthetizes pulps of molars and some second premolars but does not predictably anesthetize first premolars, canines, or lateral and central incisors.[140,141] The high tuberosity technique is preferred to the greater palatine approach, because it is easier and less painful.[140] Generally, the second division nerve block is not advocated for routine restorative procedures. An infiltration of the individual teeth is preferred.

The *palatal anterior superior alveolar (P-ASA) nerve block* has been advocated for anesthetizing all the maxillary incisors with a single palatal injection into the incisive canal.[142] However, this injection technique does not provide predictable pulpal anesthesia for the incisors and canines[143] and is often painful.[31]

The *anterior middle superior alveolar (AMSA) nerve block* has been advocated for unilaterally anesthetizing the maxillary central and lateral incisors, canines, and first and second premolars with a single palatal injection in the premolar region.[144] However, this injection technique does not provide predictable pulpal anesthesia for these maxillary teeth[145] and is often painful.[32]

Pain, Inflammation, and Anxiety

As mentioned, results differ from normal when an anesthetic is given to patients with either pain or inflammation (or both) or to those with anxiety.

SUPPLEMENTAL ANESTHESIA FOR RESTORATIVE DENTISTRY IN THE MANDIBLE AND MAXILLA

Indications

A supplemental injection is used if the standard injection is not effective. It is useful to repeat an initial injection only if the patient is not exhibiting the "classic" signs of soft tissue anesthesia. Generally, if the classic signs are present, reinjection is not very effective.[146] For example, after the inferior alveolar nerve block, the patient develops lip, chin, and tongue numbness and quadrant "deadness" of the teeth. A useful procedure is to test the pulp of the tooth with cold (cold refrigerant) or an electric pulp tester before the cavity preparation is begun.[42,43] If the patient feels pain to cold, a supplemental injection is indicated. Assuming that reinjection using the inferior alveolar nerve block approach will be successful is wishful thinking; failure the first time is usually followed by failure on the second attempt. The dentist should go directly to a supplemental technique. Three such injections are the (1) *infiltration injection,* (2) *intraosseous (IO) injection,* and (3) *periodontal ligament (PDL) injection.*

Infiltration

Additional Infiltration of Lidocaine in the Maxilla

Because the duration of pulpal anesthesia for infiltration in the maxilla is less than 60 minutes, adding a cartridge of 2% lidocaine with epinephrine at 30 minutes in the anterior teeth and at about 45 minutes in premolar and molar teeth significantly improves the duration of pulpal anesthesia and may be the best way to extend the duration of pulpal anesthesia in maxillary teeth.[131]

Infiltration of Articaine in the Mandible

An important clinical finding is that a buccal articaine infiltration of the first molar and premolars and a labial infiltration of the anterior teeth, after an inferior alveolar nerve block, should provide pulpal anesthesia for approximately 1 hour.[102,119,120] The second molar may require a supplemental intraosseous or periodontal ligament injection.

Intraosseous Anesthesia

The IO injection has been shown to be effective by substantial research and clinical usage. It is particularly useful in conjunction with a conventional injection when it is likely that supplemental anesthesia will be necessary (e.g., in mandibular second molar teeth).[121-123] The IO injection allows placement of a local anesthetic directly into the cancellous bone adjacent to the tooth. There is an IO system with two components (Stabident; Fairfax Dental, Miami, Florida; Fig. 9.6). One part is a slow-speed handpiece–driven perforator, which drills a small hole through the cortical plate (Fig. 9.7). The anesthetic solution is delivered into cancellous bone through a matching 27-gauge, ultrashort injector needle (Fig. 9.8). Another IO system uses a guide sleeve (X-tip; Dentsply, York, Pennsylvania; Fig. 9.9) that remains in the perforation (Fig. 9.10). This serves as a guide for the needle, and it may remain in place throughout the procedure in case reinjection is necessary. The perforation may be made in attached gingiva or alveolar mucosa with this system.[147]

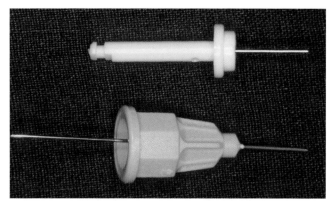

Fig. 9.6 Components of an intraosseous injection system. The perforator *(top)* is a small, sharp, latch-type drill used to make an opening through soft tissue and bone. The needle *(bottom)* is short and of small gauge to allow insertion and injection directly through the opening.

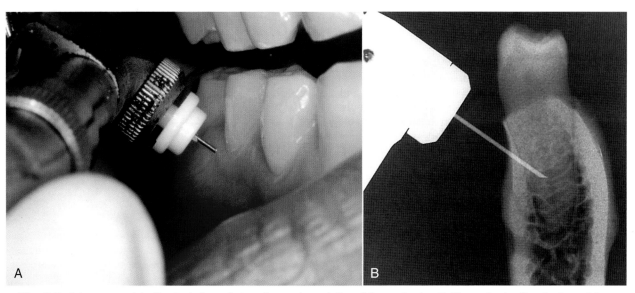

A

B

Fig. 9.7 Intraosseous injection technique. **A,** Location and angulation of the perforator. **B,** The perforator "breaks through" cortical bone into the medullary space.

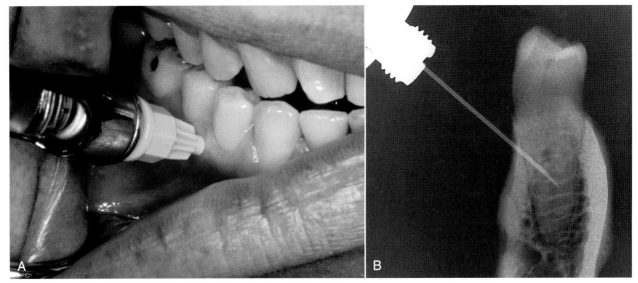

Fig. 9.8 **A,** The needle is inserted directly into the opening. **B,** Anesthetic is injected into medullary bone, where it diffuses widely to block dental nerves.

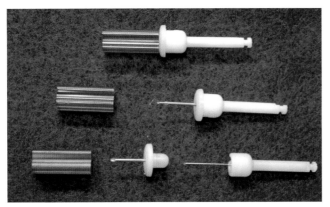

Fig. 9.9 Components of another approach to intraosseous injection: the drill and guide sleeve and cover *(top).* The drill (a special hollow needle) leads the guide sleeve through the cortical plate *(middle),* in which it is separated and withdrawn *(bottom).* The remaining guide sleeve is designed to accept a 27-gauge needle that injects the anesthetic solution.

Technique for the Stabident System

The area of perforation and injection is on a horizontal line of the buccal gingival margins of the adjacent teeth and a vertical line that passes through the interdental papilla distal to the tooth to be injected. A point approximately 2 mm below the intersection of these lines is selected as the perforation site. This site must be in attached gingiva. The soft tissue is first anesthetized by infiltration. The perforator is placed through the gingiva perpendicular to the cortical plate. With the point gently resting against bone, the clinician activates the handpiece at full speed while pushing the perforator, with light pressure, against bone and then slightly withdrawing the perforator and pushing it again against the bone (pecking motion). This action is continued until a "break through" into the cancellous bone is achieved (this takes approximately 2 to 5 seconds).[147]

The standard syringe is held in a "pen-gripping" fashion, and the needle is precisely aligned with and inserted into the

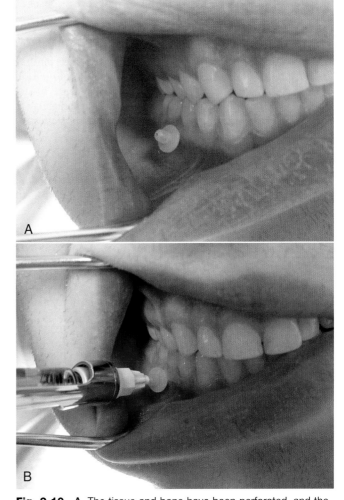

Fig. 9.10 **A,** The tissue and bone have been perforated, and the perforator now serves as a guide sleeve. **B,** The anesthetic needle is in place in the guide sleeve.

perforation. A full cartridge of anesthetic solution is *slowly* delivered over 1 to 2 minutes with light pressure. If back-pressure is encountered, the needle is rotated approximately a quarter turn and deposition is reattempted. If this attempt is unsuccessful, the needle should be removed and checked for blockage. If the needle is not blocked, it is reinserted or the site is opened with a new perforator and the injection is repeated.[147]

Perforator "Breakage"
Rarely, the metal perforator "separates" from the plastic hub. If this occurs, the perforator is easily removed with a hemostat; there are no reports of a perforator breaking into parts.[121-123,147-149]

Injection Discomfort
When the IO injection is used as a primary injection, pain is experienced about one fourth of the time.[148-150] When the IO injection is used as a supplemental injection, fewer patients experience pain.[121-123,151,152]

Selection of Perforation Site
With IO injections, distal perforation and injection to the tooth result in the best anesthesia.[121-123,147-149,151,152] The second molars are an exception; in these teeth, a mesial site is preferred.[121-123,147-149,151,152]

Anesthetic Agents
When the IO injection is used as a supplemental injection after the inferior alveolar nerve block in patients without pain, excellent success has been reported for 2% lidocaine with 1:100,000 epinephrine and 2% mepivacaine with 1:20,000 levonordefrin.[121,122] However, because of the adverse cardiovascular reactions with a long-acting anesthetic (0.5% bupivacaine with 1:200,000 epinephrine)[153] and the lack of a prolonged duration of pulpal anesthesia, this agent does not offer any advantage over lidocaine. Three percent mepivacaine plain is successful, but the duration of pulpal anesthesia is shorter.[123]

Onset of Anesthesia
Onset of anesthesia is rapid with the IO injection.[121-123,147-149,151,152] There is no waiting period for anesthesia.

Success
When the IO injection is used as a supplemental injection after an inferior alveolar nerve block in pain-free patients, success rates are very good.[121,122]

Failure
If the anesthetic solution squirts out of the perforation (back-flow) with an IO injection, anesthesia will not be obtained.[147] Reperforation or choosing another perforation site is then necessary.

Duration
With a primary IO injection, the duration of pulpal anesthesia declines steadily over 1 hour.[148,149] There is an even shorter duration with 3% mepivacaine, compared with 2% lidocaine with 1:100,000 epinephrine.[149] With a supplemental IO injection of lidocaine after the inferior alveolar nerve block in patients without pain, the duration of pulpal anesthesia is very good for 1 hour.[121,122] A solution of 3% mepivacaine, when used as a supplemental IO injection, results in a shorter anesthetic duration.[123]

Postoperative Pain and Problems
With primary and supplemental IO injection techniques, the majority of patients report no pain or mild pain postoperatively.[121-123,147-149,151,152] Fewer than 5% develop exudate and/or localized swelling at the perforation site, possibly from overheating of the bone during perforation.[121-123,147-149,151,152]

Systemic Effects
With both primary and supplemental IO injection techniques using anesthetics with a vasoconstrictor (epinephrine or levonordefrin), most patients perceive an increased heart rate.[148,149,151,152,154] When these agents are used, the patient should be informed *before the injection* of this tachycardia to lessen his or her anxiety. No significant heart rate increase occurs with 3% mepivacaine plain.[149,155] The venous plasma levels of lidocaine are the same for an IO injection as for infiltration injection.[156] Therefore, the same precautions for the maximum amount of lidocaine given for an infiltration injection apply to an IO injection.[156]

Medical Contraindications
Patients taking antidepressants, nonselective beta-blocking agents, medicine for Parkinson disease, and cocaine should not receive IO injections of solutions containing epinephrine or levonordefrin[44]; 3% mepivacaine plain is preferred.

Precautions
An IO injection should not be used with painful necrotic teeth with periapical radiolucencies or with teeth exhibiting cellulitis or abscess formation. This injection would be very painful and would likely not provide profound anesthesia.

Periodontal Ligament Injection
The PDL injection is also a useful technique if a conventional injection is unsuccessful.[157,158] The technique is clinically less effective than the IO injection[146] but still has its clinical place.

Technique
The procedure for a PDL injection (Fig. 9.11) is not difficult but does require practice and familiarity. A standard syringe or pressure syringe is equipped with a 30-gauge, ultrashort needle or a 27- or 25-gauge short needle. The needle is inserted into the mesial gingival sulcus at a 30-degree angle to the long axis of the tooth. The needle is supported by the fingers or a hemostat and is positioned with maximum penetration (wedged between the root and crestal bone). Heavy pressure is *slowly* applied on the syringe handle for approximately 10 to 20 seconds (conventional syringe), or the trigger is *slowly* squeezed once or twice with resistance (pressure syringe). *Back-pressure is important.* If there is no back-pressure (resistance)—that is, if the anesthetic readily flows out of the sulcus—the needle is repositioned, and the technique is repeated until back-pressure is attained. The injection is then repeated on the distal surface. Only a small volume of anesthetic (approximately 0.2 mL) is deposited on each surface.

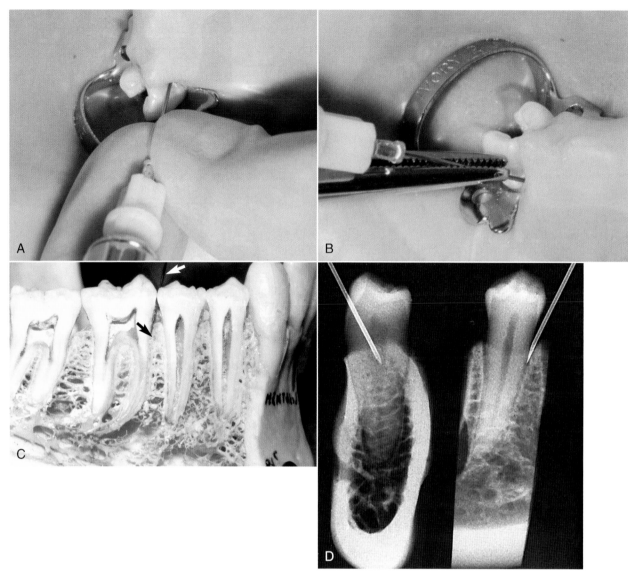

Fig. 9.11 Intraligamentary injection. **A,** Needle insertion using the fingers to prevent needle buckling. **B,** A hemostat may be substituted for the fingers to support and direct the needle. The injection may be given with or without the rubber dam in place. **C,** Note the direction and position of the needle *(arrows)*. The tip of the needle will be wedged between the crestal bone and the root surface. **D,** Angle of the needle relative to the long axis of the tooth *(left)*. With approximately a 30-degree orientation, the needle tip will be positioned close to the midline of the root.

Mechanism of Action

The PDL injection forces anesthetic solution through the cribriform plate (Fig. 9.12) into the marrow spaces and into the vasculature in and around the tooth (Figs. 9.13 and 9.14).[157-160] The primary route is not the periodontal ligament; the mechanism of action is not related to direct pressure on the nerves.[161,162]

Injection Discomfort in Asymptomatic Patients

When the PDL injection is the primary injection, needle insertion and injection may be painful about one third of the time.[161-163] In maxillary anterior teeth, the PDL injection may be quite painful[163] and should not be used. An infiltration is preferred. As a supplemental injection after an inferior alveolar nerve block, the PDL injection has a low potential to be painful.[124]

Onset of Anesthesia

The onset of anesthesia is rapid with a PDL injection; there is no waiting period to begin the clinical procedure.[161-163] If anesthesia is still not adequate, reinjection is necessary.

Success in Asymptomatic Teeth

Success rates for the PDL injection, when used as a primary injection, have been reported to be about 75% in mandibular and maxillary posterior teeth, with a duration of pulpal anesthesia of 10 to 15 minutes.[162,163] Success rates have been low in anterior teeth.[162-164] Anesthetic solutions without vasoconstrictors (3% mepivacaine) or with reduced vasoconstrictor concentrations (bupivacaine with 1:200,000 epinephrine) are not very effective.[162,165-167] Articaine is equivalent to lidocaine.[63]

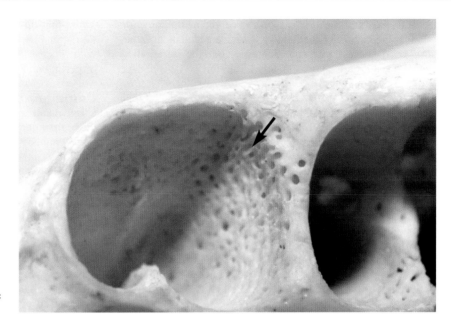

Fig. 9.12 Extraction socket of a second molar. The bone of the cribriform plate is very porous, particularly in the cervical region *(arrow)*. During the intraligamentary injection, this is the region of passage of most anesthetic solution into the medullary space.

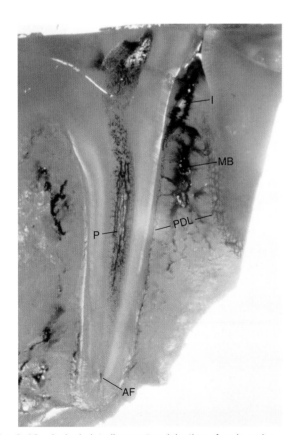

Fig. 9.13 A single intraligamentary injection of carbon dye adjacent to a dog's tooth demonstrates the distribution of dye particles. Particles are concentrated at the injection site *(I)* and in the medullary bone *(MB)*, the apical foramen *(AF)*, and the pulp *(P)* of the injected tooth. Dye particles have spread through the periodontal ligament *(PDL)* of both the injected and adjacent teeth.

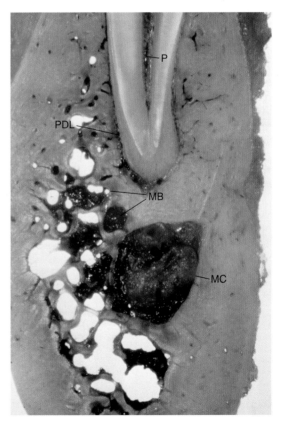

Fig. 9.14 A single injection of dye was made in the distal periodontal ligament. This frontal section, including the tooth apex and surrounding structures, shows that dye distributes to the pulp *(P)*, periodontal ligament space *(PDL)*, medullary bone space *(MB)*, and mandibular canal *(MC)*. The widespread distribution of solutions from the intraligamentary injection may anesthetize the adjacent teeth.

When the PDL injection is used as a supplemental injection (standard techniques have failed to provide adequate anesthesia), good success rates are achieved, but the duration of pulpal anesthesia is approximately 23 minutes.[124]

Duration in Asymptomatic Teeth

The duration of profound pulpal anesthesia (either primary or supplemental) with PDL injections is approximately 10 to 15 minutes.[63,124,161-163]

Postoperative Discomfort in Asymptomatic Teeth

When the PDL injection is used as a primary technique, postoperative pain occurs in one third to three fourths of patients, with a duration of 14 hours to 3 days.[63,124,161-163,168,169] There is no difference between articaine and lidocaine.[63] The discomfort is related to damage from needle insertion rather than to the pressure of depositing the solution.[168] About one third of patients report that their tooth feels "high."[162,163]

Selective Anesthesia

It has been suggested that a PDL injection may be used in the differential diagnosis of poorly localized, painful irreversible pulpitis.[170] However, adjacent teeth are often anesthetized with PDL injection of a single tooth.[161-163] Therefore, this injection is *not* useful for differential diagnosis.

Systemic Effects

Although some authors[171] have found that the PDL injection raises the heart rate, human studies have shown that these injections do not cause significant changes in heart rate.[169,172]

Other Factors

Different needle gauges (25, 27, or 30 gauge) are equally effective for PDL injections.[173] Special pressure syringes have been marketed (Fig. 9.15) but have not proved to be more effective than a standard syringe.[162,163,173]

Damage to the Periodontium

Clinical and animal studies have demonstrated the relative safety of the PDL injection.[161-163,169,174-179] Minor local damage is limited to the site of needle penetration (Fig. 9.16); this subsequently undergoes repair.[174] In some instances, periodontal infections have occurred.[162,163] The clinician should be aware that this may happen. Histologic areas of root resorption after PDL injections have also been reported, which heal with time.[178,179] Damaging effects from injecting into an area of periodontal disease are unlikely.[180]

Damage to the Pulp

Clinical and animal studies have shown no adverse effects on the pulp after PDL injections.[161-163,181,182] However, physiologic changes in the pulp do occur, including a rapid and prolonged, marked decrease in blood flow caused by epinephrine.[183] This vascular impairment has no demonstrated damaging effect, even in conjunction with restorative procedures.[184] The PDL injection probably would not result in severe pulpal injury, although this has not been studied with extensive (crown) preparations or in teeth with caries.

Damage to Primary Teeth

Minor enamel hypoplasia of succedaneous teeth has been seen after PDL injections in primary teeth.[185] However, this effect was caused by the cytotoxicity of the local anesthetic rather than by the actual injection. Therefore, this injection may be used for anesthetizing primary teeth.

Precautions

The PDL injection should not be used with necrotic pulps and periapical pathosis or with cellulitis or abscess formation. This would be very painful and likely not provide profound anesthesia.

ANESTHESIA DIFFICULTIES IN ENDODONTICS

The following is a classic scenario: The diagnosis is irreversible pulpitis. The dentist administers the standard inferior alveolar nerve block. The patient reports classic signs of anesthesia (lip numbness and a dull feeling of the tooth or

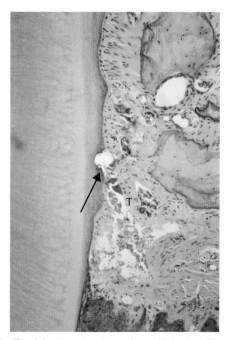

Fig. 9.16 The injection site at the time of injection. The needle tract *(T)*, which ends in a gouge in cementum *(arrow)*, is apparent in the connective tissue. No tissue changes are evident outside the penetration site, including the more apical tissues.

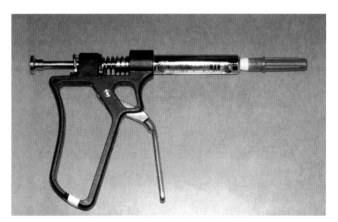

Fig. 9.15 Example of a special syringe used for the intraligamentary injection. Although these devices are capable of injecting with more pressure, they have not been shown to be superior to the standard syringe.

quadrant). After isolation, access preparation is begun. When the bur is in enamel, the patient feels nothing. Once the bur enters dentin or possibly not until the pulp is exposed, the patient feels sharp pain. Obviously, pulpal anesthesia is not profound and additional anesthetic is required. The following are some of the theories as to why this problem occurs.

1. The anesthetic solution may not completely penetrate to the sensory nerves that innervate the pulp, especially in the mandible.
2. The *central core theory* states that nerves on the outside of the nerve bundle supply molar teeth, whereas nerves on the inside supply anterior teeth (see Fig. 9.5). The anesthetic solution may not diffuse into the nerve trunk to reach all nerves to produce an adequate block, even if deposited at the correct site. This theory would explain the higher experimental failure rates in anterior teeth with the inferior alveolar nerve block.[44-55]
3. *Local tissues change* because of inflammation. This popular theory states that the lowered pH of inflamed tissue reduces the amount of the base form of the anesthetic available to penetrate the nerve membrane.[14] Consequently, there is less of the ionized form within the nerve to achieve anesthesia. Although this theory may have some validity for regions with swelling, it does not relate to anesthesia difficulties in the mandible.[44] It does not explain the major problem, which is the mandibular molar with pulpitis that is not anesthetized by an inferior alveolar injection. The injection site is distant from the area of inflammation; changes in tissue pH would be unrelated to the anesthesia problem.
4. *Hyperalgesia.* Change in nociceptor (pain receptor) pathways is a more plausible explanation. This theory states that the nerves arising in inflamed tissue have altered resting potentials and decreased excitability thresholds. These changes are not restricted to the inflamed pulp itself, but rather affect the entire neuronal membrane, extending to the central nervous system.[5,6] Local anesthetic agents are not sufficient to prevent impulse transmission, owing to these lowered excitability thresholds.[5]
5. *Apprehension.* Patients in pain often are anxious, which lowers the pain threshold. A vicious cycle may be established in which initial apprehension leads to a decreased pain threshold, which leads to anesthesia difficulties, which lead to increased apprehension, which results in loss of control and confidence, and so on. Therefore, if this cycle becomes evident, the practitioner should stop treatment immediately and regain control, schedule another appointment, or consider referral to an endodontist. Most patients will endure some pain during the initial stages of root canal treatment if they have confidence in the dentist. However, they will not tolerate being hurt repeatedly!
6. *Insufficient time allowed after injection.* The dentist may not allow adequate time for the anesthetic to diffuse and to block the sensory nerves. Onset may be very slow, particularly with the inferior alveolar block.

Success of the Inferior Alveolar Nerve Block with Symptomatic Irreversible Pulpitis

In clinical studies of mandibular posterior teeth in patients with symptomatic irreversible pulpitis, a successful inferior alveolar nerve block was achieved 15% to 57% of the time.[38-40,61,186-197] Articaine is not superior to lidocaine in this group of patients.[61,192]

Some authors have suggested that a two-cartridge volume is better than a one-cartridge volume.[195] However, some studies have used a two-cartridge volume, and success rates are similar to those for a one-cartridge volume.[38,191,196]

Success of Maxillary Molar Infiltration with Irreversible Pulpitis

Clinical studies of maxillary posterior buccal infiltrations in patients presenting with irreversible pulpitis reported successful infiltration 54% to 88% of the time.[186,198,199] Although some have found a difference between articaine and lidocaine,[200] others have not found a difference.[199,201-202]

Asymptomatic Irreversible Pulpitis versus Symptomatic Irreversible Pulpitis

Patients who have spontaneous pain (symptomatic irreversible pulpitis) have less successful anesthesia after an inferior alveolar nerve block than patients who do not have spontaneous pain or who have pain only when the tooth is stimulated (asymptomatic irreversible pulpitis).[203] It is important to distinguish between these patients when evaluating clinical success, because the success rates differ.

SUPPLEMENTAL TECHNIQUES FOR MANDIBULAR TEETH IN ENDODONTICS

Supplemental Buccal Infiltration of Articaine

Although the infiltration of articaine is effective in restorative dentistry as a supplemental technique (after the inferior alveolar nerve block), its use in endodontically involved teeth does not result in profound pulpal anesthesia.[146,190,191,196] A buccal infiltration of lidocaine is also not effective.[197] Neither buccal infiltration alone, nor buccal plus lingual infiltrations alone or after an inferior alveolar nerve block, result in successful pulpal anesthesia.[194,197,204,205]

Therefore, the IO and PDL injections are the preferred approaches; the intrapulpal (IP) injection is reserved for special endodontic situations.

Supplemental Intraosseous Injections

For use as a supplemental injection with irreversible pulpitis, high success rates (about 90%) have been reported for IO injections.[186,190,191,206] There is no difference between lidocaine and articaine.[206] Three percent mepivacaine has an 80% success rate, which increases to 98% with a second IO injection of 3% mepivacaine.[187]

Although some studies[207,208] have suggested that an IO injection alone can successfully anesthetize patients presenting with irreversible pulpitis, it is doubtful that this would be successful.[186,190,191,195]

Supplemental Periodontal Ligament Injections

Supplemental PDL injections are not as successful as supplemental IO injections.[146,209] For example, in patients with irreversible pulpitis, use of a computer-controlled local anesthetic delivery system (see Fig. 9.1) for supplemental PDL injections was successful in about half of patients with irreversible pulpitis.[210] Others have reported success in about three quarters to half of patients.[146,189] Reinjection increases the success rate.[173,189]

Supplemental Intrapulpal Injection

Besides the supplemental infiltration, IO, and PDL injections discussed previously, the IP injection is used when other methods fail.

Indications

After the inferior alveolar nerve block, on occasion IO and PDL injections do not produce profound anesthesia, even when repeated, and pain persists when the pulp is entered. This is an indication for an IP injection. However, the IP injection should not be given without first administering an inferior alveolar block plus an IO or IL injection. The IP injection is very painful without some other form of supplemental anesthesia.

Advantages and Disadvantages

Although the IP injection is somewhat popular, it has disadvantages as well as advantages, making it the last supplemental injection of choice. The major drawback is that the needle is inserted directly into a vital and very sensitive pulp; thus, the injection may be exquisitely painful. Also, the effects of the injection are unpredictable if it is not given under pressure. Once anesthesia has been obtained, the duration is short (5 to 15 minutes). Therefore, the bulk of the pulp must be removed quickly and at the correct working length to prevent recurrence of pain during instrumentation. Another disadvantage is that the pulp must be exposed to permit direct injection; often problems with anesthesia occur before pulpal exposure.

The advantage is the predictability of profound anesthesia if the IP injection is given under back-pressure. The onset of anesthesia is immediate, and no special syringes or needles are required, although different approaches may be necessary to attain the desired back-pressure.

Mechanism of Action

Strong back-pressure has been shown to be the major factor in producing anesthesia.[211,212] Depositing anesthetic passively into the pulp chamber is not adequate; the solution will not diffuse throughout the pulp. Therefore, the anesthetic agent is not solely responsible for intrapulpal anesthesia; it also depends on pressure.

Technique

The patient must be informed that a "little extra" anesthetic will ensure comfort and that there will be "a sharp sensation" as the injection is given.

One technique creates back-pressure by stoppering the access with a cotton pellet to prevent backflow of anesthetic (Fig. 9.17).[211,212] Other stoppers, such as gutta-percha, waxes, or pieces of rubber, have been used. If possible, the roof of the pulp chamber should be penetrated by a half-round bur, which allows the needle to fit snugly in the bur hole.

Another approach is an injection into each canal after the chamber has been unroofed. A standard syringe is usually equipped with a bent short needle. With fingers supporting the needle shaft to prevent buckling, the needle is positioned in the access opening and then moved down the canal, as the anesthetic is slowly expressed, to the point of wedging. Maximum pressure is then applied slowly on the syringe handle for 5 to 10 seconds. If there is no back-pressure, anesthetic flows out of the access opening. The needle is then wedged deeper or withdrawn and replaced with a larger diameter needle (or stoppered with a cotton pellet), and the injection is repeated. This may be necessary in each canal.

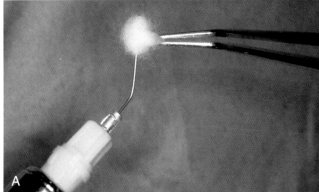

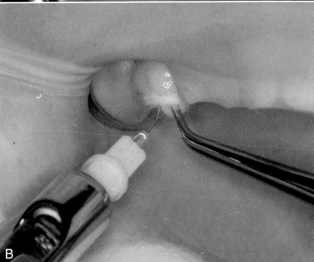

Fig. 9.17 Intrapulpal injection technique. **A,** A 45-degree bend is placed on the needle. To stopper the injection site, a cotton pellet is pulled over the needle and the needle is placed in the opening in the pulp (the patient is forewarned of discomfort!). **B,** The cotton pellet is packed *tightly* and held in the access opening, and the syringe handle is pushed *slowly*. The patient often feels sharp pain with resistance on the syringe handle; this resistance usually indicates successful anesthesia.

ANESTHETIC MANAGEMENT OF PULPAL OR PERIAPICAL PATHOSES

Symptomatic Irreversible Pulpitis

With irreversible pulpitis, the teeth most difficult to anesthetize are the mandibular molars, followed in order by the mandibular and maxillary premolars, maxillary molars, mandibular anterior teeth, and maxillary anterior teeth. The vital inflamed pulp must be instrumented and removed. Also, pulpal tissue has a very concentrated sensory nerve supply, particularly in the pulp chamber. These factors, combined with others related to inflammatory effects on sensory nerves and failures that occur with conventional techniques, make anesthetizing patients with painful irreversible pulpitis a challenge.

Different clinical situations present surprises. In some cases, inflamed vital tissue exists only in the apical canals, and the tissue in the chamber is necrotic and does not respond to the cold refrigerant or electric pulp testing. Obviously, in this situation the chamber is entered with no problem, but when the operator attempts to place a file to length, severe pain results. IO or PDL injections are helpful, and an IP injection may be used. However, irreversible pulpitis must be differentiated from a symptomatic necrotic tooth with a distinct radiographic apical abscess, because IO, PDL, and IP injections are contraindicated in the latter condition.

General Considerations

A conventional anesthetic using primary techniques is administered to the patient, and after signs of soft tissue anesthesia occur, the pain abates and the patient relaxes. Frequently, however, on access opening or when the pulp is entered, pain results because not all sensory nerves have been blocked. A useful procedure is to test the pulp of the tooth with cold (cold refrigerant) before the access is begun.[186,189] If the patient responds, an IO or PDL injection is given. However, no response does not ensure complete anesthesia.[186,189] The patient is always informed that the procedure will be immediately discontinued if pain is experienced during treatment or if there is a "premonition" of impending pain. Appropriate supplementary injections are then used. Occasionally, all attempts fail, and in that case, it is best to place a temporary restoration and refer the patient to an endodontist.

Mandibular Posterior Teeth

For mandibular posterior teeth, a conventional inferior alveolar nerve block is administered, usually in conjunction with a long buccal injection for the molars. The tooth is tested with cold refrigerant. If the result is negative, the clinician may proceed with access; if the result is positive, an IO or PDL injection is administered before access is begun. Prior to the supplemental IO injection, buccal infiltration of a cartridge of 4% articaine with 1:100,000 epinephrine is given over the tooth to reduce the pain of the injection. If pain is felt during access, the IO or PDL injection may be repeated, or an IP injection is given if the pulp is exposed. Usually, once the pulp has been removed, further pain is minimal, owing to the longer duration of mandibular anesthesia.[47-52,186]

Mandibular Anterior Teeth

For mandibular anterior teeth, an inferior alveolar injection is given. The tooth is tested with cold refrigerant. If the result is negative, the clinician may proceed with access; if the result is positive, an IO injection is administered before access is begun (the PDL injection does not work well in mandibular anterior teeth). Prior to the supplemental IO injection, labial infiltration of a cartridge of 4% articaine with 1:100,000 epinephrine is given over the tooth to reduce the pain of the IO injection. If pain is felt upon access, the IO injection is repeated. If this is unsuccessful, an IP injection is added.

Maxillary Posterior Teeth

The approaches for maxillary posterior teeth are the same as those outlined under General Considerations *except* that the initial dose of 2% lidocaine with 1:100,000 epinephrine is doubled (3.6 mL) for buccal infiltration and a palatal infiltration is given for the rubber dam retainer. The tooth is tested with cold refrigerant. If the result is negative, the clinician may proceed with access; if the result is positive, an IO or

PDL injection is administered before access is begun. If pain is felt during access, the IO or PDL injection is repeated. In some cases, an IP injection may be needed.

The duration of anesthesia in the maxilla is less than in the mandible.[126-134] Therefore, if pain is experienced during instrumentation or obturation, additional primary and/or supplemental injections are necessary.

Maxillary Anterior Teeth

In the maxillary anterior teeth, anesthetic is administered initially as a labial infiltration and occasionally as a palatal infiltration for the rubber dam retainer. The tooth is tested with cold refrigerant. If the result is negative, the clinician may proceed with access; if the result is positive, an IO injection is administered before access is begun (the PDL injection is not effective[163]). Rarely is an IO injection needed. The duration of anesthesia may be less than 1 hour, requiring additional infiltration.[126-134]

Symptomatic Pulp Necrosis

A diagnosis of symptomatic pulp necrosis indicates pain and/or swelling and therefore periapical inflammation. Because the pulp is necrotic and apical tissues are inflamed, anesthesia problems are different. These teeth may be painful when manipulated during treatment.

For the mandible, an inferior alveolar nerve block and a long buccal injection (for the molars) are administered. For maxillary teeth, if no swelling is present, the anesthetic is given with a conventional infiltration. If soft tissue swelling is present (cellulitis or abscess), infiltration is administered on either side of the swelling. Occasionally a regional block may be necessary. Access is begun *slowly*. Usually the pulp chamber is entered without discomfort if the tooth is not torqued excessively during use of the high-speed handpiece. File placement and debridement also can be performed without much pain if instruments are used gently.

Occasionally, conventional injections do not provide adequate anesthesia. IO, PDL, and IP injections are *contraindicated*. Although effective for vital pulps, these injections are painful and ineffective with apical pathosis. Rather, the patient should be informed that profound anesthesia is not present, owing to inflammation in the bone. As an alternative in maxillary molars, a PSA injection or second-division nerve block (high tuberosity technique) may be given. In anterior teeth and premolars, an infraorbital injection is administered to provide some degree of bone and soft tissue anesthesia. 9-6

In patients with severe preoperative pain without drainage from the tooth (or when no swelling can be incised), a long-acting anesthetic (e.g., bupivacaine) may help control postoperative pain in mandibular teeth; however, this is not very successful in maxillary teeth.[127,135] The duration of analgesia in the mandible is usually not so long as to preclude the prescription of oral analgesics.[52]

Asymptomatic Pulp Necrosis

Asymptomatic teeth are the easiest to anesthetize. Although it may be tempting to proceed without anesthesia, vital sensitive tissue (ingrowth of periapical tissue into canal) may be encountered in the apical portion of canals, or placement of files may cause pressure and extrusion of fluid periapically.

The conventional injections are usually administered: inferior alveolar nerve block and long buccal injection **157** (molars) for mandibular teeth and infiltration in the maxilla. Usually the patient remains comfortable. Rarely, there may be some sensitivity during canal preparation that requires an IO or IL injection. IP injection is not indicated, because bacteria and debris may be forced periapically. In the maxilla an additional infiltration may be necessary during longer procedures.

ANESTHESIA FOR SURGICAL PROCEDURES

Incision for Drainage

Patients tolerate the procedure better when some anesthesia is present before incision and drainage of a swelling. However, obtaining profound anesthesia is difficult, which should be explained to the patient. In the mandible, an inferior alveolar nerve block plus a long buccal injection (for molars) and an inferior alveolar nerve block plus labial infiltration (for premolars and anterior teeth) are administered. In the maxilla, infiltration is given mesial and distal to the swelling. For palatal swellings, a small volume of anesthetic is infiltrated over the greater palatine foramen (for posterior teeth) or over the nasopalatine foramen (for anterior teeth). With swelling over either foramen, lateral infiltration is indicated.

Injection directly into a swelling is contraindicated. These inflamed tissues are hyperalgesic and difficult to anesthetize. Traditionally it has been believed that the anesthetic solution may be affected by the lower pH of these tissues and rendered less effective and that direct injection "spreads the infection," although neither belief has been proved. Nevertheless, reasons for avoiding injection into a swelling are the pain from the injection pressure and the ineffectiveness of this technique. Theoretically, the area of swelling has an increased blood supply; therefore, the anesthetic is transported quickly into the systemic circulation, diminishing its effect. Also, edema and purulence may dilute the solution.

Periapical Surgery

Most periapical surgery should be performed by an endodontist, because these practitioners have received advanced training in surgical procedures, the periapical bone anatomy of the mandible and maxilla, the use of magnification technologies, the complex canal anatomy, and advanced microsurgical techniques for retrograde preparation and filling.

Additional considerations in periapical surgery involve anesthesia of both soft tissue and bone. Also, inflammation is usually present. In the mandible the inferior alveolar injection is reasonably effective. Additional infiltration injections in the vestibule are useful to achieve vasoconstriction, particularly in the mandibular anterior region. In the maxilla, infiltration and block injections are generally effective, and larger volumes usually are necessary to provide anesthesia over the surgical field.

If the area of operation is inflamed or the patient is apprehensive, anesthesia may not be totally successful. Additionally, the effectiveness of surgical anesthesia is decreased by half compared to anesthesia for nonsurgical procedures. With flap reflection and opening into bone, the anesthetic solution is diluted by bleeding and removed by irrigation.[213]

Use of a long-acting anesthetic has been advocated.[14,72,214] In the mandible, this is reasonably effective. In the maxilla, long-acting agents have decreased epinephrine concentrations, which result in more bleeding during surgery.[215] After periapical surgery, administration of a long-acting anesthetic has been suggested.[14] However, postsurgical pain is usually not severe and can be managed by analgesics.[215]

REFERENCES

1. Walton R, Torabinejad M: Managing local anesthesia problems in the endodontic patient, *J Am Dent Assoc* 123:97, 1992.
2. Walton R: Managing endodontic anaesthesia problems, *Endod Pract* 1:15, 1998.
3. LeClaire A, Skidmore A, Griffin J Jr, et al: Endodontic fear survey, *J Endod* 14:560, 1988.
4. Rood J, Pateromichelakis S: Inflammation and peripheral nerve sensitization, *Br J Oral Surg* 19:67, 1981.
5. Wallace J, Michanowicz A, Mundell R, et al: A pilot study of the clinical problem of regionally anesthetizing the pulp of an acutely inflamed mandibular molar, *Oral Surg Oral Med Oral Pathol* 59:517, 1985.
6. Byers M, Taylor P, Khayat B, et al: Effects of injury and inflammation on pulpal and periapical nerves, *J Endod* 16:78, 1990.
7. Weinstein P, Milgrom P, Kaufman E, et al: Patient perceptions of failure to achieve optimal local anesthesia, *Gen Dent* May-June 33:218, 1985.
8. Fiset L, Milgrom P, Weinstein P: Psychophysiological responses to dental injections, *J Am Dent Assoc* 11:4, 1985.
9. Meechan J: Intra-oral topical anaesthetics: a review, *J Dent* 28:3, 2000.
10. Rosivack R, Koenigsberg S, Maxwell K: An analysis of the effectiveness of two topical anesthetics, *Anesth Prog* 37:290, 1990.
11. Nusstein J, Beck M: Effectiveness of 20% benzocaine as a topical anesthetic for intraoral injections, *Anesth Prog* 50:159, 2003.
12. Parirokh M, Sadeghi A, Nakhaee N, et al: Effect of topical anesthesia on pain during infiltration injection and success of anesthesia for maxillary central incisors, *J Endod* 38:1553, 2012.
13. Martin M, Ramsay D, Whitney C, et al: Topical anesthesia: differentiating the pharmacological and psychological contributions to efficacy, *Anesth Prog* 41:40, 1994.
14. Malamed S: *Handbook of local anesthesia*, ed 6, St Louis, 2012, Elsevier/Mosby.
15. Martin S, Jones JS, Wynn BN: Does warming local anesthetic reduce the pain of subcutaneous injection? *Am J Emerg Med* 14:10, 1996.
16. Colaric KB, Overton DT, Moore K: Pain reduction in lidocaine administration through buffering and warming, *Am J Emerg Med* 16:353, 1998.
17. Sultan J: Towards evidence based emergency medicine: best BETs from Manchester Royal Infirmary—effect of warming local anaesthetics on pain of infiltration, *Emerg Med J* 24:723, 2007.
18. Fialkov JA, McDougall EP: Warmed local anesthetic reduces pain of infiltration, *Ann Plast Surg* 36:11, 1996.
19. Bell RW, Butt ZA, Gardner RF: Warming lignocaine reduces the pain of injection during local anaesthetic eyelid surgery, *Eye (London)* 10:558, 1996.
20. Sultan J: Towards evidence based emergency medicine: best BETs from Manchester Royal Infirmary—the effect of warming local anaesthetics on pain of infiltration, *Emerg Med J* 24:791, 2007.
21. Fuller N, Menke R, Meyers W: Perception of pain to intraoral penetration of three needles, *J Am Dent Assoc* 99:822, 1979.
22. Cooley R, Robison S: Comparative evaluation of the 30-gauge dental needle, *Oral Surg Oral Med Oral Pathol* 48:400, 1979.
23. Robison S, Mayhew R, Cowan R, et al: Comparative study of deflection characteristics and fragility of 25-, 27-, and 30-gauge short dental needles, *J Am Dent Assoc* 109:920, 1984.
24. Pogrel MA: Broken local anesthetic needles: a case series of 16 patients, with recommendations, *J Am Dent Assoc* 140:1517, 2009.
25. Kanaa H, Meechan J, Corbett P, et al: Speed of injection influences efficacy of inferior alveolar nerve blocks: a double-blind randomized controlled trial in volunteers, *J Endod* 32:919, 2006.
26. Aggarwal V, Singla M, Miglani S, et al: A prospective, randomized single-blind evaluation of effect of injection speed on anesthetic efficacy of inferior alveolar nerve block in patients with symptomatic irreversible pulpitis, *J Endod* 38:1578, 2012.
27. Saloum FS, Baumgartner JC, Marshall G, et al: A clinical comparison of pain perception to the Wand and a traditional syringe, *Oral Surg Oral Med Oral Pathol Oral Radiol Endod* 86:691, 2000.
28. Goodell GG, Gallagher FJ, Nicoll BK: Comparison of a controlled injection pressure system with a conventional technique, *Oral Surg Oral Med Oral Pathol Oral Radiol Endod* 90:88, 2000.

29. Nicholson JW, Berry TG, Summitt JB, et al: Pain perception and utility: a comparison of the syringe and computerized local injection techniques, *Gen Dent* 249:167, 2001.

30. Primosch RE, Brooks R: Influence of anesthetic flow rate delivered by the Wand local anesthetic system on pain response to palatal injections, *Am J Dent* 15:15, 2002.

31. Nusstein J, Burns Y, Reader A, et al: Injection pain and postinjection pain of the palatal anterior superior alveolar injection, administered with the Wand Plus system, comparing 2% lidocaine with 1:100,000 epinephrine to 3% mepivacaine, *Oral Surg Oral Med Oral Pathol Oral Radiol Endodon* 97:164, 2004.

32. Nusstein J, Lee S, Reader A, et al: Injection pain and postinjection pain of the anterior middle superior alveolar injection administered with the Wand or conventional syringe, *Oral Surg Oral Med Oral Pathol Oral Radiol Endod* 98:124, 2004.

33. Palm AM, Kirkegaard U, Poulsen S: The wand versus traditional injection for mandibular nerve block in children and adolescents: perceived pain and time of onset, *Pediatr Dent* 26:481, 2004.

34. Nusstein J, Steinkruger G, Reader A, et al: The effects of a two-stage injection technique on inferior alveolar nerve block injection pain, *Anesth Prog* 53:126, 2006.

35. Liddell A, Locker D: Gender and age differences in attitudes to dental pain and dental control, *Community Dent Oral Epidemiol* 25:314, 1997.

36. Fillingim R, Edwards R, Powell T: The relationship of sex and clinical pain to experimental pain responses, *Pain* 83:419, 1999.

37. Lin L, Shovlin F, Skribner J, et al: Pulp biopsies from the teeth associated with periapical radiolucency, *J Endod* 10:436, 1984.

38. Lindemann M, Reader A, Nusstein J, et al: Effect of sublingual triazolam on the success of inferior alveolar nerve block in patients with irreversible pulpitis, *J Endod* 34:1167, 2008.

39. Stanley W, Drum M, Nusstein J, et al: Effect of nitrous oxide on the efficacy of the inferior alveolar nerve block in patients with irreversible pulpitis, *J Endod* 38:565, 2012.

40. Khademi AA, Saatchi M, Minaiyan M, et al: Effect of preoperative alprazolam on the success of inferior alveolar nerve block for teeth with irreversible pulpitis, *J Endod* 38:1337, 2012.

41. Kaufman E, Weinstein P, Milgrom P: Difficulties in achieving local anesthesia, *J Am Dent Assoc* 108:205, 1984.

42. Dreven L, Reader A, Beck M, et al: An evaluation of an electric pulp tester as a measure of analgesia in human vital teeth, *J Endod* 13:233, 1987.

43. Certosimo A, Archer R: A clinical evaluation of the electric pulp tester as an indicator of local anesthesia, *Oper Dent* 21:25, 1996.

44. Reader A, Nusstein J, Drum M: *Successful local anesthesia for restorative dentistry and endodontics*, Hanover Park, Ill, 2011, Quintessence.

45. Nusstein J, Reader A, Beck M: Anesthetic efficacy of different volumes of lidocaine with epinephrine for inferior alveolar nerve blocks, *Gen Dent* 50:372, 2002.

46. Ågren E, Danielsson K: Conduction block analgesia in the mandible, *Swed Dent J* 5:81, 1981.

47. Vreeland D, Reader A, Beck M, et al: An evaluation of volumes and concentrations of lidocaine in human inferior alveolar nerve block, *J Endod* 15:6, 1989.

48. Hinkley S, Reader A, Beck M, et al: An evaluation of 4% prilocaine with 1:200,000 epinephrine and 2% mepivacaine with 1:20,000 levonordefrin compared with 2% lidocaine with 1:100,000 epinephrine for inferior alveolar nerve block, *Anesth Prog* 38:84, 1991.

49. Chaney M, Kerby R, Reader A, et al: An evaluation of lidocaine hydrocarbonate compared with lidocaine hydrochloride for inferior alveolar nerve block, *Anesth Prog* 38:212, 1992.

50. Nist R, Reader A, Beck M, et al: An evaluation of the incisive nerve block and combination inferior alveolar and incisive nerve blocks in mandibular anesthesia, *J Endod* 18:455, 1992.

51. McLean C, Reader A, Beck M, et al: An evaluation of 4% prilocaine and 3% mepivacaine compared with 2% lidocaine (1:100,000 epinephrine) for inferior alveolar nerve block, *J Endod* 19:146, 1993.

52. Fernandez C, Reader A, Beck M, et al: A prospective, randomized, double-blind comparison of bupivacaine and lidocaine for inferior alveolar nerve blocks, *J Endod* 31:499, 2005.

53. Yared GM, Dagher BF: Evaluation of lidocaine in human inferior alveolar nerve block, *J Endod* 23:575, 1997.

54. Wali M, Drum M, Reader A, et al: Prospective, randomized single-blind study of the anesthetic efficacy of 1.8 and 3.6 milliliters of 2% lidocaine with 1:50,000 epinephrine for inferior alveolar nerve blocks, *J Endod* 36:1459, 2010.

55. Dagher FB, Yared GM, Machtou P: An evaluation of 2% lidocaine with different concentrations of epinephrine for inferior alveolar nerve block, *J Endod* 23:178, 1997.

56. Malamed SF, Gagnon S, LeBlanc D: Articaine hydrochloride: a study of the safety of a new amide local anesthetic, *J Am Dent Assoc* 132:177, 2001.

57. Oertel R, Rahn R, Kirch W: Clinical pharmacokinetics of articaine, *Clin Pharmacokinet* 33:417, 1997.

58. Malamed SF, Gagnon S, Leblanc D: A comparison between articaine HCl and lidocaine HCl in pediatric dental patients, *Pediatr Dent* 22:307, 2000.

59. Malamed SF, Gagnon S, Leblanc D: Efficacy of articaine: a new amide local anesthetic, *J Am Dent Assoc* 131:635, 2000.

60. Haas DA, Harper DG, Saso MA, et al: Comparison of articaine and prilocaine anesthesia by infiltration in maxillary and mandibular arches, *Anesth Prog* 37:230, 1990.

61. Claffey E, Reader A, Nusstein J, et al: Anesthetic efficacy of articaine for inferior alveolar nerve blocks in patients with irreversible pulpitis, *J Endod* 30:568, 2004.

62. Vahatalo K, Antila H, Lehtinen R: Articaine and lidocaine for maxillary infiltration anesthesia, *Anesth Prog* 40:114, 1993.

63. Berlin J, Nusstein J, Reader A, et al: Efficacy of articaine and lidocaine in a primary intraligamentary injection administered with a computer-controlled local anesthetic delivery system, *Oral Surg Oral Med Oral Pathol Oral Radiol Endod* 99:361, 2005.

64. Mikesell P, Nusstein J, Reader A, et al: A comparison of articaine and lidocaine for inferior alveolar nerve blocks, *J Endod* 31:265, 2005.

65. Moore PA, Boynes SG, Hersh EV, et al: The anesthetic efficacy of 4 percent articaine 1:200,000 epinephrine: two controlled clinical trials, *J Am Dent Assoc* 137:1572, 2006.

66. Schertzer ER, Malamed SF: Articaine vs lidocaine, *J Am Dent Assoc* 131:1248, 2000.

67. Haas DA, Lennon D: A 21-year retrospective study of reports of paresthesia following local anesthetic administration, *J Can Dent Assoc* 61:319, 1995.

68. Gaffen AS, Haas DA: Retrospective review of voluntary reports of nonsurgical paresthesia in dentistry, *J Can Dent Assoc* 75:579, 2009.

69. Garisto GA, Gaffen AS, Lawrence HP, et al: Occurrence of paresthesia after dental local anesthetic administration in the United States, *J Am Dent Assoc* 141:836, 2010.

70. Pogrel M: Permanent nerve damage from inferior alveolar nerve blocks: an update to include articaine, *J Calif Dent Assoc* 35:271, 2007.

71. Davis W, Oakley J, Smith E: Comparison of the effectiveness of etidocaine and lidocaine as local anesthetic agents during oral surgery, *Anesth Prog* 31:159, 1984.

72. Rosenquist J, Rosenquist K, Lee P: Comparison between lidocaine and bupivacaine as local anesthetics with diflunisal for postoperative pain control after lower third molar surgery, *Anesth Prog* 35:1, 1988.

73. Dunsky J, Moore P: Long-acting local anesthetics: a comparison of bupivacaine and etidocaine in endodontics, *J Endod* 10:6, 1984.

74. Crout R, Koraido G, Moore P: A clinical trial of long-acting local anesthetics for periodontal surgery, *Anesth Prog* 37:194, 1990.

75. Cepeda MS, Tzortzopoulou A, Thackrey M, et al: Adjusting the pH of lidocaine for reducing pain on injection (review), *Cochrane Database Syst Rev* 2010.

76. Hanna MN, Elhassan A, Veloso PM, et al: Efficacy of bicarbonate in decreasing pain on intradermal injection of local anesthetics: a meta analysis, *Reg Anesth Pain Med* 34:122, 2009.

77. Bowles WH, Frysh H, Emmons R: Clinical evaluation of buffered local anesthetic, *Gen Dent* 43:182, 1995.

78. Kashyap VM, Desai R, Reddy PB, et al: Effect of alkalinisation of lignocaine for intraoral nerve block on pain during injection, and speed of onset of anaesthesia, *Br J Oral Maxillofac Surg* 49:e72, 2011.

79. Al-Sultan AF: Effectiveness of pH adjusted lidocaine versus commercial lidocaine for maxillary infiltration anesthesia, *Al-Rafidain Dent J* 4:34, 2004.

80. Al-Sultan AF, Fathie WK, Hamid RS: A clinical evaluation on the alkalization of local anesthetic solution in periapical surgery, *Al-Rafidain Dent J* 6:71, 2006.

81. Whitcomb M, Drum M, Reader A, et al: A prospective, randomized double-blind study of the anesthetic efficacy of sodium bicarbonate buffered 2% lidocaine with 1:100,000 epinephrine in inferior alveolar nerve blocks, *Anesth Prog* 57:59, 2010.

82. Primosch RE, Robinson L: Pain elicited during intraoral infiltration with buffered lidocaine, *Am J Dent* 9:5, 1996.

83. Gow-Gates G: Mandibular conduction anesthesia: a new technique using extra-oral landmarks, *Oral Surg Oral Med Oral Pathol* 36:321, 1973.

84. Akinosi J: A new approach to the mandibular nerve block, *Br J Oral Surg* 15:83, 1977.

85. Todorovic L, Stajcic Z, Petrovic V: Mandibular versus inferior alveolar dental anaesthesia: clinical assessment of 3 different techniques, *Int J Oral Maxillofac Surg* 15:733, 1986.

86. Goldberg S, Reader A, Drum M, et al: Comparison of the anesthetic efficacy of the conventional inferior alveolar, Gow-Gates, and Vazirani-Akinosi techniques, *J Endod* 34:1306, 2008.

87. Montagnese T, Reader A, Melfi R: A comparative study of the Gow-Gates technique and a standard technique for mandibular anesthesia, *J Endod* 10:158, 1984.

88. Sisk AL: Evaluation of the Akinosi mandibular block technique in oral surgery, *Oral Maxillofac Surg* 44:113, 1986.

89. Yucel E, Hutchison IL: A comparative evaluation of the conventional and closed mouth technique for inferior alveolar nerve block, *Aust Dent J* 40:15, 1995.

90. Martinez GJM, Benito PB, Fernandez CF, et al: A comparative study of direct mandibular nerve block and the Akinosi technique, *Med Oral* 8:143, 2003.

91. Joyce AP, Donnelly JC: Evaluation of the effectiveness and comfort of incisive nerve anesthesia given inside or outside the mental foramen, *J Endod* 19:409, 1993.

92. Whitworth JM, Kanaa MD, Corbett IP, et al: Influence of injection speed on the effectiveness of incisive/mental nerve block: a randomized, controlled, double-blind study in adult volunteers, *J Endod* 33:1149, 2007.

93. Batista da Silva C, Berto LA, Volpato MC, et al: Anesthetic efficacy of articaine and lidocaine for incisive/mental nerve block, *J Endod* 36:438, 2010.

94. Yonchak T, Reader A, Beck M, et al: Anesthetic efficacy of infiltrations in mandibular anterior teeth, *Anes Prog* 48:55, 2001.

95. Meechan JG, Ledvinka JI: Pulpal anesthesia for mandibular central incisor teeth: a comparison of infiltration and intraligamentary injections, *Int Endod J* 35:629, 2002.

96. Meechan JG, Kanaa MD, Corbett IP, et al: Pulpal anesthesia for permanent first molar teeth: a double-blind randomized cross-over trial comparing buccal and buccal plus lingual infiltration injections in volunteers, *Int Endod J* 39:764, 2006.

97. Kanaa MD, Whitworth JM, Corbett IP, et al: Articaine and lidocaine mandibular buccal infiltration anesthesia: a prospective randomized double-blind cross-over study, *J Endod* 32:296, 2006.

98. Jung Y, Kim JH, Kim ES, et al: An evaluation of buccal infiltrations and inferior alveolar nerve blocks in pulpal anesthesia for mandibular first molars, *J Endod* 34:11, 2008.

99. Corbett IP, Kanaa MD, Whitworth JM, et al: Articaine infiltration for anesthesia of mandibular first molars, *J Endod* 34:514, 2008.

100. Robertson D, Nusstein J, Reader A, et al: The anesthetic efficacy of articaine in buccal infiltration of mandibular posterior teeth, *J Am Dent Assoc* 138:1104, 2007.

101. McEntire M, Nusstein J, Drum M, et al: Anesthetic efficacyof 4% articaine with 1:100,000 epinephrine versus 4% articaine with 1:200,000 epinephrine as a primary buccal infiltration in the mandibular first molar, *J Endod* 37:450, 2011.

102. Nuzum FM, Drum M, Nusstein J, et al: Anesthetic efficacy of articaine for combination labial plus lingual infiltrations versus labial infiltration in the mandibular lateral incisor, *J Endod* 36:952, 2010.

103. Jaber A, Whitworth JM, Corbett IP, et al: The efficacy of infiltration anaesthesia for adult mandibular incisors: a randomized double-blind cross-over trial comparing articaine and lidocaine buccal and buccal plus lingual infiltrations, *Br Dent J* 209:E16, 2010.

104. Berns J, Sadove M: Mandibular block injection: a method of study using an injected radiopaque material, *J Am Dent Assoc* 65:735, 1962.

105. Galbreath J: Tracing the course of the mandibular block injection, *Oral Surg Oral Med Oral Pathol* 30:571, 1970.

106. Hannan L, Reader A, Nist R, et al: The use of ultrasound for guiding needle placement for inferior alveolar nerve blocks, *Oral Surg Oral Med Oral Pathol Oral Radiol Endod* 87:658, 1999.

107. Simon F, Reader A, Drum M, et al: A prospective, randomized single-blind study of the anesthetic efficacy of the inferior alveolar nerve block administered with a peripheral nerve stimulator, *J Endod* 36:429, 2010.

108. Strichartz G: Molecular mechanisms of nerve block by local anesthetics, *Anesthesiology* 45:421, 1976.

109. Cooley R, Robison S: Comparative evaluation of the 30-gauge dental needle, *Oral Surg Oral Med Oral Pathol* 48:400, 1979.

110. Davidson M: Bevel-oriented mandibular injections: needle deflection can be beneficial, *Gen Dent* 37:410, 1989.

111. Hochman MN, Friedman MJ: In vitro study of needle deflection: a linear insertion technique versus a bidirectional rotation insertion technique, *Quintessence Int* 31:33, 2000.

112. Aldous J: Needle deflection: a factor in the administration of local anesthetics, *J Am Dent Assoc* 77:602, 1968.

113. Kennedy S, Reader A, Nusstein J, et al: The significance of needle deflection in success of the inferior alveolar nerve block in patients with irreversible pulpitis, *J Endod* 29:630, 2003.

114. Steinkruger G, Nusstein J, Reader A, et al: The significance of needle bevel orientation in achieving a successful inferior alveolar nerve block, *J Am Dent Assoc* 137:1685, 2006.

115. Wilson S, Johns P, Fuller P: The inferior and mylohyoid nerves: an anatomic study and relationship to local anesthesia of the anterior mandibular teeth, *J Am Dent Assoc* 108:350, 1984.

116. Clark S, Reader A, Beck M, et al: Anesthetic efficacy of the mylohyoid nerve block and combination inferior alveolar nerve block/mylohyoid nerve block, *Oral Surg Oral Med Oral Pathol Oral Radiol Endod* 87:557, 1999.

117. Yonchak T, Reader A, Beck M, et al: Anesthetic efficacy of unilateral and bilateral inferior alveolar nerve blocks to determine cross innervation in anterior teeth, *Oral Surg Oral Med Oral Pathol Oral Radiol Endod* 92:132, 2001.

118. Droll B, Drum M, Nusstein J, et al: Anesthetic efficacy of the inferior alveolar nerve block in red-haired women, *J Endod* 38:1564, 2012.

119. Haase A, Reader A, Nusstein J, et al: Comparing anesthetic efficacy of articaine versus lidocaine as a supplemental buccal infiltration of the mandibular first molar after an inferior alveolar nerve block, *J Am Dent Assoc* 139:1228, 2008.

120. Kanaa MD, Whitworth JM, Corbett IP, et al: Articaine buccal infiltration enhances the effectiveness of lidocaine inferior alveolar nerve block, *Int Endod J* 42:238, 2009.

121. Dunbar D, Reader A, Nist R, et al: Anesthetic efficacy of the intraosseous injection after an inferior alveolar nerve block, *J Endod* 22(9):481-486, 1996.

122. Guglielmo A, Reader A, Nist R, et al: Anesthetic efficacy and heart rate effects of the supplemental intraosseous injection of 2% mepivacaine with 1:20,000 levonordefrin, *Oral Surg Oral Med Oral Pathol Oral Radiol Endod* 87:284, 1999.

123. Gallatin E, Stabile P, Reader A, et al: Anesthetic efficacy and heart rate effects of the intraosseous injection of 3% mepivacaine after an inferior alveolar nerve block, *Oral Surg Oral Med Oral Pathol Oral Radiol Endod* 89:83, 2000.

124. Childers M, Reader A, Nist R, et al: Anesthetic efficacy of the periodontal ligament injection after an inferior alveolar nerve block, *J Endod* 22:317, 1996.

125. Bunczak-Reeh M, Hargreaves K: Effect of inflammation on the delivery of drugs to dental pulp, *J Endod* 24:822, 1998.

126. Nusstein J, Wood M, Reader A, et al: Comparison of the degree of pulpal anesthesia achieved with the intraosseous injection and infiltration injection using 2% lidocaine with 1:100,000 epinephrine, *Gen Dent* 53:50, 2005.

127. Gross R, McCartney M, Reader A, et al: A prospective, randomized, double-blind comparison of bupivacaine and lidocaine for maxillary infiltrations, *J Endod* 33:1021, 2007.

128. Mikesell A, Drum M, Reader A, et al: Anesthetic efficacy of 1.8 mL and 3.6 mL of 2% lidocaine with 1:100,000 epinephrine for maxillary infiltrations, *J Endod* 34:121, 2008.

129. Evans G, Nusstein J, Drum M, et al: A prospective, randomized double-blind comparison of articaine and lidocaine for maxillary infiltrations, *J Endod* 34:389, 2008.

130. Brunetto PC, Ranali J, Ambrosano GMB, et al: Anesthetic efficacy of 3 volumes of lidocaine with epinephrine in maxillary infiltration anesthesia, *Anesth Prog* 55:29, 2008.

131. Scott J, Drum M, Reader A, et al: The efficacy of a repeated infiltration in prolonging duration of pulpal anesthesia in maxillary lateral incisors, *J Am Dent Assoc* 140:318, 2009.

132. Mason R, Drum M, Reader A, et al: A prospective, randomized, double-blind comparison of 2% lidocaine with 1:100,000 and 1:50,000 epinephrine and 3% mepivacaine for maxillary infiltrations, *J Endod* 35:1173, 2009.

133. Katz S, Drum M, Reader A, et al: A prospective, randomized, double-blind comparison of 2% lidocaine with 1:100,000 epinephrine, 4% prilocaine with 1:200,000 epinephrine and 4% prilocaine for maxillary infiltrations, *Anesth Prog* 57:45, 2010.

134. Lawaty I, Drum M, Reader A, et al: A prospective, randomized, double-blind comparison of 2% mepivacaine with 1:20,000 levonordefrin versus 2% lidocaine with 1:100,000 epinephrine for maxillary infiltrations, *Anesth Prog* 57:139, 2010.

135. Danielsson K, Evers H, Nordenram A: Long-acting local anesthetics in oral surgery: an experimental evaluation of bupivacaine and etidocaine for oral infiltration anesthesia, *Anesth Prog* March/April 32:65-68, 1985.

136. Loetscher C, Melton D, Walton R: Injection regimen for anesthesia of the maxillary first molar, *J Am Dent Assoc* 117:337, 1988.

137. Pfeil L, Drum M, Reader A, et al: Anesthetic efficacy of 1.8 milliters and 3.6 milliters of 2% lidocaine with 1:100,000 epinephrine for posterior superior alveolar nerve blocks, *J Endod* 36:598, 2010.

138. Berberich G, Reader A, Drum M, et al: A prospective, randomized, double-blind comparison of the anesthetic efficacy of 2% lidocaine with 1:100,000 and 1:50,000 epinephrine and 3% mepivacaine in the intraoral, infraorbital nerve block, *J Endod* 35:1498, 2009.

139. Karkut B, Reader A, Drum M, et al: A comparison of the local anesthetic efficacy of the extraoral versus the intraoral infraorbital nerve block, *J Am Dent Assoc* 141:185, 2010.

140. Broering R, Reader A, Drum M, et al: A prospective, randomized comparison of the anesthetic efficacy of the greater palatine and high tuberosity second division nerve blocks, *J Endod* 35:1337, 2009.

141. Forloine A, Drum M, Reader A, et al: A prospective, randomized, double-blind comparison of the anesthetic efficacy of two percent lidocaine with 1:100,000 epinephrine and three percent mepivacaine in the maxillary high tuberosity second division nerve block, *J Endod* 36:1770, 2010.

142. Friedman M, Hochman M: P-ASA block injection: a new palatal technique to anesthetize maxillary anterior teeth, *J Esthet Dent* 11:63, 1999.

143. Burns Y, Reader A, Nusstein J, et al: Anesthetic efficacy of the palatal anterior superior alveolar injection, *J Am Dent Assoc* 135:1269, 2004.

144. Friedman M, Hochman M: Using AMSA and P-ASA nerve blocks for esthetic restorative dentistry, *Gen Dent* 5:506, 2001.

145. Lee S, Reader A, Nusstein J, et al: Anesthetic efficacy of the anterior middle superior alveolar (AMSA) injection, *Anesth Prog* 51:80, 2004.

146. Kanaa MD, Whitworth JM, Meechan JG: A prospective trial of different supplementary local anesthetic techniques after failure of inferior alveolar nerve block in patients with irreversible pulpitis in mandibular teeth, *J Endod* 38:421, 2012.

147. Gallatin J, Reader A, Nusstein J, et al: A comparison of two intraosseous anesthetic techniques in mandibular posterior teeth, *J Am Dent Assoc* 134:1476, 2003.

148. Coggins R, Reader A, Nist R, et al: Anesthetic efficacy of the intraosseous injection in maxillary and mandibular teeth, *Oral Surg Oral Med Oral Pathol Oral Radiol Endod* 81:634, 1996.

149. Replogle K, Reader A, Nist R, et al: Anesthetic efficacy of the intraosseous injection of 2% lidocaine (1:100,000 epinephrine) and 3% mepivacaine in mandibular first molars, *Oral Surg Oral Med Oral Pathol Oral Radiol Endod* 83:30, 1997.

150. Gallatin J, Nusstein J, Reader A, et al: A comparison of injection pain and postoperative pain of two intraosseous anesthetic techniques, *Anesth Prog* 50:111, 2003.

151. Reitz J, Reader A, Nist R, et al: Anesthetic efficacy of the intraosseous injection of 0.9 ml of 2% lidocaine (1:100,000 epinephrine) to augment an inferior alveolar nerve block, *Oral Surg Oral Med Oral Pathol Oral Radiol Endod* 86:516, 1998.

152. Stabile P, Reader A, Gallatin E, et al: Anesthetic efficacy and heart rate effects of the intraosseous injection of 1.5% etidocaine (1:200,000 epinephrine) after an inferior alveolar nerve block, *Oral Surg Oral Med Oral Pathol Oral Radiol Endod* 89:407, 2000.

153. Bacsik CJ, Swift JQ, Hargreaves KM: Toxic systemic reactions of bupivacaine and etidocaine hydrochloride, *Oral Surg Oral Med Oral Pathol Oral Radiol Endod* 79:18, 1995.

154. Chamberlain TM, Davis RD, Murchison DF, et al: Systemic effects of an intraosseous injection of 2% lidocaine with 1:100,000 epinephrine, *Gen Dent* May-June 48:299-302, 2000.

155. Gallatin E, Stabile P, Reader A, et al: Anesthetic efficacy and heart rate effects of the intraosseous injection of 3% mepivacaine after an inferior alveolar nerve block, *Oral Surg Oral Med Oral Pathol Oral Radiol Endod* 89:83, 2000.

156. Wood M, Reader A, Nusstein JM, et al: Comparison of intraosseous and infiltration injections for venous lidocaine blood concentrations and heart rate changes after injection of 2% lidocaine with 1:100,000 epinephrine, *J Endod* 31:435, 2005.

157. Smith G, Walton R, Abbott B: Clinical evaluation of periodontal ligament anesthesia using a pressure syringe, *J Am Dent Assoc* 107:953, 1983.

158. Eriksen H, Aamdal H, Kerekes K: Periodontal anesthesia: a clinical evaluation, *Endod Dent Traumatol* 2:267, 1986.

159. Dreyer W, van Heerden J, Joubert J: The route of periodontal ligament injection of local anesthetic solution, *J Endod* 9:471, 1983.

160. Tagger M, Tagger E, Sarnat H: Periodontal ligament injection: spread of solution in the dog, *J Endod* 20:283, 1994.

161. Moore K, Reader A, Meyers W, et al: A comparison of the periodontal ligament injection using 2% lidocaine with 1:100,000 epinephrine and saline in human mandibular premolars, *Anesth Prog* 34:181, 1987.

162. Schleder J, Reader A, Beck M, et al: The periodontal ligament injection: a comparison of 2% lidocaine, 3% mepivacaine, and 1:100,000 epinephrine to 2% lidocaine with 1:100,000 epinephrine in human mandibular premolars, *J Endod* 14:397, 1988.

163. White J, Reader A, Beck M, et al: The periodontal ligament injection: a comparison of the efficacy in human maxillary and mandibular teeth, *J Endod* 14:508, 1988.

164. Meechan JG, Ledvinka JI: Pulpal anesthesia for mandibular central incisor teeth: a comparison of infiltration and intraligamentary injections, *Int Endod J* 35:629, 2002.

165. Johnson G, Hlava G, Kalkwarf K: A comparison of periodontal intraligamental anesthesia using etidocaine HCl and lidocaine HCl, *Anesth Prog* 32:202, 1985.

166. Gray R, Lomax A, Rood J: Periodontal ligament injection: alternative solutions, *Anesth Prog* 37:293, 1990.

167. Meechan JG: A comparison of ropivacaine and lidocaine with epinephrine for intraligamentary anesthesia, *Oral Surg Oral Med Oral Pathol Oral Radiol Endod* 93:469, 2002.

168. D'Souza J, Walton R, Peterson L: Periodontal ligament injection: an evaluation of extent of anesthesia and postinjection discomfort, *J Am Dent Assoc* 114:341, 1987.

169. Nusstein J, Berlin J, Reader A, et al: Comparison of injection pain, heart rate increase and post-injection pain of articaine and lidocaine in a primary intraligamentary injection administered with a computer-controlled local anesthetic delivery system, *Anesth Prog* 51:126, 2004.

170. Simon D, Jacobs L, Senia S, et al: Intraligamentary anesthesia as an aid in endodontic diagnosis, *Oral Surg Oral Med Oral Pathol* 54:77, 1982.

171. Pashley D: Systemic effects of intraligamental injections, *J Endod* 12:501, 1986.

172. Cannell H, Kerwala C, Webster K, et al: Are intraligamentary injections intravascular? *Br Dent J* 175:281, 1993.

173. Walton R, Abbott B: Periodontal ligament injection: a clinical evaluation, *J Am Dent Assoc* 103:103, 1981.

174. Walton R, Garnick J: The periodontal ligament injection: histologic effects on the periodontium in monkeys, *J Endod* 8:22, 1981.

175. List G, Meister F Jr, Nery E, et al: Gingival crevicular fluid response to various solutions using the intraligamentary injection, *Quintessence Int* 19:559, 1988.

176. Brannström M, Nordenvall K, Hedstrom K: Periodontal tissue changes after intraligamental anesthesia, *J Dent Child* 11(12):417, 1982.

177. Galili D, Kaufman E, Garfunkel A, et al: Intraligamental anesthesia: a histological study, *Int J Oral Surg* 13:511, 1984.

178. Roahen J, Marshall J: The effects of periodontal ligament injection on pulpal and periodontal tissues, *J Endod* 16:28, 1990.

179. Pertot W, Dejou J: Bone and root resorption: effects of the force developed during periodontal ligament injections in dogs, *Oral Surg Oral Med Oral Pathol* 74:357, 1992.

180. Cromley NL, Adams DF: The effect of intraligamentary injections on diseased periodontiums in dogs, *Gen Dent* 39:33, 1991.

181. Peurach J: Pulpal response to intraligamentary injection in cynomolgus monkey, *Anesth Prog* 32:73, 1985.

182. Torabinejad M, Peters D, Peckham N, et al: Electron microscopic changes in human pulps after intraligamental injection, *Oral Surg Oral Med Oral Pathol* 76:219, 1993.

183. Kim S: Ligamental injection: a physiological explanation of its efficacy, *J Endod* 12:486, 1986.

184. Plamondon T, Walton R, Graham G, et al: Pulp response to the combined effects of cavity preparation and periodontal ligament injection, *Oper Dent* 15:86, 1990.

185. Brannström M, Lindsko S, Nordenvall K: Enamel hypoplasia in permanent teeth induced by periodontal ligament anesthesia of primary teeth, *J Am Dent Assoc* 109:735, 1984.

186. Nusstein J, Reader A, Nist R, et al: Anesthetic efficacy of the supplemental intraosseous injection of 2% lidocaine with 1:100,000 epinephrine in irreversible pulpitis, *J Endod* 24:487, 1998.

187. Reisman D, Reader A, Nist R, et al: Anesthetic efficacy of the supplemental intraosseous injection of 3% mepivacaine in irreversible pulpitis, *Oral Surg Oral Med Oral Pathol Oral Radiol Endod* 84:676, 1997.

188. Kennedy S, Reader A, Nusstein J, et al: The significance of needle deflection in success of the inferior alveolar nerve block in patients with irreversible pulpitis, *J Endod* 29:630, 2003.

189. Cohen H, Cha B, Spangberg L: Endodontic anesthesia in mandibular molars: a clinical study, *J Endod* 19:370, 1993.

190. Matthews R, Drum M, Reader A, et al: Articaine for supplemental, buccal mandibular infiltration anesthesia in patients with irreversible pulpitis when the inferior alveolar nerve block fails, *J Endod* 35:343, 2009.

191. Oleson M, Drum M, Reader A, et al: Effect of preoperative ibuprofen on the success of the inferior alveolar nerve block in patients with irreversible pulpitis, *J Endod* 36:379, 2010.

192. Tortamano IP, Siviero M, Costa CG, et al: A comparison of the anesthetic efficacy of articaine and lidocaine in patients with irreversible pulpitis, *J Endod* 35:165, 2009.

193. Aggarwal V, Jain A, Kabi D: Anesthetic efficacy of supplemental buccal and lingual infiltrations of articaine and lidocaine after an inferior alveolar nerve block in patients with irreversible pulpitis, *J Endod* 35:925, 2009.

194. Aggarwal V, Singla M, Kabi D: Comparative evaluation of anesthetic efficacy of Gow-Gates mandibular conduction anesthesia, Vazirani-Akinosi technique, buccal-plus-lingual infiltrations, and conventional inferior alveolar nerve anesthesia in patients with irreversible pulpitis, *Oral Surg Oral Med Oral Pathol Oral Radiol Endod* 109:303, 2010.

195. Aggarwal V, Singla M, Miglani S, et al: Comparative evaluation of 1.8 mL and 3.6 mL of 2% lidocaine with 1:200,000 epinephrine for inferior alveolar nerve block in patients with irreversible pulpitis: a prospective, randomized single-blind study, *J Endod* 38:753, 2012.

196. Simpson M, Drum M, Reader A, et al: Effect of preoperative ibuprofen/acetaminophen on the success of the inferior alveolar nerve block in patients with symptomatic irreversible pulpitis, *J Endod* 37:593, 2011.

197. Parirokh M, Satvati SA, Sharifi R, et al: Efficacy of combining a buccal infiltration with an inferior alveolar nerve block for mandibular molars with irreversible pulpitis, *Oral Surg Oral Med Oral Pathol Oral Radiol Endod* 109:468, 2010.

198. Aggarwal V, Singla M, Miglani S, et al: A prospective, randomized, single-blind comparative evaluation of anesthetic efficacy of posterior alveolar nerve blocks, buccal infiltrations, and buccal plus palatal infiltrations in patients with irreversible pulpitis, *J Endod* 37:1491, 2011.

199. Kanaa MD, Whitworth JM, Meechan JG: A comparison of the efficacy of 4% articaine with 1:100,000 epinephrine and 2% lidocaine with 1:80,000 epinephrine in achieving pulpal anesthesia in maxillary teeth with irreversible pulpitis, *J Endod* 38:279, 2012.

200. Srinivasan N, Kavitha M, Loganathan CS, et al: Comparison of anesthetic efficacy of 4% articaine and 2% lidocaine for maxillary buccal infiltration in patients with irreversible pulpitis, *Oral Surg Oral Med Oral Pathol Oral Radiol Endod* 107:133, 2009.

201. Sherman MG, Flax M, Namerow K, et al: Anesthetic efficacy of the Gow-Gates injection and maxillary infiltration with articaine and lidocaine for irreversible pulpitis, *J Endod* 34:656, 2008.

202. Rosenberg PA, Amin KG, Zibari Y, et al: Comparison of 4% articaine with 1:100,000 epinephrine and 2% lidocaine with 1:100,000 epinephrine when used as a supplemental anesthetic, *J Endod* 33:403, 2007.

203. Argueta-Figueroa L, Arzate-Sosa G, Mendieta-Zeron H: Anesthetic efficacy of articaine for inferior alveolar nerve blocks in patients with symptomatic versus asymptomatic irreversible pulpitis, *Gen Dent* 60:e39, 2012.

204. Aggarwal V, Singla M, Rizvi A, et al: Comparative evaluation of local infiltration of articaine, articaine plus ketorolac, and dexamethasone on anesthetic efficacy of inferior alveolar nerve block with lidocaine in patients with irreversible pulpitis, *J Endod* 37:445, 2011.

205. Poorni S, Veniashok B, Senthilkumar AD, et al: Anesthetic efficacy of four percent articaine for pulpal anesthesia by using inferior alveolar nerve block and buccal infiltration techniques in patients with irreversible pulpitis: a prospective randomized double-blind clinical trial, *J Endod* 37:1603, 2011.

206. Bigby J, Reader A, Nusstein J, et al: Articaine for supplemental intraosseous anesthesia in patients with irreversible pulpitis, *J Endod* 32:1044, 2006.

207. Reemers T, Glickman G, Spears R, et al: The efficacy of the IntraFlow intraosseous injection as a primary anesthesia technique, *J Endod* 34:280, 2008.

208. Pereira LA, Groppo FC, Bergamaschi CD, et al: Articaine (4%) with epinephrine (1:100,000 or 1:200,000) in intraosseous injections in symptomatic irreversible pulpitis of mandibular molars: anesthetic efficacy and cardiovascular effects, *Oral Surg Oral Med Oral Pathol Oral Radiol Endod* 116(2):e85-91, 2013.

209. Zarei M, Ghoddusi J, Sharifi E, et al: Comparison of the anesthetic efficacy of and heart rate changes after periodontal ligament or intraosseous X-tip injection in mandibular molars: a randomized controlled clinical trial, *Int Endod J* 45:921, 2012.

210. Nusstein J, Claffey E, Reader A, et al: Anesthetic effectiveness of the supplemental intraligamentary injection, administered with a computer-controlled local anesthetic delivery system, in patients with irreversible pulpitis, *J Endod* 31:354, 2005.

211. Birchfield J, Rosenberg P: Role of the anesthetic solution in intrapulpal anesthesia, *J Endod* 1:26, 1975.

212. VanGheluwe J, Walton R: Intrapulpal injection: factors related to effectiveness, *Oral Surg Oral Med Oral Pathol Oral Radiol Endod* 83:38, 1997.

213. Yamazaki S, Seino H, Ozawa S, et al: Elevation of a periosteal flap with irrigation of the bone for minor oral surgery reduces the duration of action of infiltration anesthesia, *Anes Prog* 53:8, 2006.

214. Davis W, Oakley J, Smith E: Comparison of the effectiveness of etidocaine and lidocaine as local anesthetic agents during oral surgery, *Anesth Prog* 31:159, 1984.

215. Meechan J, Blair G: The effect of two different local anaesthetic solutions on pain experience following apicoectomy, *Br Dent J* 175:410, 1993.

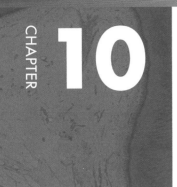

CHAPTER 10

Endodontic emergencies and therapeutics

Paul D. Eleazer, Paul A. Rosenberg

LEARNING OBJECTIVES

After reading this chapter, the student should be able to:

1. Recognize the incidence of flare-ups.
2. Describe appropriate diagnostic procedures for endodontic emergencies.
3. Describe the initial patient contact and patient management issues.
4. Describe the role of the staff in discriminating between a true emergency and a nonemergent case.
5. Recognize the categories of flare-ups: pretreatment, intervisit, and postobturation.
6. Describe appropriate nomenclature for diagnostic categories of pulpal and periapical pathologic conditions.

7. Describe the causes of flare-ups and their management.
8. Recognize anatomic factors that may lead to more rapid progression of infection.
9. Recognize the importance of profound anesthesia.
10. Describe the potential role of predisposing factors, including genetics, gender, and anxiety, in exacerbations.
11. Use preoperative, intraoperative, and postoperative pharmaceuticals (e.g., anxiolytics, anesthetics, antiinflammatories, analgesics, and antimicrobials) in emergency cases.

Endodontic emergencies represent an important and complex part of clinical practice. Proper diagnosis and treatment require a knowledge of pulp and periapical pathosis and the ability to use the appropriate diagnostic tests. Diagnostic findings must be synthesized with the patient's medical and dental history and chief complaint to select the best clinical procedures and therapeutics to address the emergency. The clinician must have an understanding of pain mechanisms, local anesthesia, the appropriate use of therapeutics, and patient management skills. Emergencies may occur prior to the inception of treatment, during treatment, or immediately after the canal or canals have been obturated.[1-6] Clinical, biologic, and predisposing factors associated with flare-ups are reviewed in this chapter.

The immediate goal of an emergency visit is to bring the case under control by eliminating the patient's primary cause of distress, which is most often pain with or without swelling. Definitions of what constitutes an endodontic emergency vary, but severe pain and swelling are the hallmarks of an emergency. A *flare-up* is often defined as severe pain and/or swelling after endodontic treatment requiring an unscheduled appointment and active treatment.[7] Traumatic injuries may also be the cause of an emergency visit (see Chapter 11).

DIAGNOSIS AND TREATMENT PLANNING

Determining the cause of the pain and/or swelling is a critical initial step in the emergency visit. Without an accurate diagnosis, treatment is unlikely to be effective. Initially, the clinician must determine whether the cause of the problem is odontogenic or nonodontogenic. Determination of the precise cause of the emergency follows. A number of potential causes must be considered, including microbial, occlusal, psychogenic, or referred pain of dental or nondental origin. Often, simply listening to the history of the chief complaint and onset of the symptoms provides sufficient information for the clinician to make a tentative diagnosis, which must then be confirmed with radiographs and clinical tests.

There are numerous classic patient narratives that provide critical information. An example is the patient who describes having had no pain until he or she bit down on something hard, which resulted in an immediate, sharp, lancinating pain and left a tooth tender to even finger pressure. Those few words are a powerful clue to causation and require investigation into a possible vertical or other type of fracture (Fig. 10.1).

By contrast, a patient who relates being awakened by pain at night but then feeling better as the day progresses, only to

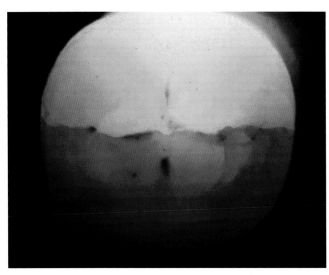

Fig. 10.1 Photograph of a brightly transilluminated tooth from the buccal aspect shows sharp difference on each side of a mesial to distal crack. Note that the light transmission is markedly reduced at the fracture line. Such illumination would gradually diminish throughout the occlusal surface in an intact tooth. The crack limits light transmission, so the diagnosis can be easily made.

have the pain return during sleep, does not fit the most common profile of an irreversible pulpitis. This patient requires a differential diagnosis for bruxism, temporomandibular joint dysfunction (TMD), or irreversible pulpitis.

The astute diagnostician must be a good listener and be able to synthesize information. Basic clinical tests include palpation, percussion, and thermal and electrical testing. Radiographs are an essential component of the diagnostic visit and may include periapicals, bitewings and cone beam computed tomography (CBCT). The clinician is cautioned against making a diagnosis based on a single radiograph (see Chapter 5 for further discussion of the diagnostic process).

Treatment planning involves a series of questions that must be answered prior to initiating treatment and may require consultation with the referring dentist and/or other health care professionals. Once the diagnosis has been made, an important question concerns the endodontic prognosis of the tooth. Factors include the restorability of the tooth, the crown-to-root ratio, the periodontal status, and the overall restorative plan, in addition to systemic health factors that could influence the plan. To determine an appropriate plan, additional information may be required from other dentists and physicians. The patient's past dental history is also a factor. A patient missing numerous teeth and with poor oral hygiene is probably not the best candidate for an endodontic procedure with a questionable prognosis. A basic question to consider is how the patient's oral health interests are best served. Should endodontic therapy be performed, or would an implant be a better approach? A review of the literature indicates that both procedures have a high rate of success when treatment is properly planned and completed.

INCIDENCE OF EXACERBATIONS

The incidence of exacerbations has been estimated to be as low as 1.5%[8] and as high as 20%.[9] This wide range of

estimates may be attributed to different definitions of exacerbations, varying study designs, and other procedural variations. A consistently high incidence of exacerbations should serve as a signal to the clinician to evaluate basic procedures, such as accuracy of measurement control and instrumentation. Breakdowns in either of those procedures could account for high rates of exacerbation.

The Initial Patient Contact

The initial emergency patient contact occurs most often by telephone prior to the initiation of endodontic treatment. The patient may report a history of long-term, low-level pain that has escalated to a more severe level. At this point the dentist must begin a basic triage, which includes determining whether the situation is truly an emergency and whether the problem seems to be odontogenic in nature. It may not be possible to clearly determine the status of the patient by telephone, and it is recommended that the clinician see such patients on an emergency basis to better determine the diagnosis and appropriate treatment.

The staff must be trained to respond appropriately to emergency calls. The person receiving the initial call should be able to differentiate between what is and is not a true emergency. However, when doubt exists about the urgency of the case, the clinician must make the final decision.

Patient Management

Patient anxiety is an important factor in achieving a satisfactory endodontic outcome, especially at an emergency visit. More than 200 studies indicate that preemptive behavioral intervention to reduce anxiety before and after surgery reduces postoperative pain intensity and intake of analgesics and accelerates recovery.[10] A clinical study determined that the higher the level of anxiety, as measured by a visual analogue anxiety scale, the less likely it was that pain would be eliminated after administration of a local anesthetics.[11] A conversation with the patient prior to treatment, in which the clinician discusses the pain-preventive strategy, including the use of profound local anesthesia, is an important element of the therapeutic approach.

Profound Anesthesia

Achieving profound local anesthesia for teeth with irreversible pulpitis is challenging and critical. Maxillary anesthesia is usually achieved by the use of infiltration or block anesthesia in the buccal and palatal areas. If profound anesthesia is defined as achieving the complete absence of pain, a single injection for a mandibular molar is usually insufficient. Intraosseous, ligamental, and intrapulpal injections are valuable supplementary injections that can help achieve this goal (see Chapter 9). It is important to note that a numb lip is not adequate proof of complete local anesthesia. The clinician is advised to recheck the chief complaint prior to initiating treatment. Absence of the chief complaint, whether it is thermal sensitivity or pain on percussion, is the best means of determining profound anesthesia.

CATEGORIES OF EMERGENCIES

Pretreatment Emergency

As mentioned, patients may present with a history of long-term, low-level discomfort that has suddenly escalated to **163** intolerable pain and swelling. It is essential that a thorough diagnosis be made prior to instituting treatment. Usually, such emergencies are accompanied by a high level of patient anxiety, which can further complicate diagnosis and treatment. Teeth that cause pretreatment emergencies may be associated with irreversible pulpitis and/or symptomatic periodontitis or pulp necrosis with or without apical pathosis and swelling. Swelling may be localized or diffused. Each of these situations requires a somewhat different clinical approach based on biologic considerations.

Management of Irreversible Pulpitis

Basic biologic processes may explain the cause of an exacerbation of a tooth with irreversible pulpitis. Irreversible pulpitis is often the result of inflammation of the pulp due to a microbial insult from caries or microleakage associated with a defective restoration. Exacerbation of a tooth with irreversible pulpitis is characterized by pain, which may be severe. The pain may occur with or without provocation and tends to increase in severity. A pulp with irreversible pulpitis is usually free of bacterial colonization in the root canal. Infection is most often confined to the coronal site of the pulp that is exposed to the oral cavity. As long as the radicular pulp remains vital, it usually protects itself against microbial invasion and colonization.[12]

It has been demonstrated that removal of the pulp from the pulp chamber (pulpotomy) is a highly predictable approach to alleviating pain at an emergency visit (Fig. 10.2).[13] It is considered preferable, if time permits, after measurement control, to remove all pulp tissue from the canal or canals. A clinical study demonstrated that partial pulpectomy resulted in a higher rate of postoperative pain (13%) compared with pulpotomy (6%). Other important factors associated with postoperative pain were female gender, younger age, and molar teeth. An emergency was defined as a visit to the dental emergency clinic within 24 hours of treatment for pain not controlled by ibuprofen, aspirin (ASA), or Tylenol.[14] It is challenging to remove inflamed tissue and infected debris from the canal system without pushing toxic material through the apical foramina into the periapical tissues. Establishing an accurate measurement control and maintaining it during instrumentation are critical in avoiding this complication.

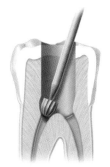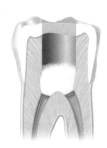

Fig. 10.2 Removal of coronal pulp. Pulpotomy and placement of a dry cotton pellet and a temporary filling result in relief of pain from irreversible pulpitis.

INTERAPPOINTMENT EMERGENCIES

Causes of Flare-Up

There are a number of hypotheses concerning the true cause of flare-ups, which have been described as multifactorial. Causes include iatrogenic mechanical irritation of the tissues beyond the apical terminus and/or the pushing of dentin chips and remnants of infected pulp tissue into the periapical tissues. A procedural accident often impedes therapy or makes it impossible for therapy to be completed, such as by preventing thorough mechanical debridement or creating a bacteria-tight seal for a root canal system. An increased risk exists when a procedural accident occurs during treatment of infected teeth.[15] There are also chemical factors, including irrigants, intracanal dressings, and sealers.[7] Endodontic procedural errors are not the direct cause of treatment failure; they increase the risk of failure because of the clinician's inability to eliminate microorganisms from the infected root canals.[16]

The number of treatment visits has also been examined as a factor in flare-ups. In a retrospective study, the flare-up rate in necrotic molars in one-visit compared with two-visit endodontic treatment was examined.[17] Treatment records of 402 consecutive patients with pulpally necrotic first and second molars were compared. One-visit treatment showed an advantage at the 95% confidence level. However, retrospective analyses do not control for the reason that a case took one or more appointments to complete, and some other studies have shown no differences between single and multiple visits in the incidence of flare-ups.[1]

Interappointment flare-ups most often occur after instrumentation of the canal system. The biologic factors resulting in pain in cases with irreversible pulpitis (vital cases) and in pain/swelling in necrotic (nonvital) cases may differ and are reviewed.

Frequently, iatrogenic errors cause problems. An example is leaving shredded pulp tissue in the canal system. After a working length measurement has been taken, the clinician should follow with complete debridement of tissue from the canal. This does not mean that the canal is fully shaped and ready for obturation, but rather that all pulp tissue in the canal has been removed.

Most important, before emergency treatment is initiated, the clinician should understand the biologic cause of the problem. For example, was there an iatrogenic component to the exacerbation, as occurs when an inaccurate measurement is used, or was an accurate measurement established but not maintained? Another reasonable possibility concerns the tooth's occlusion. Was the tooth under treatment left high in occlusion? This would exacerbate an inflamed periodontal membrane, resulting in pericementitis.

It has been determined that clean dentin chips pushed into the apical tissue did not result in a vigorous tissue reaction, whereas dentin chips contaminated by bacterial debris posed a problem and resulted in an inflammatory reaction.[18,19] In a nonvital case (necrotic, infected), debris may have been pushed into the periapical tissues, resulting in an immunologic and inflammatory response. These possibilities and others must be considered before selecting the appropriate treatment and determining whether an analgesic and/or an antibiotic are indicated. It is important to note that an antibiotic should never be used to control pain in a case with irreversible pulpitis.[20,21]

Biology of the Necrotic (Nonvital) Exacerbation

If we consider treatment of irreversible pulpitis (vital case) to be essentially a biologic challenge of removing well-innervated and inflamed tissue from a canal without causing increased pain, the necrotic (nonvital) case may be considered a microbiologic problem. Microorganisms are the most common etiologic cause of postoperative pain and post-treatment disease in the necrotic case. Exacerbation of the necrotic tooth occurs in the periapical tissues and is an immune/inflammatory reaction due to the extrusion of intracanal bacteria and tissue debris. The exacerbation may be characterized by pain with or without swelling. Swelling may be diffused or localized or may become a cellulitis.

As noted previously, clean dentin chips pushed into the apical tissue did not result in a tissue reaction, whereas those contaminated by bacterial debris resulted in an inflammatory reaction.[18]

Treatment of the necrotic exacerbation is focused on the root canal if there is no swelling. Reinstrumentation and irrigation are the basic treatments directed at reducing the intracanal level of microorganisms. If swelling exists, the clinician should consider incision and drainage followed by instrumentation and irrigation of the canal. Antibiotics alone should not be used without concomitant instrumentation and irrigation. Although incision and drainage is directed at reducing periapical tissue pressure and eliminating pus, reinstrumentation and irrigation are directed at the primary cause of the problem, which is remaining intracanal bacteria.

Postobturation Emergencies

It has been demonstrated histologically that the most favorable response of periapical tissues occurred when both instrumentation and filling were short of the apical constriction.[22] A clinical study found that the best treatment outcome in infected teeth with periradicular lesions occurred when the apical terminus of the filling was 0 to 2 mm short of the radiographic apex.[23] The same study determined that the prognosis was less favorable with significant underfill or overfill. These findings are corroborated by other research reports.[24,25]

Postobturation emergencies may include pain and diffuse swelling. Tenderness to finger pressure or percussion or an inability to comfortably bite on the tooth is often a predictor of postobturation pain. It is strongly recommended that obturation be deferred in such cases until the patient is pain free and the tooth in question can be used in function. During treatment of a postobturation exacerbation, the clinician must decide whether it is necessary to remove the root canal filling. Much depends on the condition of the tooth prior to obturation. A critical factor is the status of the tooth prior to filling. Was the tooth asymptomatic or did symptoms persist after instrumentation? Filling canals in the presence of continuing symptoms is often a predictor of postobturation complications. The nature of the swelling should also be considered. If there is swelling, is it diffuse in nature or becoming larger and fluctuant? Treatment for postobturation exacerbations may range from using pharmacotherapeutics, including analgesics and/or antibiotics, up to retreatment with or without incision for drainage. The clinician must consider the variables and then determine whether the primary cause of the patient's symptoms is inflammatory in nature, due to the procedure itself, or active infection. In most cases, if basic endodontic principles have been followed, the root canal filling does not have to be removed and postobturation pain can be treated with analgesics.

Predisposing Factors

An increasing body of evidence indicates that there may be factors that predispose a patient to pain and that could affect the outcome of treatment. Among those factors are the patient's genetics, gender, and level of anxiety.

Genetics

Findings suggest that specific markers associated with the proinflammatory mediator interleukin 1β (IL-1β), a key regulator of host response, may contribute to increased susceptibility to periapical pathosis.[25] It has also been suggested that genetic factors are associated with an individual's susceptibility to developing symptomatic dental abscesses.[26]

Gender

Evidence clearly demonstrates that women are at substantially greater risk for many clinical pain conditions. A growing body of evidence over the past 10 to 15 years has indicated that there are substantial differences in clinical and experimental pain responses between women and men.[27] It has been found that naturally redheaded women required 19% more desflurane (volatile anesthetic) than women with dark hair. It was also concluded that red hair in women was a distinct phenotype associated with anesthetic requirements in humans.[28] In 2005 it was found that there was increased thermal sensitivity and reduced subcutaneous lidocaine efficacy in redheads. Recent studies have found significant avoidance of dental care by women with red hair, probably due to increased anxiety associated with past resistance to local anesthesia. Having natural red hair or an MC1R variant, or both, could predict dental care avoidance related to anxiety.[29,30] This finding was gender specific and was not demonstrated in male patients. However, no difference in anesthetic efficacy could be demonstrated between women with red hair and those with black hair.[30]

Anxiety

Numerous studies have shown that preemptive behavioral intervention to reduce anxiety before and after surgery reduces postoperative pain intensity, intake of analgesics, and accelerates recovery.[10,31] One clinical study determined, using a visual analogue anxiety scale, that the higher the anxiety score, the less likely it was that pain would be eliminated during treatment, regardless of the number of injections.[11]

Microbiology of Flare-Ups

(This section is meant to complement Chapter 3, Endodontic Microbiology.)

When painful flare-ups occur after vital pulp extirpation, microorganisms are not likely to be involved unless iatrogenic contamination or a leaking interappointment restoration is involved. In every case, great care must be taken to avoid introducing bacteria into the canal system. When bleeding from the pulp space is observed, the cause may be periapical inflammation, probably secondary to infection or from torn tissues. Bleeding from the canal for which the diagnosis or observation is that the pulp is necrotic may be due to periradicular infection, which produces a strong inflammatory response and pressure, forcing bloody drainage outward. Many different microbial species are now appreciated as being present in necrotic pulps.[32] Viruses, bacteria, and fungi have been identified to date. The newly identified Archaea have also been identified in primary infections of the root canal space.[33] Ridding the space of bacteria within pulpal ramifications of the main canals and within dentinal tubules can be quite problematic.

Sources of Microbes in the Canal Space

In the natural history of endodontic disease, bacteria typically arrive in the canal space from caries, generally regarded as the most common source of pulpal infection. Periodontal disease, fractures, abrasion, and even trauma to a pulpally intact tooth have also been demonstrated to be avenues of entry for microbes. In their typical narrow dimension, bacteria are about 1 μm, whereas dentinal tubules approach four times that diameter. Increased peritubular dentin may impede but not eliminate bacterial ingress with age.[34]

Often the first microbes in the root canal are dependent upon oxygen for their existence. In the usual scenario, the oxygen within the pulp space is consumed within a few days, and the preponderance becomes facultative and obligate anaerobic bacteria. The majority of these organisms are gram-negative rods, although this is not universal. These bacteria often exist at low rates of reproduction, owing to their lower energy production in the absence of oxygen. Introduction of oxygen during endodontic treatment may allow facultative bacteria to shift to the much more energy efficient citric acid cycle (tricarboxylic acid cycle) and result in a flare-up.

The significance of bacteria and other microorganisms in endodontic pathology was elegantly demonstrated by Kakehashi and colleagues in their classic work from 1965.[35] With no microbial presence, simply accessing the pulp canals without pulp debridement resulted in no disease. Remaining pulp tissue remained vital in spite of food and debris impaction into the canal spaces. The control group of conventional animals showed microbial invasion through the teeth into periapical structures, as is typically seen in patients. The only difference was the absence of bacteria, clearly demonstrating that bacteria are the primary agent of endodontic disease. Therefore, practitioners should be vigilant in eliminating bacteria from the canal system and preventing their penetration into the periapical tissues.

Use of the rubber dam when performing endodontics is considered the standard of care for all dentists.[36] The dam has the dual role of preventing aspiration or swallowing of instruments and preventing bacterial leakage into the access preparation.

A great number of microbes have been found within root canal spaces, in large part due to newer genetic fingerprinting techniques. Many of these newly discovered denizens do not grow in traditional laboratory systems. Siqueira and Rocas reported that more than 460 unique bacterial taxa have been recorded to date.[37] Using other methods, the group estimated the number from nine acute and eight chronic infections to total more than 900 species.[38]

Microbial invaders can spread by direct invasion, enhanced by spreading factors, such as collagenase, hyaluronidase, gelatinase, and other enzymes. Also important is microbial motility. Chemotaxis is another trait that may aid in attracting bacteria. The theory that bacteria can be actively drawn toward an area of inflammation, known as *anachoresis*, remains poorly demonstrated. Bacterial spread by such means directly into adjacent tissues is well demonstrated, as is spreading within the circulatory system in blood and lymph.[39]

Questions have been raised about the use of water from dental units during endodontic irrigation. It is well documented that water taken from the dental unit is often contaminated and may pose a problem.

Dental unit waterlines harbor bacteria at alarming levels. This is due to two major factors. First, the narrow-diameter lines have low flow rates, and biofilms form within a few days, shedding bacterial colonies into the stream with each use. Second, the nature of the plastic material in the dental tubing aids bacterial attachment. Atlas and coworkers[40] found the pathogen *Legionella pneumophila* and other species of *Legionella* in 68% of the dental units tested by their team. Concentrations were greater than 1,000/mL in 36%, and above 10,000/mL in 19%.[40] Fotos's team noted a higher incidence of antibodies to *Legionella* in dental workers.[41] Shepherd's research team found that failure to follow the regimen of a commercial preparation of hydroperoxide ion-phase transfer catalyst cleaner/disinfectant resulted in persistence of the infection.[42] Interestingly, they found that oral streptococci were present in 80% of their samples; they interpreted this as meaning that these organisms had come from other patients, in spite of antiretraction valves on the dental units. Sterile water is readily available in sterile IV bags, and several dental equipment manufacturers have pressure chambers for expressing the water under pressure. Tubing for delivery must be sterilized, which is not currently possible with most dental units, making this an alternative for dedicated surgical irrigation.

Given these considerations, it seems unwise to use dental unit water for irrigation of the canal space. Opening the tooth creates a break in the integumentary boundary of the body, perhaps allowing the entry of pathogenic bacteria.

Intracanal Disinfectants

Proper use of disinfectants, which kill rapidly, compared to antibiotics, which need time to effect a kill, remains a keystone of endodontic therapy. Sodium hypochlorite has remained popular because it is not only very efficient and nonspecific at killing microorganisms, it also is the only common disinfectant that dissolves tissue remnants in the canal space. Higher concentrations and more time are needed for this to occur. Sufficient time to kill bacteria resident in tubules is also important. Local antibiotics placed within the canal are enjoying a resurgence, particularly in the case of pulp revascularization. There should be no bravado about how fast a clinician can perform endodontic therapy. Sufficient time for disinfectant is likely a minimum of 15 minutes after the canal has been debrided of detectable pulp tissue.

Signs and Symptoms of Infection

Early identification of an infection, followed by aggressive therapy, is important in patient care. Worsening microbial adaptability makes patient monitoring critical. It remains the responsibility of dentists to alert patients to report signs of worsening infection and to be available to their patients when infections worsen. Similarly, practitioners must train their staff to recognize signs of infection and to expedite the proper care of these patients. Such signs include swelling, malaise, pain, and fever.

Worsening signs and symptoms might indicate a need for hospitalization, perhaps under the care of an infectious disease specialist. Swelling may lead to direct invasion of adjacent tissues. Complications of this include progression into the fascial planes, leading inferiorly to the mediastinum and superiorly to the brain. Hematogenous spread may not feature frank swelling, although the infection is spreading dangerously. Malaise may be the only sign of infective endocarditis, which may occur weeks after the infection began. Pain must be carefully evaluated, because it has many causes. Pain secondary to infection can be masked by drugs and may be underreported or exaggerated. An elevated body temperature, although not always present, is an important sign that infection has spread beyond the immediate periapical area. Fever is an important objective sign that should be included in a thorough work-up. Patients presenting with fever secondary to a dental infection should be considered for systemic antimicrobial drug therapy.

Microbial Resistance

Resistance to antimicrobial drugs has seen a dramatic increase. There are many reasons for this, and practitioners may be forced to return to techniques of local drainage, as was the case prior to the antibiotic era. As we discover more and more about microbes' ability to exchange genetic material, it seems only reasonable to expect a worsening of resistance in the future. Aggressive research is under way to discover more effective drugs, but the outcome is not certain. Microorganisms likely will develop resistance to new drugs, given time.

THERAPY

Canal Debridement and Disinfection

Instrumentation of the canal space has been shown to reduce bacterial numbers, yet complete disinfection is unattainable.[43] Physical removal of the necrotic pulp contents obviously reduces numbers. Nevertheless, careful studies point out that mechanical canal debridement is not reliable in removing all tissue spaces.[44] Even with the best irrigation, bacteria may persist.[45]

Disinfectants will surely remain effective agents because of their rapid kill time, which denies microorganisms the time to adapt to these harsh chemicals. However, practitioners should recognize that disinfectants also harm host cells and are not to be used periapically. Whereas disinfectants kill quickly and indiscriminately, antibiotics target specific metabolic processes or surface structures of bacteria and spare host cells.

Drainage

Drainage of pus from an abscess can speed recovery (Figs. 10.3 and 10.4). The removal of dead lymphocytes and a preponderance of dead bacteria from the center of an infection can bring rapid resolution of symptoms and head off worsening of the infection. Return of local vascular flow aids the process of reaching and maintaining antibiotic levels and also reduces local tissue acidity, enhancing the action of local anesthetics. Chronic drainage by way of a sinus tract sharply reduces the occurrence of flare-up because of drainage. Surgical drainage can be quite helpful in treating infections. An

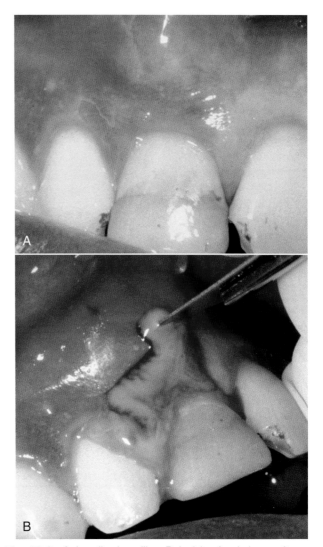

Fig. 10.3 **A,** Localized swelling. **B,** Incision for drainage after cleaning and shaping of the offending incisor. (Courtesy Dr. E. Rivera.)

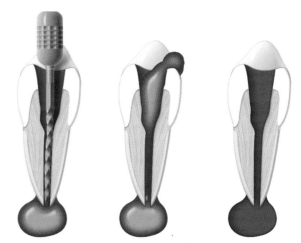

Fig. 10.4 After opening into the root canal and establishment of drainage, instrumentation should be confined to the root canal system. Release of purulence removes a potent irritant (pus) and relieves pressure.

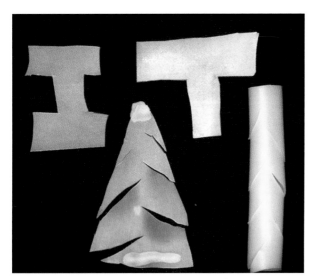

Fig. 10.5 Types of rubber drains. *Left to right,* I drain, Christmas tree drain, T drain, and Penrose drain with oblique cuts. These drains are self-retentive and do not require suturing to the incision margins.

in-dwelling drain to prevent premature closure of the epithelium is indicated in many situations (Fig. 10.5). Foreign bodies and larger amounts of necrotic tissue may call for surgical removal.[46] Mohammadi and Abbott advocate use of this approach to prevent the tissue damage characteristic of disinfectants inadvertently introduced into the periapex.[47]

PHARMACOTHERAPY FOR FLARE-UPS

Antimicrobial Drugs

Administration of antibiotics has sharply reduced morbidity and mortality from bacterial infections since the development of these drugs nearly a century ago. Currently we are experiencing a shift of bacteria toward increased levels of resistance to these drugs. The scope of this problem can be appreciated by considering the large genetic diversity of bacteria, which have a gene pool that, among all species, reaches into the millions.[48] Although bacteria can adapt by mutation, more commonly they gain a genetic advantage by obtaining new genetic material directly from their environment; from other bacteria, such as with conjugation (even beyond species lines); or by viral transfer (bacteriophage). Overuse of antibiotics, especially to enhance farm animal growth rates, has played a major role in the exposure of microbes to antibiotics, with resultant tolerance. It is important for the clinician to know the action of the antimicrobial drug; its expected spectrum, mode of action, and concentration in abscess or bone; and the site and speed of elimination and metabolism. This information must be tailored to the medical history of the patient. Close follow-up is also important to determine when it might be time to change to a different type of drug or to discontinue a drug when signs and symptoms of infection abate.

Combinations of antibiotics are becoming more useful; however, for acute infections it is still considered wise to avoid combining a drug that acts by slowing protein synthesis with one that kills actively growing bacteria. Use of broad-spectrum antibiotics and of certain combinations has been associated with higher overgrowth of the spore-forming gut pathogen *Clostridium difficile,* which may cause serious, even life-threatening, results for patients.[49] The use of antimicrobials carries the responsibilities of being aware of this and other reactions, of appropriately monitoring patients, and of being knowledgeable about their management.

There is no indication for prescribing antibiotics "in case there is an infection" or "to prevent it turning into an infection." Well-controlled research has shown that painful pulpitis is not relieved by systemic antimicrobial therapy.[21] In one study, the 40 participants experienced the same need for pain relievers, regardless of whether they took penicillin or placebo. Pain intensity scores given by the patients were similar over the 7-day study period prior to definitive endodontic treatment.[70] Another researcher noted that total pulp removal gave the most reliable pain relief.[50]

Classic antimicrobial drugs (antibiotics) have been limited to bacterial infections due to various unique metabolic and structural aspects that present a drug target. Antimicrobials can be categorized as those that kill rapidly, either by creating disruptions in the cell wall or by direct attack on the bacterial DNA, and those that kill more slowly by slowing bacterial protein synthesis at their ribosomes. The penicillins, cephalosporins, fluoroquinolones, and metronidazole are in the first category and thus kill rather rapidly. Slower acting drugs include the macrolides, tetracyclines, chloramphenicol, and clindamycin. Generally, an active infection is not treated with drugs from each group because protein synthesis interference slows growth and inhibits the so-called bactericidal rapid killers by simply delaying reproduction.

Antibiotics do not make the infection go away. They merely work as an adjunct to the patient's defenses. Most infections involve multiple bacterial species, and only elimination of the key ones in the commensal or symbiotic relationship is needed.[32]

Two main indications exist for use of antimicrobial drugs; namely, to treat active infection and to prevent infection. The use of these drugs is quite different for these different approaches. In therapy for active infections, antibiotics have been used locally and/or systemically. Grossman originally recommended intracanal antibiotics,[51] a practice that has seen a recent resurgence for elimination of all canal bacteria prior to stimulation of periapical stem cells in pulp regeneration. Most often, oral antibiotics are prescribed for systemic infection. Clearly, we are witnessing a failure of these drugs due to overuse, both in patients and in farm animals. Research is under way to develop new types, but they will surely be overcome in time, given the powerful resources of the huge variety of microorganisms. As mentioned, in addition to mutation, bacterial cells can share genetic material with each other, even across species. The astute practitioner avoids use of antibiotics when not clearly indicated. Such conservation warrants education of patients and follow-up after their treatment.

For treatment of active infection, the ideal drug focuses only on the pathogens for a particular patient, and therapy should last only until the host defenses are in control. The concepts of culturing and antibiotic sensitivity testing should become part of this approach.[52]

Prophylaxis is indicated for several heart conditions and for prosthetic joints. The protocol for this application is high-dose, short-term, broad-spectrum coverage during the time of therapy to aid the host in defeating bacteria that penetrate into the body.[53]

No antibiotic can be relied upon as a certain cure. The patient with worsening infection should be aware of how to reach help. Significant aftereffects of antibiotic therapy can occur, such as an overgrowth of the spore-forming anaerobe *C. difficile* in the large bowel, which currently is increasing in incidence, with a significant mortality rate.[54,55] Brain abscess is a known sequela of dental infection and has a high mortality rate.[56] Mortality from cavernous sinus infection, often caused by a dental infection, is alarmingly high. Similarly, Lemierre's disease is characterized by the occasional endodontic pathogen *Fusobacterium necrophorum* penetrating the jugular vein wall and progressing into the lungs. Familiarity with fascial planes as a means of direct spread of infection is important, as is awareness of hematogenous or lymphatic metastasis of infection.

It has also been found that lower antibiotic concentrations encouraged antibiotic resistance,[57] a finding that signals practitioners to use adequate concentrations when drug therapy is indicated and to instruct patients not to skip doses.[57]

More than ever, all health care providers must take care to prevent the unnecessary exposure of bacteria to drugs, thereby worsening the resistance problem. Antibiotics should be reserved for active infections; yet, they should not spared in cases where truly needed. Important questions must be resolved prior to writing a prescription. Is the patient is febrile or are there signs and symptoms that the infection is ranging beyond the tooth? Is the patient immunocompromised? The balance of potential good versus potential harm should be weighed. **If** the signs and symptoms indicate that the infection is localized and **if** the patient is immunocompetent, then local debridement and disinfection of the pulp space may be sufficient, inasmuch as this procedure eliminates most of the pulp contents, removes a large percentage of the bacteria, and perhaps enables drainage. However, if the infection invades the tissues beyond the immediate root end area, systemic drug therapy is indicated.[58]

Analgesics

Patient communication is quite important in dealing with pain. Researchers in Canada found that patients who received a reassuring telephone call after surgery needed less analgesic.[59] Reassurance may be all that is needed in some circumstances.

Pain is an indicator to the patient of trouble in the body. Although individual variability modulates this symptom, pain is part of the definition of flare-up. Patient discomfort is usually the motivating factor in seeking treatment. Management of this symptom is important for the dentist and the patient. Typically the pain threshold can be elevated by drugs, and/or the cause of the pain from infection can be treated with local and perhaps systemic drugs.

Opioids, Acetaminophen, and Nonsteroidal Antiinflammatory Drugs

Full knowledge of the principles of pharmacology is import for prescribers, and the reader is referred to a pharmacology text for review. Important considerations include the drug's half-life, the dosing interval, the compatibility of a proposed drug with food, the patient's allergic reaction history, and potential interactions with drugs the patient takes on a regular basis. This discussion is limited to specific principles of drug therapy for flare-up.

Drugs to diminish pain perception can be divided into two broad categories, opioids and others. Whether bacterial in origin or otherwise, almost all dental pain arises from inflammation. Opioids and acetaminophen are considered to act primarily on the central nervous system (CNS). In contrast, inflammation-suppressing drugs, such as corticosteroids and nonsteroidal antiinflammatory drugs (NSAIDs), are very effective in reducing pain through their action at the site of injury.[60] The combination of NSAIDs with acetaminophen, which apparently acts centrally, is even more effective.[61,62]

A recent dental extraction study found the combination of acetaminophen and ibuprofen superior to either ibuprofen plus an opioid or acetaminophen plus an opioid.[63] It has long been known that classic opioids (e.g., codeine and hydrocodone), although often prescribed, are less effective than drugs directed specifically at inflammation.[64] Also, opioids have harsh side effects, including sedation, diminution of protective reflexes, and an additive effect with all CNS depressants, in addition to addiction.

A simplified strategy for the use of these analgesic medications is shown in Fig. 10.6.

Corticosteroid Drugs

Corticosteroids, a class of drugs introduced in the 1950s, are potent inhibitors of inflammation and its pain, blocking both the proinflammatory pathway that produces prostaglandins and the path to leukotrienes. Because inflammation is reduced, it was originally thought that lessened phagocytosis would handicap the patient's ability to clear an infection promptly. However, in 1974 Olds and colleagues found that normally administered levels of supplemental corticosteroid had little effect on phagocytosis.[65]

Holland found that pulpal inflammation was limited when steroids were present systemically at the time of pulpectomy in animals. The area of periapical inflammation was one third as large, and the amount of nerve sprouting at the neurotomy site was graded as reduced.[66]

Pain of irreversible pulpitis has been shown to be sharply reduced prior to definitive treatment of pulpectomy.[67] Inasmuch as the onset of action is a matter of hours, the practitioner may consider a long-acting local anesthetic.[68]

In the risk versus reward determination, pain reduction from the wound of pulpectomy may be a factor, along with more widespread inflammation associated with periapical infection. Corticosteroid-reduced inflammation may also retard the natural disease history, leading to pulp necrosis for several days.[67]

Steroids (more accurately termed *glucocorticosteroids*) are normally produced by the adrenal cortices, along with a host of other chemicals. Chronic high steroid production, such as occurs with an adrenal tumor, results in Cushing's syndrome. Long-term steroid dosing for various medical conditions may have a similar effect. Such patients do not tolerate stress well, and consideration should be given to increasing their normal steroid dose for a physically or psychologically stressful procedure. Typically steroids are given in gradually reduced daily doses to allow adrenal function to return to baseline. If a single bolus of drug is given, adrenal suppression gradually rebounds, negating the need for tapered dosing. Langeland and coworkers were unable to demonstrate differences from control, using the light microscope, when a corticosteroid was applied directly to the pulp.[69]

Flexible Analgesic Strategy

	Aspirin-like drugs indicated	Aspirin-like drugs contraindicate
Mild Pain	Ibuprofen 400-600 mg	Acetaminophen 325 mg
Moderate Pain	Ibuprofen 400-600 mg + Acetaminophen 325 mg	Acetaminophen 650 mg
Severe Pain	Ibuprofen 400-600 mg + Hydrocodone 7.5 mg & Acetaminophen 300 mg	Acetaminophen 325 mg & Oxycodone 10 mg

Fig. 10.6 Simplified analgesic strategy to guide drug selection based on the patient history and level of present or anticipated post-treatment pain. (Courtesy Dr. A. Fouad.)

REFERENCES

1. Walton R, Fouad A: Endodontic interappointment flare-ups: a prospective study of incidence and related factors, *J Endod* 18:172, 1992.
2. Mor C, Rotstein I, Friedman S: Incidence of interappointment emergency associated with endodontic therapy, *J Endod* 18:509, 1992.
3. Marshall JG, Liesinger AW: Factors associated with endodontic posttreatment pain, *J Endod* 19:573, 1993.
4. Albashaireh ZS, Alnegrish AS: Postobturation pain after single- and multiple-visit endodontic therapy: a prospective study, *J Dent* 26:227, 1998.
5. Glennon JP, Ng YL, Setchell DJ, et al: Prevalence of and factors affecting postpreparation pain in patients undergoing two-visit root canal treatment, *Int Endod J* 37(1):29-37, 2004.
6. Ng YL, Glennon JP, Setchell DJ, et al: Prevalence of and factors affecting post-obturation pain in patients undergoing root canal treatment, *Int Endod J* 37(6):381-391, 2004.
7. Tsesis I, Faivishevsky V, Fuss Z, et al: Flare-ups after endodontic treatment: a meta-analysis of literature, *J Endod* 34:1177-1181, 2008.
8. Imura N, Zuolo ML: Factors associated with endodontic flare-ups: a prospective study, *Int Endod J* 29(6):382-386, 1995.
9. Morse DR, Koren LZ, Esposito JV, et al: Asymptomatic teeth with necrotic pulps and associated periapical radiolucencies: relationship of flare-ups to endodontic instrumentation, antibiotic usage and stress, in three separate practices at three different time periods. Part 1, *Int J Psychosom* 33:5-17, 1986.
10. Carr DB, Goudas LC: Acute pain, *The Lancet* 353:2051-2058, 1999.
11. DiBernardi J, Fisch G, Rosenberg PA: Preoperative levels of anxiety as a predictor of successful local anesthesia, *J Endod* 35:432, 2009.
12. Siqueira JF: Reaction of periradicular tissues to root canal treatment: benefits and drawbacks, *Endod Topics* 10:123-147, 2005.
13. Hasselgren G, Reit C: Emergency pulpotomy: pain relieving effect with and without sedative dressings, *J Endod* 15:254, 1989.
14. Oguntebi BR, Deshepper EJ, Taylor TS, et al: Postoperative pain incidence related to the type of emergency treatment of symptomatic pulpitis, *Oral Surg Oral Med Oral Pathol* 73:479-483, 1992.
15. Siqueira JF Jr: Aetiology of root canal treatment failure: why well-treated teeth can fail, *Int Endod J* 34(1):1-10, 2001.
16. Lin LM, Rosenberg PA, Lin J: Do procedural errors cause endodontic treatment failure? *J Am Dent Assoc* 136:187-191, 2005.
17. Eleazer PD, Eleazer KR: Flare-up rate in pulpally necrotic molars in one-visit versus two-visit endodontic treatment was examined, *J Endod* 24:614-616, 1998.
18. Tronstad L: Tissue reactions following apical plugging of the root canal with dentin chips in monkey teeth subjected to pulpectomy, *Oral Surg Oral Med Oral Pathol* 45:297-304, 1978.
19. Rosenberg PA, Babick PJ, Schertzer L, et al: The effect of occlusal reduction on pain after endodontic instrumentation, *J Endod* 24:492, 1998.
20. Walton R: Interappointment flare-ups: incidence, related factors, prevention and management, *Endod Topics* 67, 2002.
21. Keenan JV, Farman AG, Fedorowicz Z, et al: Antibiotic use for irreversible pulpitis, *Cochrane Database Syst Rev* 2:CD004969, 2005.
22. Ricucci D, Langeland K: Apical limit of instrumentation and obturation. Part 2. A histological study, *J Int Endod* 31:394-409, 1998.
23. Sjogren U, Hagglund B, Sundqvist G, et al: Factors affecting the long term results of endodontic treatment, *J Endod* 16:498-504, 1990.
24. Strindberg LZ: The dependence of the results of pulp therapy on certain factors, *Acta Odontol Scand* 14(Suppl 21):1-175, 1956.
25. Morsani JM, Aminoshariae A, Han YW, et al: Genetic predisposition to persistent apical periodontitis, *J Endod* 37:4:455-459, 2011.
26. De Sá AR, Moreira PR, Xavier GM, et al: Association of CD14, IL1B, IL6, IL10 and TNFA functional gene polymorphisms with symptomatic dental abscesses, *Int Endod J* 40:563-572, 2007.
27. Fillingim RB, King CD, Ribeiro-Dasilva MC: Sex, gender, and pain: a review of recent clinical and experimental findings, *J Pain* 10:5, 447-485, 2009.
28. Liem EB, Lin CM, Suleman MI, et al: Increased anesthetic requirement in redheads, *Anesthesiology* 101:279-283, 2004.
29. Binkley CJ, Beacham A, Neace W: Genetic variations associated with red hair color and fear of dental pain: anxiety regarding dental care and avoidance of dental care, *J Am Dent Assoc* 140:896-905, 2009.
30. Droll B, Drum M, Nusstein J, et al: Anesthetic efficacy of the inferior alveolar nerve block in red-haired women, *J Endod* 38(12):1564-1569, 2012.
31. Eli I, Schwartz-Arad D, Baht R, et al: Effect of anxiety on the experience of pain in implant insertion, *Clin Oral Implant Res* 14:1, 115-118, 2003.
32. Siqueira J, Alves FR, Rocas IN: Pyrosequencing analysis of the apical root canal microbiota, *J Endod* 37(11):1499-1503, 2011.
33. Vianna ME, Conrads G, Gomes BPFA, et al: Identification and quantification of Archaea involved in primary endodontic infections, *J Clin Microbiol* 44(4):1274-1282, 2006.
34. Kakoli P, Nandakumar R, Romberg E, et al: The effect of age on bacterial penetration of radicular dentin, *J Endod* 35(1):78-81, 2009.
35. Kakehashi S, Stanley JR, Fitzgerald RJ: The effects of surgical exposures of dental pulps in germ-free and conventional laboratory rats, *Oral Surg Oral Med Oral Pathol* 20:340-349, 1965.
36. Cohen S, Schwartz S: Endodontic complications and the law, *J Endod* 13(4):191-197, 1967.
37. Siqueira JF, Rocas IN: Diversity of endodontic microbiota revisited, *J Dent Res* 88(11):969-981, 2009.
38. Santos AL, Siqueira JF, Rocas IN, et al: Comparing the bacterial diversity of acute and chronic dental root canal infections, *PLoS One* 6(11):e28088, doi:10.1371/journal.pone.0028088, 2011.
39. Mims C, Dimmock N, Nash A, et al, editors: *Mims' pathogenesis of infectious disease*, ed 4, pp 106-135, London, 1995, Academic Press.
40. Atlas RM, Williams JF, Huntington MK: *Legionella* contamination of dental unit waters, *Appl Environ Microbiol* 61(4):1208-1213, 1995.
41. Fotos PG, Westfall HN, Snyder IS, et al: Prevalence of *Legionella*-specific IgG and IgM antibody in dental clinic population, *J Dent Res* 64(12):1382-1385, 1985.
42. Shepherd PA, Shojaei MA, Eleazer PD, et al: Clearance of biofilms from dental unit waterlines through the use of hydroperoxide ion-phase transfer catalysts, *Quintessence Int* 32:755-761, 2001.
43. Dalton BC, Orstavik D, Phillips C, et al: Bacterial reduction with nickel-titanium rotary instrumentation, *J Endod* 24(11):763-767, 1998.
44. Peters OA, Boessler C, Paque F: Root canal preparation with a novel nickel-titanium instrument evaluated with micro-computed tomography: canal surface preparation over time, *J Endod* 36(6):1068-1072, 2010.
45. Zehnder M: Root canal irrigants, *J Endod* 32(5): 389-398, 2006.
46. Marshall JC, al Naqqbi A: Principles of source control in management of sepsis, *Crit Care Clin* 25(4):753-768, 2009.
47. Mohammadi Z, Abbott PV: On the local applications of antibiotics and antibiotic-based agents in endodontics and dental traumatology, *Int Endod J* 42:555-567, 2009.

48. Qin J, Li R, Raes J, et al: A human gut microbial gene catalogue established by metagenomic sequencing, *Nature* 464:59-67, 2010.

49. Blondeau JM: What have we learned about antimicrobial use and the risks for *Clostridium difficile*–associated diarrhoea? *J Antimicrob Chemother* 63(2):238-242, 2009.

50. Foaud AF: Are antibiotics effective for endodontic pain? *Endod Topics* 2:52-66, 2002.

51. Grossman LI: Polyantibiotic treatment of pulpless teeth, *J Am Dent Assoc* 43:265-278, 1951.

52. Harris T, Crawford PJM: Case report: teeth and tonsils—the use of culture and sensitivity testing for antibiotic prescribing in dental infection, *Br Dent J* 202(8):463-464, 2007.

53. Gutierrez JL, Bagan JV, Bascones A, et al: Consensus document on the use of antibiotic prophylaxis in dental surgery and procedures, *Med Oral Patol Oral Cir Bucal* 111:e188-e205, 2006.

54. Armbruster S, Goldkind L: A 5-year retrospective review of experience with *Clostridium difficile*–associated diarrhea, *Mil Med* 177(4):456-459, 2012.

55. Noren T: *Clostridium difficile* and the disease it causes, *Methods Mol Biol* 646:9-35, 2010.

56. Li X, Tronstad L, Olsen I: Brain abscesses caused by oral infection, *Endod Dent Traumatol* 15(3):95-101, 1999.

57. Zhang Q, Lambert B, Lio D, et al: Acceleration of emergence of bacterial antibiotic resistance in connected microenvironments, *Science* 333(6050):1764-1767, 2011.

58. Skucaite N, Peciuliene V, Maciulskiene V: Microbial infection and its control in cases of symptomatic apical periodontitis: a review, *Medicina* 45(5):343-350, 2009.

59. Touyz LZ, Marchand S: The influence of postoperative telephone calls on pain perception: a study of 118 periodontal surgical procedures, *J Orofac Pain* 12:219-225, 1998.

60. Keiser K, Hargreaves KM: Building effective strategies for the management of endodontic pain, *Endod Topics* 3:92-104, 2002.

61. Mehlisch DR, Aspley S, Daniels SE, et al: Comparison of the analgesic efficacy of concurrent ibuprofen and paracetamol with ibuprofen and paracetamol alone in the management of moderate to severe acute postoperative dental pain in adolescents and adults: a randomized, double-blind, placebo-controlled, parallel-group, single-dose, two-center, modified factorial study, *Clin Ther* 32(5):882-895, 2010.

62. Menhinick KA, Gutmann JL, Regan JD, et al: The efficacy of pain control following nonsurgical root canal treatment using ibuprofen or a combination of ibuprofen and acetaminophen in a randomized double-blind, placebo-controlled study, *Int Endod J* 37(8):531-541, 2004.

63. Daniels SE, Goulder MA, Aspley S, et al: A randomized, five-parallel-group, placebo-controlled trial comparing the efficacy and tolerability of analgesic combinations, including a novel single-tablet combination of ibuprofen/paracetamol, for postoperative dental pain, *Pain* 152:632-642, 2011.

64. Beaver WT: Mild analgesics: a review of their clinical pharmacology, *Am J Med Sci* 251:576-599, 1966.

65. Olds JW, Reed WP, Eberle B, et al: Corticosteroids, serum, and phagocytosis: in vitro and in vivo studies, *Infect Immun* 9(3):524-529, 1974.

66. Holland GR: Steroids reduce the periapical inflammatory and neural changes after pulpectomy, *J Endod* 22(9):455-458, 1996.

67. Gallatin E, Reader A, Nist R, et al: Pain reduction in untreated irreversible pulpitis using an intraosseous injection of Depo-Medrol, *J Endod* 26:633-638, 2000.

68. Glassman G, Krasner P, Morse DR, et al: A prospective randomized double-blind trial on efficacy of dexamethasone for endodontic interappointment pain in teeth with asymptomatic inflamed pulps, *Oral Surg Oral Med Oral Pathol* 67:96-100, 1989.

69. Langeland K, Langeland LK, Anderson DM: Corticosteroids in dentistry, *Int Dent J* 27(3):217-251, 1977.

70. Nagle D, Reader A, Beck M, et al: Effect of systemic penicillin on pain in untreated irreversible pulpitis, *Oral Surg Oral Med Oral Pathol Oral Radiol Endod* 90(5):636-640, 2000.

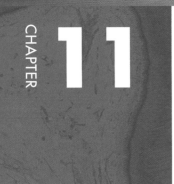

Management of traumatic dental injuries

Nestor Cohenca

LEARNING OBJECTIVES

After reading this chapter, the student should be able to:

1. Describe the clinical and radiographic features of enamel fractures, uncomplicated crown fractures, complicated crown fractures, crown-root fractures, root fractures, concussion, subluxation, luxations (lateral, extrusive, and intrusive), avulsions, and alveolar fractures.
2. Describe possible short- and long-term responses of pulp, periradicular tissues, and hard tissues to the injuries listed previously.
3. List pertinent information needed when examining patients with dental injuries (health history, nature of injury, and symptoms).
4. Describe the diagnostic tests and procedures used in examining patients with dental injuries and interpret the findings.

5. Describe appropriate treatment strategies (immediate and long term) for various types of traumatic injuries.
6. Recognize outcomes of traumatic dental injuries.
7. Recognize pulp space obliteration and describe management considerations.
8. Recognize surface resorption, inflammatory (infection-related) resorption, and replacement (ankylosis-related) resorption, and describe their respective treatment strategies.
9. Describe the differences in treatment strategies for traumatic dental injuries in primary and permanent dentition.

Trauma to teeth involves the dental pulp and the periodontium either directly or indirectly; consequently, endodontic considerations are important in evaluating and treating traumatic dental injuries. The purpose of this chapter is to describe the incidence of dental trauma, etiologic factors, examination procedures, emergency care, treatment options, and possible sequelae in traumatized teeth. Because injuries occur to primary teeth also, a separate section has been included for these teeth. The recommendations for managing traumatic dental injuries are based on the guidelines published by the International Association of Dental Traumatology, which publishes updated guidelines on its Web site *(www.iadt-dentaltrauma.org)*.

Epidemiologic studies have shown that the incidence of dental trauma ranges from 25% to 58%, and the most common age group affected is children 8 to 12 years.[1-5] Sgan-Cohen and colleagues reported a total prevalence of 29.6%.[4] Severe trauma, at least involving the dentin, was found among 13.5% and was more prevalent among children with an incisal overjet and incompetent lip. Falls were the main cause of dental trauma (44.9%), but sports and violence also were important causes. Fractures of enamel or enamel and dentin are the most common sequelae of dental trauma. The teeth most often traumatized are the maxillary central incisors (88%), maxillary laterals (7%), and mandibular incisors (5%). Among sports, basketball is associated with the highest injury rate, with an incidence of 10.6 injuries per 100 athlete-seasons among men and 5 injuries per 100 athlete-seasons among women.[6] The incidence for basketball players was five times higher than that for football players, for whom mouthguard use is mandatory.

Age is an important factor in trauma to teeth. By age 14, about 25% of children will have had an injury involving their permanent teeth.[1,7] The significance of age is a "good news/bad news" situation. The good news is that pulps in children's teeth have a better blood supply than those in adults and better repair potential. The bad news is that root development is interrupted in teeth with damaged pulps, leaving the roots thin and weak. Cervical fractures often occur either spontaneously or from even minor injuries because of thin dentin walls. Therefore, when dental injuries occur in children, every effort must be made to preserve pulp vitality.

Box 11.1   Classification of Dental Injuries

- *Enamel fracture:* Involves the enamel only and includes enamel chipping and incomplete fractures or enamel cracks.
- *Crown fracture without pulp exposure:* An uncomplicated fracture involving the enamel and dentin with no pulp exposure.
- *Crown fracture with pulp exposure:* A complicated fracture involving the enamel and dentin and exposure of the pulp.
- *Crown-root fracture:* Tooth fracture that includes the enamel, dentin, and root cementum and may or may not include the pulp.
- *Root fracture:* Fracture of the root only involving the cementum, dentin, and pulp; also referred to as a *horizontal root fracture.*
- *Luxation injuries:* Tooth luxations include concussion, subluxation, extrusive luxation, lateral luxation, and intrusive luxation.
- *Avulsion:* Complete displacement of a tooth out of its socket.
- *Fracture of the alveolar process (mandible or maxilla):* Fracture or comminution of the alveolar socket or of the alveolar process.

Table 11.1   Radiographic classification of odontogenic development

Classification	Description
0	No crypt
1	Presence of a crypt
2	Initial calcification
3	One-third crown completed
4	Two-thirds crown complete
5	Crown almost completed
6	Crown completed
7	One-third root completed
8	Two-thirds root competed
9	Root almost open (open apex)
10	Root apex completed

Classification of traumatic injuries promotes better communication and dissemination of information. The system used in this chapter is based on Andreasen and Andreasen's modification of the World Health Organization classification (Box 11.1).[1,8] Feliciano and de Franca Caldas evaluated 164 articles and 54 different classifications and concluded that, according to the literature, the Andreasens' model was the most frequently used classification system (32%).[9] Treatment recommendations are based on the official guidelines of the International Association of Dental Traumatology (IADT).[10-12]

EXAMINATION AND DIAGNOSIS

Examination of a patient with dental injuries should include the history (chief complaint, history of present illness, pertinent medical history) and a clinical examination. The emphasis in this chapter is on those aspects of the examination that specifically relate to dental trauma.[13]

Stage of Root Development and Dental Trauma

Knowledge of the developmental stages of permanent teeth is essential for clinical practice in several dental specialties because it may influence diagnosis, treatment planning, and outcomes. In 1960 Nolla published a classification system for odontogenic development based on radiographic interpretation (Table 11.1).[14] This system has been widely used,[15,16] and it is particularly important for appropriate diagnosis and treatment of traumatized teeth. In 1976 Fulling and Andreasen demonstrated that the late differentiation of Aδ nerve fibers in the dental pulp could explain the lack of a reliable and predictable response of erupting and undeveloped teeth to thermal and electrical stimulation.[17] In young patients with immature teeth, carbon dioxide (CO_2) snow and dichlorodifluoromethane (DDM) are the most reliable sensitivity tests, followed by electrical pulp testing and ethyl chloride and

ice.[18] Therefore, in the absence of reliable clinical tests, radiographic evidence of root development and dentin maturation during follow-up examination may be critical for providing the clinician with reliable information about the presence of a vital dental pulp.

History

Pertinent information about traumatic injuries should be obtained expeditiously by following a system.

Chief Complaint

The chief complaint is simply a statement, in the patient's (or parents') own words, of the current problem; for example, "I broke my tooth," or "My tooth feels loose." It may also be unstated, as in a patient with obvious injuries.

History of Present Illness

To obtain the history of the present illness (injury), the dentist can ask a few specific questions, such as the following.

- *When and how did the injury occur?* The date and time of the accident are recorded. The record should include *how* the injury took place (i.e., bicycle accident, playground, sports, violence, or other). Such information is useful in the search for avulsed teeth and embedded tooth fragments, assessment of possible contamination, determination of the time factor with respect to the choice of treatment and the healing potential, and completion of accident reports.
- *Have you had any other injuries to your mouth or teeth in the past?* Individuals may have repeated traumatic injuries if they are accident prone or participate in contact sports.[13] Crown or root fractures may have occurred as a result of an earlier injury but are observed at a later time. A history of previous episodes of trauma may affect the healing potential of the pulp and periodontium. It should also raise concern about the possibility of physical abuse of a child.

- *What problems are you now having with your tooth or teeth?* Pain, mobility, and occlusal interference are common symptoms. The patient's description of symptoms aids diagnosis.

Medical History

The patient's medical history is often significant. For example, the patient may have an allergy to prescribed medication, may be taking medications that interact with proposed new medications, or may have a medical condition that affects treatment. The patient's tetanus immunization status should be recorded; a booster may be indicated with contaminating injuries, such as avulsions and penetrating lip and soft tissue lesions.[19]

The need for neurologic evaluation should always be considered and ruled out. Concussion is a disturbance in brain function caused by direct or indirect force to the head.[20] It is a functional, rather than structural, injury that results from shear stress to brain tissue caused by rotational or angular forces; direct impact to the head is not required. Headache is the most common symptom of concussion, although a variety of clinical domains (e.g., somatic, cognitive, affective) can be affected (Box 11.2). Signs and symptoms are nonspecific; therefore, a temporal relationship between an appropriate mechanism of injury and the symptoms must be determined.[20] In cases in which a head concussion is suspected, the patient should be immediately referred for a full neurologic examination.

Clinical Examination

The lips, oral soft tissues, and facial skeleton should be examined, in addition to the teeth and supporting structures.

Soft Tissues

The purpose of the soft tissue evaluation is to determine the extent of tissue damage and to identify and remove foreign objects from wounds. In crown fractures with adjacent soft tissue lacerations, wounds are examined visually and radiographically for tooth fragments. Lips are likely areas for a foreign body impaction. Also, severe lacerations require suturing (Fig. 11.1).

Facial Skeleton

The facial skeleton is evaluated for possible fractures of the jaw or alveolar process. Such fractures, when they involve tooth sockets, may produce pulpal necrosis in teeth associated with fracture lines.[21,22] Alveolar fractures are suspected when several teeth are displaced or move as a unit; when tooth displacement is extensive; when occlusal misalignment is present; or when there is continuous bleeding from gingival tissues.

Teeth and Supporting Tissues

Examination of teeth and supporting tissues should provide information about damage that may have occurred to dental hard tissues, pulps, periodontal ligaments, and bony sockets. The following sections present guidelines for a method of collecting information systematically.

Mobility

The clinician examines the teeth (gently) for mobility, noting whether adjacent teeth also move when one tooth is moved

---

Box 11.2 Selected Symptoms of Concussion

Affective/emotional symptoms
- Anxiety/nervousness*
- Clinginess
- Depression
- Emotional distress
- Irritability*
- Personality changes
- Sadness

Cognitive symptoms
- Amnesia
- Confusion
- Delayed verbal and other responses
- Difficulty concentrating*
- Difficulty remembering*
- Disorientation*
- Feeling foggy*
- Feeling slowed down*
- Feeling stunned
- Inability to focus
- Loss of consciousness
- Slurred speech
- Vacant stare

Sleep
- Decreased sleep
- Difficulty initiating sleep
- Drowsiness*
- Increased sleep*

Somatic/physical symptoms
- Blurred vision
- Convulsions
- Dizziness/poor balance
- Fatigue
- Headache
- Lightheadedness
- Light sensitivity
- Nausea
- Noise sensitivity
- Numbness/tingling
- Tinnitus
- Vomiting

*Most commonly seen symptoms
From Scorza KA, Raleigh MF, O'Connor FG: Current concepts in concussion: evaluation and management, *Am Fam Physician* 85:123-132, 2012.

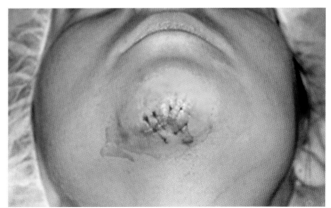

Fig. 11.1 Laceration of soft tissues requiring sutures.

(indicating an alveolar fracture). The degree of horizontal mobility is recorded: 0 for normal mobility; 1 for slight mobility (less than 1 mm), 2 for marked mobility (1 to 3 mm); and 3 for severe mobility (greater than 3 mm), both horizontally and vertically. If there is no mobility, the teeth are percussed for sounds of ankylosis (metallic sound). Absence of normal mobility may indicate ankylosis or "locking" of the tooth in bone, such as with intrusion and lateral luxation.

Displacement

A displaced tooth has been moved from its normal position. If this occurs as a result of a traumatic injury, it is referred to as *luxation* (discussed later in the chapter).

Periodontal Damage

Injury to the supporting structures of teeth may result in swelling and bleeding involving the periodontal ligament. The involved teeth are sensitive to percussion, even light tapping. Apical displacement with injury to vessels entering the apical foramen may lead to pulp necrosis if the blood supply is compromised.[23]

The use of *percussion* can help identify periodontal injury. This testing procedure must be done gently because traumatized teeth are often exquisitely painful to even light tapping. In a combined histologic, bacteriologic, and radiographic study, Andreasen showed that only tenderness to percussion at the time of diagnosis of pulp necrosis was related to an infected, necrotic pulp.[24] Therefore, special attention should be given to this test, especially when the tooth consistently and reliably shows an abnormal tenderness to percussion. Uninjured teeth should be examined first to enhance the patient's confidence and understanding of the procedures. In addition to testing the tooth or teeth involved in the patient's complaint, it is important to include several adjacent and opposing teeth. This permits recognition of other dental injuries of which the patient may not be aware and that may not be obvious clinically. If later complications develop involving one of these adjacent or opposing teeth, previous information aids diagnosis.

Pulpal Injury

The ideal pulpal response to injury is complete recovery after a traumatic injury. Two other potential outcomes may occur: calcific metamorphosis, in which the pulp tissue is gradually replaced with calcified tissue (recognized clinically as a yellowing effect on the crown) or pulp necrosis, which can result in external inflammatory (infection-related) root resorption.[25] Rarely, resorption may occur in the pulp space (internal resorption). In any case, a tooth may undergo resorption without any clinical symptoms, which emphasizes the need for follow-up controls.

The status of the pulp may be determined by the symptoms, history, and clinical tests (see Chapter 5). However, two clinical tests deserve consideration here because of their applicability to traumatized teeth: the electrical pulp test (EPT) and the cold test with dichlorodifluoromethane (DDM) (Endo-Ice; Hygenic Corp., Akron, Ohio). These test the neural tissue (specifically Aδ nerves) within the pulp chamber and are generally reliable for evaluating and monitoring pulpal status except in teeth with incomplete root development.[7,23] Nevertheless, evaluating the vascular supply to the pulp is the ultimate test to determine vitality of the tissue. Current evidence demonstrates that pulpal blood flow can be accurately assessed with laser Doppler flowmetry (LDF)[26-28] and with pulse oximetry (Fig. 11.2).[29-32] Gopikrishna and colleagues[31] compared the efficacy of a custom-made pulse oximeter dental probe with EPT and thermal testing for measuring the pulp vitality status of recently traumatized permanent teeth. The results demonstrated a positive responsiveness to thermal and electrical pulp tests that increased from no response on day 0 to 29.4% teeth on day 28, 82.35% of teeth at 2 months, and 94.11% teeth at 6 months. However, the pulse oximeter gave positive vitality readings that remained constant over the study period from day 0 to 6 months in all patients.

Radiographic Examination

Radiographs can reveal fractures of bone and teeth and the stage of root development. Horizontal root fractures and lateral luxations are often overlooked because the conventional angle may miss irregularities that are not parallel with the x-ray beam. Therefore, multiple exposures should be routine for examination of traumatized teeth to ensure complete disclosure and diagnosis of the injury.[7,23]

The film size should be such that it can accommodate two incisors without bending or distorting the image. It is also important to use a film holder whenever possible to achieve standardized radiographic images, especially for subsequent comparisons.

Recent improvements in three-dimensional (3D) digital radiographic imaging have introduced a new perspective, allowing us to evaluate the anatomic structures, both hard and soft tissue, in three spatial planes.[33] The traditional projection

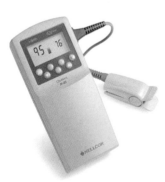
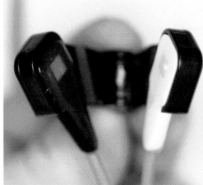
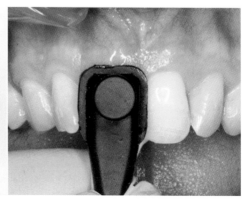

Fig. 11.2 Pulse oximetry unit with a commercially available sensor that fits dental tissues. (Courtesy of Covidien.)

(plain film) radiograph is a two-dimensional shadow of a three-dimensional object; 3D imaging overcomes this major limitation by providing a true representation of the anatomy while eliminating superimpositions. Several studies have reported the use of computed tomography (CT) and digital radiography for differential diagnosis,[34-36] assessment of treatment outcomes,[37,38] endodontics,[39] oral and maxillofacial surgery,[40-42] implantology,[43,44] and orthodontics, with reliable linear measurements for reconstruction and imaging of dental and maxillofacial structures.[45-47] The indications for cone beam computed tomography (CBCT) in dental traumatology were first described in 2007.[48,49] Cases that may appear straightforward on periapical radiographs (Fig. 11.3) may reveal a different and more complex situation when evaluated three-dimensionally (Fig. 11.4).

A thorough examination and accurate records form the basis for an appropriate treatment plan. The information gathered also provides content for accident reports that may be

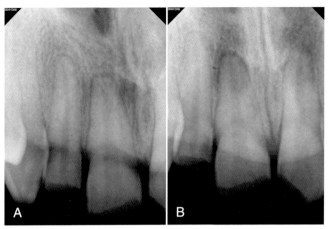

Fig. 11.3 Complicated crown fracture of the maxillary right central and lateral incisors and maxillary left central incisor. **A** and **B,** Periapical radiographs at different horizontal angles.

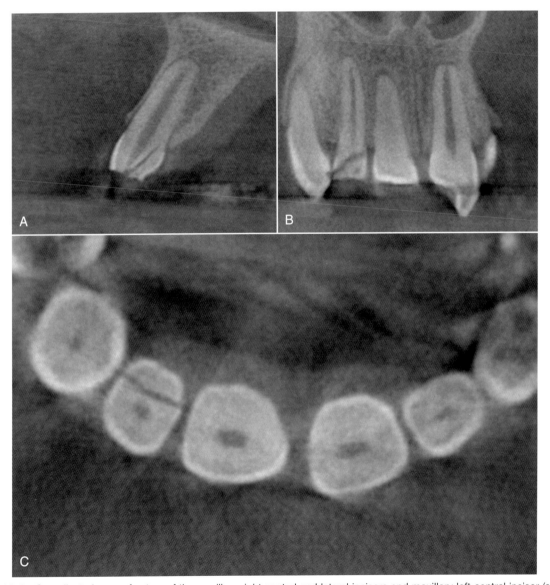

Fig. 11.4 Complicated crown fracture of the maxillary right central and lateral incisors and maxillary left central incisor (same case as in Fig. 11.5).

requested either immediately or later for legal or insurance purposes.

INJURIES TO THE HARD DENTAL TISSUES AND THE PULP

Enamel Fractures

Chips and cracks confined to enamel do not in themselves constitute a hazard to the pulp. The prognosis is good; however, the injury that produced the fracture may also have displaced (luxated) the tooth and damaged the blood vessels supplying the pulp. If the tooth is sensitive to percussion or if there are other signs of injury, the clinician should follow the recommended guidelines, according to the type of trauma (i.e., subluxation, luxation) (presented later in the chapter). Grinding and smoothing the rough edges or restoring lost tooth structure may be all that is necessary.

Uncomplicated Crown Fractures
Description

Uncomplicated crown fractures involve enamel and dentin without pulpal exposure. Such injuries are usually not associated with severe pain and generally do not require urgent care. The prognosis is good unless there is an accompanying luxation injury, in which case the tooth may be sensitive to percussion.[23] If it is, the outlined recommendations should be followed according to the diagnosis and type of trauma (presented later in the chapter) must be followed.

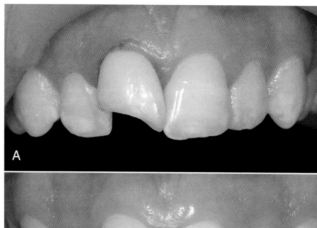
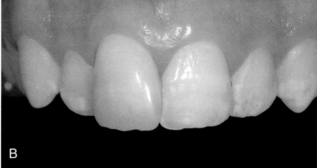

Fig. 11.5 Uncomplicated crown fracture of the maxillary right central incisor. Preoperative **(A)** and postoperative **(B)** views of restoration with composite resins. (Courtesy Dr. Gabriela Ibarra.)

Treatment

Since the advent of the acid-etch technique, conservative restoration of crown-fractured incisors with composite resin has become possible without endangering the pulp (Fig. 11.5). More conservative yet is reattachment of the separated enamel-dentin fragment. This requires application of a dentin bonding agent after the enamel has been acid-etched to improve the fracture strength of the restored incisor. Both clinical experiments and bonding studies have indicated that reattachment of dentin-enamel crown fragments is an acceptable restorative procedure and does not threaten pulp vitality.[50] In general, fracture bonding represents an advance in the treatment of anterior fractures. The dental anatomy is restored with a normal tooth structure that abrades at a rate identical to that of the adjacent non-injured teeth. Also, pulpal status may be reliably monitored.

Chair time for the restorative procedure is minimal. The use of indirect veneering techniques at a later date to reinforce bonding or to restore the fractured incisor is a conservative approach to improving esthetics and function.[51]

Complicated Crown Fractures
Description

Complicated crown fractures involve the enamel, dentin, and pulp. Because the pulp is exposed, the fracture is considered complicated. The extent of fracture, the stage of root development, and the length of time since injury are noted.

Considering the extent of fracture helps to determine pulpal treatment and restorative needs; a small fracture may undergo vital pulp therapy and can be restored by an acid-etched composite restoration. An extensive fracture may require root canal treatment with a post and core–supported crown, depending on the age of the patient (Fig. 11.6).

The stage of root maturation is an important factor in choosing between pulpotomy and pulpectomy. Immature teeth have thin-walled roots; every effort should be made to preserve the pulp to allow continued root development. The best technique for achieving this goal is a *shallow (partial) pulpotomy* (described later in the chapter). Vital pulp therapy followed by acid-etched composite restoration or reattachment of the fractured segment also is often feasible in mature teeth. However, if the extent of tooth loss dictates restoration with a crown, root canal treatment is recommended.[10]

The time lapse between injury and examination may directly affect pulpal health. In general, the sooner a tooth is treated, the better the prognosis for preserving the pulp. However, as a rule, pulps that have been exposed for less than a week can be treated by pulpotomy. Successful pulpotomy procedures after pulp exposure of several weeks' duration have been reported.[52-54]

Treatment of Crown Fractures

Teeth with crown fractures and exposed pulps can be treated by pulp capping, pulpotomy (vital pulp therapy), or root canal therapy before restoration of lost tooth structure. If vital pulp therapy is planned, it is important to perform treatment as soon after the injury as possible.

Vital Pulp Therapy

The main reason for recommending vital pulp therapy in a tooth with an exposed pulp is to preserve the vitality of the pulp. This is particularly important in immature teeth, in

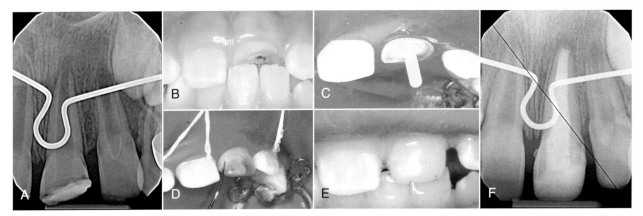

Fig. 11.6 Preoperative periapical radiograph **(A)** and clinical photograph **(B)** of a complicated crown fracture of the maxillary left central incisor. **C** and **D,** Upon completion of the endodontic therapy, a fiber post was placed, followed by the coronal restoration. The results are shown in a postoperative clinical photograph **(E)** and a final periapical radiograph **(F).**

which continued root development results in a stronger tooth that is more resistant to fractures than one with thin root walls.

In the past, pulpotomy meant removal of pulp tissue to or below the cervical level. Loss of pulp tissue in that area prevents dentin formation, which results in a weakened tooth that is more prone to fracture. In recent years, a more conservative and shallow pulpotomy has been popularized by Cvek and has sometimes been referred to as the *Cvek technique.*[52] This shallow, or partial, pulpotomy preserves all the radicular and most of the coronal pulp tissue, allowing more hard tissue to develop in the root.

The pulp may need to be removed to or below the cervical level when the entire crown of an immature tooth fractures. Pulpotomy then is performed to encourage enough additional root development to allow subsequent crown restoration or post and core construction to support a crown. These situations are relatively uncommon. In recent years, the technique has been modified to use mineral trioxide aggregate (MTA; e.g., ProRoot MTA [Tulsa Dental Products, Tulsa, Oklahoma]) instead of calcium hydroxide.[55,56]

Case Selection
Both immature and mature teeth that can subsequently be restored with acid-etched composite can be treated with a shallow (partial) pulpotomy. In general, immature teeth are more likely to be involved for the reasons stated previously.

Technique
The shallow (partial) pulpotomy procedure (Fig. 11.7) starts with induction of anesthesia and rubber dam isolation. The exposed dentin is washed with saline or sodium hypochlorite solution. Extruding granulation tissue is removed with a spoon excavator from the pulp wound site; this provides an opportunity to determine more accurately the size and location of the exposure. Next, pulp tissue is removed to a depth of about 2 mm below the exposure. This relatively small amount of pulp removal is the reason the procedure is called a *shallow* or *partial pulpotomy.*

The procedure is accomplished using a water-cooled small round diamond (about the size of a No. 2 or No. 4 round bur) in the high-speed handpiece. Gently and gradually, the surface layers of pulp tissue are wiped away, beginning at the exposure site and extending into the pulp to a depth of about 2 mm below the exposure site.

After the pulp has been amputated to the desired level, a dentin shelf is created surrounding the pulp wound. The wound is gently washed with sterile saline, and hemostasis can usually be expected within 5 minutes. Then the wound is washed again to remove the clot and is dressed with calcium hydroxide. The remainder of the cavity is carefully sealed with hard-setting cement, such as glass ionomer. When the cement has set, the tooth may be restored with acid-etched composite.

Because calcium hydroxide liners disintegrate with time, whenever possible the tooth should be reentered after 6 to 12 months to remove the initial calcium hydroxide layer and replace it with a dentin bonding material. This prevents microleakage at the site where the initial calcium hydroxide has deteriorated and produced a space between the new dentin bridge and the covering restoration.

If MTA is used in place of calcium hydroxide, it is not necessary to wait for bleeding to stop completely. The material requires moisture for curing and can be placed directly onto the pulp tissue. Care must be taken to reduce the risk of forcing the material into the pulp proper; the clinician should gently dab small increments of the material onto the pulp using a moist cotton pellet. The pulpotomy space is filled with MTA white powder so that it is completely flush with the fractured dentin surface. The material is then allowed to cure, which may take 4 to 6 hours. During the curing time, it is not necessary to protect the material with a restoration, but the patient must avoid using the tooth. After curing, the tooth may be restored either with a composite resin or by bonding the fractured crown segment back onto the tooth.[55] It is not necessary to subsequently reenter the tooth, because MTA is stable and does not break down in the manner of calcium hydroxide.

Treatment Evaluation
Treatment is evaluated after 6 months and then yearly. Successful shallow pulpotomy procedures may be considered definitive treatment and have a very good long-term success rate (Fig. 11.8).[54,57]

Root Canal Therapy
Teeth with mature roots may undergo either pulpotomy or root canal therapy; root canal therapy is usually necessary to accommodate prosthetic requirements. For example, if the

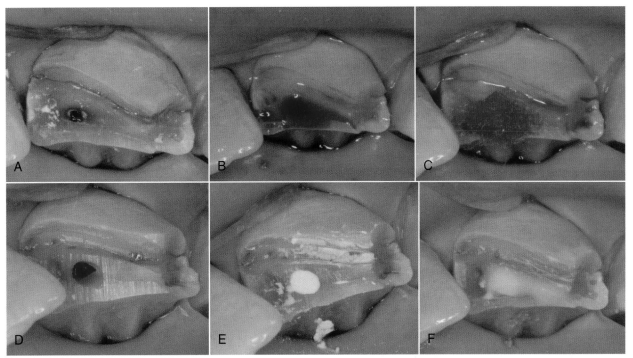

Fig. 11.7 Complicated crown fracture of the maxillary right central incisor. The partial pulpotomy procedure is clinically illustrated in the following steps: **A,** Pulp is exposed; **B,** pulpal tissue is excised 2 mm below the exposure; **C,** bleeding is controlled by pressure only (cotton pellet moistened with saline); **D,** hemostasis is obtained; **E,** white mineral trioxide aggregate (MTA) seal is applied; **F,** protection of the MTA is achieved using a layer of glass ionomer lining.

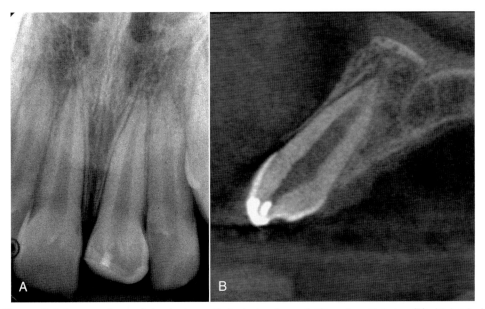

Fig. 11.8 Six-month follow-up after partial pulpotomy. Periapical radiograph **(A)** and sagittal view **(B)** obtained with cone beam computed tomography (CBCT).

crown has fractured in the gingival margin region, root canal treatment allows post and core and crown placement.

Crown-Root Fractures
Description
Crown-root fractures are usually oblique and involve both the crown and the root. Anterior teeth show the so-called chisel-type fracture, which splits the crown diagonally and extends subgingivally to a root surface. This type of fracture resembles a crown fracture but is more extensive and more serious because it includes the root. Another variation is the fracture that shatters the crown (Fig. 11.9). The pieces are held in place only by the part of a fractured segment still attached to the periodontal ligament. In all of these fractures, the pulp is usually exposed.

In contrast to other traumatic injuries, in which posterior teeth are rarely involved, crown-root fractures often include **179**

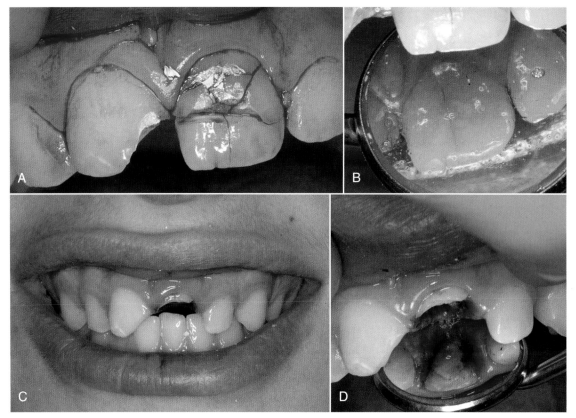

Fig. 11.9 **A** and **B,** Buccal and lingual photographs of a crown and root fracture immediately upon presentation. **C** and **D,** Images after removal of the fractured segments.

the molars and premolars. Cusp fractures that extend subgingivally are common. Diagnostically, however, they may be difficult to identify in the early stages of development. Similarly, vertical fractures along the long axis of roots are difficult to detect and diagnose.

Crown-root fractures in posterior teeth cannot always be associated with a single traumatic incident, although bicycle or automobile accidents at times may produce these results. The risk is increased with a sharp blow to the chin, causing the jaws to slam together; skin abrasions under the chin may be a sign of such an impact. Also, all posterior teeth should be examined with a sharp explorer to detect movement of loose fragments.

Examination

Crown-root fractures are complex injuries that are difficult both to evaluate and to treat. Until recently, it was recommended that all loose fragments be removed to evaluate the extent of injury. This may still be necessary in some instances; however, with the availability of newer bonding agents, it is now possible to bond loose fragments at least temporarily. The current recommendation is to attempt to bond loose fragments together, particularly if the tooth is immature and still developing.[10] Clinical judgment must be used to decide which course of action to follow.

In a tooth with a crown that has been broken into several pieces, it is not unusual to find that this shattering effect also has extended to the root. Additional radiographs at different angles and CBCT imaging may help to identify radicular fracture lines (Fig. 11.10).[7,48]

Emergency Care

Teeth with crown-root fractures are often painful; such injuries frequently require urgent care. This may consist of bonding loose tooth fragments but often includes pulp therapy (Fig. 11.11). If the root is immature, pulpotomy is preferable to pulpectomy, whereas pulpectomy is the treatment of choice in patients with fully developed teeth (Fig. 11.12). Definitive treatment should be postponed until an overall endodontic and restorative treatment plan has been developed.[10]

Treatment Planning

Crown-root fractures are often complicated by pulp exposures and extensive loss of tooth structure. In the development of a treatment plan, many questions must be considered:

- Which is better for this tooth, pulpotomy or pulpectomy?
- After all loose fragments have been removed, will there be enough tooth structure to support a restoration? Or, if the loose fragments are bonded in an immature tooth, will it last until the alveolus has developed enough for placement of an implant?
- Is the subgingival fracture below a level at which a restorative margin can be placed, thus necessitating root extrusion or gingivoplasty or alveoplasty?
- Should the tooth be extracted and replaced with a bridge or implant? Or, if extraction is chosen, can the space be closed orthodontically?

These are but a few of the many questions that must be answered, not only for crown-root fractures, but also in other complicated trauma situations. Because of the complexity of

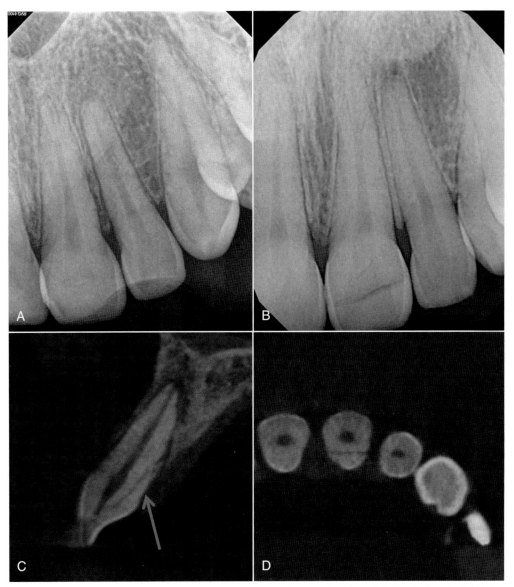

Fig. 11.10   **A** and **B,** Periapical radiographs demonstrating a crown fracture line. **C** and **D,** Sagittal and axial slides confirming the presence and extension of the fractures lines *(arrow).*

these cases, a team approach involving specialists in pediatric dentistry, endodontics, periodontics, orthodontics, oral and maxillofacial surgery, and prosthodontics is beneficial in the development of a treatment plan.

Root Fractures
Description
Fractures of roots have been called *intraalveolar root fractures, horizontal root fractures,* and *transverse root fractures.* They do not occur often and may be difficult to detect.[1,7,13,58] Radiographically, a root fracture is visualized if the x-ray beam passes through the fracture line. Because these fractures often are transverse-to-oblique (involving pulp, dentin, and cementum), they may be missed if the central beam's direction is not parallel or close to parallel to the fracture line. For this reason, a steep vertical angle view is obtained, in addition to the normal parallel angle, whenever a root fracture is suspected. This additional angle (i.e., foreshortened, or occlusal, view [approximately 45 degrees]) detects many fractures,

particularly in the apical regions of the roots (Fig. 11.13).[58,59] Recently, May and colleagues demonstrated that CBCT is most useful in cases in which conventional radiography yields inconclusive results or shows a fracture in the middle third of a root.[60] In such cases CBCT may rule out or confirm an oblique course of fracture involving the cervical third in the labiolingual dimension (Fig. 11.14).

Clinically, root fractures may present as mobile or displaced teeth with pain on biting. Symptoms are typically mild. If mobility and displacement of the coronal segment are absent or slight, the patient may have no chief complaint and may not seek treatment.[61] In general, the more cervical the fracture, the more mobility and displacement of the coronal segment and the greater the likelihood of pulp necrosis of this segment if it is not promptly repositioned. Splinting is indicated in cervical and middle third root fractures.[10,62,63] Root fractures in the apical third usually require no immediate treatment but must be observed long term.[62]

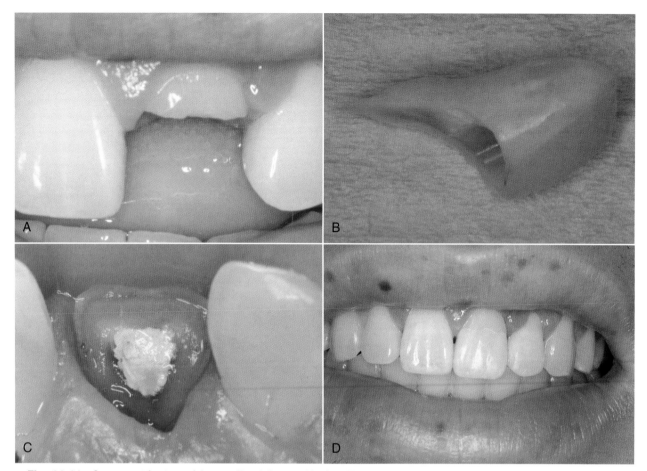

Fig. 11.11 Crown-root fracture of the maxillary left central incisor. Emergency procedure for stabilization of the coronal fragment using acid etch/resin applied to the remaining tooth structure.

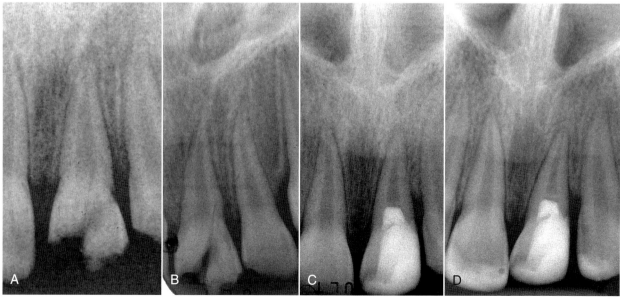

Fig. 11.12 Crown-root fracture of the maxillary left central incisor treated with cervical pulpotomy. **A** and **B,** Periapical radiographs at different horizontal angles. **C,** Two-month follow-up. **D,** Six-month follow-up.

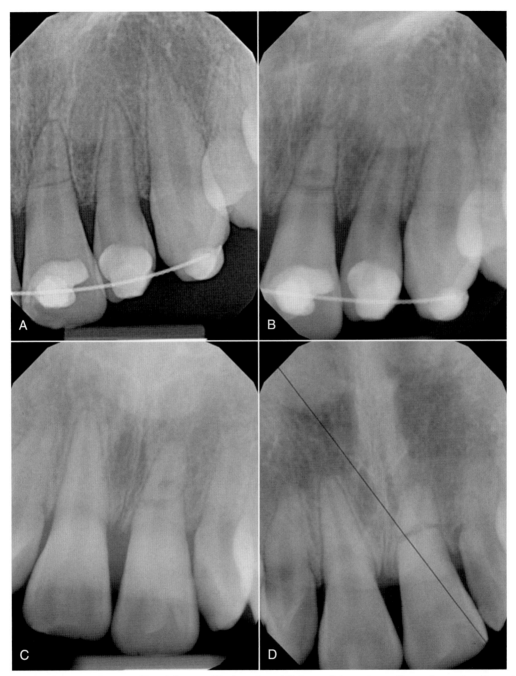

Fig. 11.13 Root fracture of the maxillary left central incisor. **A** and **B,** Immediate postoperative radiographs after reduction and splinting. **C,** Six-month follow-up. **D,** Follow-up at 18 months.

Emergency Care

Initial treatment for root fractures—repositioning and stabilization—should be of acute priority for best results (Fig. 11.15). Repositioning of displaced coronal tooth segments is easier if performed soon after the injury; delayed repositioning may require orthodontic intervention to allow movement of the coronal segment into a desirable position.

After repositioning, the coronal tooth segment must be splinted to allow repair of the periodontal tissues (see Fig. 11.15). Four to 6 weeks of stabilization are usually sufficient, unless the fracture location is close to the crest of the alveolar bone, in which case longer splinting periods may be advisable.[62] The outcome of the emergency care must be monitored periodically.

Sequelae of Root Fractures

Root fractures are often characterized by the development of calcific metamorphosis (radiographic obliteration) in one segment (usually the coronal) or both segments; therefore, EPT readings may be very high or absent. However, in the absence of other evidence of pulp necrosis (bony lesions laterally at the level of the fracture or symptoms of irreversible pulpitis or necrosis), lack of response to EPT by itself does not indicate a need for root canal treatment. The majority of **183**

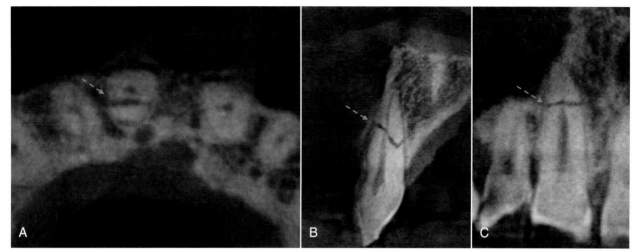

Fig. 11.14 Root fracture of the maxillary left central incisor. Cone beam computed tomography demonstrates the fracture in all three planes: axial **(A)**, sagittal **(B)**, and coronal **(C)**.

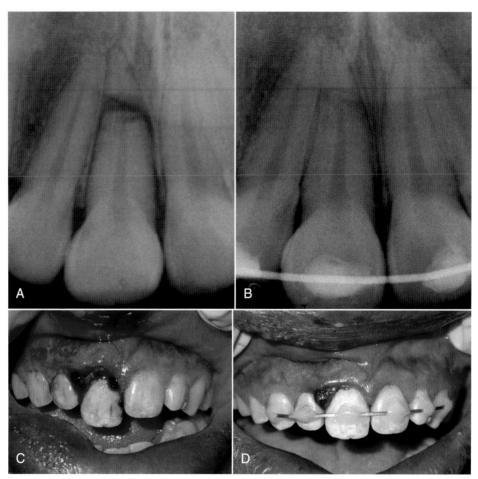

Fig. 11.15 Root fracture of the maxillary right central incisor. **A** and **B**, Periapical radiograph and clinical photograph of the tooth when the patient arrived at the emergency department. **C** and **D**, Reduction, repositioning, and splinting.

root fractures heal either spontaneously or after splint therapy[64-66] (see Fig. 11.13).

Root Canal Treatment

Root canal treatment is indicated when pathosis is evident, usually owing to the development of pulp necrosis in the coronal portion that subsequently leads to inflammatory lesions adjacent to the fracture lines (Fig. 11.16).[66] The endodontic procedure, when necessary, usually is complex, and referral to a specialist should be considered. In contrast to root canal treatment in most other endodontic situations, when it is indicated for teeth with horizontal root fractures, the

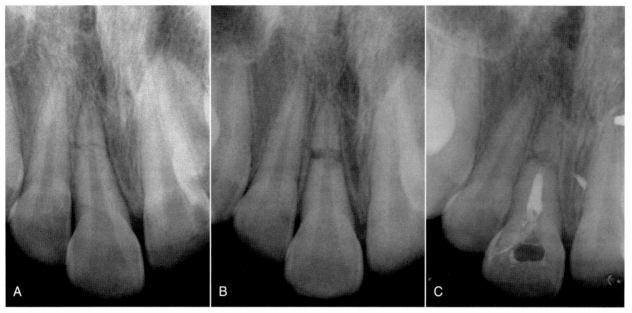

Fig. 11.16 Root fracture of the maxillary right central incisor. **A,** Preoperative periapical radiograph. **B,** One month later, after removal of the splint. Note the separation of the coronal and apical fragments. Endodontic therapy of the coronal fragment was initiated. **C,** Two-year follow-up.

Table 11.2 Differential diagnosis for the most common injuries to the periodontium

	Sensitivity to percussion	Mobility	Displacement
Concussion	Yes	No	No
Subluxation	Yes	Yes	No
Luxation	Yes	Yes	Yes

treatment is usually limited to the root canal in the coronal segment to the fracture line. The pulp in the apical segment usually remains vital.[66-69]

INJURIES TO THE PERIODONTIUM

Injuries to the periodontium involve trauma to the supporting structures of teeth and often affect the neural and vascular supply to the pulp. The cause is usually a sudden impact, such as a blow or striking a hard object in a fall.[70] In general, the more severe the degree of displacement, the greater the damage to the periodontium and to the dental pulp. Table 11.2 provides a summary of the typical clinical and radiographic findings associated with different types of injuries to the periodontium.

Concussion

With concussion, the tooth is sensitive to percussion only. There is no increase in mobility, and the tooth has not been displaced. The pulp may respond normally to testing, and no radiographic changes are found.[10]

Subluxation

Teeth with subluxation injuries are sensitive to percussion and also have increased mobility. Although sulcular bleeding might be present, this clinical finding does not provide a diagnosis. The teeth are not displaced, and the pulp may respond normally to testing, sometimes after initially failing to respond. Radiographic findings are unremarkable.[10]

Luxation

Luxation is an injury to the supporting structures with loosening of the tooth and clinical or radiographic displacement. The injury may displace the tooth in three possible directions: extrusive, lateral, or intrusive.

Extrusive Luxation

With extrusive luxation, teeth are partially displaced from the socket along the long axis. Extruded teeth have greatly increased mobility, and radiographs show displacement. The pulp usually does not respond to testing.[10,17,18]

Lateral Luxation

By definition, with lateral luxation the teeth may be displaced lingually, buccally, mesially, or distally (i.e., away from their normal position in a horizontal direction). However, because the impact always comes from the facial aspect, the crown is displaced lingually and the apex buccally, creating a subsequent alveolar fracture. If the apex has been displaced into the surrounding alveolar bone, the tooth may be quite firm. A metallic sound on percussion might indicate that the root tip has been forced into the alveolar bone.

Intrusive Luxation

With intrusive luxation the teeth are forced into their sockets in an axial (apical) direction, at times to the point of not being clinically visible. They have no mobility, resembling ankylosis.[71]

Examination and Diagnosis

The clinical descriptions of the five types of luxation injuries should be sufficient to make the initial diagnosis. Pulpal status must be continually monitored until a definitive diagnosis can be made, which in some cases may require several months or years. DDM and EPT are used in monitoring pulpal status.[72]

Concussion injuries generally respond to pulp testing. Because the injury is less severe, the pulpal blood supply is more likely to return to normal.

Teeth in the *subluxation* injury group also tend to retain or recover pulpal responsiveness but less predictably than teeth with concussion injuries. In both cases, an immature tooth with an open apex usually has a good prognosis.

Extrusive, lateral, and *intrusive luxation* injuries involve displacement of the teeth and therefore more damage to apical vessels and nerves. Pulp responses in teeth with extrusive, lateral, or intrusive luxations are often absent. These pulps often do not recover responsiveness even if the pulp is vital (has blood supply) because sensory nerves may be permanently damaged. Exceptions are immature teeth with wide-open apices; these teeth often regain or retain pulp vitality (responsiveness to sensitivity tests) even after severe injuries.[23,72]

Monitoring of pulpal status requires a schedule of pulp testing and radiographic evaluations for a long enough period to permit determination of the outcome with a degree of certainty (this may take 2 years or longer). Pulpal status is best monitored with pulp testing, radiographic findings, and observation for developing symptoms and for crown color changes.[23,25,72]

Pulp Testing

Sensitivity tests, including cold (DDM) and EPT, are used to evaluate the sensory response of teeth that have been injured; several adjacent and opposing teeth are included in the test. An initial lack of response is not unusual, nor is a high reading on the pulp tester. Retesting is done in 4 to 6 weeks, and the results are recorded and compared with the initial responses. If the pulp responds in both instances, the prognosis for pulp survival is good. A pulp response that is absent initially and present at the second visit indicates a probable recovery of vitality, although cases of subsequent reversals have been noted.[31,73-75] If the pulp fails to respond both times, the prognosis is questionable and the pulp status uncertain. In the absence of other findings indicating pulp necrosis, the tooth is retested in 3 to 4 months. Continued lack of response may indicate pulp necrosis by infarct, but lack of response may not be enough evidence to make a diagnosis of pulp necrosis. That is, the pulp may permanently lose sensory nerve supply but retain its blood supply. After some time, the pulp often responds to testing if it recovers.[72]

Radiographic Evaluation

The initial radiograph made after the injury will not disclose the pulpal condition. However, it is important for evaluation of the general injury to the tooth and alveolus and serves as a basis for comparison for subsequent radiographs. As demonstrated by Cohenca and colleagues,[48] the use of CBCT is vital in luxation injuries, particularly lateral luxations in which a concomitant alveolar fracture is common. The 3D imaging allows for better diagnosis of alveolar fractures and confirms the correct position of the tooth within the socket. In the case presented in Figs. 11.17 and 11.18, the patient was diagnosed with a lateral luxation. Although three different periapical radiographs failed to reveal the position of the tooth in relation to its alveolus (Fig. 11.17), the CBCT scan clearly demonstrated a cortical bone fracture and displacement of the apex toward the buccal aspect (Fig. 11.18).

Radiographs are also indicated for early diagnosis and treatment of external resorptions and periradicular bony changes. Resorptive changes, particularly external changes, may occur soon after injury; if no attempt is made to arrest the destructive process, much of the root may be rapidly lost. Inflammatory (infection-related) resorption can be intercepted by timely endodontic intervention.[23,72]

Periodic radiographs show whether the root of a developing tooth is continuing to grow (a positive sign indicating recovery of the pulp). Another finding may be pulp space

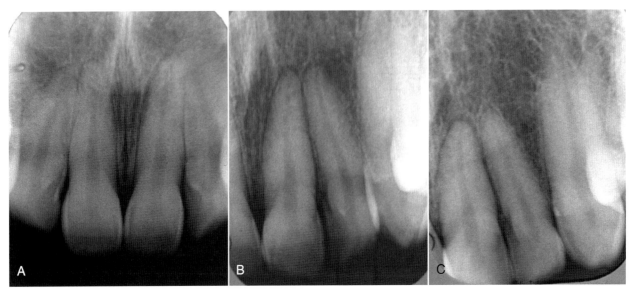

Fig. 11.17 **A** to **C,** Periapical radiographs failed to reveal the position of the tooth in relation to its alveolus.

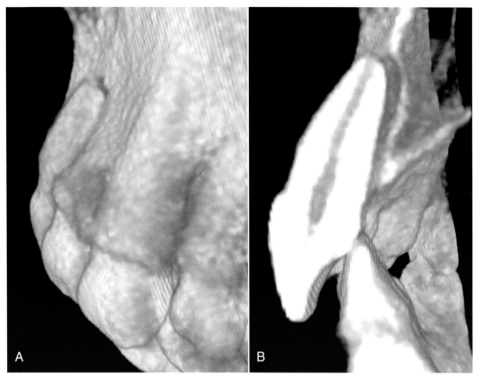

Fig. 11.18 Cone beam computed tomography. Transaxial volumetric reconstruction **(A)** and sagittal plane view **(B)** demonstrating lateral luxation of the maxillary left central incisor with a concomitant alveolar fracture.

calcification or obliteration, a common finding after luxation injuries in immature teeth.[76] Also called *calcific metamorphosis,* this canal obliteration may be partial or nearly complete (after several years) and does not indicate a need for root canal treatment except when other signs and symptoms suggest pulp necrosis.[76]

Crown Color Changes

Pulpal injury may cause discoloration, even after only a few days. Initial changes tend to be pink. Subsequently, if the pulp does not recover and becomes necrotic, there may be a grayish darkening of the crown, often accompanied by a loss in translucency (Fig. 11.19). In addition, color changes may take place as a result of calcific metamorphosis of the pulp. Such color changes are likely to be yellow to brown and do not indicate pulp pathosis. Other signs, findings, or symptoms are necessary to diagnose pulp necrosis.[72,76]

Discoloration may be reversed. This usually happens relatively soon after the injury and indicates that the pulp is vital. Because of unpredictable changes associated with traumatized teeth, long-term evaluation is recommended.[72]

Treatment of Luxation Injuries

Luxation injuries, regardless of type, often present diagnostic and treatment complexities that require consultation with specialists. For *concussion* injuries, no immediate treatment is necessary. A soft diet is recommended for 2 weeks, and if possible the patient should avoid biting until sensitivity has subsided. Pulpal status is monitored as described. *Subluxation* may likewise require no treatment unless mobility is moderate; if grade 2 mobility is present, stabilization may be necessary for a short period (1 to 2 weeks).[77,78]

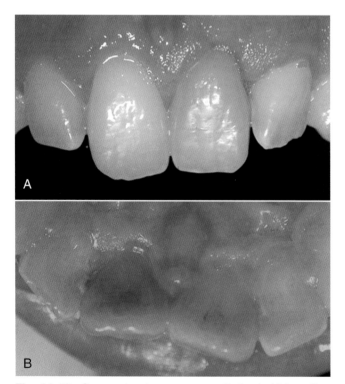

Fig. 11.19 Crown color changes as a result of pulpal injury after a luxation injury: buccal view **(A)** and lingual view **(B).**

Extrusive and *lateral luxation* injuries require repositioning and splinting. The duration of splinting varies with the severity of injury. Extrusions may need only 2 weeks, whereas lateral luxations that involve bony fractures need 4 weeks.[10] Professional judgment dictates variations from these recommendations. Root canal treatment is indicated for teeth with a diagnosis of irreversible pulpitis or pulp necrosis. Such a diagnosis often requires a combination of signs and symptoms, such as discoloration of the crown, lack of pulp response to pulp testing, and a periradicular lesion seen radiographically.[10] However, severe cases of either extrusive or lateral luxation of mature teeth might require endodontic therapy within the first 2 weeks (Fig. 11.20).

Treatment of *intrusive luxation* injuries depends on root maturity.[79,80] If the tooth is incompletely formed with an open apex, it may reposition spontaneously. A clinical study revealed that in young patients 12 to 17 years old who have complete root formation, spontaneous re-eruption is possible and was found to be the best treatment with regard to marginal periodontal healing.[80] In older patients (i.e., older than 17 years) with complete root formation, either surgical or orthodontic extrusion should be attempted. Root canal treatment is indicated for intruded teeth with the exception of those with immature roots, in which case the pulp may revascularize.[81] The patient must be monitored carefully because complications, such as failure of pulpal healing, usually are symptomless. If radiographic evidence indicates pulp necrosis (lack of continued root development), root canal treatment should be performed.[10]

Root canal therapy is indicated for luxated teeth in which the pulps become necrotic. Often in luxated teeth there has been damage to the root cementum; if the pulps become infected, external resorption is stimulated by the presence of bacteria in the pulp space. To arrest any ongoing resorption and to prevent additional resorption, it is important to make every effort to disinfect the root canal system during root canal treatment. It has been recommended that calcium hydroxide be placed in the canal for up to 2 weeks to aid disinfection before the root canals are filled.[82]

Avulsion
Description
An avulsed tooth is one that has been totally displaced from its alveolar socket. If the tooth is replanted soon after avulsion (immediate replantation), the periodontal ligament has a good chance of healing. Time out of socket and the storage medium used are the critical factors in successful replantation. It is important to preserve the periodontal ligament cells and the fibers attached to the root surface by keeping the tooth moist and minimizing handling of the root.[11,83-86]

Treatment
Three situations involving avulsions may arise: (1) an individual may telephone for advice about an avulsed tooth, presenting an opportunity for immediate replantation (within minutes); (2) a patient may be brought to the office with a tooth that has been kept in a physiologic storage medium or osmolality-balanced medium and/or stored dry (the extraoral dry time has been less than 60 minutes); or (3) the tooth has been out for *longer* than 1 hour and has not been kept in a storage medium.

Immediate Replantation
The prognosis is improved by replantation immediately after avulsion.[83-86] Many individuals (e.g., parents, athletic instructors, and others) are aware of this emergency procedure and can replant on-site. Some may ask for advice by phone.

When a patient who has had a tooth replanted at the accident site comes to the dental office, the replantation should be examined both clinically and radiographically. The dentist looks for additional injuries to adjacent or opposing teeth, and evaluates the replanted tooth for stability and alignment. The procedure outlined in the next section is followed, with the exception of the replantation step.

Replantation Within 1 Hour of Avulsion—Tooth with a Closed Apex
If replantation is not feasible at the place of injury, the injured person should be brought to the dental office and the tooth transported in such a way as to keep it moist.[11,87,88] The most common storage medium is Hanks Balanced Salt Solution (HBSS),[89] which is commercially available as a kit (Save-a-Tooth; Phoenix-Lazerus, Pottstown, Pennsylvania). However, if this is not available, milk is an excellent alternative.[89-92] Saliva is acceptable, whereas water is not good for maintaining root-surface cell vitality.[83-86]

When the patient arrives, the following steps are recommended:
1. Place the tooth in a cup of physiologic saline while preparing for replantation.
2. Take radiographs of the area of injury to look for evidence of alveolar fracture. Consider the use of CBCT, if indicated.
3. Examine the avulsion site carefully for any loose bone fragments that may be removed. If the alveolus is collapsed, spread it open gently with an instrument.

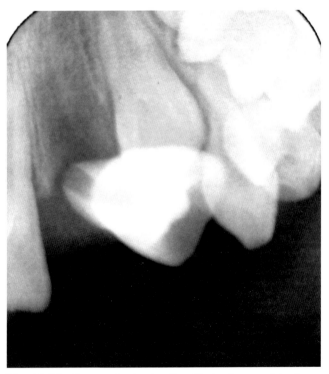

Fig. 11.20 Severe extrusive luxation. The tooth was retained only by soft tissue.

4. Irrigate the socket gently with saline to remove contaminated coagulum.
5. Grasp the crown of the tooth with extraction forceps to avoid handling the root.
6. Examine the tooth for debris and, if present, gently remove it with saline from a syringe.
7. Using the forceps, partially insert the tooth into the socket; gentle finger pressure can be used for complete seating of the tooth, or the patient can bite on a piece of gauze to accomplish the seating.
8. Check for proper alignment and correct any hyperocclusion. Soft tissue lacerations should be tightly sutured, particularly cervically.
9. Stabilize the tooth for 2 weeks with a flexible splint; nylon, stainless steel, or nickel-titanium wires up to 0.016 inch (0.4 mm) in diameter are significantly more flexible.[93]

Replantation Within 1 Hour of Avulsion—Tooth with an Open Apex

When the patient arrives, the following steps are recommended:

1. Place the tooth in a cup of physiologic saline while preparing for replantation.
2. Administer a local anesthetic.
3. Examine the alveolar socket, looking for fracture of the socket wall.
4. If available, cover the root surface topically with a tetracycline-based antibiotic before replanting the tooth.[11,94-98]
5. Replant the tooth with slight digital pressure.
6. Suture gingival lacerations, especially in the cervical area.
7. Verify normal position of the replanted tooth.
8. Apply a flexible splint (wires up to 0.016 inch [0.4 mm]) for 2 weeks.

For children younger than 9 years, Amoxicillin to 50 mg/kg in divided doses every 8 hours for 7 days can be prescribed. A tetanus booster injection is recommended if the previous one was administered more than 5 years earlier.

Root canal treatment is indicated for mature teeth and should be done optimally after 1 week and before the splint is removed (the splint stabilizes the tooth during the procedure). Timing is crucial in preventing the onset and progression of external inflammatory root resorption. The exceptions to routine root canal therapy are immature teeth with wide-open apices; they may revascularize but must be evaluated at regular intervals of 2, 6, and 12 months after replantation. If subsequent evaluations indicate pulp necrosis, root canal treatment, probably including apexification, is indicated.[11,94]

Replantation with Dry Time Longer Than 60 Minutes—Tooth with a Closed Apex

If a tooth has been out of the alveolar socket for longer than 1 hour (and has not been kept moist in a suitable medium), periodontal ligament cells and fibers will not survive, regardless of the stage of root development. Replacement root resorption (characterized by ankylosis) is likely to be the eventual sequela of replantation. Therefore, treatment efforts before replantation include treating the root surface with fluoride to slow the resorptive process.[84]

When the patient arrives, the following steps are recommended:

1. Examine the area of tooth avulsion and examine the radiographs for evidence of alveolar fractures.
2. Remove debris and pieces of soft tissue adhering to the root surface using a dry piece of gauze.
3. In cases of delayed replantation, root canal treatment should be carried out on the tooth either prior to replantation or 7 to 10 days later, as in other replantation situations.
4. Suction the alveolar socket carefully to remove the blood clot and irrigate the socket with saline.
5. Replant the tooth gently into the socket, checking for proper alignment and occlusal contact.
6. Apply a flexible splint (wires up to 0.016 inch [0.4 mm]) for 4 weeks.

Soaking the tooth in a 2.4% solution of sodium fluoride (acidulated to a pH of 5.5) for 20 minutes has been suggested to slow down osseous replacement,[99] but this should not be seen as an absolute recommendation.

Patient Instructions

Antibiotics are recommended for patients with replanted avulsed teeth.[100] In patients 12 years of age or older, doxycycline 100 mg two times per day for 7 days is the current recommendation. Alternatively, amoxicillin 500 mg three times per day for 7 days can be prescribed. For children under the age of 12, penicillin V 25 to 50 mg/kg of body weight in divided doses every 6 hours for 7 days can be prescribed.[11] A tetanus booster injection is recommended if the previous one had been administered more than 5 years earlier.[19] Supportive care is important. Instruct the patient (and parents) to use a soft diet for up to 2 weeks, to brush with a soft toothbrush after every meal, and to use a chlorhexidine mouth rinse (0.12%) twice a day for a week.

Sequelae of Dental Trauma
Pulp Necrosis

When the pulp is diagnosed as necrotic, the main factor to be considered is the stage of root development. If the root is fully matured, root canal therapy is the treatment of choice. In immature teeth with open apexes, treatment options include apexification and pulp revascularization.

Classic apexification refers to long-term use of calcium hydroxide, for up to 18 months. However, such a long treatment process may result in crown-root fracture at the cervical area (thin, weak dentinal walls), and lack of a an immediate permanent and esthetic restoration.

Several procedures and materials have been used to induce root-end barrier formation. In 2001, Witherspoon and Ham reported promising results when using MTA in single-visit apexification treatment of immature teeth with necrotic pulps.[101] Moreover, the use of an intracanal medication is not necessary when MTA is used as an apical plug.

Pulp revascularization procedures for the treatment of immature teeth with necrotic pulps and apical periodontitis have gained much attention as a result of encouraging results seen from numerous in vitro and in vivo studies.[102,103] The advantage of revascularization procedures over apexification procedures is that the former allow continued maturation of the root.[104,105]

Pulp Canal Obliteration (Calcific Metamorphosis)

The complete or partial calcification of the root canal space is a common finding after luxation injuries in immature teeth with a well vascularized pulp.[76] This canal obliteration may be partial or nearly complete (after several years) and does not indicate a need for root canal treatment except when other signs and symptoms suggests pulp necrosis.[76]

Root Resorption

External root resorption is a frequent occurrence in replanted avulsed teeth. Three types have been identified: surface, inflammatory, and replacement.[106,107]

Surface Resorption

Also called "repair-related resorption," surface resorption is transient and shows as lacunae of resorption in the cementum of replanted teeth. They are not usually visible on radiographs. If resorption does not continue, the lacunae are repaired by deposition of new cementum.

Inflammatory (Infection-Related) Resorption

Inflammatory resorption occurs as a response to the presence of infected necrotic pulp tissue in conjunction with injury to the periodontal ligament. It occurs with replanted teeth (Fig. 11.21) in addition to other types of luxation injuries. It is characterized by loss of tooth structure and adjacent alveolar bone. Resorption usually subsides after removal of the necrotic, infected pulp, so the prognosis is good. Root canal treatment is therefore recommended routinely for replanted teeth with closed apices to prevent the occurrence of inflammatory resorption.

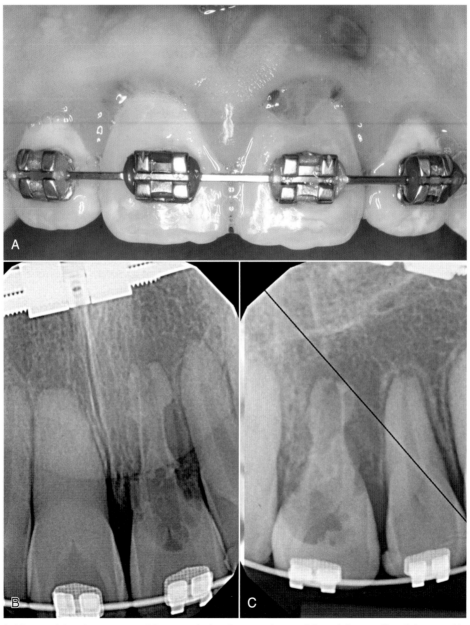

Fig. 11.21 A 14-year-old patient presented for consultation 5 years after avulsion of the maxillary left central incisor. A clinical photograph **(A)** and radiographic examination **(B** and **C)** revealed the presence of external inflammatory root resorption.

External Replacement (PDL-Related) Resorption

In replacement resorption, the tooth structure is resorbed and replaced by bone (Fig. 11.22), resulting in ankylosis in which bone fuses directly to the root surface. The characteristics of ankylosis are lack of physiologic mobility, failure of the tooth to erupt along with adjacent teeth (leading to infraocclusion in young individuals), and a "solid" metallic sound on percussion. Currently no treatment is available for replacement resorption, which tends to be continuous until the root is replaced by bone. In teeth that have had long extraalveolar dry periods, the resorptive process is apparently slowed (but not halted) by immersing the tooth in fluoride before replantation.[88,106]

Root Canal Treatment

Mature avulsed teeth, when replanted, cannot be expected to reestablish pulpal blood supply.[85] Revascularization may occur in immature teeth with wide open apices, but it is unpredictable and must be monitored carefully. These teeth must be monitored radiographically over time to watch for evidence of pulp necrosis.

In the mature replanted tooth, root canal treatment is definitely indicated and ideally should be started 7 to 10 days after replantation. The splint may remain during treatment for stability. The use of calcium hydroxide as an antimicrobial intracanal inter-appointment medicament may be helpful.[82,106] It is particularly beneficial if the root canal is infected, a condition that would be likely to occur when root canal treatment is delayed more than a few weeks after replantation. Long-term use calcium hydroxide is not recommended due to the effect on dental structures.[108] Rosenberg and colleagues demonstrated that root canal filling with calcium hydroxide weakened dentin by 23% to 43.9% compared to filling with gutta-percha, resulting in a significant decrease in fracture strength with increasing dressing time.[109]

The procedure consists of cleaning and shaping, followed by calcium hydroxide placement for a minimum of 1 to 2 weeks.[82] Obturation is then accomplished with gutta-percha and sealer. Long-term evaluation is necessary to monitor for possible resorption.

Restoration of the coronal access opening, both temporary and permanent, is a key to success. It is important to prevent bacterial leakage into the root canal system. For long-term stability, a dentin bonding agent with acid-etch composite is indicated.

Alveolar Fractures

Pulp necrosis is often associated with alveolar fractures, which may in turn be associated with other major facial injuries.[21,22] The initial need is to diagnose the presence of the fracture (Fig. 11.23) and then proceed with management, which consists of reduction and splinting of the segment to the adjacent teeth. If available, the use of CBCT is highly recommended. Oral and maxillofacial surgeons usually perform this procedure. When the patient is able to have the teeth examined, those in the line of fracture and adjacent teeth are evaluated. Lack of response to pulp testing, if not reversed within 3 to 6 months, may indicate pulp necrosis, but the presence of other indicators (apical radiolucency or symptoms) is necessary before root canal treatment is recommended.[110]

MANAGEMENT OF TRAUMATIC INJURIES IN THE PRIMARY DENTITION

A traumatic dental injury in a child is always a stressful situation both for the patient and the parents. After clinical and radiographic examination, a careful diagnosis should be made in order to recommend conservative, biologically based emergency treatment and to avoid taking any risk that may damage the developing permanent successors (Fig. 11.24).[12,111]

Luxation injuries are common in the primary dentition; most of them are left untreated, to await spontaneous reposition influenced by physiologic forces of the tongue and lips. Injuries requiring emergency care are crown fractures with pulp exposure and those in which displacement occurs, resulting in occlusal interference: root fractures, alveolar fractures, extrusions, and lateral luxations (Fig. 11.25). The ability of the dentist to cope with a very young child, which may include the safe use of sedative agents; dealing with the close relationship between the apex of the primary tooth and its developing permanent successor; and the degree of root resorption of the primary tooth all are factors to be considered when selecting an appropriate treatment.[12,111]

Crown Fractures Without Pulp Exposure

Crown fractures become urgent care cases when very young children have broken teeth with sharp edges. Primary teeth may be restored with glass ionomer or composite, or the fracture sites may be smoothed without restoring them.

Crown Fractures with Pulp Exposure

A crown fracture with pulp exposure is a difficult emergency situation, especially when a very young child is affected. **191**

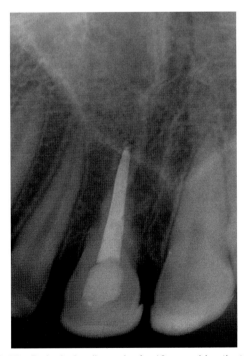

Fig. 11.22 Periapical radiograph of a 12-year-old patient 2 years after replantation of the maxillary right central incisor. Note the presence of replacement root resorption (dentin replaced by bone) in the absence of radiolucencies.

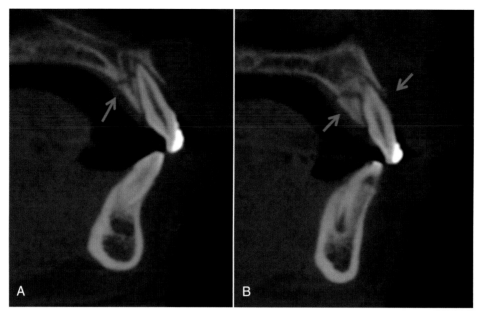

Fig. 11.23 Alveolar fractures of the lingual (**A** and **B**) and buccal (**B**) cortical plates.

Treatment includes partial pulpotomy with calcium hydroxide, pulpotomy, or extraction, depending on the patient's age and cooperation. If vital pulp therapy is possible, the fractured crown may be restored with composite resins.

Crown-Root Fractures
A crown-root fracture in primary teeth usually exposes the pulp, and extraction is indicated.

Root Fractures
Removing the coronal segment and leaving the root apex in situ is the treatment of choice for root fractures with marked coronal displacement. Any attempt to remove the root apex may damage the subjacent permanent tooth bud. Root fractures not accompanied by mobility usually require no treatment unless problems develop subsequently.

Alveolar Fractures
Alveolar fractures are severe injuries that may dictate treatment under general anesthesia. The displaced segment should be repositioned and splinted to adjacent teeth for up to 4 weeks.

Luxation Injuries
Concussion and *subluxation* injuries require no treatment other than promoting good oral hygiene to prevent healing complications. Crown color changes are usually the main complaint for seeking treatment. Because it has not been possible to relate discolored teeth to pulpal status,[112-114] persistent gray discoloration of the crown is not considered an indication for root canal treatment[115] unless a sinus tract or an abscess develops. Discolored primary teeth may return to normal color, probably indicating recovery of the pulp (Fig. 11.26). Pulp canal obliteration is common after luxation injuries.[116] This changes the primary crown to a darker yellow color, which is not pathologic and requires no treatment.

Teeth with *lateral* and *extrusive luxations* may be left untreated; they may be repositioned if there is occlusal interference; or they may be extracted, depending on the severity of injury.

Teeth with *intrusive luxation* should be carefully evaluated to determine the direction of intrusion. Radiographs provide valuable information to confirm the intruded position of the tooth and its proximity to the permanent successor.[117] If the intruded tooth appears foreshortened on the film, the apex is oriented toward the x-ray cone. Therefore, these teeth should present no danger to the permanent successor and may be left to reerupt. If the tooth appears elongated, the apex is oriented toward the permanent successor and may pose a risk to the permanent tooth bud. The tooth should be carefully extracted if it impinges on the permanent successor. The permanent tooth buds should also be evaluated for symmetry.

Avulsions
Replantation of avulsed primary teeth is not recommended because of the risk of damage to the permanent successor (Fig. 11.27). Severe impacts resulting in avulsions may cause damage at the time of injury, so treatment that may inflict an additional injury to the succedaneous teeth must be avoided. Furthermore, the parents should be asked to bring in the avulsed tooth to ensure that the tooth is not intruded. A radiographic examination confirms tooth avulsion and reveals the stage of development of the permanent tooth bud.

Patient Instructions
Parents should receive information on how to brush their children's teeth after an injury. Careful oral hygiene after each meal, in addition to topical use of chlorhexidine twice a day for 1 week, keeps plaque away. Also, restricted use of pacifiers is indicated.

PREVENTION

Dental trauma frequently results in the need for lifelong follow-up treatment. A comprehensive practice in contemporary dentistry must include prevention of oral injuries. Such

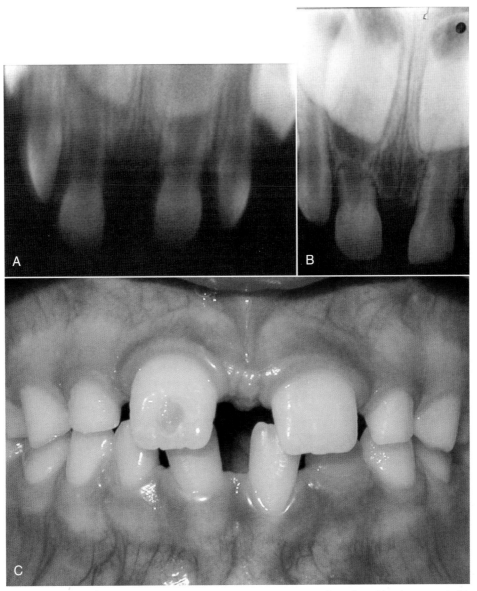

Fig. 11.24 Hypoplasia in a permanent incisor after avulsion and subsequent replantation of a primary central incisor. A 1-year-old boy fell and struck the central incisors against a table. The primary right central incisor was avulsed and replanted. The patient followed a 7-day course of amoxicillin. **A,** Radiograph at the time of injury shows the replanted immature central incisor. **B,** At the 3-year, 5-month follow-up control, the root has been almost completely resorbed. The contralateral tooth shows complete root formation. **C,** Crown hypoplasia of the right permanent successor at 7-year follow-up control.

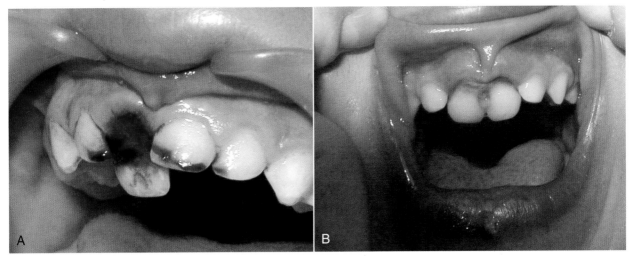

Fig. 11.25 Treatment priorities after traumatic injuries in the primary dentition include urgent care to alleviate pain and enable recovery of masticatory function. **A,** Severe tooth displacement. **B,** Extrusive luxation of both primary central incisors.

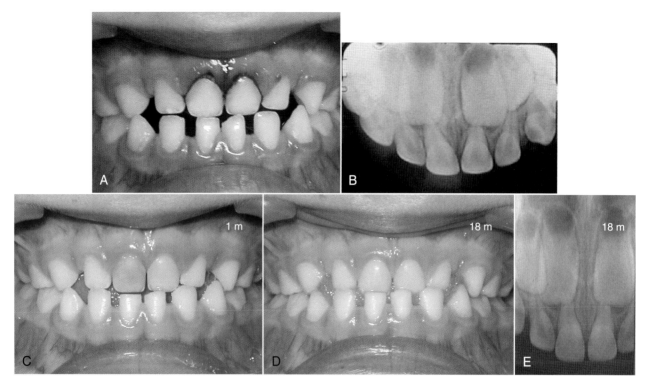

Fig. 11.26 Color changes in primary teeth after a subluxation injury. A 5-year-old girl fell while playing and struck her front teeth against the floor. **A,** The girl arrived in the clinic within 1 hour for clinical examination. Both central incisors were mobile but not displaced. Bleeding from the gingival crevice was observed. Because of minor occlusal interference, slight grinding of the opposite teeth was performed. Oral hygiene instructions given to the mother included topical use of chlorhexidine. **B,** Radiograph at the time of injury shows no radiographic changes. **C,** After 1 month, there is no occlusal interference, but gray discoloration is seen in both central incisors. **D,** At 18-month follow-up control, the color of the crowns has returned to normal. **E,** Periapical radiograph shows pulp canal obliteration in both traumatized teeth.

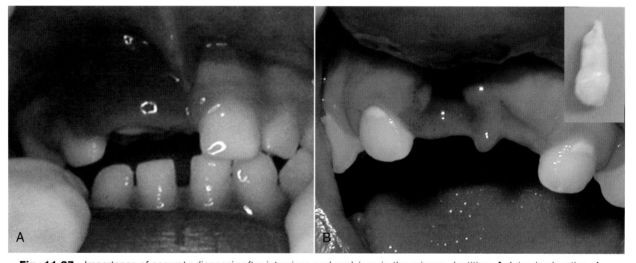

Fig. 11.27 Importance of accurate diagnosis after intrusions and avulsions in the primary dentition. **A,** Intrusive luxation. A maxillary right central incisor has been deeply intruded in the alveolar socket, giving the appearance of having been avulsed. **B,** Avulsion. The avulsed tooth was brought into the clinic, confirming that it was not intruded.

a preventive approach involves education, early orthodontic treatment in predisposed children, and protective devices for contact sports. Education should focus not only on the prevention of dental trauma, but also on the implementation of therapeutic guidelines at the site of injury. Several studies have reported the need of such an education campaign among lay people,[118] teachers,[119] coaches,[119,120] physicians,[121] nurses, paramedics,[122] and even dentists.[123] Dental trauma has been found to be more prevalent among children with an incisal overjet of more than 7 mm and/or with incompetent lips.[4,124] In these patients, the maxillary anterior teeth are directly exposed to any impact without interposition of soft tissue.

Thus, early orthodontic treatment is also highly recommended to prevent dental trauma.

Dental professionals have the responsibility to educate patients and the public about mouthguard protection for contact sports. It is also imperative to provide inexpensive devices that are easily accessible to the athletes or their parents. Athletic mouthguards have been recommended for decades with varying levels of athlete acceptance. Current research supports the fact that custom-made mouthguards had no negative effect on athletic performance and strength and were reported as being comfortable and not causing breathing difficulty in collegiate athletes.[125,126]

REFERENCES

1. Andreasen JO, Andreasen FM: Classification, etiology and epidemiology of traumatic dental injuries. In Andreasen JO, Andreasen FM, editors: *Textbook and color atlas of traumatic injuries to the teeth*, ed 3, Copenhagen, 1994, Munksgaard.
2. Gutmann JL, Gutmann MS: Cause, incidence, and prevention of trauma to teeth. *Dent Clin North Am* 39:1-13, 1995.
3. Camp JH: Management of sports-related root fractures, *Dent Clin North Am* 44:95-109, vi-vii, 2000.
4. Sgan-Cohen HD, Megnagi G, Jacobi Y: Dental trauma and its association with anatomic, behavioral, and social variables among fifth and sixth grade schoolchildren in Jerusalem, *Community Dent Oral Epidemiol* 33:174-180, 2005.
5. Hecova H, Tzigkounakis V, Merglova V, et al: A retrospective study of 889 injured permanent teeth, *Dent Traumatol* 26:466-475, 2010.
6. Cohenca N, Roges RA, Roges R: The incidence and severity of dental trauma in intercollegiate athletes, *J Am Dent Assoc* 138:1121-1126, 2007.
7. Andreasen JO, Andreasen FM, Bakland L, et al: *Traumatic dental injuries: a manual*, ed 2, Oxford, UK, 2003, Blackwell Munksgaard.
8. World Health Organization: Application of the international classification of diseases to dentistry and stomatology, In. 3 ed. Geneva, 1993, ICD-DA.
9. Feliciano KM, de Franca Caldas A Jr: A systematic review of the diagnostic classifications of traumatic dental injuries, *Dent Traumatol* 22:71-76, 2006.
10. Diangelis AJ, Andreasen JO, Ebeleseder KA, et al: International Association of Dental Traumatology guidelines for the management of traumatic dental injuries. Part 1. Fractures and luxations of permanent teeth, *Dent Traumatol* 28:2-12, 2012.
11. Andersson L, Andreasen JO, Day P, et al: International Association of Dental Traumatology guidelines for the management of traumatic dental injuries. Part 2. Avulsion of permanent teeth, *Dent Traumatol* 28:88-96, 2012.
12. Malmgren B, Andreasen JO, Flores MT, et al: International Association of Dental Traumatology guidelines for the management of traumatic dental injuries. Part 3. Injuries in the primary dentition, *Dent Traumatol* 28:174-182, 2012.
13. Bakland LK, Andreasen JO: Examination of the dentally traumatized patient, *J Calif Dent Assoc* 24:35-37, 40-44, 1996.
14. Nolla CM: The development of the permanent teeth, *J Dent Child* 27:254-266, 1960.
15. de Oliveira DM, de Souza Andrade ES, et al: Correlation of the radiographic and morphological features of the dental follicle of third molars with incomplete root formation, *Int J Med Sci* 5:36-40, 2008.
16. Pioto NR, Costa B, Gomide MR: Dental development of the permanent lateral incisor in patients with incomplete and complete unilateral cleft lip, *Cleft Palate Craniofac J* 42:517-520, 2005.
17. Fulling HJ, Andreasen JO: Influence of maturation status and tooth type of permanent teeth upon electrometric and thermal pulp testing, *Scand J Dent Res* 84:286-290, 1976.
18. Fuss Z, Trowbridge H, Bender IB, et al: Assessment of reliability of electrical and thermal pulp testing agents, *J Endod* 12:301-305, 1986.

19. Arnon SS: Tetanus. In Behrman R, Kleigman R, Arvin AM, editors: *Nelson's textbook of pediatrics*, ed 15, Philadelphia, 1995, Saunders.
20. Scorza KA, Raleigh MF, O'Connor FG: Current concepts in concussion: evaluation and management, *Am Fam Physician* 85:123-132, 2012.
21. Kamboozia AH, Punnia-Moorthy A: The fate of teeth in mandibular fracture lines: a clinical and radiographic follow-up study, *Int J Oral Maxillofac Surg* 22:97-101, 1993.
22. Oikarinen K, Lahti J, Raustia AM: Prognosis of permanent teeth in the line of mandibular fractures, *Endod Dent Traumatol* 6:177-182, 1990.
23. Andreasen FM, Andreasen JO: Diagnosis of luxation injuries: the importance of standardized clinical, radiographic and photographic techniques in clinical investigations, *Endod Dent Traumatol* 1:160-169, 1985.
24. Andreasen FM: Histological and bacteriological study of pulps extirpated after luxation injuries, *Endod Dent Traumatol* 4:170-181, 1988.
25. Andreasen FM, Pedersen BV: Prognosis of luxated permanent teeth: the development of pulp necrosis, *Endod Dent Traumatol* 1:207-220, 1985.
26. Setzer FC, Challagulla P, Kataoka SH, et al: Effect of tooth isolation on laser Doppler readings, *Int Endod J* 46(6):517-522, 2013.
27. Emshoff R, Moschen I, Strobl H: Use of laser Doppler flowmetry to predict vitality of luxated or avulsed permanent teeth, *Oral Surg Oral Med Oral Pathol Oral Radiol Endod* 98:750-755, 2004.
28. Emshoff R, Emshoff I, Moschen I, et al: Laser Doppler flow measurements of pulpal blood flow and severity of dental injury, *Int Endod J* 37:463-467, 2004.
29. Radhakrishnan S, Munshi AK, Hegde AM: Pulse oximetry: a diagnostic instrument in pulpal vitality testing, *J Clin Pediatr Dent* 26:141-145, 2002.
30. Schnettler JM, Wallace JA: Pulse oximetry as a diagnostic tool of pulpal vitality, *J Endod* 17:488-490, 1991.
31. Gopikrishna V, Tinagupta K, Kandaswamy D: Comparison of electrical, thermal, and pulse oximetry methods for assessing pulp vitality in recently traumatized teeth, *J Endod* 33:531-535, 2007.
32. Gopikrishna V, Tinagupta K, Kandaswamy D: Evaluation of efficacy of a new custom-made pulse oximeter dental probe in comparison with the electrical and thermal tests for assessing pulp vitality, *J Endod* 33:411-414, 2007.
33. Scarfe WC: Imaging of maxillofacial trauma: evolutions and emerging revolutions, *Oral Surg Oral Med Oral Pathol Oral Radiol Endod* 100:S75-S96, 2005.
34. Simon JH, Enciso R, Malfaz JM, et al: Differential diagnosis of large periapical lesions using cone beam computed tomography measurements and biopsy, *J Endod* 32:833-837, 2006.
35. Trope M, Pettigrew J, Petras J, et al: Differentiation of radicular cyst and granulomas using computerized tomography, *Endod Dent Traumatol* 5:69-72, 1989.
36. Shrout MK, Hall JM, Hildebolt CE: Differentiation of periapical granulomas and radicular cysts by digital radiometric analysis, *Oral Surg Oral Med Oral Pathol* 76:356-361, 1993.
37. Cotti E, Vargiu P, Dettori C, et al: Computerized tomography in the management and follow-up of extensive periapical lesion, *Endod Dent Traumatol* 15:186-189, 1999.
38. Camps J, Pommel L, Bukiet F: Evaluation of periapical lesion healing by correction of gray values, *J Endod* 30:762-766, 2004.
39. Cotton TP, Geisler TM, Holden DT, et al: Endodontic applications of cone beam volumetric tomography, *J Endod* 33:1121-1132, 2007.
40. Ziegler CM, Woertche R, Brief J, et al: Clinical indications for digital volume tomography in oral and maxillofacial surgery, *Dentomaxillofac Radiol* 31:126-130, 2002.
41. Danforth RA, Peck J, Hall P: Cone beam volume tomography: an imaging option for diagnosis of complex mandibular third molar anatomical relationships, *J Calif Dent Assoc* 31:847-852, 2003.
42. Eggers G, Mukhamadiev D, Hassfeld S: Detection of foreign bodies of the head with digital volume tomography, *Dentomaxillofac Radiol* 34:74-79, 2005.
43. Hatcher DC, Dial C, Mayorga C: Cone beam CT for presurgical assessment of implant sites, *J Calif Dent Assoc* 31:825-833, 2003.
44. Sato S, Arai Y, Shinoda K, et al: Clinical application of a new cone beam computerized tomography system to assess multiple two-dimensional images for the preoperative treatment planning of maxillary implants: case reports, *Quintessence Int* 35:525-528, 2004.
45. Maki K, Inou N, Takanishi A, et al: Computer-assisted simulations in orthodontic diagnosis and the application of a new cone beam x-ray computed tomography, *Orthod Craniofac Res* 6(Suppl 1):95-101; discussion, 79-82; 2003.
46. Baumrind S, Carlson S, Beers A, et al: Using three-dimensional imaging to assess treatment outcomes in orthodontics: a progress report from the University of the Pacific, *Orthod Craniofac Res* 6(Suppl 1):132-142, 2003.
47. Danforth RA, Dus I, Mah J: 3-D volume imaging for dentistry: a new dimension, *J Calif Dent Assoc* 31:817-823, 2003.
48. Cohenca N, Simon JH, Roges R, et al: Clinical indications for digital imaging in dento-alveolar trauma. Part 1. Traumatic injuries, *Dent Traumatol* 23:95-104, 2007.
49. Cohenca N, Simon JH, Mathur A, et al: Clinical indications for digital imaging in dento-alveolar trauma. Part 2. Root resorption, *Dent Traumatol* 23:105-113, 2007.
50. Farik B, Munksgaard EC, Kreiborg S, et al: Adhesive bonding of fragmented anterior teeth, *Endod Dent Traumatol* 14:119-123, 1998.
51. Andreasen FM, Flugge E, Daugaard-Jensen J, et al: Treatment of crown fractured incisors with laminate veneer restorations: an experimental study, *Endod Dent Traumatol* 8:30-35, 1992.
52. Cvek M: A clinical report on partial pulpotomy and capping with calcium hydroxide in permanent incisors with complicated crown fracture, *J Endod* 4:232-237, 1978.
53. Fuks AB, Cosack A, Klein H, et al: Partial pulpotomy as a treatment alternative for exposed pulps in crown-fractured permanent incisors, *Endod Dent Traumatol* 3:100-102, 1987.
54. Mejare I, Cvek M: Partial pulpotomy in young permanent teeth with deep carious lesions, *Endod Dent Traumatol* 9:238-242, 1993.

55. Bakland LK: Management of traumatically injured pulps in immature teeth using MTA, *J Calif Dent Assoc* 28:855-858, 2000.

56. Ford TR, Torabinejad M, Abedi HR, et al: Using mineral trioxide aggregate as a pulp-capping material, *J Am Dent Assoc* 127:1491-1494, 1996.

57. Fuks AB, Gavra S, Chosack A: Long-term followup of traumatized incisors treated by partial pulpotomy, *Pediatr Dent* 15:334-336, 1993.

58. Andreasen JO, Andreasen FM: Root fractures. In Andreasen JO, Andreasen FM, editors. *Textbook and color atlas of traumatic injuries to the teeth*. ed 3, Copenhagen, 1994, Munksgaard.

59. Bender IB, Freedland JB: Clinical considerations in the diagnosis and treatment of intra-alveolar root fractures, *J Am Dent Assoc* 107:595-600, 1983.

60. May J, Cohenca N, Peters OA: Contemporary management of horizontal root fractures to the permanent dentition: diagnosis—radiologic assessment to include cone beam computed tomography, *J Endod* 39:S20-S25, 2013.

61. Andreasen FM, Andreasen JO, Bayer T: Prognosis of root-fractured permanent incisors: prediction of healing modalities, *Endod Dent Traumatol* 5:11-22, 1989.

62. Andreasen JO, Andreasen FM, Mejare I, et al: Healing of 400 intra-alveolar root fractures. Part 2. Effect of treatment factors such as treatment delay, repositioning, splinting type and period and antibiotics, *Dent Traumatol* 2004;20:203-211, 2004.

63. Andreasen JO, Andreasen FM, Mejare I, et al: Healing of 400 intra-alveolar root fractures. Part 1. Effect of pre-injury and injury factors such as sex, age, stage of root development, fracture type, location of fracture and severity of dislocation, *Dent Traumatol* 20:192-202, 2004.

64. Herweijer JA, Torabinejad M, Bakland LK: Healing of horizontal root fractures, *J Endod* 18:118-122, 1992.

65. Zachrisson BU, Jacobsen I: Long-term prognosis of 66 permanent anterior teeth with root fracture, *Scand J Dent Res* 83:345-354, 1975.

66. Andreasen JO, Hjorting-Hansen E: Intraalveolar root fractures: radiographic and histologic study of 50 cases, *J Oral Surg* 25:414-426, 1967.

67. Cvek M, Andreasen JO, Borum MK: Healing of 208 intra-alveolar root fractures in patients aged 7-17 years, *Dent Traumatol* 17:53-62, 2001.

68. Welbury R, Kinirons MJ, Day P, et al: Outcomes for root-fractured permanent incisors: a retrospective study, *Pediatr Dent* 24:98-102, 2002.

69. Cvek M, Mejare I, Andreasen JO: Conservative endodontic treatment of teeth fractured in the middle or apical part of the root, *Dent Traumatol* 20:261-269, 2004.

70. Crona-Larsson G, Noren JG: Luxation injuries to permanent teeth: a retrospective study of etiological factors, *Endod Dent Traumatol* 5:176-179, 1989.

71. Andreasen JO, Bakland LK, Matras RC, et al: Traumatic intrusion of permanent teeth. Part 1. An epidemiological study of 216 intruded permanent teeth, *Dent Traumatol* 22:83-89, 2006.

72. Andreasen FM: Pulpal healing after luxation injuries and root fracture in the permanent dentition, *Endod Dent Traumatol* 1989;5:111-131, 1989.

73. Cohenca N, Karni S, Rotstein I: Transient apical breakdown following tooth luxation, *Dent Traumatol* 19:289-291, 2003.

74. Andreasen FM: Transient root resorption after dental trauma: the clinician's dilemma, *J Esthet Restor Dent* 15:80-92, 2003.

75. Andreasen FM: Transient apical breakdown and its relation to color and sensibility changes after luxation injuries to teeth, *Endod Dent Traumatol* 2:9-19, 1986.

76. Andreasen FM, Zhijie Y, Thomsen BL, et al: Occurrence of pulp canal obliteration after luxation injuries in the permanent dentition, *Endod Dent Traumatol* 3:103-115, 1987.

77. Mandel U, Viidik A: Effect of splinting on the mechanical and histological properties of the healing periodontal ligament in the vervet monkey (Cercopithecus aethiops), *Arch Oral Biol* 34:209-217, 1989.

78. Nasjleti CE, Castelli WA, Caffesse RG: The effects of different splinting times on replantation of teeth in monkeys, *Oral Surg Oral Med Oral Pathol* 53:557-566, 1982.

79. Humphrey JM, Kenny DJ, Barrett EJ: Clinical outcomes for permanent incisor luxations in a pediatric population. I. Intrusions, *Dent Traumatol* 19:266-273, 2003.

80. Andreasen JO, Bakland LK, Andreasen FM: Traumatic intrusion of permanent teeth. Part 3. A clinical study of the effect of treatment variables such as treatment delay, method of repositioning, type of splint, length of splinting and antibiotics on 140 teeth, *Dent Traumatol* 22:99-111, 2006.

81. Andreasen JO, Bakland LK, Andreasen FM: Traumatic intrusion of permanent teeth. Part 2. A clinical study of the effect of preinjury and injury factors, such as age, stage of root development, tooth location, and extent of injury including number of intruded teeth on 140 intruded permanent teeth, *Dent Traumatol* 22:90-98, 2006.

82. Trope M, Moshonov J, Nissan R, et al: Short- vs long-term calcium hydroxide treatment of established inflammatory root resorption in replanted dog teeth, *Endod Dent Traumatol* 11:124-128, 1995.

83. Andreasen JO, Borum MK, Andreasen FM: Replantation of 400 avulsed permanent incisors. Part 3. Factors related to root growth, *Endod Dent Traumatol* 11:69-75, 1995.

84. Andreasen JO, Borum MK, Jacobsen HL, et al: Replantation of 400 avulsed permanent incisors. Part 4. Factors related to periodontal ligament healing, *Endod Dent Traumatol* 11:76-89, 1995.

85. Andreasen JO, Borum MK, Jacobsen HL, et al: Replantation of 400 avulsed permanent incisors. Part 2. Factors related to pulpal healing, *Endod Dent Traumatol* 11:59-68, 1995.

86. Andreasen JO, Borum MK, Jacobsen HL, et al: Replantation of 400 avulsed permanent incisors. Part 1. Diagnosis of healing complications, *Endod Dent Traumatol* 11:51-58, 1995.

87. Trope M: Avulsion and replantation, *Refuat Hapeh Vehashinayim* 19:6-15, 76, 2002.

88. Trope M: Clinical management of the avulsed tooth: present strategies and future directions, *Dent Traumatol* 18:1-11, 2002.

89. Blomlof L: Storage of human periodontal ligament cells in a combination of different media, *J Dent Res* 60:1904-1906, 1981.

90. Blomlof L, Lindskog S, Hammarstrom L: Periodontal healing of exarticulated monkey teeth stored in milk or saliva, *Scand J Dent Res* 89:251-259, 1981.

91. Blomlof L, Otteskog P, Hammarstrom L: Effect of storage in media with different ion strengths and osmolalities on human periodontal ligament cells, *Scand J Dent Res* 89:180-187, 1981.

92. Blomlof L: Milk and saliva as possible storage media for traumatically exarticulated teeth prior to replantation, *Swed Dent J Suppl* 8:1-26, 1981.

93. Kwan SC, Johnson JD, Cohenca N: The effect of splint material and thickness on tooth mobility after extraction and replantation using a human cadaveric model, *Dent Traumatol* 28:277-281, 2012.

94. Kling M, Cvek M, Mejare I: Rate and predictability of pulp revascularization in therapeutically reimplanted permanent incisors, *Endod Dent Traumatol* 2:83-89, 1986.

95. Cvek M, Cleaton-Jones P, Austin J, et al: Effect of topical application of doxycycline on pulp revascularization and periodontal healing in reimplanted monkey incisors, *Endod Dent Traumatol* 6:170-176, 1990.

96. Cvek M, Cleaton-Jones P, Austin J, et al: Pulp revascularization in reimplanted immature monkey incisors: predictability and the effect of antibiotic systemic prophylaxis, *Endod Dent Traumatol* 6:157-169, 1990.

97. Yanpiset K, Trope M: Pulp revascularization of replanted immature dog teeth after different treatment methods, *Endod Dent Traumatol* 16:211-217, 2000.

98. Ritter AL, Ritter AV, Murrah V, et al: Pulp revascularization of replanted immature dog teeth after treatment with minocycline and doxycycline assessed by laser Doppler flowmetry, radiography, and histology, *Dent Traumatol* 20:75-84, 2004.

99. Shulman LB, Gedalia I, Feingold RM: Fluoride concentration in root surfaces and alveolar bone of fluoride-immersed monkey incisors 3 weeks after replantation, *J Dent Res* 52:1314-1316, 1973.

100. Hammarstrom L, Pierce A, Blomlof L, et al: Tooth avulsion and replantation: a review, *Endod Dent Traumatol* 2:1-8, 1986.

101. Witherspoon DE, Ham K: One-visit apexification: technique for inducing root-end barrier formation in apical closures, *Pract Proced Aesthet Dent* 13:455-460; quiz, 62; 2001.

102. Bose R, Nummikoski P, Hargreaves K: A retrospective evaluation of radiographic outcomes in immature teeth with necrotic root canal systems treated with regenerative endodontic procedures, *J Endod* 35:1343-1349, 2009.

103. Iwaya SI, Ikawa M, Kubota M: Revascularization of an immature permanent tooth with apical periodontitis and sinus tract, *Dent Traumatol* 17:185-187, 2001.

104. Yamauchi N, Nagaoka H, Yamauchi S, et al: Immunohistological characterization of newly formed tissues after regenerative procedure in immature dog teeth, *J Endod* 37:1636-1641, 2011.

105. Yamauchi N, Yamauchi S, Nagaoka H, et al: Tissue engineering strategies for immature teeth with apical periodontitis, *J Endod* 37:390-397, 2011.

106. Trope M, Yesilsoy C, Koren L, et al: Effect of different endodontic treatment protocols on periodontal repair and root resorption of replanted dog teeth, *J Endod* 18:492-496, 1992.

107. Andreasen JO, Andreasen FM: Root resorption following traumatic dental injuries, *Proc Finn Dent Soc* 88(Suppl 1):95-114, 1992.

108. Andreasen JO, Farik B, Munksgaard EC: Long-term calcium hydroxide as a root canal dressing may increase risk of root fracture, *Dent Traumatol* 18:134-137, 2002.

109. Rosenberg B, Murray PE, Namerow K: The effect of calcium hydroxide root filling on dentin fracture strength, *Dent Traumatol* 23:26-29, 2007.

110. Andreasen JO: Fractures of the alveolar process of the jaw: a clinical and radiographic follow-up study, *Scand J Dent Res* 78:263-272, 1970.

111. Flores MT: Traumatic injuries in the primary dentition, *Dent Traumatol* 18:287-298, 2002.

112. Soxman JA, Nazif MM, Bouquot J: Pulpal pathology in relation to discoloration of primary anterior teeth, *ASDC J Dent Child* 51:282-284, 1984.

113. Croll TP, Pascon EA, Langeland K: Traumatically injured primary incisors: a clinical and histological study, *ASDC J Dent Child* 54:401-422, 1987.

114. Holan G, Fuks AB: The diagnostic value of coronal dark-gray discoloration in primary teeth following traumatic injuries, *Pediatr Dent* 18:224-227, 1996.

115. Holan G: Long-term effect of different treatment modalities for traumatized primary incisors presenting dark coronal discoloration with no other signs of injury, *Dent Traumatol* 22:14-17, 2006.

116. Borum MK, Andreasen JO: Sequelae of trauma to primary maxillary incisors. I. Complications in the primary dentition, *Endod Dent Traumatol* 14:31-44, 1998.

117. Holan G, Ram D: Sequelae and prognosis of intruded primary incisors: a retrospective study, *Pediatr Dent* 21:242-247, 1999.

118. Stokes AN, Anderson HK, Cowan TM: Lay and professional knowledge of methods for emergency management of avulsed teeth, *Endod Dent Traumatol* 8:160-162, 1992.

119. Holan G, Cohenca N, Brin I, et al: An oral health promotion program for the prevention of complications following avulsion: the effect on knowledge of physical education teachers, *Dent Traumatol* 22:323-327, 2006.

120. Perunski S, Lang B, Pohl Y, et al: Level of information concerning dental injuries and their prevention in Swiss basketball: a survey among players and coaches, *Dent Traumatol* 21:195-200, 2005.

121. Holan G, Shmueli Y: Knowledge of physicians in hospital emergency rooms in Israel on their role in cases of avulsion of permanent incisors, *Int J Paediatr Dent* 13:13-19, 2003.

122. Lin S, Levin L, Emodi O, et al: Physician and emergency medical technicians' knowledge and experience regarding dental trauma, *Dent Traumatol* 22:124-126, 2006.

123. Cohenca N, Forrest JL, Rotstein I: Knowledge of oral health professionals of treatment of avulsed teeth, *Dent Traumatol* 22:296-301, 2006.

124. Brin I, Ben-Bassat Y, Heling I, et al: Profile of an orthodontic patient at risk of dental trauma, *Endod Dent Traumatol* 16:111-115, 2000.

125. Duddy FA, Weissman J, Lee RA Sr, et al: Influence of different types of mouthguards on strength and performance of collegiate athletes: a controlled-randomized trial, *Dent Traumatol* 28:263-267, 2012.

126. Kececi AD, Cetin C, Eroglu E, et al: Do custom-made mouth guards have negative effects on aerobic performance capacity of athletes? *Dent Traumatol* 21:276-280, 2005.

Endodontic radiography

Richard E. Walton, Ashraf F. Fouad

CHAPTER OUTLINE

LEARNING OBJECTIVES

After reading this chapter, the student should be able to:

1. Describe the importance of radiographs in endodontic diagnosis, treatment, and postoperative evaluation.
2. Discuss special applications of radiography to endodontics.
3. Discuss reasons for limiting the number of exposures.
4. Identify normal anatomic features in the maxilla and mandible on radiographs.
5. Describe radiographic characteristics to differentiate between endodontic and nonendodontic (normal and pathologic) radiolucencies and radiopacities.
6. Describe the reasons for varying horizontal and vertical cone angulations on working radiographs to create image shift.
7. Describe how to determine the third dimension on angled radiographs (i.e., faciolingual structures [SLOB] rule).
8. Describe structural elements of the tooth as visualized on both facial and angled projections.

9. Discuss how to detect the presence of and locate undiscovered canals or roots on angled working radiographs.
10. Describe techniques for making "working" radiographs (i.e., film/sensor placement and cone alignment with dental dam in place).
11. Describe specific details of film/sensor placement and cone alignment for each tooth on working radiographs.
12. Describe the limitations of rapid processing of working films.
13. Describe the radiographic technique for locating a "calcified" canal.
14. Discuss the limitations of radiographic interpretation.
15. Describe some new technologies and their application to endodontic radiography now and in the future.
16. Describe the technique for extraoral positioning of the film and cone.
17. Describe the specific indications of cone beam computed tomography (CBCT) in endodontics.

We are sick of the roentgen ray . . . you can see other people's bones with the naked eye, and also see through eight inches of solid wood. On the revolting indecency of this there is no need to dwell. But what we seriously put before the attention of the Government . . . that it will call for legislative restriction of the severest kind. Perhaps the best thing would be for all civilized nations to combine to burn all works on the roentgen rays, to execute all the discoverers, and to corner all the tungstate in the world and whelm it in the middle of the ocean.

Editorial in the *Pall Mall Gazette*, London, 1896

Obviously (and fortunately), the concern expressed by the editorial in this London publication did not become the popular view of radiography. Radiographs are essential; they are a second set of "eyes" for the dentist. This is particularly true in endodontics, in which so many diagnostic and treatment decisions are based on radiographic findings. Because most structures of concern are not visible to the naked eye, there is considerable dependence on radiographs, which are an obvious necessity and a blessing. But they also may be somewhat of a liability from the standpoint of both safety and time, and unfortunately, radiographs are often overinterpreted or underinterpreted.

A radiographic exposure is an irreversible procedure; therefore, only necessary exposures should be made. With the increasing emphasis and justifiable concern for radiation safety, overall radiation exposure must be minimized.[1] However, the radiation dosage to oral and other tissues has been calculated to be very low and to cause minimal (but some) risk.[2,3]

Another concern is the time required to make and process individual radiographs—time is money. Therefore, in the interests of both safety and time, only the radiographs necessitated by the procedure should be made.

This chapter discusses radiography as applied to endodontic procedures. Radiography as a discipline in dentistry has become increasingly important with advances in technology and has recently been granted specialty status, thereby replacing endodontics as the youngest dental specialty.[4] Technology has exploded in recent years, with new devices and approaches that require special training and experience. How these new devices and approaches apply to diagnosis and treatment in endodontics is discussed later in this chapter.

IMPORTANCE OF RADIOGRAPHY IN ENDODONTICS

Radiographs perform essential functions in three areas: diagnosis, treatment, and postoperative evaluation or follow-up. Each of these has limitations that require its own special approach. A single radiograph is but a two-dimensional shadow of a three-dimensional (3D) object. For maximum information, the third dimension must be visualized and interpreted.[5] The advent of 3D radiographic techniques, such as CBCT (discussed later in the chapter), has highlighted this concept.

Digital Radiography
The use of digital radiography is becoming more common in dentistry. Although there are technical advantages over conventional approaches, the same limitations apply. Overall, digital radiographs are equivalent to conventional radiographs with regard to diagnostic and treatment-related accuracy. These factors and other considerations are discussed further throughout this chapter.

Diagnosis
Diagnostic radiology involves not only identifying the presence and nature of pathosis, but also determining root and pulp anatomy and characterizing and differentiating other normal structures.

Identifying Pathosis
Radiographs must be studied carefully by someone with a working knowledge of the changes that indicate pulpal, periapical, periodontal, or other bony lesions. Many changes are obvious, but some are subtle.

Determining Root and Pulpal Anatomy
Determining the anatomy involves not only identifying and counting the roots and canals, but also identifying unusual tooth anatomy, such as dens invaginatus and a C-shaped configuration,[6] and determining curvatures, canal relationships, and canal location.[7,8] Identification also includes characterizing the cross-sectional anatomy of individual roots and canals (Fig. 12.1).

Characterizing Normal Structures
Numerous radiolucent and radiopaque structures often lie in close proximity. Frequently, these structures are superimposed over and obscure crowns and roots.[9] These must be

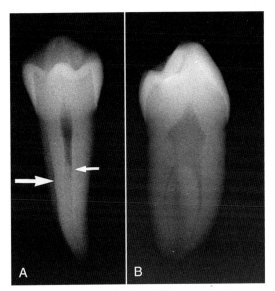

Fig. 12.1 **A,** The facial projection of this premolar gives some limited information about pulp/root morphology. "Fast break" *(small arrow)* usually indicates canal bifurcation. A double root prominence on the mesial surface *(large arrow)* indicates two bulges and a concavity; its absence on the distal surface indicates a flat or convex root surface. **B,** The same premolar from the proximal view. The presence of two definitive canals, each in its own "root bulge," is confirmed.

distinguished and differentiated from pathosis and from normal dental structures.

Treatment
"Working" radiographs are made while the dental dam is in place, which creates problems in film placement and cone positioning. These radiographs are exposed *during* the treatment phase and have special applications.

Determining Working Lengths
The distance from a reference point to the radiographic apex is determined precisely. This establishes the distance from the apex at which the canal is to be prepared and obturated.[10]

Moving Superimposed Structures
Radiopaque anatomic structures often overlie and obscure roots and apices. Using special cone angulations, these radiopaque structures can be "moved" to give a clear image of the apex.

Locating Canals
Canal location is obviously essential to success. Standard and special techniques allow the practitioner to determine the position of canals not located during access.

Differentiating Canals and Periodontal Ligament Spaces
Canals end in the chamber and at the apex. A periodontal ligament space ends on a surface and in a furcation (molars) and demonstrates an adjacent lamina dura (Fig. 12.2).

Evaluating Obturation
Postoperative radiographs provide considerable information on canal preparation and obturation. The length from the **199**

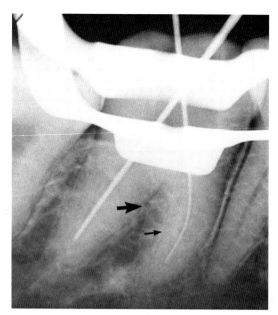

Fig. 12.2 This distal angulation shows the root surface outline *(large arrow)* and a periodontal ligament space *(small arrow)* with an adjacent lamina dura. The file is in the mesiobuccal canal (same lingual, opposite buccal [SLOB] rule).

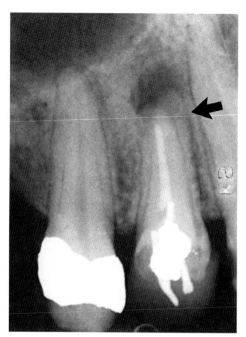

Fig. 12.3 Failed root canal treatment because of missed root or canal. This mesial-angled radiograph clearly shows the untreated lingual root *(arrow).* (Courtesy Dr. L. Wilcox.)

apex, density, taper, preservation of original canal shape, and general quality of obturation in each canal are determined from these radiographs.

Follow-up Evaluation (Recall)

Ultimate success is verified at specified intervals of months or years after treatment. Because failures often occur without signs or symptoms, radiographs are essential to evaluate periapical status.[11]

Identifying New Pathosis

The presence and nature of lesions that arise after treatment are best detected on radiographs. These lesions may be periapical, periodontal, or nonendodontic. It is important to remember that such lesions frequently present with no overt signs or symptoms and are detectable only on radiographs (Fig. 12.3).

Evaluating Healing

Pretreatment lesions should be resolving or should have resolved. In a successful (healed) treatment, restitution of generally normal structures should be evident on recall radiographs (Fig. 12.4).

Special Applications

Radiographs should be used to their maximum advantage. The following alternative techniques greatly enhance the ability to make an accurate and definitive diagnosis and to control treatment procedures.

Cone-Image Shift

Varying either the vertical or, particularly, the horizontal cone angulation from parallel alters images and enhances interpretation.[5,12] These shifts reveal the third dimension and superimposed structures. Shifts also permit identification and positioning of objects that lie in the faciolingual plane.

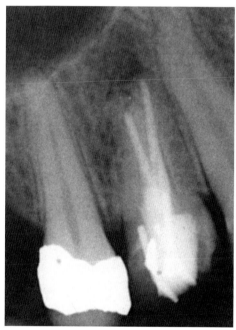

Fig. 12.4 Same tooth as shown in Fig. 12.3. Recall radiograph after 9 months shows almost complete regeneration of bone, indicating a healing lesion. A permanent restoration must be placed as soon as possible. (Courtesy Dr. L. Wilcox.)

Working Radiographs

Working radiographs are essential aids to treatment and are exposed when necessary but with discretion.

RADIOGRAPHIC SEQUENCE

Radiographs are made in a recommended order and number for each procedure. The minimum number is described here, although special situations may require additional exposures.

Diagnostic Radiographs
Number
The number of exposures depends on the situation. For diagnosis in most cases, only a single exposure is necessary. A properly positioned film and cone (usually a parallel projection is best) permits visualization at least 3 to 4 mm beyond the apex. The initial diagnostic radiograph is used primarily to detect pathosis and to provide general information on root and pulp anatomy. A bitewing radiograph may aid in determining the extent of caries or in detecting caries or an open margin of a crown. Usually, it is not necessary at this time to make additional films for identification of additional canals except in endodontically treated teeth, in which missed canals can be identified by using a shift.

If other films are at hand, each gives a slightly different view of the same tooth (Fig. 12.5). *Examine the tooth on each film in which it appears.*

Angulation
Unquestionably, the most accurate radiographs are made using a paralleling technique.[13] The advantages are (1) less distortion and more clarity and (2) reproducibility of film and cone placement with preliminary and subsequent radiographs. Reproducibility is important when assessing whether changes occurring in the periapex indicate healing or nonhealing. Paralleling devices enhance reproducibility.

There may be special situations in which the paralleling technique is not feasible, such as a low palatal vault, maxillary tori, exceptionally long roots, or an uncooperative or gagging patient; these circumstances may necessitate an alternative technique. A second choice is the modified paralleling technique; the least accurate technique is the bisecting angle.

Working Radiographs
Special situations require special considerations. Although the basic principles of doing everything possible to obtain the best quality radiograph are followed, there are definite limitations in making working films. These require cooperation by the patient if he or she holds the film or sensor in position.

These radiographs are usually neither parallel nor bisecting angle. The technique used is called *modified paralleling.*[14] Essentially, the film is not parallel to the tooth, but the central beam is oriented at right angles to the film surface. In endodontic working radiographs, a further modification is made by varying the horizontal cone angle. Specific details of film/sensor and cone placement and radiographic interpretation are discussed later in this chapter.

Working Length
In general, establishment of working length should require only a single exposure. If a root contains or may contain two superimposed canals, either a mesial or distal angle projection is absolutely necessary; the straight facial view is not particularly helpful.[15] Additional working length radiographs may be required later for confirmation of working lengths to detect the presence or lengths of newly discovered canals (Fig. 12.6) or for reexposure if an apex has been cut off in the first radiograph.

Master Cone
The same principles used with working length films apply. With proper technique, only one radiograph is necessary to evaluate the length of the master gutta-percha cone. The master cones should extend to, or very close to, the corrected working length. (Procedures for the fitting of master cones are discussed in Chapter 18.)

Other Considerations
Additional working radiographs are often required. For example, they are useful as aids in locating a canal or in determining the occurrence of procedural accidents (perforations, separated instruments, or ledges). Variations in cone positioning and angulation are made as required. When there is doubt about the accuracy of the master cone fit, an intermediary fill radiograph may be exposed after the master cone has been condensed with sealer but before the obturation is finalized. Errors in length or density can be corrected at this stage.

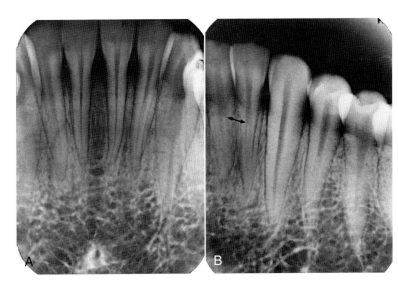

Fig. 12.5 **A,** Facial projection of incisors suggests a single canal and a single root. **B,** Distal (canine) projection gives a different perspective. The canals of the lateral and central incisors are seen to bifurcate in the middle third of the root *(arrow)* and reunite in the apical third.

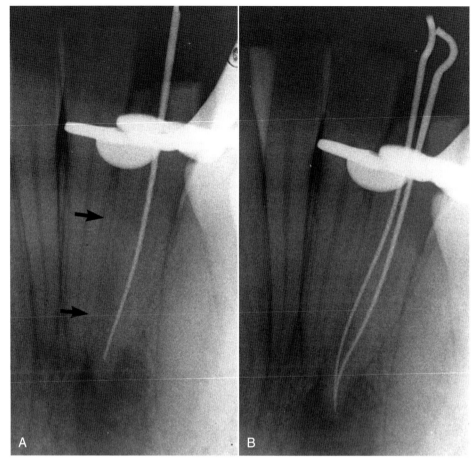

Fig. 12.6 Identifying and locating a canal. This incisor was rotated, requiring mesially angled working radiographs. **A,** The file is off-center, as indicated by the mesial root surface *(arrows)*. Therefore, the file is in the facial canal. **B,** A search to the lingual locates the lingual canal. There is a common canal apically.

Obturation

The same basic principles used for diagnostic radiographs apply. At least a parallel projection should be made. In teeth with multiple canals, it is desirable to supplement this with an angled projection to visualize separate superimposed canals for separate evaluation of each. However, the radiograph gives only a rough indication of obturation length and quality.[16,17]

Follow-up Evaluation (Recall)

The same principles used for diagnostic and obturation radiographs (parallel projection and exposure factors) apply to recall radiographs. There is one exception. If treatment is deemed to be questionable or a failure, additional angled radiographs are often required to search for a previously undetected canal or other abnormality.

EXPOSURE CONSIDERATIONS

Proper x-ray machine settings and careful film processing are important for maximal quality and interpretative diagnostic and working radiographs. D film (Ultraspeed) and E film (Ektaspeed) have been used and compared. Although D film has been shown to have slightly better contrast, overall suitability is equivalent for the two film types.[18] The newer Ektaspeed Plus film produces an image similar in quality to Ultraspeed film but requires only half the radiation of Ultraspeed.[19]

The optimal setting for maximal contrast between radiopaque and radiolucent structures is 70 kV. Exposure time and milliamperage should be set individually on each machine. Therefore, the preferred film types are E and Ektaspeed Plus to minimize x-ray irradiation at 70 kV and to maximize clarity.

Digital radiographs require much less exposure time than conventional radiographs, which is a definite advantage. In general, there does not appear to be a significant difference in clinical accuracy between conventional and digital radiography[20] or among different digital radiography systems.[21]

CONE-IMAGE SHIFT

The cone-image shift reveals the third dimension.

Principles
Image Shift
Superimposed Structures
The cone-image shift technique separates and identifies the facial and lingual structures.[5] An example is the mesiobuccal

root of a maxillary molar that contains two superimposed canals. The cone shift separates and permits visualization of both canals.

Faciolingual Determination

Principles of relative movement of structures and film orientation are applied to the differentiation of object position (Figs. 12.7 and 12.8).

SLOB Rule

When two objects and the film or sensor are in a fixed position buccal and lingual from each other, and the radiation source (cone) is moved in a horizontal or vertical direction, images of the two objects move in the opposite direction (Fig. 12.9). The facial (buccal) object shifts farthest away; the lingual object moves in the direction of the cone movement. The resulting radiograph shows a lingual object that moved

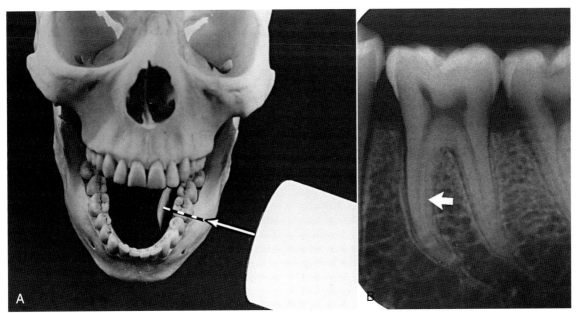

Fig. 12.7 **A,** The film is positioned parallel to the plane of the arch. The cone has the central ray *(arrow)* directed toward the film at right angles. This is the basic cone-film relationship used for horizontal or vertical angulations. **B,** There is a clear outline of the first molar but limited information about superimposed structures (canals that lie in the buccolingual plane). The arrow points to a periodontal ligament space adjacent to a superimposed root bulge, not to a second canal. (From Walton R: Endodontic radiographic techniques, *Dent Radiogr Photogr* 46:51, 1973.)

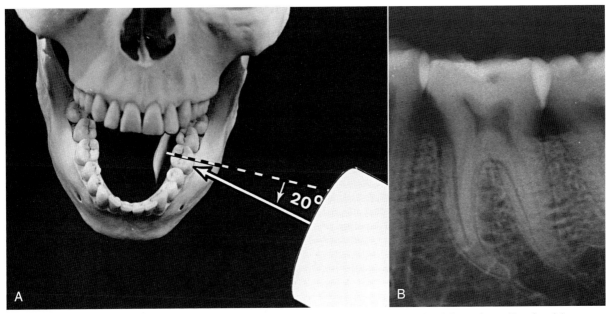

Fig. 12.8 **A,** The horizontal angulation of the cone is 20-degrees mesial from the parallel, right-angle position (mesial projection). **B,** The resultant radiograph demonstrates the morphologic features of the root or canal in the third dimension. For example, two canals are now visible in the distal root of the first molar. (From Walton R: Endodontic radiographic techniques, *Dent Radiogr Photogr* 46:51, 1973.)

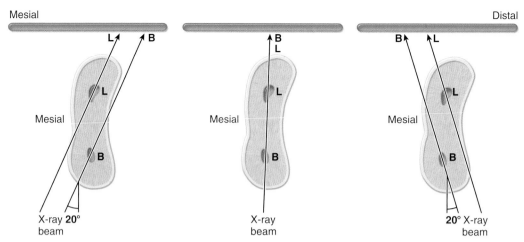

Mesial   Distal

Mesial   Mesial   Mesial

X-ray **20°**   X-ray   **20°** X-ray
beam   beam   beam

Fig. 12.9 Central (x-ray) beam passing directly through a root containing two canals superimposes the canals on the film. When the cone is shifted to the mesial or distal aspect, the lingual object moves in the same direction as the cone; the buccal object moves in the opposite direction (SLOB rule). (Courtesy Dr. A. Goerig.)

relatively in the same direction as the cone and a buccal object that moved in the opposite direction.[22] This principle is the origin of the acronym SLOB (same lingual, opposite buccal).

One way to visualize this is to close one eye and hold two fingers directly in front of the open eye so that one finger is superimposed on the other. By moving the head one way and then the other, the position of the fingers relative to each other shifts. The same effect is produced with two superimposed roots (the fingers) and the way in which they move relative to the radiation source (the eye) and the central beam (the line of sight). When the cone-shift technique is used, it is critical to know in which direction the shift was made and to determine what is facial and what is lingual. Otherwise, serious errors may occur.

Indications and Advantages
Separation and Identification of Superimposed Canals
Separation and identification of superimposed canals is necessary in all teeth that may contain two canals lying in a faciolingual plane. All teeth have this likelihood in at least one of their roots, except maxillary anterior teeth, which have one canal except in rare situations.

Movement and Identification of Superimposed Structures
Occasionally, a radiopaque object may overlie a root. An example is the zygomatic process, which often obscures the apices of maxillary molars. Because this dense structure lies facial to the roots, a mesial shift of the cone "pushes" the zygoma distally (Fig. 12.10). In addition, a decrease in vertical angulation of the cone "pushes" the zygoma superiorly.

Determination of Working Length
Individual superimposed canals may be traced from orifice to apex (Fig. 12.11).

Determination of Curvatures
The SLOB rule applies when determining curvatures. Depending on the direction of movement of the curvature relative to the cone, it can be determine whether this curvature is facial

or lingual. The severity of the curvature can also be determined.

Determination of Faciolingual Locations
The SLOB principle is applied to locating something on a root surface or within a canal. One example might be the site of a perforation or external resorption: to which surface does it extend, facial or lingual? Two radiographs at different horizontal angles readily disclose this (Fig. 12.12).

Identification of Undiscovered Canals
The SLOB procedure applies during access. An anatomic axiom is that *if a root contains only a single canal, that canal will be positioned close to the center of the root.* If a single canal is discovered initially on access preparation, an instrument is placed in the canal. Then a radiograph *must* be made either mesial or distal because another canal may be present. If the instrument is skewed considerably off center, another canal must be present (Fig. 12.13). The location of the missed canal is determined by applying the SLOB rule.

Location of "Calcified" Canals
Locating "calcified" canals also applies during access preparation. Another endodontic anatomic axiom is that *a root always contains a canal.* The canal may be very tiny, or it may be difficult or impossible to find or negotiate, but it is present. Also, canals are frequently not visible on radiographs. A single canal will lie in the center of the root. Therefore, when searching for an elusive canal by penetrating progressively deeper with a bur or an ultrasonic tip, occasionally two working radiographs must be made. One is made from the straight facial view and the other from either the mesial or distal view. The straight facial radiograph gives the mesiodistal location of the access penetration; the mesial- or distal-angled radiograph indicates the faciolingual angulation of the access preparation. The direction is adjusted accordingly toward the center of the root, where the canal surely lies (Fig. 12.14). Newer technologies, such as cone beam computed tomography (CBCT), may allow the identification of canals that could not be easily identified clinically (Fig. 12.15).

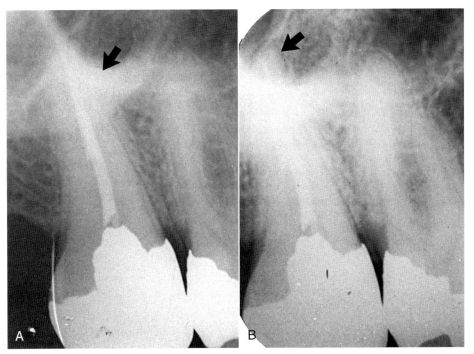

Fig. 12.10 **A,** Malar process of maxillary zygoma *(arrow)* obscures the apex and blocks the view of the obturation. **B,** Slight mesial shift of the cone "pulls" the lingually positioned root apex *(arrow)* to the mesial for visibility.

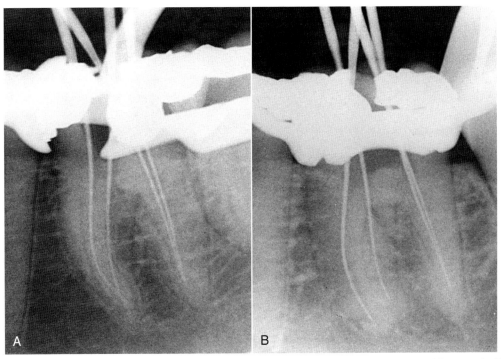

Fig. 12.11 **A,** Mesial project gives limited information about morphologic features and relationship of four canals. **B,** Correct distal projection for mandibular molars "opens up" roots. Mesial canals are easily visualized for their entire length. The distal canal is a single wide canal because instruments are close and parallel.

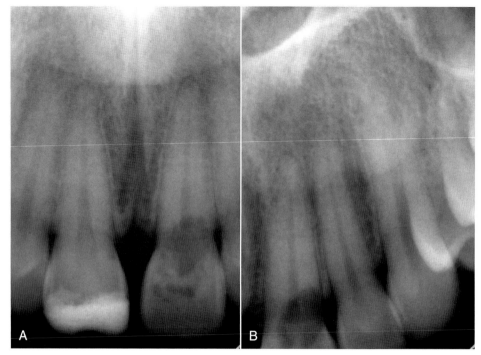

Fig. 12.12 **A,** Resorptive lesion is superimposed on the canal and appears to be external because the outline of the canal is still visible through a portion of it. **B,** Distal shift reveals a palatal extension of the resorptive defect because it has moved in the direction of the shift.

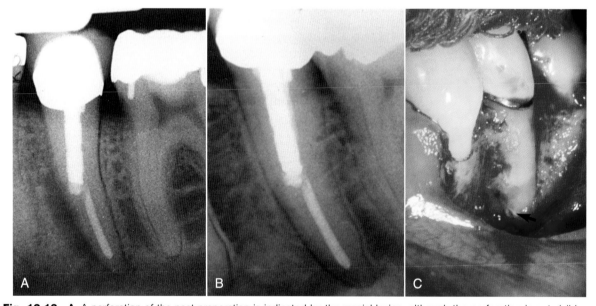

Fig. 12.13 **A,** A perforation of the post preparation is indicated by the mesial lesion, although the perforation is not visible on this facial projection. The perforation is visible toward the buccal or lingual aspect and is revealed on an additional angled radiograph. **B,** The tip of the post has moved slightly distal on this mesial projection, and the perforation therefore is located toward the buccal aspect (SLOB rule). **C,** The perforation site *(arrow)*.

Disadvantages

The cone-image shift has inherent problems and therefore on occasion should not be used, or the angulation of the cone should be minimized.

Decreased Clarity

The clearest radiograph with the most definition is a parallel or modified parallel projection.[23] When the central beam changes direction relative to object and film (passing through the object and striking the film at an angle), the object becomes blurred (Fig. 12.16). Distinctions between radiolucent and radiopaque objects show less contrast. This blurred or fuzzy appearance increases as the cone angle increases, and other structures are more likely to be superimposed. Therefore, for maximum clarity, the cone angle should deviate only to the extent necessary to obtain sufficient shift for interpretive purposes.

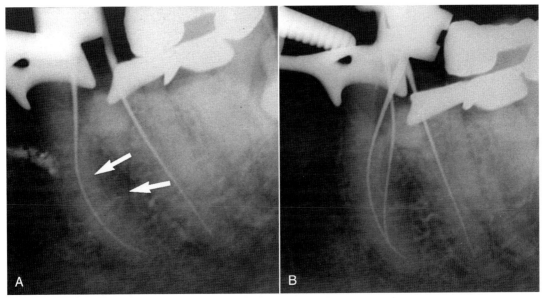

Fig. 12.14 Technique for locating a canal missed during access preparation and searching of the chamber. **A,** Distal radiograph with a single file in the mesial root shows the file skewed buccally. Therefore, another canal would be located toward the lingual aspect. The vertical radiolucent lines *(arrows)* are periodontal ligament spaces of the mesial root. **B,** A careful search toward the lingual aspect reveals the canal.

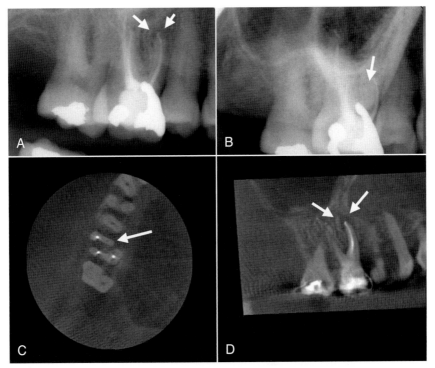

Fig. 12.15 **A,** Endodontically treated tooth #3 with possible periapical radiolucency related to the mesial buccal root. The patient is having recurrence of symptoms. **B,** Distal shift shows possible missed mesiolingual (MB2) canal in that root. **C,** Axial plane view on a CBCT shows the location of the missed canal. **D,** Clear view of the periapical radiolucency on the sagittal plane view of the CBCT.

Superimposition of Structures

Objects that ordinarily have a natural separation on parallel radiographs may, with cone shift, move relative to each other and become superimposed. One example is the roots of a maxillary molar. A parallel radiograph generally shows three separate roots and separate apices. A mesial- or distal-angled radiograph moves the palatal root over the distobuccal or mesiobuccal root, reducing the ability to distinguish the apices clearly (Fig. 12.17). Another example is an increase in the vertical angulation of the cone in the maxillary incisor region; this may "pull" the apices "into" the radiodense anterior nasal spine.

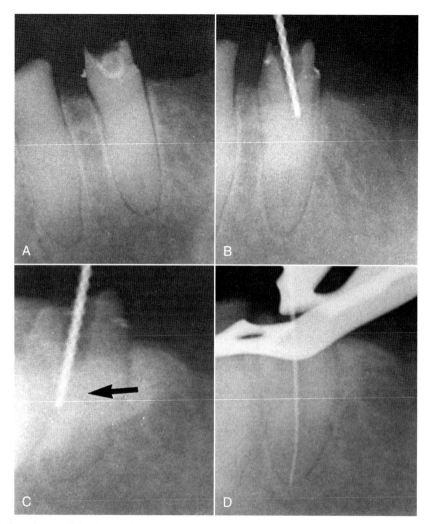

Fig. 12.16 Location of a canal that has undergone severe calcific metamorphosis. Initial searching is done without a rubber dam. **A,** A small, receded canal and missing crown make orientation and canal search difficult. **B,** Facial radiograph taken during access shows that preparation is mesial to the canal. (Remember, the canal occupies the center of the root.) **C,** Mesial radiograph shows that access is also misdirected to the buccal aspect; the canal is centered *(arrow)*. Therefore, the subsequent search must be to the distal and lingual aspects. **D,** When the bur is redirected, the single canal is discovered in the center of the root. Now the rubber dam is placed.

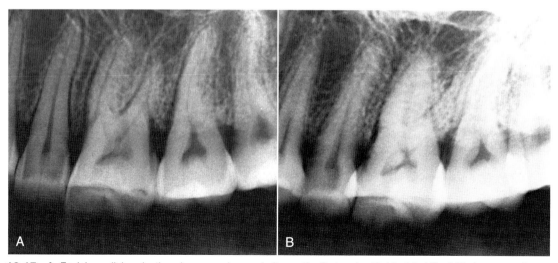

Fig. 12.17 **A,** Facial parallel projection shows maximum clarity on the first molar. **B,** Mesial shift of 30 degrees reduces contrast and the distinction between radiopaque and radiolucent objects. Also, roots are now superimposed, making interpretation more difficult.

ENDODONTIC RADIOGRAPHIC ANATOMY

Interpretation

Radiographs can be termed *the great pretenders;* they often are as misleading as they are helpful.[24,25] There is a definite tendency to try to extract more information from a radiograph than is present. The practitioner must remember that only hard tissues, not soft tissues, are visible. For example, pulpitis by itself is not associated with any radiographic changes. Thus a radiograph of a patient with irreversible pulpitis may not be helpful in diagnosing this condition, although it may reveal periapical bony changes, possible etiologic factors, possible internal or external resorption, and/or root canal anatomy.

Limitations

Studies of interpretation of bony lesions have shown that considerable bone must be resorbed before the lesion is clearly visible.[26,27] This, of course, varies with root location and thickness of the overlying cortical bone. In most regions, a periapical lesion tends to be most evident radiographically if cortical bone has resorbed. However, resorption of only medullary bone may be sufficient for visualization.[28,29] In either case, a periapical inflammatory lesion must be well developed and fairly extensive before an obvious radiolucency can be seen.

DIFFERENTIAL DIAGNOSIS

Endodontic Pathosis
Radiolucent Lesions

Radiolucent lesions have the following four distinguishing characteristics, which aid in differentiating them from non-endodontic pathoses (Fig. 12.18):

1. The apical/radicular lamina dura is absent, having been resorbed.
2. A "hanging drop of oil" shape is characteristic of the radiolucency, although this is a generalization because these lesions may have a variety of appearances.
3. The radiolucency "stays" at the apex, regardless of cone angulation.
4. A cause of pulpal necrosis is usually (but not always) evident.

A common concept is that an endodontic granuloma can be distinguished from a radicular cyst. The supposed differential is that the cyst is outlined radiographically by a "corticated" or radiopaque lamina. It has been demonstrated that this is *not* a reliable indicator.[30]

The ultimate differentiation is not the radiograph but the pulp test. If a developed, sizable radiolucency is an endodontic lesion, it *must* result from a necrotic (hence nonresponsive) pulp.

Radiopaque Lesions

Radiopaque lesions are better known as *condensing osteitis.* Such lesions have an opaque, diffuse appearance, and histologically they represent an increase in trabecular bone.[31] The radiographic pattern is one of diffuse borders and a roughly concentric arrangement around the apex (Fig. 12.19). Pulpal necrosis and a radiolucent inflammatory lesion may or may not be present. Frequently, condensing osteitis and apical peri-

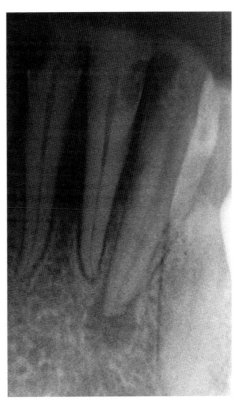

Fig. 12.18 Characteristics of apical radiolucency strongly suggest endodontic pathosis. Lamina dura is not present, and the lesion has a "hanging drop of oil" appearance. The cause of pulpal necrosis is also evident.

odontitis are present together. The pulp is often vital and inflamed.

Nonendodontic Pathosis
Radiolucent Lesions

Radiolucent lesions are varied but infrequent. Bhaskar lists 38 radiolucent lesions of the jaws, 35 of which are nonendodontic and have a variety of configurations and locations,[32] and many are positioned at or close to the apexes and radiographically mimic endodontic pathosis. Again, the pulp test provides the cardinal differentiation—nonendodontic lesions are associated with a responsive tooth. With previously endodontically treated teeth, the diagnosis may be challenging.[33] In these cases the practitioner should examine carefully the patient's medical history and assess for a possible endodontic etiology; the shape, location, and history of the radiolucency; associated unusual symptoms, such as numbness of the lip; and signs such as ulceration, soft tissue induration, or fixed lymph nodes.

Radiopaque Lesions

Frequently, interpretive errors are made in identifying radiopaque structures located in the apical region of the mandibular posterior teeth. Unlike condensing osteitis, these are not pathologic and have a more well-defined border and a homogeneous structure. They are not associated with pulpal pathosis (Fig. 12.20).

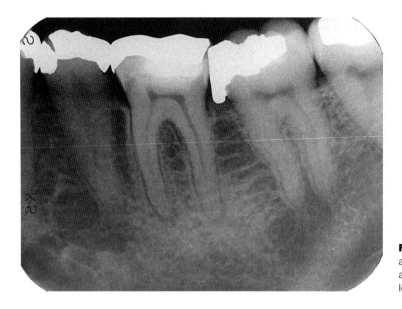

Fig. 12.19 Condensing osteitis. There is diffuseness and a concentric arrangement of increased trabeculation around the apex. Close inspection shows a radiolucent lesion at the apices also.

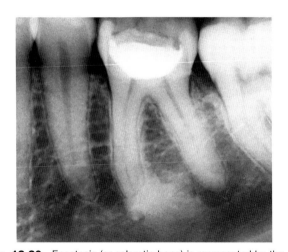

Fig. 12.20 Enostosis (or sclerotic bone) is represented by the dense, homogeneous, defined radiopacity. This is not pathosis and is common in the posterior mandible near the apices, although it may occur in any region. This radiodense area would have appeared on earlier radiographs.

Anatomic Structures

Several anatomic entities are superimposed on or may be confused with endodontic pathosis. Although most radiology courses cover identification of these structures, it is not uncommon for a practitioner to fail to identify these normal structures when there is an existing or suspected endodontic problem. Common sources of confusion are the areas created by sparse trabecular patterns, particularly in the mandible. Another problem area is the apical region of the maxillary anterior teeth. One must remember to look *through* these radiolucencies for an apical lamina dura.

Mandible

The classic example of a radiolucency that may overlie an apex is the mental foramen over a mandibular premolar.[34] This is easily identified by noting movement on angled radiographs and by identifying the lamina dura (Fig. 12.21).[35]

Maxilla

The maxilla region contains several structures (both radiolucent and radiopaque) that may be confused with endodontic pathosis. Examples are the maxillary sinus, incisive canals, nasal fossa, zygomatic process, and anterior nasal spine. As mentioned, the characteristics of the structure and pulp responsiveness to tests are important in differentiation.

SPECIAL TECHNIQUES

Bitewing Projections

Although not truly a "special technique," bitewing projections are often helpful in diagnosis and treatment planning. The relationships of film, cone, and tooth give a more consistent parallel orientation (Fig. 12.22).

Film/Sensor-Cone Placement
Film and Sensor Selection

Posterior packet film should be used for every projection in all patients except children. The anterior (narrow) films are unnecessary and in fact are frequently not wide enough to pick up an apex on an angled radiograph. Use of wider packet film obviously requires special placement for anterior projections (Fig. 12.23). The film type recommended for diagnostic radiographs is E (Ektaspeed) film.[36]

A charged couple device (CCD) or complementary metal-oxide semiconductor (CMOS) digital sensors generally follow the same dimensions as film except for width. Most sensors are bulky in thickness and therefore less comfortable for patients than film. It may be necessary to use the size 1 digital sensor in some situations to avoid gagging and permit reasonably parallel projections, more so than the equivalent sizes of film as discussed before. Alternatively, photostimulable phosphor (PSP) plates could be used. These have the exact same dimensions as film and require that the latent image be processed so that it can be recognized by the computer.

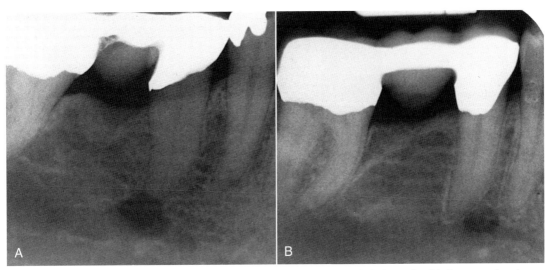

Fig. 12.21 **A,** Radiolucent area over the apex could be mistaken for pathosis. **B,** Pulp testing (vital response) and a more distal angulation show the radiolucency to be a buccally placed (SLOB rule) mental foramen.

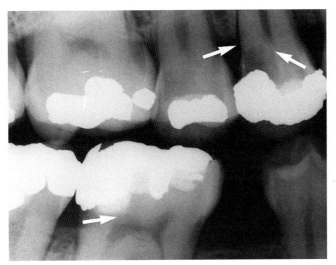

Fig. 12.22 Bitewing radiograph shows important features clearly: relationship of bone to gingival extent of caries *(arrows)* and depth of caries and restorations relative to the pulp *(lower arrow).* (Courtesy Dr. C. Koloffon.)

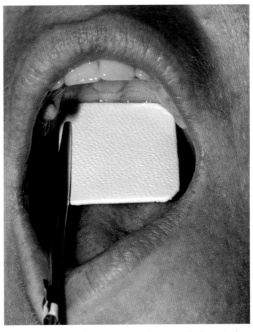

Fig. 12.23 Narrow palate requires placement of posterior packet film distally. Note that the superior edge of the film is distal to the tuberosities.

Film and Sensor Holders

Special adaptations of paralleling devices can be used for endodontic working films.[37] However, with some practice, nothing is more effective than a hemostat for ease and adaptability for film or sensor holders with tabs that allow hemostat positioning. The hemostat also is conveniently placed and sterilized in a kit with other instruments. The hemostat handle aligns the cone in both the vertical and horizontal planes (Fig. 12.24). Having the patient hold the film or sensor with direct finger pressure is discouraged. This is awkward and in the case of film, frequently results in a bent film with a distorted radiographic image (Fig. 12.25). *The film surface must remain flat.*

The hemostat-positioned film or sensor is placed by the operator. Then the patient holds the hemostat in the same position. The cone is aligned parallel to the hemostat in the frontal plane (vertical angulation; Fig. 12.26) and at 90 degrees to the handle (horizontal plane; Fig. 12.27). Because

the handle is at an angle of 90 degrees to the film surface, the central beam strikes the target surface at the same 90-degree angle. This is the modified parallel technique because the film or sensor often is not parallel to the tooth. However, with the modified parallel technique, distortion is minimal and is not significant in working radiographs.[14]

Holders are currently available that can allow sensors to be positioned in a paralleling or modified paralleling projection even with the dental dam in place (Fig. 12.28).

Film/Sensor Placement

Usually, films and sensors are positioned in the standard periapical projection. However, there are exceptions. Because of the relative narrowness of the arches, maxillary and **211**

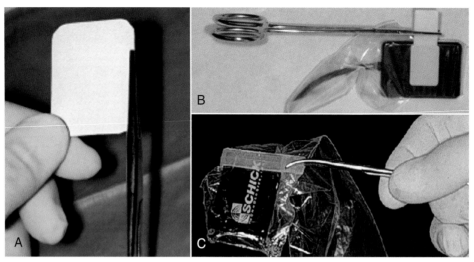

Fig. 12.24 **A,** A hemostat is used for grasping the film and as a cone positioning and orientation device. A hemostat holds an adhesive tab **(B)** and a plastic holder **(C)** of digital sensors.

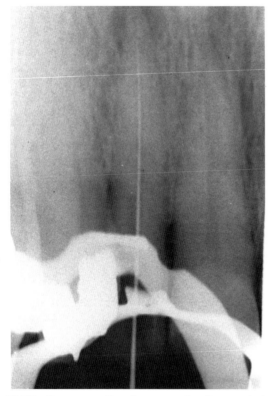

Fig. 12.25 Pressure on film often causes bending, producing a distorted image. This bent film "stretches" the apical half of the root, making accurate interpretation and length determination impossible.

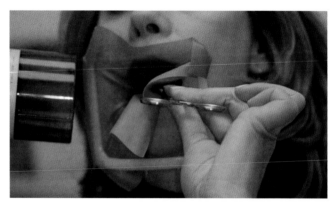

Fig. 12.26 Vertical angulation of the cone is set by aligning the long axis of the cone with the end of the hemostat handle.

mandibular anterior projections require film or sensor placement farther posteriorly.

In the maxillary posterior region, particularly when molars are imaged, the film or sensor is placed on the side of the median raphe opposite the teeth to be radiographed; this has the effect of positioning the top of the film in a more superior position relative to the apices (Fig. 12.29).

In the mandibular posterior region, the film or sensor is positioned toward the midline (under the tongue). Also, if the

mouth is closed slightly, the mylohyoid muscle relaxes and permits them to drop inferiorly.

The radiolucent dental dam frame is not removed during film placement. A lower corner or edge of the dental dam is released to allow insertion and positioning of the hemostat and film or sensor (see Fig. 12.26).

Cone Alignment
Indicated cone positions (facial, mesial, or distal) are discussed in the following sections (Figs. 12.30 and 12.31).

Facial Projection
Maxillary anterior teeth rarely have more than a single root and a single canal, thus only a facial (straight-on) projection is required. This is also true for maxillary molars unless a second mesiobuccal (mesiolingual) canal is detected and negotiated during access. The straight facial projection provides maximum resolution and clarity (which is difficult at best with maxillary molars).

Mesial Projection
The mesial projection is indicated for maxillary and mandibular premolars and for mandibular canine teeth. A mesial

To summarize, angled working radiographs are made for maxillary premolars and molars with a mesiolingual canal and for all mandibular teeth. The maxillary projections are mesial and the mandibular projections are as follows: incisor—distal, canine—mesial, premolar—mesial, and molar—distal. An acronym for the cone angles on the mandible is DMMD.

Digital Working Radiographs
The same principles apply as with conventional analogue working films, including similar positioning of both the cone and the image-capturing device. The charged storage phosphor system and the direct digital systems use a rigid sensor that can be positioned and then held in place with the patient's finger. A preferred approach is to use a simple device that has been developed specifically for digital sensors. It is a tab with a sticky portion that attaches to the sensor. An extending tab end can be held with a hemostat. The cone is then aligned using the handle of the hemostat, as previously described.

Rapid Processing
With the conventional analogue technique, there are special approaches, and solutions are available for fast processing (less than 1 minute) of working films; this may be beneficial for speed viewing. However, if these rapid processing techniques are used, films may not retain their quality with time unless they are thoroughly fixed and washed.[38] Therefore, if a film is to be processed rapidly, a double-packet film should be used, with the duplicate processed in the routine manner.

Extraoral Film/Cone Positioning
Some patients cannot tolerate radiographs intraorally, usually because of gagging problems. Acceptable diagnostic and working films can be obtained with special positioning of the film and cone (Fig. 12.32).[39]

NEW TECHNOLOGY

New approaches to radiography have been and are being developed. These approaches are unique, and some will improve existing techniques in addition to reducing the radiation dose to patients. This new technology includes digital radiography, digital subtraction radiology, and tomography.[40-42]

Digital Radiography
A variety of digital radiographic systems have been compared, although none has been shown to be significantly superior in image quality.[43] These systems are of considerable interest, offering the advantages of reduced radiation to the patient, increased speed of obtaining the image, ability to be transmitted, computer storage and enhancement, and a system that does not require a darkroom or x-ray processor.[44] However, these systems generally show no superiority to conventional radiographs for diagnosis or working films.[45-50] Furthermore, computer image enhancement does not seem to improve diagnostic interpretation significantly.[51]

Cone Beam Computed Tomography
CBCT is a form of computed tomography in which only a focused, cone-shaped beam of x-rays is projected at the imaged tissues. The diameter of the exposed tissues ranges from 40×40 mm to 170×120 mm (or more in certain

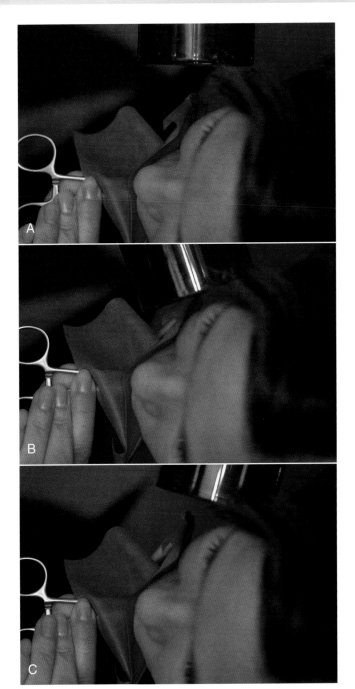

Fig. 12.27 Horizontal angulation is determined by looking down from the top of the patient's head. **A,** The position is set by aligning the long axis of the cone (central beam) 90 degrees to the long axis of the hemostat handle. Mesial **(B)** and distal **(C)** horizontal angulations are then varied accordingly.

projection is used for maxillary molars to identify and treat a mesiolingual (MB2) canal.

Distal Projection
The distal projection is used for mandibular incisors and mandibular molars. The distal is preferred to the mesial projection for mandibular molars because of the relative position of the canals. In general, the distal angle more effectively "opens up" the mesial root.

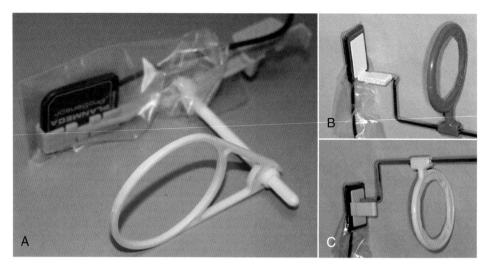

Fig. 12.28 A, Sensor holder that allows sensor placement in a paralleling device with the dental dam in place. The other side of the holder has a tab that allows the patient to bite for positioning when the dental dam is removed. B and C, XCP-style holders with adhesive to the sensor.

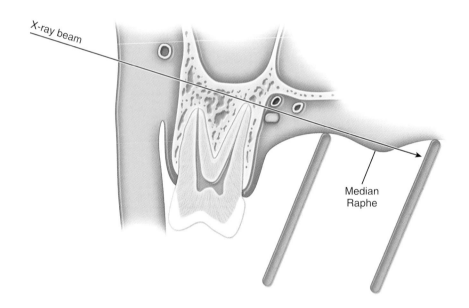

X-ray beam

Median Raphe

Fig. 12.29 Positioning the film on the opposite side of the median raphe has the effect of "pulling" the upper edge of the film more superior relative to the apices.

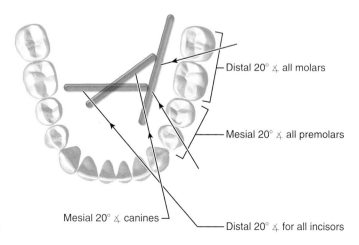

Distal 20° ⅄ all molars

Mesial 20° ⅄ all premolars

Mesial 20° ⅄ canines

Distal 20° ⅄ for all incisors

Fig. 12.30 Correct film-cone placement on the mandible.

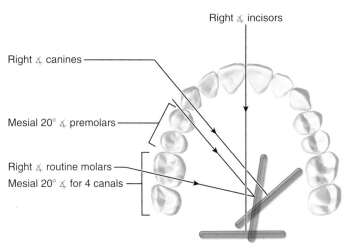

Right ∡ incisors

Right ∡ canines

Mesial 20° ∡ premolars

Right ∡ routine molars
Mesial 20° ∡ for 4 canals

Fig. 12.31 Correct film-cone placement on the maxilla.

machines); however, the limited volume significantly reduces the amount of radiation compared with traditional computed tomography. Moreover, the resolution of the CBCT image volume can be as low as 76 μm, which allows visualization of very small objects, such as difficult to find canals (see Fig. 12.15). Although the radiation exposure from one periapical digital radiograph is estimated to be equivalent to 1 day of background radiation, the exposure from a CBCT image varies from 0.7 to 8 days, and equivalent exposure from a full mouth series of F-speed film is about 21 days.[52-54]

Because CBCT provides 3D imaging, it is very useful in special situations. Examples are diagnosis of and treatment planning for teeth with a complex anatomy or extensive resorptive lesions (Fig. 12.33). In cases in which previous

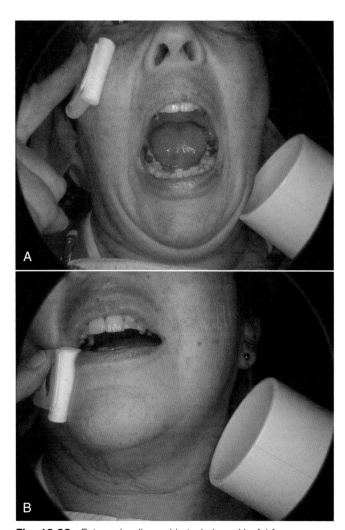

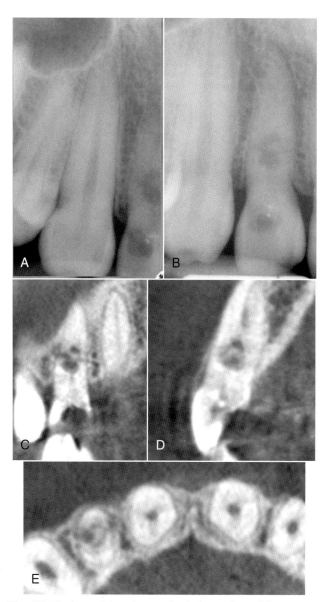

Fig. 12.32 Extraoral radiographic technique. Useful for gaggers, this technique involves placing the film or sensor on the cheek. Increasing the exposure time is usually necessary. **A,** Maxillary posterior: cone is positioned −45 degrees to the occlusal plane. **B,** Mandibular posterior: cone is positioned −35 degrees.

Fig. 12.33 Large internal resorptive lesion and possible perforation. **A** and **B,** Conventional radiographs with two angles did not provide enough information on the extent of the lesion. CBCT imaging in the coronal **(C),** sagittal **(D),** and axial **(E)** planes provides important additional information for treatment planning.

treatment was not successful, there is a need to identify the etiology of failure and to determine whether retreatment or surgery is more appropriate (see Fig. 12.15). This is also useful in assessing the diagnosis or treatment outcome if the patient has symptoms but no apparent etiology can be determined. The sensitivity of CBCT is higher than that of periapical radiography in detecting periapical lesions[55,56] and identifying vertical root fractures.[57] CBCT is also superior to digital radiographs in assessing healing (lesion resolution) on follow-up examination.[56] In addition, it is useful for identifying and localizing bony structures, such as the mandibular canal.[58]

All available clinical diagnostic tests and conventional imaging modalities are used before CBCT is selected, so as to conform to the "as low as reasonably achievable" (ALARA) principle. Routine use of CBCT for all cases or for all cases in which previous treatment may require retreatment or surgery is not justified at this time.[59]

REFERENCES

1. Bengtsson G: Maxillo-facial aspects of radiation protection focused on recent research regarding critical organs, *Dentomaxillofac Radiol* 7:5, 1978.
2. Danforth R, Torabinejad M: Estimated radiation risks associated with endodontic radiography, *Endod Dent Traumatol* 6:21, 1990.
3. Torabinejad M, Danforth R, Andrews K, et al: Absorbed radiation by various tissues during simulated endodontic radiography, *J Endod* 15:249, 1989.
4. Berry J: Oral and maxillofacial radiology arrives; first new dental specialty in 36 years, *Am Dent Assoc News* 30:1, 1999.
5. Walton R: Endodontic radiographic techniques, *Dent Radiogr Photogr* 46:51, 1973.
6. Lambrianidis T, Lyroudia K, Pandelidou O, et al: Evaluation of periapical radiographs in the recognition of C-shaped mandibular second molars, *Int Endod J* 34:458, 2001.
7. Serman N, Hasselgren G: The radiographic incidence of multiple roots and canals in human mandibular premolars, *Int Endod J* 25:234, 1992.
8. Sion A, Kaufman B, Kaffe I: The identification of double canals and double rooted anterior teeth by Walton's projection, *Quintessence Int* 15:747, 1984.
9. Tamse A, Kaffe I, Fishel D: Zygomatic arch interference with correct radiographic diagnosis in maxillary molar endodontics, *Oral Surg Oral Med Oral Pathol* 50:563, 1980.
10. Stein TJ, Corcoran JF: Radiographic "working length" revisited, *Oral Surg Oral Med Oral Pathol* 74:796, 1992.
11. Zakariasen K, Scott D, Jensen J: Endodontic recall radiographs: how reliable is our interpretation of endodontic success or failure and what factors affect our reliability? *Oral Surg Oral Med Oral Pathol* 57:343, 1984.
12. Slowey R: Radiographic aids in the detection of extra root canals, *Oral Surg Oral Med Oral Pathol* 37:762, 1974.
13. Bhakdinaronk A, Manson-Hing LR: Effect of radiographic technique upon prediction of tooth length in intraoral radiography, *Oral Surg Oral Med Oral Pathol* 51:100, 1981.
14. Forsberg J: Radiographic reproduction of endodontic "working length" comparing the paralleling and the bisecting-angle techniques, *Oral Surg Oral Med Oral Pathol* 64:353, 1987.
15. Klein R, Blake S, Nattress B, et al: Evaluation of x-ray beam angulation for successful twin canal identification in mandibular incisors, *Int Endod J* 30:58, 1997.
16. Kersten H, Wesselink P, VanVelzen T: The diagnostic reliability of the buccal radiograph after root canal filling, *Int Endod J* 20:20, 1987.
17. Eckerbom M, Magnusson T: Evaluation of technical quality of endodontic treatment: reliability of intraoral radiographs, *Endod Dent Traumatol* 13:259, 1997.
18. Kleier D, Benner S, Averbach R: Two dental x-ray films compared for rater preference using endodontic views, *Oral Surg Oral Med Oral Pathol* 59:201, 1985.

19. Brown R, Hadley J, Chambers D: An evaluation of Ektaspeed Plus film versus Ultraspeed film for endodontic working length determination, *J Endod* 24:54, 1998.
20. Kullendorff B, Petersson K, Rohlin M: Direct digital radiography for the detection of periapical bone lesions: a clinical study, *Endod Dent Traumatol* 13:183-189, 1997.
21. Folk RB, Thorpe JR, McClanahan SB, et al: Comparison of two different direct digital radiography systems for the ability to detect artificially prepared periapical lesions, *J Endod* 31:304-306, 2005.
22. Richards AG: The buccal object rule, *Dent Radiogr Photogr* 53:37, 1980.
23. Biggerstaff RH, Phillips JR: A quantitative comparison of paralleling long-cone and bisection-of-angle periapical radiography, *Oral Surg Oral Med Oral Pathol* 41:673, 1976.
24. Goldman M, Pearson AH, Darzenta N: Endodontic success: who's reading the radiograph? *Oral Surg Oral Med Oral Pathol* 33:432, 1972.
25. Reit C, Hollender L: Radiographic evaluation of endodontic therapy and the influence of observer variation, *Scand J Dent Res* 91:205, 1983.
26. Bender I, Seltzer S: Roentgenographic and direct observation of experimental lesions of bone, *J Am Dent Assoc* 62:153, 1961.
27. Schwartz S, Foster J: Roentgenographic interpretation of experimentally produced bony lesions. I, *Oral Surg Oral Med Oral Pathol* 32:606, 1971.
28. Pitt Ford T: The radiographic detection of periapical lesions in dogs, *Oral Surg Oral Med Oral Pathol* 57:662, 1984.
29. Lee S, Messer H: Radiographic appearance of artificially prepared periapical lesions confined to cancellous bone, *Int Endod J* 19:64, 1986.
30. Ricucci D, Mannocci F, Ford T: A study of periapical lesions correlating the presence of a radiopaque lamina with histological findings, *Oral Surg Oral Med Oral Pathol Oral Radiol Endod* 101:389, 2006.
31. Maixner D, Green T, Walton R, et al: Histologic examination of condensing osteitis, *J Endod* 18:196, 1992 (abstract).
32. Bhaskar SN: *Radiographic interpretation for the dentist*, ed 6, St Louis, 1981, Mosby.
33. Nevins A, Ruden S, Pruden P, et al: Metastatic carcinoma of the mandible mimicking periapical lesion of endodontic origin, *Endod Dent Traumatol* 4(5):238-239, 1988.
34. Phillips JL, Weller RN, Kulild JC: The mental foramen. II. Radiographic position in relation to the mandibular second premolar, *J Endod* 18:271, 1992.
35. Fishel D, Buchner A, Hershkowith A, et al: Roentgenologic study of the mental foramen, *Oral Surg Oral Med Oral Pathol* 41:682, 1976.
36. Powell-Cullingford A, Pitt Ford T: The use of E-speed film for root canal length determination, *Int Endod J* 26:268, 1993.

37. Gound T, DuBois L, Biggs S: Factors that affect rate of retakes for endodontic treatment radiographs, *Oral Surg Oral Med Oral Pathol* 77:514, 1994.
38. Pestritto ST: Comparison of diagnostic quality of dental radiographs produced by five rapid processing techniques, *J Am Dent Assoc* 89:353, 1974.
39. Newman M, Friedman S: Extraoral radiographic technique: an alternative approach, *J Endod* 29:419, 2003.
40. Hedrick R, Dove SB, Peters D, et al: Radiographic determination of canal length: direct digital radiography versus conventional radiography, *J Endod* 20:320, 1994.
41. Pascon E, Introcaso J, Langeland K: Development of predictable periapical lesion monitored by subtraction radiography, *Endod Dent Traumatol* 3:192, 1987.
42. Kullendorf B, Grondahl K, Rohlin M, et al: Subtraction radiology of interradicular bone lesions, *Acta Odontol Scand* 50:259, 1992.
43. Almeida S, Oliveira A, Ferreira R, et al: Image quality in digital radiographic systems, *Braz Dent J* 14:2, 2003.
44. Baker W, Loushine R, West L, et al: Interpretation of artificial and in vivo periapical bone lesions comparing conventional viewing versus a video conferencing system, *J Endod* 26:39, 2000.
45. Akdeniz B, Sogur B: An ex vivo comparison of conventional and digital radiography for perceived image quality of root fillings, *Int Endod J* 38:397, 2005.
46. Bhaskaran V, Qualtrough A, Rushton VE, et al: A laboratory comparison of three imaging systems for image quality and radiation exposure characteristics, *Int Endod J* 38:645, 2005.
47. Kositbowornchai S, Hanwachirapong D, Somsopon R, et al: Ex vivo comparison of digital images with conventional radiographs for detection of simulated voids in root canal filling material, *Int Endod J* 30:287, 2006.
48. Burger C, Mork T, Hutter J, et al: Direct digital radiography versus conventional radiography for estimation of canal length in curved canals, *J Endod* 25:260, 1999.
49. Holtzmann D, Johnson W, Southard T, et al: Storage-phosphor computed radiography versus film radiography in the detection of pathologic periradicular bone loss in cadavers, *Oral Surg Oral Med Oral Pathol* 86:90, 1998.
50. Sullivan J, Di Fiore P, Koerber A: radiovisiography in the detection of periapical lesions, *J Endod* 26:32, 2000.
51. Scarfe W, Czerniejewski W, Farman A, et al: In vivo accuracy and reliability of color-coded image enhancements for the assessment of periradicular lesion dimensions, *Oral Surg Oral Med Oral Pathol Oral Radiol Endod* 88:603, 1999.
52. Ludlow JB, Davies-Ludlow LE, Brooks SL, et al: Dosimetry of three CBCT devices for oral and maxillofacial radiology, *Dentomaxillofac Radiol* 35:219-226, 2006.
53. White SC, Pharoah MJ: *Oral radiology: principles and interpretation*, St Louis, 2009, Mosby.

54. American Association of Endodontists: Cone beam computed tomography, *Endodontics: Colleagues for Excellence* [newsletter], summer 2011, Chicago, 2011, The Association.

55. de Paula-Silva FW, Wu MK, Leonardo MR, et al: Accuracy of periapical radiography and cone-beam computed tomography scans in diagnosing apical periodontitis using histopathological findings as a gold standard, *J Endod* 35(7):1009-1012, 2009.

56. Patel S, Wilson R, Dawood A, et al: The detection of periapical pathosis using digital periapical radiography and cone beam computed tomography. Part 1. Preoperative status, *Int Endod J* 45:702, 2012.

57. Edlund M, Nair MK, Nair UP: Detection of vertical root fractures by using cone-beam computed tomography: a clinical study, *J Endod* 37(6):768-772, 2011.

58. Kim T, Caruso J, Christensen H, et al: A comparison of cone-beam tomography and direct measurement in the examination of the mandibular canal and adjacent structures, *J Endod* 36:1191, 2010.

59. American Association of Endodontists and American Academy of Oral and Maxillofacial Radiology: Joint position statement of the American Association of Endodontists and the American Academy of Oral and Maxillofacial Radiology: use of cone-beam computed tomography in endodontics, *Oral Surg Oral Med Oral Pathol Oral Radiol Endod* 111(2):234-237, 2011.

Endodontic instruments

Van T. Himel, Kent A. Sabey

LEARNING OBJECTIVES

After reading this chapter, the student should be able to:

1. Define a basic set of instruments appropriate for diagnosis, emergency treatment, canal preparation, obturation, and bleaching.
2. Describe the general physical properties of endodontic instruments and show how these characteristics are related to their use.
3. Describe the basic design (longitudinal, cross-sectional, and tip configuration) of the more common canal preparation instruments and their mode of use.
4. Explain the basis for sizing and taper (standardization) of hand-operated instruments.
5. Describe and differentiate between conventional files and files of alternative designs.
6. Define the differences between stainless steel and

nickel-titanium intracanal instruments, including physical properties and usage characteristics.
7. Describe the action and use of rotary instruments for both cleaning and shaping canals.
8. Describe the proper use of instruments to prevent breakage within the canal.
9. Recognize visible changes that predispose instruments to breakage.
10. Describe techniques for sterilization and disinfection of instruments.
11. Select appropriate sterilization methods for each instrument type.
12. Identify procedures and chemicals that might cause deterioration of files and explain how to recognize such deterioration.

This text is directed toward the basics of clinical endodontics; therefore, the instruments described in this chapter are not all inclusive. A clinician's knowledge of the purpose, composition, design, function, proper technique, safety guidelines, and maintenance for each instrument is critical to treatment success. Using the correct instrument for each step is a basic rule for success and prevention of procedural errors.

Some hand instruments are common to many dental procedures (mirror, explorer, spoon excavator), but others have been designed to adapt to the requirements of root canal treatment. Originally, these instruments were few in number and crude in design.[1] Early hand-operated files had long handles that were best suited for preparation of anterior teeth. As root canal treatment diversified, smaller "finger" instruments were developed for posterior teeth. In addition to being more adaptable, these provided improved tactile sense for the operator.[2] As hand-operated instruments underwent changes, mechanized instruments, such as rotary, reciprocating, and ultrasonic devices, were finding their way into the specialty. New instrument designs continue to evolve (and to be marketed),

always with the hope of improving efficiency and treatment outcomes.

This chapter reviews a basic armamentarium for various procedures and systems for effective sterilization. The different designs of endodontic intracanal instruments are introduced, including types of metals and important aspects of their physical properties and usage characteristics. Detailed information about all aspects of manufacturing and testing of intracanal instruments is beyond the scope and intent of this chapter; however, certain essential facts, as identified in the learning objectives, are presented to enable effective instrument use (and prevent abuse).

INSTRUMENTS FOR DIFFERENT PROCEDURES

Examination and Diagnosis Kit

A basic kit for examination and diagnosis includes items found in routine restorative kits, such as a cassette to hold instruments during sterilization and storage, mouth mirror, general purpose explorer, and periodontal probe. Cotton

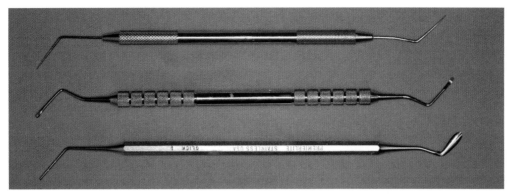

Fig. 13.1 Specialized endodontic instruments. *Top,* D16 explorer. *Center,* 31L spoon excavator. *Bottom,* Glick #1. The plugger end *(left)* is for heating and removal of gutta-percha; the paddle *(right)* is for placing temporary materials.

forceps are used for various functions during the exam procedure, including holding cotton pellets for cold testing or cotton rolls when controlling moisture for electric pulp tests.

Although not necessarily considered instruments, other materials usually required are isolation materials: gauze, cotton rolls, Dri-Angles, a rubber dam, cotton pellets, occlusion paper, bite stick, wooden stick or Tooth Slooth, evacuation devices (high speed and saliva ejector), and devices for radiographs.

Routine Endodontic Procedure Kit

Instruments for local anesthesia, radiographs, isolation, endodontic access, and length determination are described in other chapters. For the majority of visits in which routine endodontic therapy (cleaning, shaping, and obturation) is delivered, a kit includes any special instruments, in addition to those in the examination and diagnosis kit mentioned previously.

A number of instruments have been specially adapted for endodontics (Fig. 13.1). For example, the DL16 explorer is double ended and has long, tapered tines at varying angles to the handle. Explorers should never be heated. Debris is removed from the pulp chamber and canals with a specialized spoon excavator, which has an extra-long shank compared to the more standard spoon used in restorative dentistry. The Glick #1 instrument has a "paddle" end (for placement of materials such as temporary restorations) and a "plugger" end (for removal or condensation of gutta-percha). The plugger end may be heated. The rod-shaped plugger may have markings to indicate 5-mm increments. Other root canal long-shanked pluggers (flat end) and spreaders (pointed end) are used during placement of various materials into root canal systems.

Specific techniques for these instruments are discussed in other chapters of this text. For other aspects of many procedures, a spatula, millimeter ruler, device for holding files, scissors, hemostats, bur block with burs, and syringes (anesthetic and irrigation) are usually included.

A common method of irrigating canals, called "needle irrigation," usually uses a 5- or 10-cc Luer-Lok syringe with a 27- to 30-gauge needle. The safest needle delivery method uses a non-open-ended device that is side vented and/or closed ended, causing the irrigant to be expressed laterally, thus reducing the risk of apical extrusion.[3]

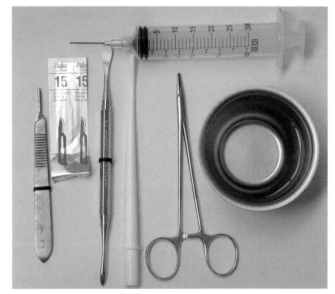

Fig. 13.2 Basic emergency kit for an incision for drainage includes (1) scalpel handle and (2) blade, (3) periosteal elevator, (4) suction tip, (5) needle holder, (6) irrigating syringe with an 18-gauge needle, and (7) sterile saline. A rubber dam drain is a frequent addition.

Sonic or ultrasonic agitation devices, negative apical pressure systems (EndoVac),[4] and laser photon-initiated photoacoustic streaming (PIPS)[5] have been shown to provide improved effectiveness in some situations. The scope of this chapter does not allow full descriptions of all these devices and methods.

Emergency Kit

Required instruments are dictated by diagnosis. Procedures may vary and may include pulpotomy, pulpectomy, occlusal adjustment, or incision for drainage of an acute apical abscess.

Most emergency situations can be managed with a typical examination or routine procedure kit. If an incision for drainage is required, other devices should be available: scalpel handle and blade; periosteal elevator; small, curved hemostat; latex drain, needle holder, suture material, 25-cc irrigation syringe, 18-gauge irrigation needle, sterile saline, and surgical suction tip (Fig. 13.2).

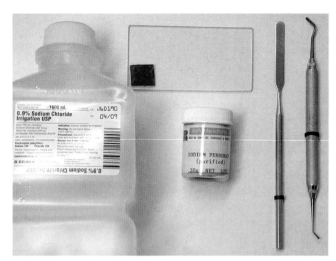

Fig. 13.3 Equipment for internal bleaching. Sterile saline for mixing with sodium perborate. Spatula for mixing and plastic instrument for paste and temporary placement.

Instruments for Bleaching

Instruments for bleaching are included with the cleaning and shaping tray, with the addition of the paste ingredients and a plastic instrument (Fig. 13.3). The plastic instrument is used to place the bleaching mixture (usually sodium perborate and sterile water) in the pulp chamber, followed by a temporary restoration.

INTRACANAL PREPARATION INSTRUMENTS

The purpose of canal preparation (cleaning and shaping) is to mechanically debride and allow chemical disinfection, followed by sealing of the spaces. Shaping of the canals is partially dictated by the method of obturation to be used. Various instruments have been designed to reduce risks while increasing efficiency and effectiveness. The clinician must become knowledgeable about the materials, design principles, and manufacturer's recommendations for the instruments.

To mechanically debride a region of the canal space completely, an instrument must contact and plane all walls.[6] Despite continual improvements in design and physical properties, there are still no instruments or techniques that totally mechanically prepare and shape all root canal spaces.[7] Irregular spaces do not correspond to, and cannot always be well prepared by, an instrument with a regular (round) shape. These incongruences between reality and ideal shape require judicious and skillful use of canal preparation instruments to maximize debridement while avoiding procedural errors.[8]

Other instrument systems are activated using ultrasonic or sonic energy and are diverse in design. Some resemble barbed broaches or files, and others are diamond-coated wires. All insert into a dedicated vibratory handpiece that energizes the instrument. Again, none of these special designs or techniques has been shown to be superior in achieving treatment outcomes.

Physical Properties

Currently two basic categories of metal are used to construct root canal–shaping instruments: stainless steel and nickel-titanium. Individual compositions of the metals and handling during fabrication vary among manufacturers, resulting in instruments with different properties. Many of these changes are proprietary knowledge. The clinician should select the instrument type based on the physical properties needed for the procedure (e.g., stiffness, flexibility, cutting efficiency, memory, durability) and cost.[9]

Stainless steel instruments are primarily composed of carbon, iron, and nickel (traces of manganese [Mn], chromium [Cr], and molybdenum [Mo] may be added to achieve specific properties). Stainless steel instruments are relatively inflexible, which renders them less adaptable to canal curvatures.

New metal alloys have been incorporated to attempt to improve the quality of files. Nickel-titanium instruments are composed of approximately 55% nickel and 45% titanium, which can vary by manufacturer. Besides specific elemental content, during the manufacturing process variables are manipulated, such as temperature or heating and cooling phases, resulting in instruments with significantly different properties. Nickel-titanium instruments are more flexible and adapt more readily to fine, curved canals[10] but have no advantage over stainless steel files in straight and irregular canal spaces.[11-13]

Nickel-titanium does not conform to the normal rules of metallurgy. Because it is a superelastic metal, external stresses transform the austenitic crystalline form of nickel-titanium into the martensitic crystalline structure, which can accommodate greater stress without increasing the strain.

Due to the unique crystalline structure and phase-change capability of nickel-titanium, most of these files have shape memory; that is, they are able return to their original shape after being deformed. This is an important ability; shape memory gives nickel-titanium alloys the flexibility and toughness necessary for routine use as effective rotary endodontic files in curved canals.[14] Nevertheless, when torsional strength was tested, stainless steel proved more resistant than nickel-titanium to fracture by twisting.[9,15]

Besides traditional Ni-Ti instruments, alterations of composition, processing, and design have led to other new "models," including M-Wire (Dentsply, Tulsa, Oklahoma), CM wire (DS Dental, Johnson City, Tennessee), and the Twisted File (Sybron, Culver City, California). It has been shown that by controlling the memory of nickel-titanium, the number of cycles to fracture increased three to five times.[16] Nickel-titanium has been adapted for both hand instruments and rotary applications, and many designs have been developed.

Instrument Fabrication

Recent developments with metal composition and processing allow files to be fabricated from a blank wire by grinding, twisting, or a combination of these processes. This process can be highly variable between brands and results in different instrument designs, physical characteristics, and working properties.[17] A "ground" instrument is produced by placing a blank wire in a lathe and grinding it to a specific design (e.g., stainless steel Hedstrom files [Fig. 13.4] and stainless steel K-type files [Fig. 13.5]). K-type files are made by twisting or grinding a square or triangular tapered wire to form cutting edges along the length of the shaft (Fig. 13.6).

To produce a twisted file, one end of the blank is fixed in a lathe, and the other end is allowed to rotate until the desired

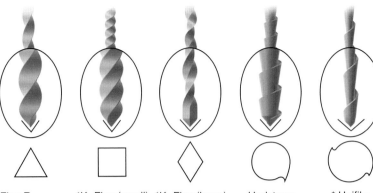

Fig. 13.4 Longitudinal and cross-sectional shapes of various hand-operated instruments. Note that small sizes of K-reamers, K-files, and the K-Flex have a different shape than the larger sizes.

*Flex R
K–Reamer
(large)
K–File (large)

*K–Flex (small)
K–Reamer
(small)
K–File (small)

*K–Flex (large)

Hedstrom

* Unifile
* S–File

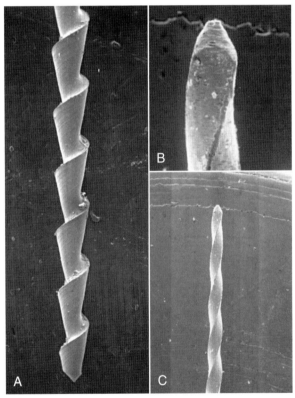

Fig. 13.5 A, Hedstrom file, machined by rotating a wire on a lathe. Note the spiral shape. These are efficient cutters (on the pull stroke) but are more susceptible to separation when locked and twisted. **B** and **C,** A machined K-type file. Note that the transition angle at the leading edge of the tip is rounded, rendering it noncutting.

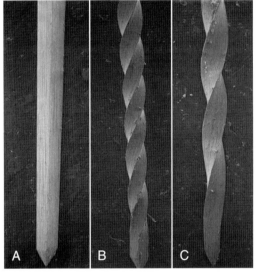

Fig. 13.6 Ground-twisted instruments. **A,** A square file blank ground from wire. After counterclockwise twisting, the appearance of a file (more flutes **[B]**) and a reamer (fewer flutes **[C]**).

design shape is achieved. A ground-twisted wire is fabricated by first grinding a wire into tapered geometric blanks of various shapes (square, triangular, rhomboid) and then twisting it to produce helical cutting edges.

Physical Characteristics

Several factors inherent to stainless steel and nickel-titanium wire instruments must be considered. How is adequate flexibility maintained without instrument fatigue? How much

abuse can the files endure before fatigue and failure ensue? When has a file been fatigued to a critical point? How can an efficient cutting edge be maintained while avoiding the creation of new, nonanatomic canal spaces? Although these metals may have different physical properties and different use characteristics, both can fatigue and separate when used incorrectly.[7]

Nickel-titanium alloy has a modulus of elasticity that is one-fourth to one-fifth that of stainless steel, allowing a wide range of elastic deformation.[18] An advantage of this increased flexibility is that a file can better follow a canal curvature with less deformation (transportation) during enlargement.

Materials researchers and manufacturers hold various theories about file properties, such as "flexibility may be increased by increasing length or decreasing cross-sectional diameter" and "a more acute cutting angle can mean more efficient substance removal by a blade."[19,20] Bench-top research has identified certain important limits to specific physical properties and incorporated these findings into a series of standards for the manufacture of instruments. However, clinical behavior may not directly relate to such in vitro testing.[21]

221

Instrument nomenclature follows International Organization for Standardization (ISO). Hand-operated instruments include K-type reamers and files, broaches, and Hedstrom-type files. Other instruments can be engine-driven, thus have a latch that inserts into a slow-speed handpiece. These include rotary (Gates-Glidden and Peeso) engine-driven reamers and files, and reciprocating files or reamers.

American National Standards/American Dental Association (ANSI/ADA) specification No.101 has established torsional standards for all nickel-titanium and stainless steel rotary instruments.[22] The term *torsional limits* refers to the amount of rotational torque that can be applied to a "locked" instrument to the point of breakage (separation). Obviously, an instrument should have sufficient strength to be rotated and reasonably worked without separating.[23,24] *Fatigue* also occurs as a file is rotating in a curved canal. For this reason, rotary files should never rotate in a canal for more than a few seconds, especially if no movement to withdraw occurs. Under cyclic fatigue test conditions, nickel-titanium files have increased resistance to fracture compared with stainless steel files.[24]

Efforts to enhance the properties of nickel-titanium alloy are ongoing; it has been demonstrated that altering surface characteristics and the process of manufacturing may increase the durability and flexibility of these instruments. Electropolishing, surface coatings, and surface implantation have been used for this purpose.[25,26]

Sharpness and corrosion resistance are properties related to metal and design. Traditional metals have included stainless or carbon steel. Although these are similar in some respects, many carbon steel instruments have been shown to cut somewhat more efficiently than stainless steel instruments.[27] However, carbon steel is no longer used because it is more susceptible to corrosion caused by autoclaving and irrigating solutions.[28]

Instrument Design and Standardization

Many variables in the design of instruments can affect their function, efficacy, and efficiency. By changing the cross-sectional design from square to triangular or rhomboid and decreasing the number of flutes per millimeter, greater flexibility is gained. To improve the consistency of treatment, the ADA has established several specifications (No. 28, 58, 95, and 101) that cover various types of instruments and characteristics such as dimensions, stiffness, corrosion resistance, acceptable tolerances in manufacturing, color code, taper, tip geometry, size, fatigue resistance, and torsional resistance.[22,29-33]

Despite reported sizes and shapes, it should be noted that hand-operated instruments do not demonstrate reliable and consistent dimensional standardization. This should always be a consideration when preparing canal spaces.[34]

Color Coding

Color coding of file handles designates size, thereby simplifying instrument selection during treatment (Fig. 13.7). Stripes on the file shank, which vary in number, color, and location, indicate the size and taper of many rotary instruments. Color coding may vary according to the manufacturer.

Dimensions

Dimensions of files and reamers are designated according to the diameters of the instrument at specified positions along its

File #	D0 diameter (in mm)	Handle Color
06	0.06	
08	0.08	
10	0.10	
15	0.15	
20	0.20	
25	0.25	
30	0.30	
35	0.35	
40	0.40	
45	0.45	
50	0.50	
55	0.55	
60	0.60	
70	0.70	
80	0.80	
90	0.90	
100	1.00	
110	1.10	
120	1.20	
130	1.30	
140	1.40	

Fig. 13.7 Color coding specifications for standardization of files and reamers.

length (ADA specification No. 28) (Fig. 13.8). File tip diameters increase in 0.05-mm increments up to size 60 files (0.60 mm at D0), and then by 0.10-mm increments up to size 140.

The spiral cutting edge of the instrument has traditionally been at least 16 mm long, and the diameter at the end of the cutting edges is D16. A considerable number of variations exists, and several brands have shorter lengths of cutting edges. This decrease allows a narrower shank and increased flexibility.

Length

Files are usually available in many lengths, the most common being 21, 25, and 31 mm. The shorter instruments afford improved operator control and easier access to posterior teeth, where limited opening can impair access. The appropriate length should be selected based on the location of the tooth in the mouth, access, and individual root length.

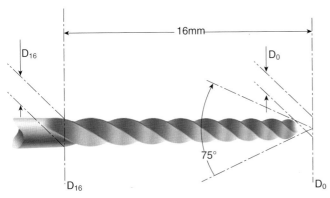

Fig. 13.8 Specifications for standardization of files and reamers.

Taper

Taper can be defined as the rate of change of cross-sectional diameter. A file with a taper of 0.02 (2%) increases in diameter at a rate of 0.02 mm per running millimeter of length beginning at D0 through D16. Likewise, a file with a taper of 0.04 (4%) increases in diameter at a rate of 0.04 mm per running millimeter of length beginning at D0 through D16. For example, a 0.02 taper No. 20 file is 0.20 mm in diameter at D0, tapers 0.32 mm over 16 mm, and has a diameter of 0.52 mm at D16.

Files may have constant, variable, or no taper along their length, depending on the instrument's design. Hand stainless steel files are traditionally 0.02 (2%) taper, whereas nickel-titanium files are available in many tapers (e.g., 0.00, 0.02, 0.04, 0.06). Files with greater taper create canal preparations with increased flaring; however, these have not been demonstrated to be superior.[35] The choice of file taper is driven by the provider's preference, the root canal anatomy, and the demands of the desired root canal preparation shape.

Tip Design

Early files had a 75-degree tip angle that was meant to provide cutting efficiency without an excessively sharp transition angle. Today's instruments have tips that vary from sharp to noncutting (see Fig. 13.5, *B*); noncutting tips may involve less engagement of dentin than sharp tips. The intent is to "guide" the file through the curve rather than cutting only the outer canal wall.[36,37]

As the tip area transitions into the cutting area, instruments incorporate a design feature called a *land*. When the instrument is rotated, the cutting edges plane the canal wall while the land area adds strength and keeps the instrument centered; this centering is important in fine, curved canals.[10,38]

Hand-Operated Instruments

Barbed broaches are stainless steel instruments with plastic handles. Manufacturers create barbs on tapered wire broaches by scoring and prying a tag of metal away from the long axis of the wire (Fig. 13.9). The barbs entangle and allow removal of canal contents. This instrument should be neither bound in the canal nor aggressively forced around a canal curvature because the barbs may engage the canal wall, resulting in instrument fracture. Barbed broaches should never be reused. The use of broaches has decreased in popularity.

Besides their configuration, a difference between files and reamers is their intended use. For root canal preparation, two

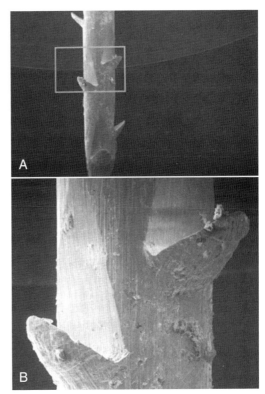

Fig. 13.9 A barbed broach showing the barbs pulled away from the instrument shaft.

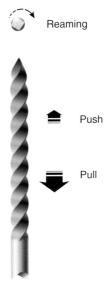

Fig. 13.10 Filing and reaming motions. Tooth structure is removed primarily on the pull stroke with filing and on rotation with reaming.

types of motion are common, reaming and filing (Fig. 13.10).[39] Files can be effective when used in both filing (pulling and planing) and reaming (twisting and cutting) motions; reamers are least effective when used in a filing motion.

The reamer configuration is achieved by creating fewer twists; this results in increased flute spacing, which tends to prevent clogging of the cutting edge.[40] In use, reamers are twisted and withdrawn; therefore, cutting occurs during **223** rotation. This motion consists of rotating the instrument clockwise in a preexisting hole or patent canal and scribing an arc from one cutting edge to the next.

Files are manipulated with a rasping, or push-pull planing motion. This is more efficient when there are many flutes or spirals making contact with the canal walls. First, the instrument is advanced to its full length using a passive "twiddling" (teasing without planing) motion. Next, the file is rotated (a quarter turn or more) and then withdrawn from the canal space while the tip is pushed firmly against a wall, much as a paintbrush is applied to a wall when painting. The twiddling, reaming, and withdrawal motions are repeated with the file tip pushed against a different portion of the canal wall on each outstroke until all walls have been planed (circumferential filing).

Hedstrom files and files of a similar design (S or U files) are used only with a filing motion; they are very effective at smoothing walls. Hedstrom-type files are more prone to separation because of their decreased cross-sectional core diameter compared to equivalent-sized instruments of other designs; they should not be used with a reaming motion, which would introduce torsional stress and fracture.

Mechanically Operated Instruments

Mechanically operated instruments (e.g., rotary, reciprocating, vibratory, and lasers) can introduce several additional actions in the canal space to assist in the shaping procedure.

Rotary

Some preparation techniques require slow-speed rotary instruments to facilitate preparation, primarily in establishing straight-line access (Fig. 13.11) or in flaring the coronal third of the canal spaces. These instruments are variable in length

and usually fabricated from stainless steel, although some are available in nickel-titanium.

Gates-Glidden rotary drills are elliptical (flame-shaped) burs with a thin shank and latch attachment; they are used to open the orifice. They also achieve straight-line access by removing the dentin shelf and rapidly flaring the coronal third of the canal. Gates-Glidden drills are designed to break high in the shank region. This allows easier removal of the broken instrument from a tooth; fracture near the cutting head may block a canal.[33,41,42] It is important to note that these drills must be continuously rotated. If they stop, the head may lock in the canal, resulting in torsional failure and fracture.

Peeso rotary reamers (originally designed for post preparation) are similar to Gates-Glidden drills but have longer cutting sides with or without safe tips, which are parallel rather than elliptical in shape. Peeso reamers have been suggested as a means of improving straight-line access, although they are less well-controlled than Gates-Glidden drills.[42]

Gates-Glidden and Peeso instruments are aggressive and can rapidly overenlarge a canal. Their use should be restricted to orifice opening and initial coronal flaring. Both are available in various sizes (Table 13.1) and lengths.

Lentulo spirals are twisted wire instruments used in a slow-speed handpiece (Fig. 13.12) to spin pastes (e.g., calcium hydroxide preparations), sealers, or cements into canal spaces. They must be used passively to avoid screwing into canals, "throwing" quantities of unset material beyond the apical foramen, and separation.

Many *engine-driven nickel-titanium files* used for canal preparation rely on rotational motion, a reaming action, which affords substantial control in small, curved canals. These instruments are usually designed without an actively cutting tip and have less tendency to transport the apical preparation.[43,44] The files are available in a large variety of shapes, designs, and material composition (Fig. 13.13). Use of these instruments by dental students in laboratories has demonstrated fewer preparation errors compared with the use of stainless steel hand instruments.[45-47]

One innovative nickel-titanium instrument, the rotary Lightspeed (Fig. 13.14), incorporates three distinct features: a noncutting pilot tip; a small, paddle-shaped cutting area (fabricated in a "stamping" process); and a relatively thin, flexible shaft. These instruments tend to stay centered in curved canals and allow for larger apical preparation sizes.[10,48-50]

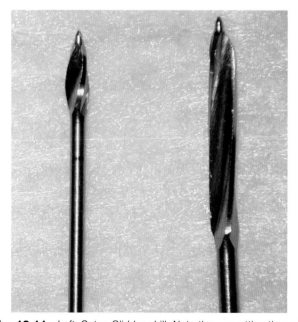

Fig. 13.11 *Left,* Gates-Glidden drill. Note the noncutting tip and the elliptical shape. *Right,* Peeso reamer. Note the noncutting "safe" tip and parallel sides. These are stiffer and more aggressive than the Gates-Glidden drill. Both are used for straight-line access preparation.

Table 13.1	Rotary flaring instruments*	
Size	**Gates-Glidden drills**	**Peeso reamers**
No. 1	0.4 mm	0.7 mm
No. 2	0.6 mm	0.9 mm
No. 3	0.8 mm	1.1 mm
No. 4	1.0 mm	1.3 mm
No. 5	1.2 mm	1.5 mm
No. 6	1.4 mm	1.7 mm

*Size varies by manufacturer.

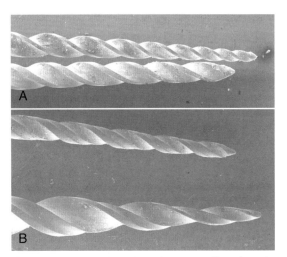

Fig. 13.13 Examples of nickel-titanium rotary files of varying design. **A,** 0.04 and greater taper (GT) titanium files (ProFile). **B,** Quantec files. Note the aggressive taper of the file on the bottom.

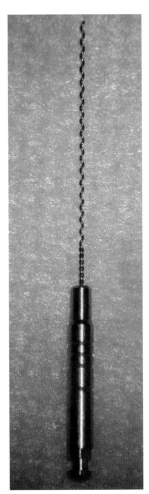

Fig. 13.12 The Lentulo spiral drill is used to spin calcium hydroxide into canals.

Reciprocating

Recent innovations include systems that use a mechanically operated reciprocal filing motion rather than the traditional complete rotary motion. Studies are ongoing regarding the potential advantages, efficacy, and safety of such instrument systems.[51]

Vibratory

Another mechanically driven instrument motion is vibratory (ultrasonic or sonic) motion. The intent is to create instrument motion and activity with sonic or ultrasonic frequencies. A variety of tips and configurations are available for conservatively removing dentin during apical root-end preparations and for searching for and negotiating small canals.

Lasers

Lasers have been introduced for root canal preparation, with mixed results. Currently, the most promise seems to be in disinfection.[5]

Avoidance of Instrument Separation

Signs that instrument separation may occur are *unwinding* of the flutes (clockwise twisting and opening of the flutes), *roll-up* of the flutes (excessive continued clockwise twisting after unwinding), tip distortion (excessively bent tip), wear, and corrosion (Fig. 13.15). If any of these signs are observed, the file should be discarded.

Each instrument is engineered and designed to be used at a specific rotational speed and with a suggested amount of maximum torque. The manufacturer of the nickel-titanium rotary files suggests using them in high-torque, slow-speed handpieces that rotate at 150 to 500 rpm.

Studies have suggested that lower speeds reduce the likelihood of instrument fracture.[52-54] Fig. 13.16 shows instrument fatigue, roll-up, and breakage of nickel-titanium instruments after use in canals. Preflaring (passive step-back) of canals has been shown to allow more uses of rotary instruments before separation.[54]

The Lightspeed nickel-titanium instruments are also used in high-torque, slow-speed handpieces at 750 to 2,000 rpm. Within this limit, faster rotational speed does not appear to increase the likelihood of fracture.[55] If fracture should occur, these instruments are designed to fracture at the most coronal aspect. The number of canals that can be prepared with any nickel-titanium instrument varies, depending on the size and curvature of the canals and the pressure used with the files. The smaller and more curved the canal, the more wear and tear. Files must be discarded if any deformation occurs. Some manufacturers suggest and label their files as "single use only" or "single patient use."

INTRACANAL OBTURATION INSTRUMENTS

After cleaning, shaping, disinfection, and drying, the canal spaces are hermetically sealed. Most techniques require the placement of sealer prior to, or in conjunction with, the main obturation material. The sealer can be applied in several ways, such as with an endodontic file or spreader, a paper point, or a Lentulo spiral; by injection; or with gutta-percha cone.

Once the sealer has been properly applied in the canal spaces, any of various acceptable obturation methods can be used. Depending on the selected materials and technique, the required armamentarium may vary. The basic instruments used for two common techniques, cold lateral compaction and warm vertical compaction, are described here.

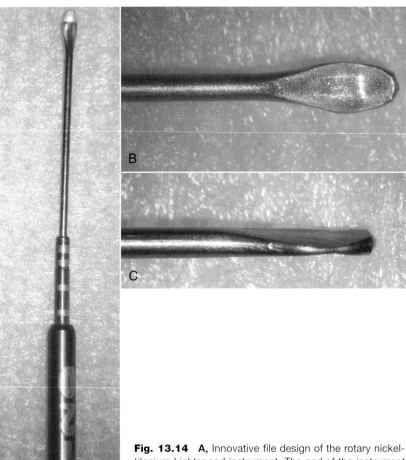

Fig. 13.14 **A,** Innovative file design of the rotary nickel-titanium Lightspeed instrument. The end of the instrument does the work, and the noncutting tip and small, flexible shaft tend to stay centered during preparation of the canal. **B** and **C,** Magnified views of the tip of the Lightspeed instrument.

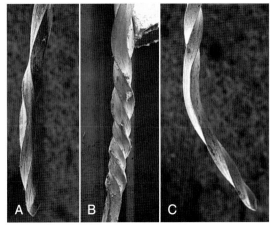

Fig. 13.15 Defects created during instrumentation. Each file shown must be discarded because of possible breakage. **A,** Unwinding of the flutes. **B,** "Roll-up" of the flutes. **C,** Unwound and bent instrument.

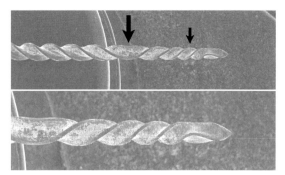

Fig. 13.16 Overused rotary nickel-titanium files showing "roll-up" *(small arrow)*, and "unwinding" *(large arrow)*.

Lateral Compaction

The main instrument used for cold lateral compaction is the spreader, which is used to laterally compact and adapt gutta-percha and create space for accessory cones. Two types of spreaders are handled spreaders and finger spreaders (Fig. 13.17). The handled instruments, made of annealed stainless steel, are stiffer.

As with canal preparation instruments, spreaders come in various tip sizes and tapers. Standard spreaders increase diameter at the same rate as a file with 0.02 taper; highly tapered spreaders increase at a higher rate. The greater the taper, the more the canal space must be enlarged or flared to facilitate spreader penetration.

Both stainless steel and nickel-titanium spreaders are available. The obvious advantage of nickel-titanium over stainless

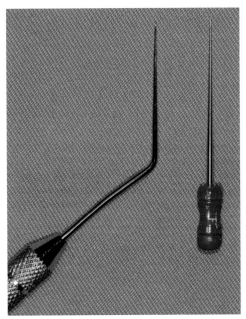

Fig. 13.17 D11 handled spreader *(left)* and a fine finger spreader *(right)*. Both are designed for lateral condensation. The finger spreader (or plugger) is more versatile and safer.

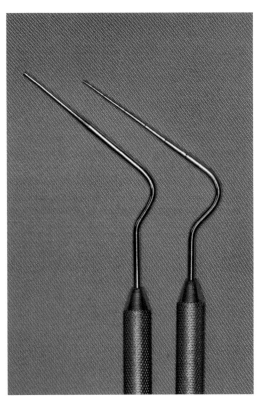

Fig. 13.19 Heat transfer *(left)* and condenser (heater-plugger) *(right)* for vertical condensation of gutta-percha.

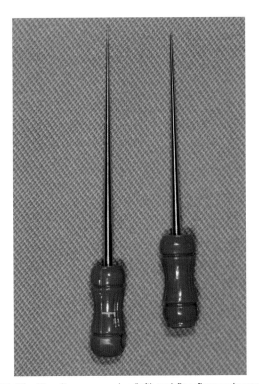

Fig. 13.18 Fine finger spreader *(left)* and fine finger plugger *(right)*. The two are used similarly for lateral condensation. Spreaders are pointed, and pluggers are flat at the tip.

steel is greater spreader penetration in highly curved canals.[56] Nickel-titanium spreaders also create less stress in curved canals compared with stainless steel.[57] Handled instruments are capable of generating more force within a canal space during obturation, so finger spreaders should be considered when obturating curved canals (Fig. 13.18). All spreaders should be used cautiously with regard to the amount of applied force.

Warm Vertical Compaction

For warm vertical condensation, instruments can be divided into two categories: those that transfer heat to the gutta-percha, and those that compact the gutta-percha (pluggers) (Fig. 13.19). In this procedure, the filling material is alternately heated and then vertically compacted with pluggers. These pluggers are available in sets of varying sizes, which allows an appropriate fit in the various diameters of the prepared canal space. The pluggers push softened gutta-percha filling material into all the crevices of a canal space. Care must be taken in this process because warming of the material may result in less apical control than with lateral condensation.

If an obturation method requires the application of heat, this can be done either manually with a heated plugger (e.g., the Glick #1) or with other pluggers suitably sized for the prepared canal. Also available are several electronic devices that automatically generate heat along the portion of the instrument that will enter the canal space. These heat-generation devices have device-specific tips with sizes and tapers that correspond to the size and taper of the shaped canal space or the obturation technique.

Most pluggers also have handles; however, finger pluggers may be used in lieu of handled instruments. Pluggers are usually available in sets and may be single ended or double ended, depending on the manufacturer. In the apical portions of the canal, smaller diameter instruments are required. In the more coronal aspects, larger diameter pluggers function best to compact the obturation material vertically.

After the "down-packing" of the warmed gutta-percha, the remaining unfilled canal space can be obturated effectively and efficiently with warmed, injectable gutta-percha.

Some manufacturers offer a combination system: a heat source device with a method of injecting warm gutta-percha into a single unit. There are also cordless or battery-operated devices for most obturation functions that can facilitate space restrictions and efficiency. These are transferable between treatment rooms.

Other obturation techniques include carrier-based and injection methods. Every instrument cannot be described here. Likewise, new sealers and specific obturation materials and techniques are continually being introduced, some of which may require a specialized armamentarium specific to that material or method of obturation. There is considerable marketing of these devices and materials, and frequently no substantive data or clinical testing is available to verify claims of effectiveness.

DISINFECTION AND STERILIZATION

The term *clean* indicates that an object is visibly free of debris, stain, or potential contaminants. *Disinfection* is an attempt, to any degree, to reduce microbial contamination; this may not necessarily result in an object being sterile. A *sterile* object is completely free of all bacteria, viruses, fungi, or other living organisms.

Files and other instruments are likely contaminated, even when new. Sterilization is recommended prior to initial or subsequent use. During endodontic procedures, instruments are exposed to and may retain blood, soft and hard tissue remnants, and viruses and bacteria and their byproducts. Therefore, they must be cleaned and disinfected and then sterilized.

As procedures are ongoing, surface disinfection and cleaning of instruments can be performed with a gauze or sponge soaked in 70% isopropyl alcohol or other approved solution. Instruments can be wiped thoroughly or files can be thrust briskly in and out of a sponge to dislodge debris and contact the disinfectant. This cleans but does not sterilize the instrument.

Ideally, all instruments should be able to withstand heat sterilization. For objects that cannot be sterilized, disposable or "single-use" items are recommended. To facilitate organization, sterilization, and storage of instruments, the use of commercially available cassettes is helpful for larger examination and procedure kits. Fewer instrument numbers, such

as for emergencies or bleaching, may be managed with bagging.

Different sterilization techniques are available. A few concepts are presented here. For a complete discussion of sterilization principles, techniques, and protocols, the reader should consult a textbook or manual on the subject.

Cold sterilization requires that objects be immersed for a sufficient period in solutions (e.g., glutaraldehyde), usually for at least 24 hours. Because this method is not verifiable with biologic indicators, it is the least desirable.

A common method of sterilizing all files and other endodontic hand instruments is the steam or chemical autoclave. Instruments that have been wrapped in gauze should be autoclaved for 20 minutes at 121°C and 15 psi.[58] This kills all bacteria, spores, and viruses.

Pressure sterilizers using a chemical rather than water have the advantage of causing less rusting. However, both steam and chemical autoclaving dull the edges of all cutting instruments, owing to expansion with heat and contraction with cooling, resulting in some degree of permanent edge deformation.

Dry heat is superior for sterilizing sharp-edged instruments, such as scissors, to best preserve their cutting edge. The time cycle for dry heat sterilization is temperature dependent. After the temperature reaches 160°C, the instruments should be left undisturbed for 60 minutes. The disadvantage of this method is the substantial time required, both for sterilization and subsequently for cooling. If the temperature falls below 160°C, the full 60-minute heat cycle must be repeated.[58]

There is some debate as to which method is most effective for sterilizing endodontic files. Most studies use nickel-titanium rotary files.

Several papers agree that although cleaning files is difficult, it can be done effectively with adequate attention to detail. Perhaps the best protocol would include mechanical, chemical, and ultrasonic cleaning of instruments.[59,60] Others have demonstrated that if an ultrasonic bath is used, the files should be placed loosely within the unit[61] or that perhaps a nanobased foam product could be beneficial.[62]

There is also some debate about whether these instruments can actually be adequately sterilized between uses; some suggest that they be considered single-patient use only.[63,64] Each manufacturer has guidelines for each instrument type.

Certain physical properties of some nickel-titanium rotary files are unaffected by sterilization processing.[65-67] The effects of the disinfection and sterilization processes on some physical properties have not been tested. Therefore, caution should be exercised when using files in a multiple-use protocol.

REFERENCES

1. Weinberger B: *An introduction to the history of dentistry*, St Louis, 1948, Mosby.
2. Luks S, Bolatin L: The myth of standardized root canal instruments, *N Y J Dent* 43:109, 1973.
3. Vinothkumar TS, Kavitha S, Gomathi LLNS, et al: Influence of irrigating needle tip designs in removing bacteria inoculated into instrumented root canals measured by single tube luminomitor, *J Endod* 33:746-748, 2007.
4. Nielsen B, Baumgartner C: Comparison of the EndoVac system to needle irrigation of root canals, *J Endod* 33:611-615, 2007.
5. Peters OA, Bardsley S, Fong J, et al: Disinfection of root canals with photon-initiated photoacoustic streaming, *J Endod* 37:1008-1012, 2011.
6. Walton RE: Histologic evaluation of different methods of enlarging the pulp canal space, *J Endod* 2:304, 1976.
7. Peters OA, Laib A, Goering TN, et al: Changes in root canal geometry after preparation assessed by high-resolution computed tomography, *J Endod* 27:1-6, 2001.
8. Peters OA: Current challenges and concepts in the preparation of root canal systems: a review, *J Endod* 30:559, 2004.
9. McSpadden JT: *Mastering endodontic instruments*, Chattanooga, Tenn, 2007, Cloudland Institute.
10. Short JA, Morgan LA, Baumgartner JC: A comparison of canal centering ability of four instrumentation techniques, *J Endod* 23:503, 1997.
11. Peters OA, Peters CI, Schönenberger K, et al: ProTaper rotary root canal preparation: effects of canal anatomy on final shape analyzed by micro CT, *Int Endod J* 36:86, 2003.
12. Peters OA, Schönenberger K, Laib A: Effects of four Ni-Ti preparation techniques on root canal geometry assessed by micro computed tomography, *Int Endod J* 34:221, 2001.

13. Rhodes JS, Pitt Ford TR, Lynch JA, et al: A comparison of two nickel-titanium instrumentation techniques in teeth using micro computed tomography, *Int Endod J* 33:279, 2000.

14. Kazemi RB, Stenman E, Spangberg LW: A comparison of stainless steel and nickel-titanium H-type instruments of identical design: torsional and bending tests, *Oral Surg Oral Med Oral Pathol Oral Radiol Endod* 90:500-506, 2000.

15. Kazemi RB, Stenman E, Spångberg LSW: Machining efficiency and wear resistance of NiTi endodontic files, *Oral Surg Oral Med Oral Pathol Oral Radiol Endod* 81:596, 1996.

16. Shen Y, Qian W, Abtin H, et al: Fatigue testing of controlled memory wire nickel-titanium rotary instruments, *J Endod* 37:997-1001, 2011.

17. Braga LC, Magalhaes RR, Nakagawa RK, et al: Physical and mechanical properties of twisted or ground nickel-titanium instruments, *Int Endod J* 46:458, 2012.

18. Walia HM, Brantley WA, Gerstein H: An initial investigation of the bending and torsional properties of nitinol root canal files, *J Endod* 14:346, 1988.

19. Miserendino LJ, Moser JB, Heuer MA, et al: Cutting efficiency of endodontic instruments. Part I. A quantitative comparison of the tip and fluted regions, *J Endod* 11:435, 1985.

20. Miserendino LJ, Moser JB, Heuer MA, et al: Cutting efficiency of endodontic instruments. Part II. Analysis of tip design, *J Endod* 12:8, 1986.

21. Zinelis S, Magnissalis EA, Margelos J, et al: Clinical relevance of standardization of endodontic file dimensions according to the ISO 3630-1 specification, *J Endod* 28:367, 2002.

22. American Dental Association: *American National Standard/American Dental Association specification no. 101, root canal instruments: general requirements*, Chicago, 2001, The Association.

23. Seto BG, Nicholls JI, Harrington GW: Torsional properties of twisted and machined endodontic files, *J Endod* 16:355, 1990.

24. Yared GM, Bou Dagher FE, Machtou P: Cyclic fatigue of ProFile rotary instruments after clinical use, *Int Endod J* 33:204, 2000.

25. Lee DH, Park B, Saxena A, et al: Enhanced surface hardness by boron implantation in nitinol alloy, *J Endod* 22:543, 1996.

26. Rapisarda E, Bonaccorso A, Tripi TR, et al: Wear of nickel-titanium endodontic instruments evaluated by scanning electron microscopy: effect of ion implantation, *J Endod* 27:588-592, 2001.

27. Oliet S, Sorin SM: Cutting efficiency of endodontic reamers, *Oral Surg Oral Med Oral Pathol* 36:243, 1973.

28. Mueller HJ: Corrosion determination techniques applied to endodontic instruments: irrigating solutions systems, *J Endod* 8:246, 1982.

29. American Dental Association Council on Dental Materials: New American Dental Association specification No. 28 for endodontic files and reamers, *J Am Dent Assoc* 93:813, 1976.

30. American Dental Association Council on Dental Materials Instruments and Equipment: Revised ADA specification No. 28 for endodontic files and reamers, *J Am Dent Assoc* 104:506, 1982.

31. American National Standards Institute/American Dental Association: Specification No. 58 for root canal files, type H (Hedstrom), *J Am Dent Assoc* 104:88, 1982.

32. American Dental Association Council on Dental Materials Instruments and Equipment: Revised ANSI/ADA specification No. 28 for root canal files and reamers, type K and No. 58 for root canal files, type H (Hedstrom), *J Am Dent Assoc* 118:239, 1989.

33. American Dental Association: *American National Standard/American Dental Association specification No. 95, root canal enlargers*, Chicago, 2003, The Association.

34. Stenman E, Spangberg LS: Root canal instruments are poorly standardized, *J Endod* 19:327, 1993.

35. Peters OA, Barbakow F, Peters CI: An analysis of endodontic treatment with three nickel-titanium rotary root canal preparation techniques, *Int Endod J* 37:849, 2004.

36. Powell SE, Simon JH, Maze BB: A comparison of the effect of modified and nonmodified instrument tips on apical canal configuration, *J Endod* 12:293, 1986.

37. Card SJ, Sigurdsson A, Orstavik D, et al: The effectiveness of increased apical enlargement in reducing intracanal bacteria, *J Endod* 28:779, 2002.

38. Kosa DA, Marshall G, Baumgartner JC: An analysis of canal centering using mechanical instrumentation techniques, *J Endod* 25:441, 1999.

39. Webber J, Moser JB, Heuer MA: A method to determine the cutting efficiency of root canal instruments in linear motion, *J Endod* 6:829, 1980.

40. Felt RA, Moser JB, Heuer MA: Flute design of endodontic instruments: its influence on cutting efficiency, *J Endod* 8:253, 1982.

41. Luebke NH, Brantley WA: Torsional and metallurgical properties of rotary endodontic instruments. Part 2. Stainless steel Gates Glidden drills, *J Endod* 17:319, 1991.

42. Luebke NH, Brantley WA, Sabri ZI, et al: Physical dimensions, torsional performance, and metallurgical properties of rotary endodontic instruments. Part 3. Peeso drills, *J Endod* 18:13, 1992.

43. Coleman CL, Svec TA: Analysis of Ni-Ti versus stainless steel instrumentation in resin simulated canals, *J Endod* 23:232, 1997.

44. Kuhn WG, Carnes DL Jr, Clement DJ, et al: Effect of tip design of nickel-titanium and stainless steel files on root canal preparation, *J Endod* 23:735, 1997.

45. Himel VT, Ahmed KM, Wood DM, et al: An evaluation of nitinol and stainless steel files used by dental students during a laboratory proficiency exam, *Oral Surg Oral Med Oral Pathol Oral Radiol Endod* 79:232, 1995.

46. Pettiette MT, Metzger Z, Phillips C, et al: Endodontic complications of root canal therapy performed by dental students with stainless-steel K-files and nickel-titanium hand files, *J Endod* 25:230, 1999.

47. Baumann MA, Roth A: Effect of experience on quality of canal preparation with rotary nickel-titanium files, *Oral Surg Oral Med Oral Pathol Oral Radiol Endod* 88:714, 1999.

48. Glossen CR, Haller RH, Dove SB, et al: A comparison of root canal preparations using Ni-Ti hand, Ni-Ti engine-driven, and K-Flex endodontic instruments, *J Endod* 21:146, 1995.

49. Pruett JP, Clement DJ, Carnes DL Jr: Cyclic fatigue testing of nickel-titanium endodontic instruments, *J Endod* 23:77, 1997.

50. Ramirez-Salomon M, Soler-Bientz R, de la Garza-Gonzalez R, et al: Incidence of Lightspeed separation and the potential for bypassing, *J Endod* 23:586, 1997.

51. Gambarini G, Rubini AG, Al Sudani D, et al: Influence of Different angles of reciprocation on the cyclic fatigue of nickel-titanium endodontic instruments, *J Endod* 38:1408, 2012.

52. Gabel WP, Hoen M, Steiman HR, et al: Effect of rotational speed on nickel-titanium file distortion, *J Endod* 25:752, 1999.

53. Schrader C, Peters OA: Analysis of torque and force with differently tapered rotary endodontic instruments in vitro, *J Endod* 31:120, 2005.

54. Roland DD, Andelin WE, Browning DF, et al: The effect of preflaring on the rates of separation for 0.04 taper nickel-titanium rotary instruments, *J Endod* 28:543, 2002.

55. Martin B, Zelada G, Varela P, et al: Factors influencing the fracture of nickel-titanium rotary instruments, *Int Endod J* 36:262, 2003.

56. Berry KA, Loushine RJ, Primack PD, et al: Nickel-titanium versus stainless-steel finger spreaders in curved canals, *J Endod* 24:752, 1998.

57. Joyce AP, Loushine RJ, West LA, et al: Photoelastic comparison of stress induced by using stainless-steel versus nickel-titanium spreaders in vitro, *J Endod* 24:714, 1998.

58. Council on Dental Therapeutics: Sterilization or disinfection of dental instruments. In the American Dental Association: *Accepted dental therapeutics*, ed 40, Chicago, 1984, The Association.

59. Popovic J, Gasic J, Zivkoyic S, et al: Evaluation of biological debris on endodontic instruments after cleaning and sterilization procedures, *Int Endod J* 43:336-341, 2010.

60. Parashos P, Linsuwanont P, Messer HH: A cleaning protocol for rotary nickel-titanium endodontic instruments, *Aust Dent J* 49:20-27, 2004.

61. Van Eldik DA, Zilm PS, Rogers AH, et al: A SEM evaluation of debris removal from endodontic files after cleaning and steam sterilization procedures, *Aust Dent J* 9:128-135, 2004.

62. Saghiri MA, Karamifar K, Mehvazfar P, et al: The efficacy of foam cleaners in removing debris from two endodontic instruments, *Quintessence Int* 43:811-817, 2012.

63. Aasim SA, Mellor AC, Qualtrough AJ: The effect of pre-soaking and time in the ultrasonic cleaner on the cleanliness of sterilized endodontic files, *Int Endod J* 39:143-149, 2006.

64. Morrison A, Conrod S: Dental burs and endodontic files: Are routine sterilization procedures effective? *J Can Dent Assoc* 75:39, 2009.

65. Plotino G, Costanzo A, Grande NM, et al: Experimental evaluation on the influence of autoclave sterilization on the cyclic fatigue of new nickel-titanium rotary instruments. *J Endod* 38:222-225, 2012.

66. King JB, Roberts HW, Bergeron BE, et al: The effect of autoclaving on torsional moment of two nickel-titanium endodontic files, *Int Endod J* 45:156-161, 2012.

67. Casper RB, Roberts MD, Himel VT, et al: Comparison of autoclaving effects on torsional deformation and fracture resistance of three innovative endodontic file systems *J Endod* 37:1572-1575, 2011.

Internal anatomy

Richard E. Walton, Eric J. Herbranson

CHAPTER OUTLINE

Methods of Determining Pulp Anatomy
General Considerations
Alterations in Internal Anatomy

Components of the Pulp System
Variations of Root and Pulp Anatomy

LEARNING OBJECTIVES

After reading this chapter and studying the Appendix, the student should be able to:

1. Recognize errors that may cause difficulties or failures in root canal treatment owing to lack of knowledge of pulp anatomy.
2. List techniques that help determine the type of pulp canal system.
3. Draw the four most common canal types (I to IV), the shapes of roots in cross section, and common canal configurations in these roots.
4. Describe the most common root and pulp anatomy of each tooth.
5. For each tooth type, list the average length, number of roots, and most common root curvatures.
6. Characterize the more frequent variations in root and pulp anatomy of each tooth.
7. Explain why standard periapical radiographs do not present the complete picture of root and pulp anatomy.
8. Draw a representative example of the most common internal and external anatomy of each tooth and root in the following planes: (1) sagittal section of mesiodistal and faciolingual planes and (2) cross section through the cervical, middle, and apical thirds.

9. Suggest methods for determining whether roots and canals are curved and the severity of the curvature.
10. State the tenet of the relationship of pulp-root anatomy.
11. List each tooth and the root or roots that require a search for more than one canal.
12. List and recognize the significance of iatrogenic or pathologic factors that may cause alterations in pulp anatomy.
13. Define the pulp space and list and describe its major components.
14. Describe variations in the pulp system in the apical third, including the apical foramen region.
15. Describe how to determine clinically the distance from the occlusal-incisal surface to the roof of the chamber.
16. Discuss the location, morphology, frequency, and importance of accessory (lateral) canals.
17. Describe relationships between the anatomic apex, radiographic apex, and actual location of the apical foramen.
18. Describe common variations in pulp anatomy resulting from developmental abnormalities and state their significance.
19. Explain why many root curvatures are not apparent on standard radiographs.

In terms of success of treatment, a knowledge of pulp anatomy is critical. As a cause of treatment failures, lack of a working knowledge of pulp anatomy ranks second only to errors in diagnosis and treatment planning. Success in treatment depends on knowing the normal or usual configurations of the pulp and to be aware of variations. Special techniques are required to determine the internal anatomy of the tooth under treatment.

True knowledge of the pulp anatomy requires a three-dimensional understanding (Fig. 14.1). The pulp cavity must be mentally visualized both longitudinally (from coronal aspect to apical foramen) and in cross section. In addition to general morphologic features, irregularities and "hidden"

regions of pulp are present within each canal. To clean and shape the pulp system maximally, intracanal instruments must reach as many of these regions as possible to plane the walls to loosen tissue and tissue remnants.[1] Lack of attention to this important principle may lead to treatment failure.

METHODS OF DETERMINING PULP ANATOMY

Textbook Knowledge

Knowledge of anatomy gained from textbooks is the most important and most useful method. Common and frequent variations *must* be memorized for each tooth. This means

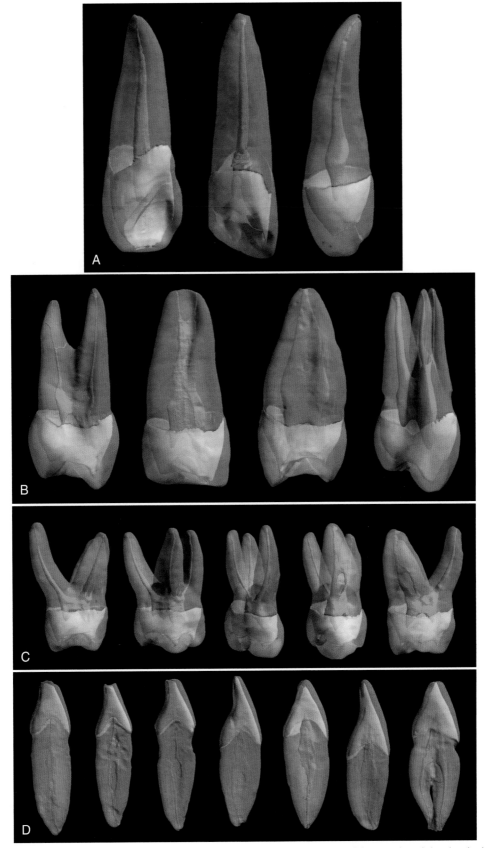

Fig. 14.1 Examples of each of the major tooth groups. These images were produced from real teeth by developing polygon computer models from research-grade micro-CT scans. The models were then segmented into pulp, dentin, and enamel. Once segmented, they were placed in an interactive computer program, and screen shots were taken of the desired view. The end result is a "transparent" image that shows both the surface and internal anatomies. **A,** Maxillary central incisor; the canal tends to be more regular in shape. **B,** Maxillary premolars, showing variations in root and internal anatomy. **C,** Maxillary molars. **D,** Mandibular incisor variations.

Continued

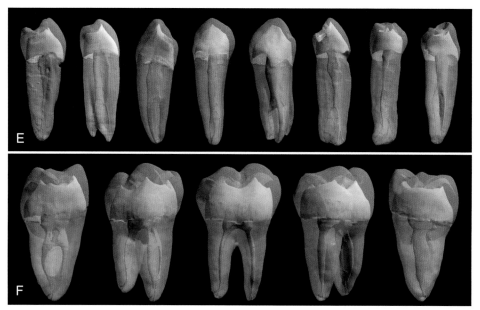

Fig. 14.1, cont'd **E,** Mandibular premolars, demonstrating the wide range of possible root and canal anatomies. **F,** Mandibular molars; a number of variations are possible. (Courtesy Eric Herbranson, images derived from the Tooth Atlas produced by eHuman.)

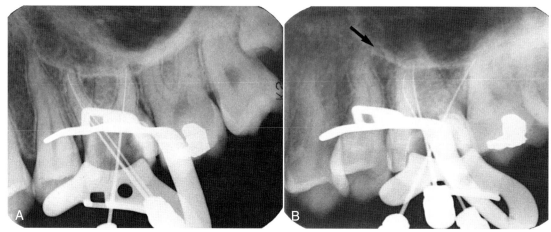

Fig. 14.2 **A,** Facial projection. Both the second premolar and the first molar appear to have fairly straight buccal roots and an uncomplicated anatomy. **B,** Mesial-angled projection. The more proximal view shows severe "bayonet" dilaceration of the second premolar with a marked buccal curve in the apex *(arrow)*. Sharp curves in the molar roots and two definitive canals in the mesiobuccal root are now evident. Both are difficult problems to treat.

having a working knowledge of the number of roots, number of canals per root and their location, longitudinal and cross-sectional shapes, most frequent curvatures (particularly in the faciolingual plane), and root outlines in all dimensions.[2-6] It is useful to know the approximate percentage of each. Anatomic features are diagrammed in the Appendix.

Radiographic Evidence

Certainly radiographs are useful, but they are somewhat over-rated for this purpose, particularly conventional periapical films.[7] The standard parallel facial projection gives just two dimensions; a common error is to examine only this view, overlooking the important third dimension (Fig. 14.2). In addition, radiographs tend to make the canals look relatively uniform in shape and taper. In fact, the aberrations often present are generally not visible (Fig. 14.2).

Standard projections indicate general anatomic features. Special radiographic techniques disclose missed canals and determine curvatures.[8-10] These techniques are discussed in detail in Chapter 12.

Exploration

Additional determinations of pulp anatomy are made during access preparation and when searching for canals. These methods also have limitations because canals often are neither readily apparent nor easily discovered with instruments.[11]

GENERAL CONSIDERATIONS

A basic tenet in pulp-root anatomy is *the shape of the pulp system reflects the surface outline of the crown and root.*[12,13]

Root shape

Canal shape

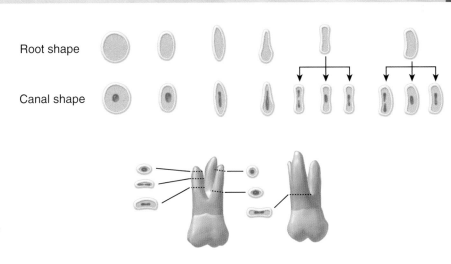

Fig. 14.3 Common variations in root or pulp cross-sectional anatomy. Note that the pulp outline tends to reflect the root outline. Deep concave roots have a greater variety of pulp anatomies.

In other words, because the pulp tends to form the surrounding dentin uniformly on opposite walls, the pulp is generally a miniature version of the tooth and conforms to the tooth surface.[14]

Root and Canal Anatomy

Although root shape in cross section is variable, there are seven general configurations: *round, oval, long oval, bowling pin, kidney bean, ribbon,* and *hourglass* (Fig. 14.3). The shape and location of canals are governed by the root shape (in cross section). Different shapes may appear at any level in a single root. For example, a root may be hourglass shaped in cross section at the cervical third, taper to a deep oval in the middle third, and blend to oval in the apical third; the number and shape of canals in each level will vary accordingly.[15] It is important to note that a canal is seldom round at any level. Assuming that it is round may result in improper canal preparation.

A knowledge of the more common variations in internal anatomy is helpful but does not give the final answer; this ultimately is determined during treatment. Root canals take various pathways to the apex. The pulp canal system is complex; canals may branch, divide, and rejoin. Traditionally canal systems have been categorized into four basic types (Fig. 14.4).[16]

However, using precise techniques, Vertucci and colleagues[17] found a complex canal system and identified four more complex and unusual variations, for ; total of eight pulp space configurations. Other investigators[18-23] have carefully studied canal morphologies in different tooth groups and examined gender and racial variations. The findings have consistently verified the results of Vertucci's study.[17]

Both gender and ethnic origin should be considered during the preoperative evaluation. Specific types of canal morphology occur in different racial groups. For example, African Americans have a higher number of mandibular premolars with extra canals. In one study, these patients had more than one canal in 33% of first premolars and 8% of second premolars; in contrast, Caucasians had multiple canals in 14% of first premolars and 3% of second premolars.[24] Asians and those of Asian descent have more variations than Caucasians and other races, such as C-shaped canals, a distolingual (third) root on mandibular first molars, and dens invaginatus.

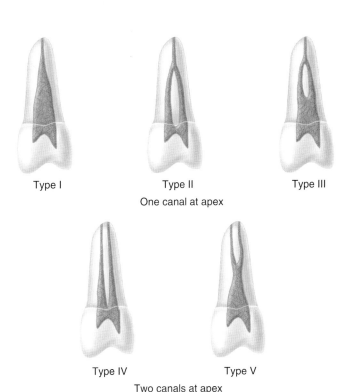

Type I   Type II   Type III

One canal at apex

Type IV   Type V

Two canals at apex

Fig. 14.4 Four basic types of canal systems. **A,** Type I—single canal from pulp chamber to apex. **B,** Type II—two separate canals from the chamber that merge short of the apex to form a single canal. **C,** Type III—two separate canals from the chamber that exit the apex in two separate foramina. **D, E,** Type IV—single canal from the chamber that divides short of the apex into two separate and distinct canals, each with its own apical foramen.

Identification of Canals and Roots

Differentiation and identification of canal orifices is facilitated by following certain procedures and by identifying anatomic features. Obviously, to clean, shape, and obturate a canal, it must first be located. In roots that *may* contain two canals, a basic rule is to *assume that the root contains two canals until it is proved otherwise.* Rather than memorize roots that often contain two canals, it is easier to remember those few that are unlikely to have two canals. Maxillary teeth contain roots that rarely have two canals: anteriors, premolars with two or three **233** roots, and distobuccal and lingual roots of molars. *All* other maxillary roots and *all* mandibular roots require a careful search for two (or possibly more) canals. The mesiobuccal roots of maxillary molars frequently contain two canals[25]; the ML (or MB2) may be difficult to locate and treat.

ALTERATIONS IN INTERNAL ANATOMY

As mentioned, the initial pulp shape reflects the root shape. However, because pulp and dentin react to their environment, changes in size (volume) and shape occur with increasing tooth age and in response to irritation.

Age

Although dentin formation occurs with age on all surfaces, it predominates in certain areas. For example, in molars, the roof and floor of the chamber show more dentin formation, eventually making the chamber almost disklike in configuration (Fig. 14.5). The treatment implications (difficulty locating chamber and canals) are obvious.[26]

Irritants

Anything that exposes dentin to the oral cavity may stimulate increased dentin formation at the base of tubules in the underlying pulp.[14] Causes of such dentin exposure include caries, periodontal disease, abrasion, erosion, attrition, cavity preparations, root planing, and cusp fractures (Fig. 14.6). Vital pulp therapy, such as pulpotomy, pulp capping, or placement of irritating materials in a deep cavity, may cause an increase in dentin formation, occlusion, calcific metamorphosis, resorption, or other unusual configurations in the chamber or canals. These tertiary (irregular secondary) dentin formations tend to occur directly under the involved tubules. Radiographs should be carefully examined to identify factors that may cause alterations in internal anatomy. Failure to do so may result in serious errors, lost time, and inadequate treatment.

Calcifications

Calcifications take two basic forms in the pulp: pulp stones (denticles) and diffuse calcifications. Although pulp stones are usually found in the chamber and diffuse calcifications in the radicular pulp, the reverse may also occur. These calcifications may form either normally or in response to irritation. Pulp stones are often seen on radiographs[27]; diffuse calcifications may obscure a pulp space but are visible only histologically.

Pulp stones in the chamber may reach considerable size and can markedly alter the internal chamber anatomy (Fig. 14.7). Although they do not totally block a canal orifice, pulp stones often make the process of locating an orifice challenging. These large pulp stones may be attached or free and are often removed during access preparation. Although pulp stones are not common in canals, if present, they are usually attached or embedded in the canal wall in the apical region. Rarely do they form a barrier to instrument passage.

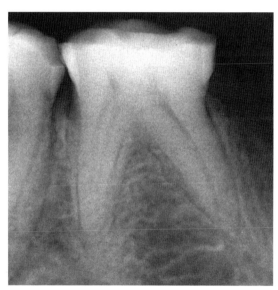

Fig. 14.6 Severe attrition has resulted in tertiary dentin formation on the roof and floor, resulting in flattening of the chamber.

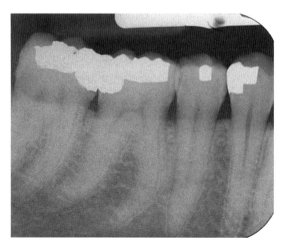

Fig. 14.5 Note the disklike configuration of the pulp chamber in the first molar, the result of the predominance of dentin formation in the roof and floor of the chamber. These chambers are difficult to locate during access preparation.

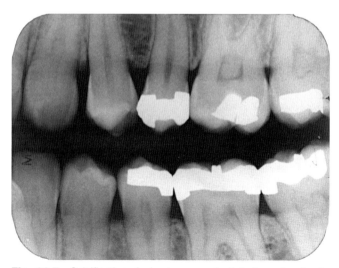

Fig. 14.7 Calcifications (pulp stones, or denticles) are visualized in the chambers. Their discrete appearance surrounded by radiolucent spaces shows these calcifications to be natural and not formed in response to irritation. (Courtesy Dr. T. Gound.)

Internal Resorption

Internal resorptions are uncommon and when present are usually not extensive. They also are a response to irritation that is sufficient to cause inflammation. Most resorptions are small and are not detectable on radiographs or during canal preparation. When visible radiographically, they are usually extensive and often perforate. Perforating internal resorptions usually create operative difficulties (Fig. 14.8).

COMPONENTS OF THE PULP SYSTEM

The pulp cavity is divided into a coronal portion (the pulp chamber) and a radicular portion (the root canal). Other features include the *pulp horns, canal orifices, accessory (lateral) canals,* and *apical foramen* (Fig. 14.9). The internal anatomy of these pulp components is altered by secondary dentin or cementum formation.

Pulp Horns

The pulp horns represent what the dentist does not want to encounter during restorative procedures but does want to locate during access preparation. Although they vary in height and location, a single pulp horn tends to be associated with each cusp in a posterior tooth, and mesial and distal horns tend to be in incisors. In general, the occlusal height of the pulp horns corresponds to the height of contour in a younger tooth, but because of continued dentin formation,

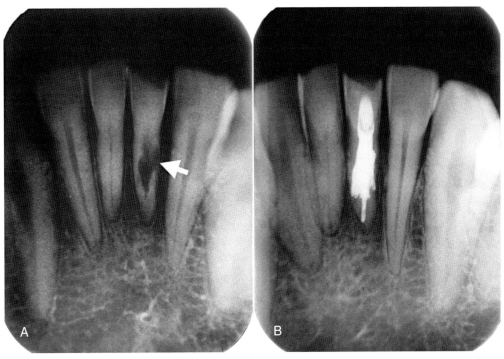

Fig. 14.8 **A,** Extensive internal resorption defect *(arrow).* **B,** Four years after treatment. Special cleaning, shaping, and obturating techniques (lateral condensation plus thermoplasticization) were required, resulting in successful treatment.

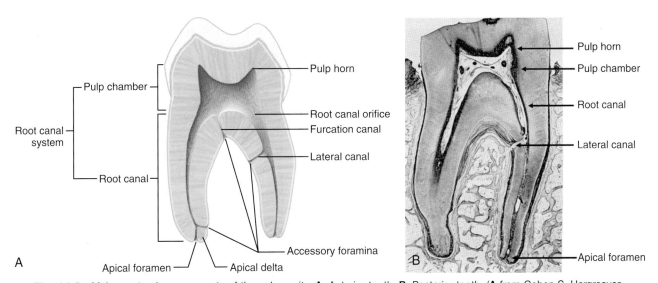

Fig. 14.9 Major anatomic components of the pulp cavity. **A,** Anterior tooth. **B,** Posterior tooth. (**A** from Cohen S, Hargreaves K, Keiser K: *Pathways of the pulp,* ed 9, St Louis, 2006, Mosby.)

the pulp horns lie closer to the cervical margin in an older tooth.

To determine the estimated depth of access on an analogue film, the height and location of the pulp horns is determined by measuring from cusp tip to pulp horn or chamber roof using a bur and a handpiece (Fig. 14.10). On a digital radiograph, the estimated depth of access is measured with the "ruler" icon.

Pulp Chamber

The pulp chamber occupies the center of the crown and trunk of the root. As mentioned, its shape, in both longitudinal and cross-sectional dimensions, depends on the shape of the crown and trunk; this configuration varies with tooth age and/ or irritation.[12] In mature molars, the roof of the chamber is usually at the level of the cementoenamel junction.[28]

Root Canals

Root canals extend the length of the root, beginning as a funneled orifice and exiting as the apical foramen. Significantly, most canals are curved, often in a facial-lingual direction.[29,30] Therefore, a curved canal is often undetectable on facial projection radiographs. As a result, the uninitiated or uninformed clinician may assume that a canal is straight and may overenlarge what in fact is a facial or lingual curvature, resulting in ledging or perforation. *The operator should always assume that a canal is curved.*

Canal shape varies with root shape and size, degree of curvature, and the age and condition of the tooth (see Figs. 14.2 and 14.3). As a rule, when two canals occur in a root, they tend to be more oval. In the deep facial-lingual root with mesial or distal (or both) concavities (hourglass or kidney bean shaped), a single canal may have a bowling pin, kidney bean, hourglass, or ribbon shape. Regardless of the shape in the cervical third, in the apical curvature the root (and canal) tends to become more oval but may be somewhat flattened.[31] A canal that is oval in the cervical one third usually is oval or ribbon shaped in the apical few millimeters.

The shape and number of canals in a root reflect the facial-lingual depth and shape of the root at each level (Fig. 14.11); the deeper the root, the greater the likelihood of two separate, definitive canals. If the root tapers toward the apical third, there is a likelihood that the canals will converge to exit as a single canal.

Irregularities and aberrations are common, particularly in posterior teeth. Such aberrations include hills and valleys (bulges and concavities) in canal walls and roots,[32] intercanal communications (isthmuses between two canals), cul-de-sacs, fins, and other variations.[33] These aberrations usually are neither accessible to instruments or irrigants nor consistently obturated.[34]

The chamber tends to occupy the center of the crown; a canal occupies the center of the root. When there are two canals in a root, each often occupies the center of its own root "bulge."

Accessory Canals

Accessory (or lateral) canals are lateral branches of the main canal that form a communication between the pulp and periodontium. They contain connective tissue and vessels and may be located at any level from furcation[35-38] to apex; however, they tend to be more common in the apical third and in posterior teeth.[38] In other words, the more apical and the farther posterior the tooth, the more likely it is that accessory canals will be present. The relationship of accessory canals to pulp health and disease, and to treatment, is debatable.[39] These

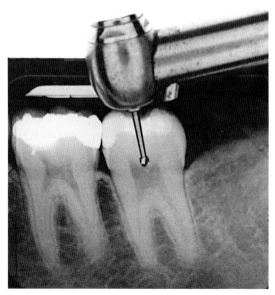

Fig. 14.10 A technique for determining the distance from the occlusal surface to the roof of the pulp chamber. This is of obvious benefit during access preparation to prevent perforation.

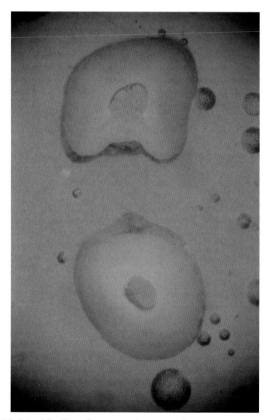

Fig. 14.11 Maxillary first premolar roots. Cross section through the buccal and lingual roots shows a concavity on the lingual surface and an irregularly shaped canal in the middle third of the buccal root. This is a common finding. (Courtesy Dr. A. Tamse.)

canals do not supply collateral circulation and therefore contribute little to pulp function; they probably represent an anomaly that occurred during root formation.

Accessory canals provide an exit for irritants from the pulp space to the lateral periodontium. They probably cannot be debrided during cleaning and shaping,[1] but they are occasionally filled with obturating materials (primarily sealer) during canal filling (Fig. 14.12). Debridement and obturation of lateral canals are unimportant for success of root canal treatment.[24,40]

Apical Region
Development
The apex is the root terminus. It is relatively straight in the young mature tooth but tends to curve more distally with time. This curvature results from continued apical-distal apposition of cementum in response to continued mesial-occlusal eruption. Alterations in the apical region may also result from resorption and irregular cementum apposition. For these reasons, apical anatomy tends to be nonuniform and unpredictable.[41-44]

Apical Foramen
The apical foramen varies in size and configuration with maturity. Before maturation, the apical foramen is open. With time and deposition of dentin and cementum, it becomes smaller and funneled. Significantly, the foramen usually does not exit at the true (anatomic) root apex[45,46]; rather, it is offset approximately 0.5 mm (seldom more than 1 mm from) the true apex.[47] The degree of deviation is unpredictable and may vary considerably from the average, particularly in the older tooth that has undergone cementum apposition (Fig. 14.13). For this reason, root canal preparation and obturation end short of the anatomic root apex, as shown in Fig. 14.14.[48] Usually, the apical foramen is not visible radiographically. The clinician relies on averages[41] or on electronic measuring devices to determine the extent of canal preparation and obturation.

Variations in Anatomy
The only consistent aspect of the apex region is its inconsistency.[39] The canal may take twists and turns, divide into several canals to form a delta with ramifications on the apical root surface, or exhibit irregularities in the canal wall (Fig. 14.15). In general, these aberrations are neither detectable nor predictably negotiable and are neither well debrided nor obturated.

A common concept is that canals round out in this apical region; this is usually not true. Canals are frequently a long oval or even ribbon shaped apically.[49] These nonround canals cannot be enlarged to a round shape without perforating or weakening the roots.[49]

Apical Constriction
The apical constriction typically has been used as an anatomic landmark for preparation and obturation. The reality is that the presence of an apical constriction is unpredictable. Frequently there is no apical constriction and, when present, it can vary shape.[50] It has been proposed that the cementodentinal junction forms the apical constriction; this is an incorrect concept. In fact, the cementodentinal junction cannot be determined clinically with accuracy,[45] and the intracanal extent of cementum is variable. If an apical constriction is present, it is not visible on a radiograph and usually is not detectable with tactile sense using a file, even by the most skilled practitioner.

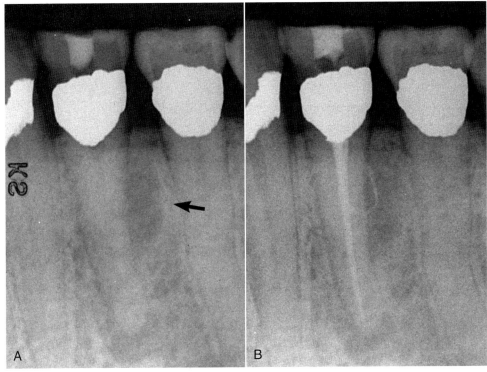

Fig. 14.12 **A,** Resorptive bony lesion *(arrow)*; this usually indicates an accessory canal (not visible) that is a pathway for irritants. **B,** The accessory canal is obvious after obturation.

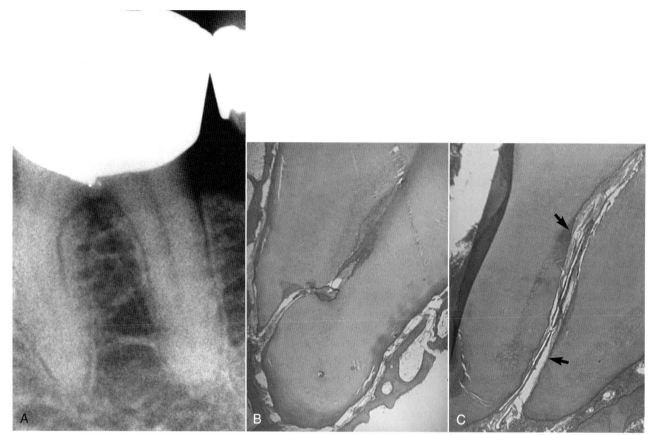

Fig. 14.13 Variations in apical canal anatomy. **A,** The radiograph often does not demonstrate the size, shape, or curvature of canals apically. **B,** Mesial root apex showing an abrupt curve and the apical foramen exiting on the mesial, well short of the anatomic apex. **C,** Distal root apex showing a uniform canal with no constriction and variable levels *(arrows)* of cementodentinal junctions; these variabilities are common. (Cadaver specimen courtesy Dr. D. Holtzmann.)

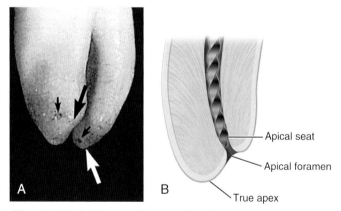

Fig. 14.14 **A,** The apical foramina *(small arrows)* do not correspond to the true anatomic apex *(large arrows).* **B,** In most situations the apical terminus or seat of the preparation will vary from the apical foramen and radiographic apex. (**A** courtesy Dr. D. Melton.)

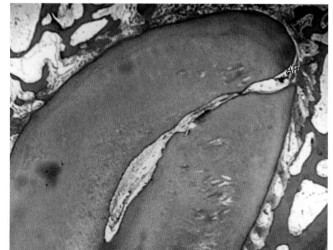

Fig. 14.15 The apical region of the canal and apical foramen *(AF)* are often very irregular.

VARIATIONS OF ROOT AND PULP ANATOMY

Representative examples of the tooth groups are diagrammed in the Appendix, where both cross-sectional and longitudinal aspects are outlined. In addition, the pulp anatomy of each is shown in relation to the design of the access preparation.

Occasionally, teeth vary significantly in root or, more likely, in pulp anatomy. Such variations and abnormalities are most common in the maxillary lateral incisors, maxillary[51-53] and mandibular premolars,[54] and maxillary molars.[55,56] Unusual root morphology tends to be bilateral.[57]

Dens Invaginatus (Dens in Dente)

Dens invaginatus is most common in maxillary lateral incisors[58]; it results from an infolding of the enamel organ during proliferation and is an error in morphodifferentiation (Fig. 14.16). It often results in an early pulp–oral cavity communication requiring root canal treatment.[59] Dens invaginatus is most common in the maxillary lateral incisor and shows varying degrees of severity and complexity.[60,61] The more severe cases should be referred to a specialist because special treatment, such as surgery, is frequently required. The prognosis of any treatment often is questionable. The invagination is usually visible on radiographs; however, it is often small and obscure. The lingual pit on maxillary anterior teeth represents a minor form of dens invaginatus.

Dens Evaginatus

A variation of invaginatus,[62] dens evaginatus is most common in mandibular premolars and in individuals of Asian ancestry (this includes Native Americans and Hispanics). Clinically, dens evaginatus initially appears as a small tubercle "bulge" on the occlusal surface, but it may not be obvious radiographically (Fig. 14.17). These tubercles often contain an extension of the pulp. When these fragile tubercles fracture off in the immature tooth, the pulp is exposed and becomes necrotic, requiring apexification. There are different treatment measures to prevent this accidental exposure of the pulp. One method, before the tubercle fractures, is to remove the tubercle with a bur and then cap, followed by a good sealing restoration with amalgam.[62]

High Pulp Horns

Occasionally, a pulp horn extends far into a cusp region, resulting in premature exposure by caries or accidental exposure during cavity preparation. These high pulp horns are often not visible on radiographs. This is most common in the mesiobuccal aspect of first molars.

Lingual Groove

Usually found in maxillary lateral incisors, a lingual groove appears as a surface infolding of dentin oriented from the cervical toward the apical direction (Fig. 14.18).[63] Frequently, this results in a deep, narrow periodontal defect that occasionally communicates with the pulp, causing a true combined endodontic/periodontal lesion (Fig. 14.19). Because treatment is difficult and unpredictable, the prognosis is poor. Usually these teeth require extraction.

Dilaceration

By definition, dilaceration is a severe or complex root curvature (see Fig. 14.1). During root formation, structures such as the cortical bone of the maxillary sinus or the mandibular canal or nasal fossa may deflect the epithelial diaphragm, resulting in the formation of a root curvature. Many of these curvatures are found in a facial-lingual plane and are not obvious on standard radiographic projections.

Other Variations

Many other pulp and root anomalies may occur.[64-67] Some occur in association with genetic disorders,[68] such as

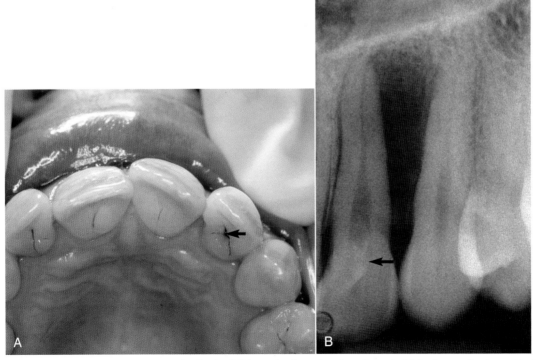

Fig. 14.16 Dens invaginatus. **A,** The invagination is visible on the lingual surface *(arrow)* of this abnormally shaped incisor. **B,** The invagination is lined internally by enamel *(arrow).* Because of communication with the pulp, the exposure resulted in pulp necrosis and apical pathosis. These situations are difficult to treat. (Courtesy Dr. W. Johnson.)

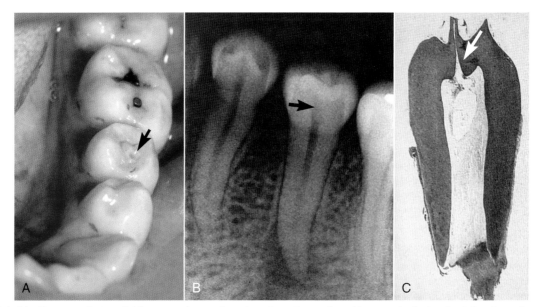

Fig. 14.17 Dens evaginatus. **A,** The second premolars show two stages; the wide arrow indicates the tubercle on the occlusal surface. **B,** The tubercle has fractured *(narrow arrow)*, exposing the pulp. **C,** Histologic section demonstrates the extension of the pulp into the evagination tubercle *(arrow)*. (**A** and **B** courtesy Dr. W. Johnson.)

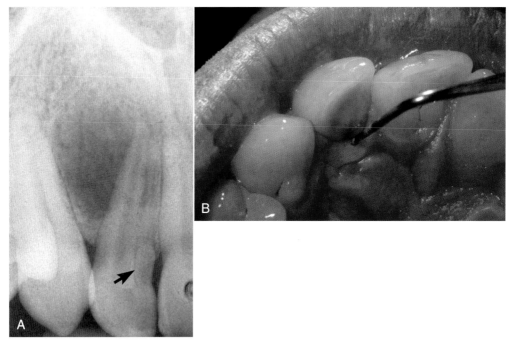

Fig. 14.18 A lingual groove, an apparent infolding during root and crown formation. **A,** The groove is faintly visible on the periapical radiograph *(arrow)*. **B,** The groove is often detected on the surface with probing and is usually untreatable. (Courtesy Dr. K. Baumgartner.)

variations in the number of canals or roots (Fig. 14.20). Teeth with unusual chamber and root canal configurations have an impact on treatment.[69,70] The astute clinician is alert to these possibilities and studies radiographs and occlusal anatomy carefully. A common abnormality is the C-shaped canal (see Appendix and Fig. 14.21). This usually occurs in mandibular second molars and is more common in Asian individuals.[71] Because of the complex internal anatomy, the prognosis for root canal treatment is questionable, owing to difficulty with

adequate debridement and obturation.[72] Additional treatment measures may be required, and patients with such teeth should be considered for referral.

Other unusual chamber and root morphologies are the occasional four-rooted maxillary second molar[73] and the three-rooted maxillary premolar (see Appendix and Fig. 14.22).[74] Another departure from the usual is the distolingual third root on mandibular first molars (see Appendix and Fig. 14.23), which can occur in any race but is seen most frequently in

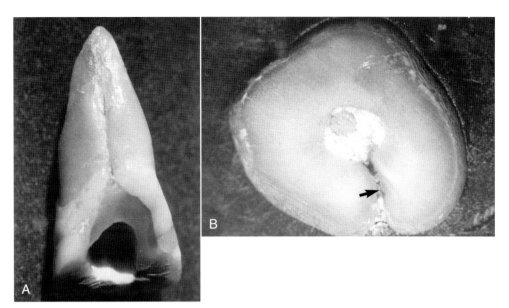

Fig. 14.19 **A,** Lingual groove defect that proved untreatable periodontally or endodontically. **B,** Cross section shows that the groove invagination *(arrow)* communicates with the pulp.

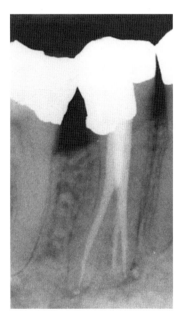

Fig. 14.20 Premolar with three canals; this is a challenge to treat.

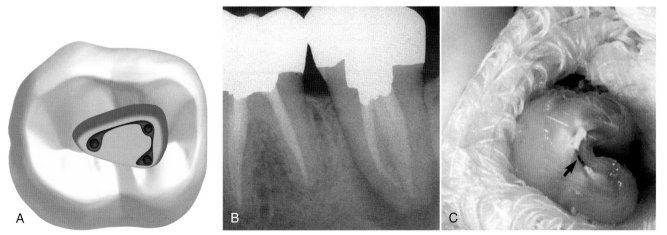

Fig. 14.21 **A,** C-shaped pulp chamber. The C-space may be continuous throughout the length of the root but is variable anatomically. More commonly, three separate canal orifices may be found within the groove. **B,** C-shaped molar shows failed treatment. **C,** After extraction and resection of the apical one third, the undebrided and unobturated groove is evident *(arrow)*.

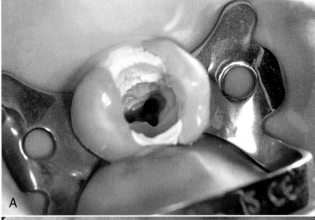

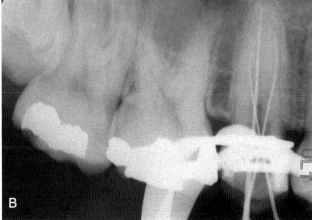

Fig. 14.22 Premolar with three roots and three canals. **A,** The access shows three distinct orifices. **B,** The radiographic appearance is similar to that of a maxillary molar.

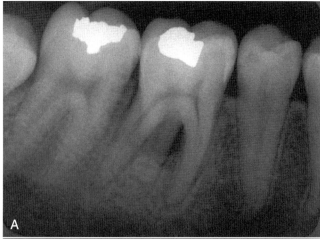

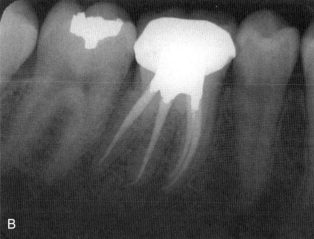

Fig. 14.23 Three-rooted mandibular molar. **A,** Pulp necrosis has caused apical and furcal bony lesions. **B,** Several months post-treatment. The resorptive lesions have resolved. (Courtesy Dr. Alan Law.)

Asian individuals. These variations may be a challenge to treat.[75,76]

New technologies using computer reconstruction of microtomography are able to provide three-dimensional morphology information on tooth and pulp anatomy. These data sets combined with interactive computer viewing software can give the student accurate study material to learn anatomy based on real teeth (Fig 14.1). In addition, some of the new narrow field clinical cone beam CT machines have resolution that is just high enough to visualize the tooth anatomy in a clinical patient. They are proving to be an important adjunct in endodontic practice.[77]

REFERENCES

1. Walton RE: Histologic comparison of different methods of pulp canal enlargement, *J Endod* 2:304, 1976.
2. Pineda F, Kuttler Y: Mesiodistal and buccolingual roentgenographic investigation of 7,275 root canals, *Oral Surg Oral Med Oral Pathol* 33:101, 1972.
3. Mueller AH: Anatomy of the root canals of the incisors, cuspids and bicuspids of the permanent teeth, *J Am Dent Assoc* 20:1361, 1933.
4. Vertucci F: Root canal anatomy of the human permanent teeth, *Oral Surg Oral Med Oral Pathol* 58:589, 1984.
5. Vertucci FJ: Root canal anatomy of the mandibular anterior teeth, *J Am Dent Assoc* 89:369, 1974.
6. Green D: Morphology of the pulp cavity of the permanent teeth, *Oral Surg Oral Med Oral Pathol* 8:743, 1955.
7. Kaffe I, Kaufman A, Littner MM, et al: Radiographic study of the root canal system of mandibular anterior teeth, *Int Endod J* 18:235, 1985.
8. Walton RE: Endodontic radiographic techniques, *Dent Radiogr Photog* 46:51, 1973.
9. Skidmore A: The importance of pre-operative radiographs and determination of root canal configuration, *Quintessence Int* 10:55, 1979.
10. Yoshioka T, Villegas J, Kobayashi C, et al: Radiographic evaluation of root canal multiplicity in mandibular first premolars, *J Endod* 30:73, 2004.
11. Johnson WT: Difficulties in locating the mesiobuccal canal in molars, *Quintessence Int* 16:169, 1985.
12. Stambaugh RV, Wittrock JW: The relationship of the pulp chamber to the external surface of the tooth, *J Prosthet Dent* 37:537, 1977.
13. Bjorndal L, Carlsen O, Thuesen G, et al: External and internal macromorphology in 3D-reconstructed maxillary molars using computerized x-ray microtomography, *Int Endod J* 32:3, 1999.
14. Bhaskar S: *Orban's oral histology*, ed 10, St Louis, 1986, Mosby.
15. Mauger M, Schindler W, Walker W III: An evaluation of canal morphology at different levels of root resection in mandibular incisors, *J Endod* 24:607, 1998.
16. Weine F, *Endodontic therapy*, ed 5, p 243, St Louis, 1996, Mosby.
17. Vertucci F, Seelig A, Gillis R: Root canal morphology of the human maxillary second premolar, *Oral Surg Oral Med Oral Pathol Oral Radiol Endod* 38:456, 1974.
18. Caliskan MK, Pehlivan Y, Sepetcioglu F, et al: Root canal morphology of human permanent teeth in a Turkish population, *J Endod* 21:200, 1995.
19. Kartal N, Yanikoglu FC: Root canal morphology of mandibular incisors, *J Endod* 18:562, 1992.
20. Gulabivala K, Aung T, Alavi A, et al: Root and canal morphology of Burmese mandibular molars, *Int Endod J* 34:359, 2001.
21. Sert S, Bayirli GS: Evaluation of the root canal configurations of the mandibular and maxillary

permanent teeth by gender in Turkish population, *J Endod* 30:391, 2004.

22. De Pablo OV, Estevez R, Peix Sanchez M, et al: Root anatomy and canal configuration of the permanent mandibular first molar: a systematic review, *J Endod* 36:1919, 2010.

23. Degerness RA, Bowles WR: Dimension, anatomy and morphology of the mesiobuccal root canal system in maxillary molars, *J Endod* 36:985, 2010.

24. Trope M, Elfenbein L, Tronstad L: Mandibular premolars with more than one root canal in different race groups. *J Endod* 12:343, 1986.

25. Weine F, Healey H, Gerstein H, et al: Canal configuration in the mesiobuccal root of the maxillary first molar and its endodontic significance (reprinted), *J Endod* 38:1305, 2012.

26. Krasner P, Randow HJ: Anatomy of the pulp chamber floor, *J Endod* 30:5, 2004.

27. Tamse A, Kaffe I, Littner MM, et al: Statistical evaluation of radiologic survey of pulp stones, *J Endod* 8:81, 1982.

28. Deutsch A, Musikant B: Morphological measurements of anatomic landmarks in human maxillary and mandibular molar pulp chambers, *J Endod* 30:388, 2004.

29. Schafer E, Diez C, Hoppe W, et al: Roentgenographic investigation of frequency and degree of canal curvatures in human permanent teeth, *J Endod* 28:211, 2002.

30. Willershausen B, Tekyatan H, Kasaj A, et al: Roentgenographic in vitro investigation of frequency and location of curvatures in human maxillary premolars, *J Endod* 32:307, 2006.

31. Gani O, Visvisian C: Apical canal diameter in the first upper molar at various ages, *J Endod* 25:689, 1999.

32. Lammertyn P, Rodrigo S, Brunotto M, et al: Furcation groove of maxillary first premolar, thickness, and dentin structures, *J Endod* 35:814, 2009.

33. von Arx T: Frequency and type of canal isthmuses in first molars detected by endoscopic inspection during periradicular surgery, *Int Endod J* 38:160, 2005.

34. Fan B, Pan Y, Gao Y, et al: Three-dimensional morphologic analysis of isthmuses in the mesial roots of mandibular molars, *J Endod* 36:1866, 2010.

35. Guttman J: Prevalence, location, and patency of accessory canals in the furcation of molars, *J Periodontol* 49:21, 1978.

36. Vertucci FJ, Anthony RL: A scanning electron microscopic investigation of accessory foramina in the furcation and pulp chamber floor of molar teeth, *Oral Surg Oral Med Oral Pathol* 62:319, 1986.

37. Haznedaroglu F, Ersev H, Odabasi H, et al: Incidence of patent furcal accessory canals in permanent molars of a Turkish population, *Int Endod J* 36:515, 2003.

38. DeDeus WD: Frequency, location, and direction of the lateral, secondary, and accessory canals, *J Endod* 1:361, 1975.

39. Sinai IH, Soltanoff W: The transmission of pathologic changes between the pulp and the periodontal structures, *Oral Surg Oral Med Oral Pathol* 36:558, 1973.

40. Barthel C, Zimmer S, Trope M: Relationship of radiologic and histologic signs of inflammation in human root-filled teeth, *J Endod* 30:75, 2004.

41. Kuttler Y: Microscope investigation of root apexes, *J Am Dent Assoc* 50:544, 1955.

42. Mjor IA, Smith MR, Ferrari M, et al: The structure of dentine in the apical region of human teeth, *Int Endod J* 34:346, 2001.

43. Ponce EH, Vilar Fernandez JA: The cemento-dentino-canal junction, the apical foramen, and the apical constriction: evaluation by optical microscopy, *J Endod* 29:214, 2003.

44. Marroquin BB, El-Sayed MA, Willerhausen-Zonnchen B: Morphology of the physiological foramen. I. Maxillary and mandibular molars, *J Endod* 30:321, 2004.

45. Dummer PM, McGinn JH, Rees DG: The position and topography of the apical canal constriction and apical foramen, *Int Endod J* 17:192, 1984.

46. Miyashita M, Kasahara E, Yasuda E, et al: Root canal system of the mandibular incisor, *J Endod* 23:479, 1997.

47. Martos J, Ferrer-Luque C, Gonzalea-Rodriguez MP, et al: Topographical evaluation of the major apical foramen in permanent teeth, *Int Endod J* 42:329, 2009.

48. Wu M, Wesselink P, Walton R: Apical terminus location of root canal treatment procedures, *Oral Surg Oral Med Oral Pathol Oral Radiol Endod* 89:99, 2000.

49. Wu M, R'Oris A, Barkin D: Prevalence and extent of long oval canals in the apical third, *Oral Surg Oral Med Oral Pathol Oral Radiol Endod* 89:739, 2000.

50. Meder-Cowherd L, Williamson A, Walton R, et al: Apical anatomy of the palatal roots of maxillary molars by using micro-computed tomography, *J Endod* 37:1162, 2011.

51. Tamse A, Katz A, Pilo R: Furcation groove of buccal root of maxillary first premolars: a morphometric study, *J Endod* 26:359, 2000.

52. Li J, Li L, Pan Y: Anatomic study of the buccal root with furcation groove and associated root canal shape in maxillary first premolars by using micro-computed tomography, *J Endod* 39:265, 2013.

53. Katz A, Wasenstein-Kohn S, Tamse A, et al: Residual dentin thickness in bifurcated maxillary premolars after root canal and dowel space preparation, *J Endod* 32:202, 2006.

54. Baisden MK, Kulild JC, Weller RN: Root canal configuration of the mandibular first premolar, *J Endod* 18:505, 1992.

55. Libfeld H, Rotstein I: Incidence of four-rooted maxillary second molars: literature review and radiographic survey of 1,200 teeth, *J Endod* 15:129, 1989.

56. Jung I-Y, Seo M-A, Fouad A, et al: Apical anatomy in mesial and mesiobuccal roots of permanent first molars, *J Endod* 31:364, 2005.

57. Sabala CL, Benenati FW, Neas BR: Bilateral root or root canal aberrations in a dental school patient population, *J Endod* 20:38, 1994.

58. Hulsmann M: Dens invaginatus: aetiology, classification, prevalence, diagnosis, and treatment considerations, *Int Endod J* 30:79, 1997.

59. Piatelli A, Trisi P: Dens invaginatus: a histological study of undemineralized material, *Endod Dent Traumatol* 9:191, 1993.

60. Oehlers F: Dens invaginatus. I. Variations of the invagination process and associated crown forms, *Oral Surg Oral Med Oral Pathol* 10:1204, 1957.

61. Gound TG: Dens invaginatus: a pathway to pulpal pathology—a literature review, *Pract Periodontics Aesthet Dent* 9:585, 1997.

62. Levitan ME, Himel VT: Dens evaginitus: literature review, pathophysiology, and comprehensive treatment regimen, *J Endod* 32:1, 2006.

63. Lara V, Consolaro A, Bruce R: Macroscopic and microscopic analysis of the palato-gingival groove, *J Endod* 26:345, 2000.

64. Yang Z-P, Yang S-F, Lee G: The root and root canal anatomy of maxillary molars in a Chinese population, *Endod Dent Traumatol* 4:215, 1988.

65. Sieraski SM, Taylor GN, Kohn RA: Identification and endodontic management of three canalled maxillary premolars, *J Endod* 15:29, 1989.

66. Manning SA: Root canal anatomy of mandibular second molars, *Int Endod J* 23:34, 1990.

67. Melton DC, Krell KV, Fuller MW: Anatomical and histological features of C-shaped canals in mandibular second molars, *J Endod* 17:384, 1991.

68. Kelsen A, Love R, Kieser J, et al: Root canal anatomy of anterior and premolar teeth in Down's syndrome, *Int Endod J* 32:211, 1999.

69. Sharma R, Pecora J, Lumley P, et al: The external and internal anatomy of human mandibular canine teeth with two roots, *Endod Dent Traumatol* 14:88, 1998.

70. Ferreira C, Gomes de Moraes I, Bernardineli N: Three-rooted maxillary second premolar, *J Endod* 26:105, 2000.

71. Jin G-C, Lee S-J, Roh B-D: Anatomical study of C-shaped canals in mandibular second molars by analysis of computed tomography, *J Endod* 32:10, 2006.

72. Solomonov M, Paque F, Fan B, et al: The challenge of C-shaped canal systems: a comparative study of the self-adjusting file and Pro Taper, *J Endod* 38:209. 2012.

73. Versiani L, Pecora G, de Sousa-Neto R: Root and root canal morphology of four-rooted maxillary second molars: a micro-computed tomography study, *J Endod* 38:977, 2012.

74. Vier-Pelisser FV, Dummer PMH, Bryant S, et al: The anatomy of the root canal system of three-rooted maxillary premolars analysed using high resolution computed tomography, *Int Endod J* 43:1122, 2010.

75. DeMoor RJ, Deroose CA, Calberson F: The radix entomolaris in mandibular first molars: an endodontic challenge, *Int Endod J* 37:789, 2004.

76. Gu Y, Lu Q, Wang H, et al: Root canal morphology of permanent three rooted mandibular first molars-part i: pulp floor and root canal system, *J Endod* 35:990, 2010.

77. Villas-Boas S, Bernardineli F, Cavenago S, et al: Micro-computed tomography study of the internal anatomy of mesial root canals of mandibular molars, *J Endod* 37:1682, 2011.

Isolation, endodontic access, and length determination

William T. Johnson, Anne E. Williamson

CHAPTER OUTLINE

Isolation

Access Openings

Access Openings and Canal Location

Errors in Access

Length Determination

LEARNING OBJECTIVES

After reading this chapter and studying the Appendix, the student should be able to:

1. Describe the reasons for rubber dam isolation during endodontic procedures.
2. List a rubber dam clamp selection for anterior, premolar, and molar teeth.
3. Identify clamps that have several applications and state which two are "universal."
4. Describe techniques for application of the clamp and rubber dam in single-tooth isolation.
5. Describe techniques to stop salivary or hemorrhagic seepage into the operative field.
6. Recognize situations in which special isolation approaches are necessary.
7. Describe techniques used in special isolation situations.
8. Identify patients with difficult isolation situations who should be considered for referral.
9. Identify major objectives of access preparation in both anterior and posterior teeth.
10. Explain why straight-line access is critical.
11. Explain the importance of pulp horn removal in anterior teeth.
12. Relate reasons and indications for removing caries or restorations during access preparation.
13. Explain the reason and technique for removing the dentin shelf in anterior and posterior teeth.

14. Describe the procedure, burs used, and sequence of operations to start and complete access preparations on various teeth.
15. Identify common errors for specific teeth that may occur during access preparation.
16. Recognize when these errors occur and know how to correct them (if correctable).
17. Describe techniques for locating difficult to find chambers or canals.
18. Demonstrate the step-by-step technique for obtaining estimated and final working lengths.
19. Account for conditions under which the working length (distance from radiographic apex) varies.
20. Describe how to designate and maintain (and create, when necessary) a stable reference point.
21. Describe electronic apex locators: how they function and when they are useful.
22. Diagram the portions of the tooth that must be removed to attain straight-line access to the canals. Illustrate this on sagittal sections of both anterior and posterior teeth.
23. Diagram the outline form of the access preparation for all teeth.
24. Show the location of each canal orifice relative to the occlusal or lingual surface.

Chapters 15, 16, and 18 deal with the technical aspects of nonsurgical root canal treatment. Areas presented include isolation, access, length determination, cleaning and shaping, and obturation. A number of instruments and techniques are advocated for treatment procedures. These chapters introduce concepts and principles that are important for successful treatment. These building blocks are based on the best available evidence and provide a basis for incorporating more complex and alternative techniques.

ISOLATION

Rubber Dam Application

Application of the rubber dam for isolation during endodontic treatment has many distinct advantages and is mandatory for legal considerations.[1] Failure to use a rubber dam indicates that the clinician does not understand the microbial nature of the disease process, the need to protect the patient from aspiration or swallowing instruments, the protection afforded the dental staff from contaminated aerosols, and the decreased success rate for treatment when strict asepsis is not used. The use of the rubber dam in the United States is considered the standard of care; thus expert testimony is not required in cases involving patients who swallowed or aspirated instruments or materials because juries are considered competent to determine negligence. Evidence exists that many general dentists unnecessarily place themselves at risk by not using the rubber dam when performing endodontic procedures.[2]

The rubber dam provides protection for the patient[3] and creates an aseptic environment; it enhances vision, retracts tissues, and makes treatment more efficient. Soft tissues are protected from laceration by rotary instruments, chemical agents, and medicaments. Irrigating solutions are confined to the operating field. Most important, rubber dam isolation protects the patient from swallowing or aspirating instruments and materials (Fig. 15.1).[4] An additional advantage is that the dentist and auxiliary employees are also protected.[5-7] The risk from aerosols is minimized,[8,9] and the dam provides a barrier

against the patient's saliva and oral bacteria. Application of the rubber dam may also reduce the potential for transmission of systemic diseases such as acquired immunodeficiency syndrome (AIDS), hepatitis, and tuberculosis.[5,9]

The rubber dam is manufactured from latex; however, non-latex rubber dam material is available for patients with latex allergy (Fig. 15.2).[10] The rubber dam can be obtained in a variety of colors that provide contrast to the tooth. The thickness also varies (light, medium, heavy, and extra heavy). A medium-weight dam is recommended because a lightweight dam is easily torn during the application process. Also, the medium material fits better at the gingival margin and provides good retraction.

The design of the rubber dam frames is also variable. For endodontics, plastic frames are recommended; they are radiolucent and do not require complete removal during exposure of interim films such as the working length and master cone radiographs and digital images.

Rubber Dam Retainers

Rubber dam clamps fit the various tooth groups. During routine treatment, metal clamps are adequate; however, they may damage tooth structure[11] or existing restorations. Some have serrated edges to enhance retention when minimal coronal tooth structure remains. Plastic clamps are manufactured and have the advantage of being radiolucent. This is an advantage in difficult cases in which the pulp chamber and canal cannot be located. Metal clamps often must be removed when exposing a radiograph or digital image for orientation purposes. When using a plastic clamp, the rubber dam can remain in place. The plastic clamps are less likely to damage tooth structure or existing restorations.[12]

Types

Different styles and shapes of rubber dam clamps are available for specific situations. The following selection is recommended: *anterior teeth:* Ivory No. 9 or 212; *premolars:* No. 0 and 2; and *molars:* No. 14, 14A, and 56. Clamps that will manage most isolation situations during root canal treatment are shown in Fig. 15.3. Winged clamps permit the application of the rubber dam as a single unit during single-tooth isolation (Fig. 15.4).[13]

Universal Clamp Designs

Two designs (see Fig. 15.3), the "butterfly" Ivory No. 9 and the Ivory No. 56, are suitable for most isolations. The butterfly design (No. 9) has small beaks, is deep reaching, and can be

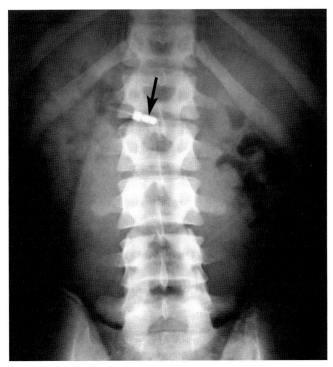

Fig. 15.1 A file *(arrow)* that a patient swallowed during endodontic treatment.

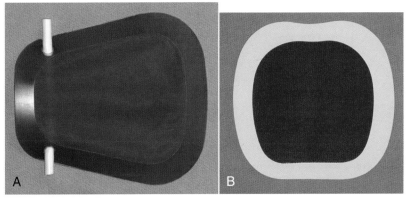

Fig. 15.2 **A** and **B,** Disposable rubber dam systems.

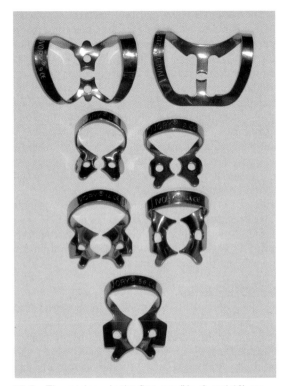

Fig. 15.3 The retainers in the first row (No. 9 and 12) are designed for anterior teeth but are useful for premolars. The two clamps in the second row (No. 0 and 2) are for premolars and anterior teeth. The third row clamps (No. 14 and 4A) are for molars. No. 14 and 14A are deeper reaching than the No. 56. The bottom row clamp (No. 56) is more universal and is used for most molars.

applied to most anterior and premolar teeth. The No. 56 clamp can isolate most molars.

With teeth that are smaller, reduced in crown preparation, or abnormally shaped, a clamp with smaller radius beaks (No. 0, 9, or 14) is necessary. Small-radius beaks can be positioned farther apically on the root, which stretches the dam cervically in the interproximal space.

Additional Designs

Clamps that may be most useful when little coronal tooth structure remains have beaks that are inclined apically. These are termed *deep-reaching clamps.* Clamps with serrated edges are also available for cases involving minimal coronal structure. These clamps should not be placed on porcelain surfaces because damage may occur.[11]

For stability, the clamp selected must have four-point contact between the tooth and beaks. Failure to have a stable clamp may result in damage to the gingival attachment and coronal structure,[11,14] or the clamp may be dislodged. Clamps may also be modified by grinding to adapt to unusual situations.[15]

Placement of the rubber dam as a single unit is fast and efficient. Once in place the dam is flossed through the contacts, and the facial and lingual portions of the dam are flipped under the wings.

Identification of the tooth requiring treatment is usually routine. However, if no caries or restorations are present, the operator may clamp the wrong tooth. This can be avoided by marking the tooth before rubber dam application or by beginning the access after placement of a throat pack without the rubber dam in place.

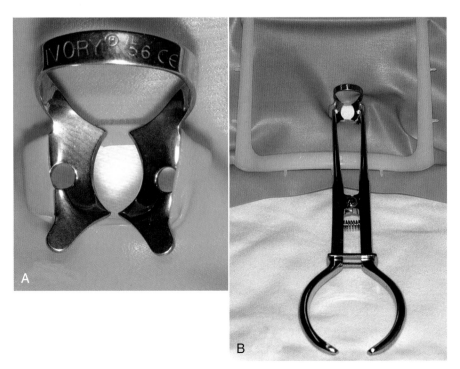

Fig. 15.4 **A,** Placement of the rubber dam as a single unit requires the use of a winged clamp. A hole is punched in the rubber dam and then stretched over the wings of the appropriate clamp. **B,** The rubber dam is attached to a plastic radiolucent frame, and the rubber dam forceps is then used to carry the unit to the tooth.

Preparation for Rubber Dam Placement

Before treatment is initiated, the degree of difficulty in obtaining adequate isolation must be assessed. Often, teeth requiring root canal treatment have large restorations, caries, or minimal remaining tooth structure that may present complications during isolation and access. Adequate isolation requires that caries, defective restorations, and restorations with leaking margins be removed before treatment. This preparation ensures an aseptic field of operation, allows assessment of tooth restorability, and permits temporization between visits.

Once the treatment plan has been finalized, it may be necessary to perform ancillary procedures to allow for placement of the rubber dam.[16,17]

Isolation of Teeth with Inadequate Coronal Structure

Ligation, the use of deep-reaching clamps, bonding, and clamping of the gingiva are the major methods of isolating teeth without adequate coronal tooth structure. Surgical management may also be required (Fig. 15.5).

Ligation

Inadequate coronal structure is not always the cause of lack of retention. In young patients the tooth may not have erupted sufficiently to make the cervical area available for clamp retention. In these cases, ligation with floss or the use of interproximal rubber Wedjets is indicated (see Fig. 15.15, *D*). Another approach is multiple tooth isolation.

Deep-Reaching Clamps

When the loss of tooth structure extends below the gingival tissues but there is adequate structure above the crestal bone, a deep-reaching clamp is indicated. It may be necessary to use a caulking material around the clamp to provide an adequate seal (Fig. 15.6). Another option is the use of an anterior retainer regardless of the tooth type.

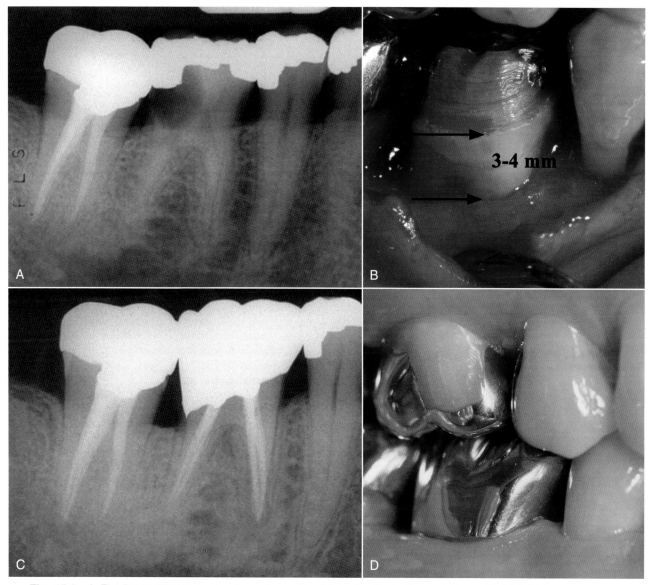

Fig. 15.5 **A,** The first molar shows extensive caries on the distal extending to the crestal bone. **B,** A full-thickness mucoperiosteal flap and osseous reduction are performed after caries excavation and preparation for a provisional crown; then, 3 to 4 mm of tooth structure coronal to the osseous crest restores the biologic width. **C,** Root canal treatment and placement of the crown. **D,** The definitive restoration.

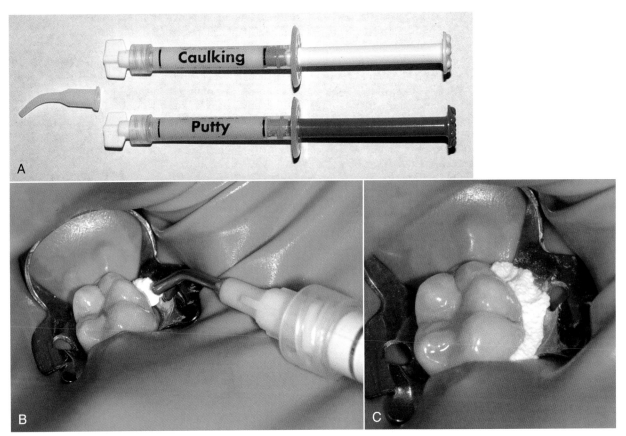

Fig. 15.6 **A,** Caulking and putty materials are available to prevent leakage after rubber dam application. **B,** Application of the caulk. **C,** The sealed dam.

Bonding

When there is missing tooth structure, including the natural height of contour, retention can be increased by bonding resin on the facial and lingual surfaces of the remaining tooth structure.[18] The clamp is placed apical to the resin undercut. After treatment the resin is easily removed. This technique is preferred over the more invasive technique of cutting horizontal grooves in the facial and lingual surfaces for the prongs of the clamp.

Clamping of the Gingiva

When the loss of tooth structure extends below the gingival tissues or below the crestal bone, clamping the gingival tissues is an option. This produces minimal damage, and the tissues heal. Postoperative discomfort is minimal (see Fig. 15.16, *D*).

Replacement of Coronal Structure
Temporary Restorations

When there is missing tooth structure but adequate retention, missing structure can be restored with reinforced intermediate restorative material (IRM) containing zinc oxide–eugenol, glass ionomers, or resins. These materials provide an adequate coronal seal and are stable until the definitive restoration is placed. Bonded materials provide a better seal with improved strength and esthetics, but placement is more time-consuming.

Coronal Buildups

Coronal buildups replace missing structure when the tooth exhibits inadequate retention for a temporary.[15,19] They are

rarely required and are time-consuming. Materials include amalgam and resins. Special retention is required, and anatomic landmarks are often lost.

Band Placement

Placement of orthodontic bands is a better option if a buildup is being considered. The bands are available in various sizes and are appropriately contoured. A band can be cemented and the missing tooth structure replaced with IRM (see Fig. 15.39). During the placement procedure, it is important to protect the canals and pulp chamber.

Provisional Crowns

Placement of temporary crowns is an option; however, they reduce visibility, result in the loss of anatomic landmarks, and may change the orientation for access and canal location. Often temporary crowns are displaced during treatment by the rubber dam clamp. In general, when provisional crowns are placed, they should be removed prior to endodontic treatment to provide the correct orientation and maintain the remaining tooth structure.

Corrective Surgery
Gingivectomy

Gingivectomy before root canal treatment is an option when the loss of tooth structure extends below the gingival tissues but there is adequate structure above the crestal bone.[20] It can also be used when the gingival tissues have grown into a carious defect. In general, the biologic width requires a minimum of 3 mm of sound tooth structure above the crestal bone: 1 mm for the epithelial attachment, 1 mm for the connective tissue attachment, and 1 mm for the margin of the final restoration.[21] If there is less than the required 3 mm of tooth structure, crown lengthening should be considered. Gingivectomy removes excessive gingival tissue and exposes the coronal root structure; however, osseous reduction is not possible. Electrosurgery is an option to the traditional scalpel because it provides a bloodless operating site. The small surgical electrodes make it easy to reach difficult areas, and the coagulating property provides hemostasis and enhances vision.[22] Care must be taken not to contact the alveolar bone because irreversible damage and necrosis will occur.[23,24]

Crown Lengthening

Crown lengthening is a procedure requiring an intrasulcular incision and flap reflection before osseous recontouring.[25-27] Enough osseous tissue is removed to provide at least 3 to 4 mm of sound tooth structure coronal to the crestal bone (see Fig. 15.5).[21,28,29] An additional factor is the ability to complete the root canal treatment adequately. Performing the surgical procedure and then discovering that the endodontic treatment cannot be accomplished is not in the best interest of the patient. For this reason, the procedures are often performed concurrently.

Orthodontic Extrusion

Orthodontic extrusion (forced eruption) is indicated when there is inadequate tooth structure for isolation and subsequent restoration and crown lengthening is contraindicated.[24,30] Criteria to consider during the treatment planning process include the resulting crown-root ratio after extrusion and esthetics (narrowing of the root form). The tooth must be extruded so that the biologic width is restored (3 mm of root coronal to the crestal bone). The minimum crown-root ratio after the extrusion is a 1 : 1 ratio.

Rubber Dam Placement
Placement as a Unit

Placement of the rubber dam, clamp, and frame as a unit is preferred (see Fig. 15.4). This is most efficient and is applicable in most cases. A traditional dam and frame can be used, or proprietary disposable systems are available (see Fig. 15.2). The steps in this process are as follows:

1. The dam is placed on the frame so that it is stretched tightly across the top and bottom but has slack horizontally in the middle.
2. A hole is punched in the dam, and then the clamp wings are attached to the dam.
3. The dam, frame, and clamp are placed as a unit to engage the tooth near the gingival margin.
4. The dam is released apically off the clamp wings to allow it to constrict around the tooth neck. The dam is then flossed through the contacts.

Placement of a Clamp, Followed by the Dam and Then the Frame

Placement of a clamp followed by the dam and frame is seldom used but may be necessary when an unobstructed view is required while the clamp is positioned. The clamp is first placed on the tooth and secured. The rubber dam is then stretched over the clamp and the frame affixed.[5]

Placement of the Rubber Dam and Frame and Then the Clamp

The preferred method for applying a butterfly clamp that does not have wings (No. 212) is to place the dam and frame and then the clamp. Better visualization is possible when the hole is stretched over the tooth and gingiva first by the operator or dental assistant, and the clamp is then placed. The No. 212 clamp has narrow beaks and is often used in situations in which wing clamps are unstable or cannot be retained.

Rubber Dam Leakage

Several proprietary products are available for placement around the rubber dam at the tooth-dam interface should leakage occur (see Fig. 15.6). These caulklike materials are easily applied and removed after treatment and are especially useful for isolation of an abutment for a fixed partial denture or for a tooth that is undergoing active orthodontic treatment.

The caulk can be placed on the gingival tissues before dam placement or at the dam-tooth interface after isolation. Both the caulking and putty materials adhere to wet surfaces, although the putty has a stiffer consistency.

Disinfection of the Operating Field

Various methods and techniques are used to disinfect the tooth, clamp, and surrounding rubber dam after placement. These include alcohol, quaternary ammonium compounds, sodium hypochlorite, organic iodine, mercuric salts, chlorhexidine, and hydrogen peroxide. An effective technique is as follows: (1) plaque is removed by rubber cup and pumice; (2) the rubber dam is placed; (3) the tooth surface, clamp, and surrounding rubber dam are scrubbed with 30% hydrogen peroxide; and (4) the surfaces are swabbed with 5% tincture of iodine or with sodium hypochlorite.[31]

ACCESS OPENINGS

Endodontic access openings are based on the anatomy and morphology of each individual tooth group. In general, the pulp chamber morphology dictates the design of the access preparation. The internal anatomy is projected onto the external surface. Internal pulp chamber morphology varies with the patient's age and secondary or tertiary dentin deposition. In anterior teeth and premolars with a single root, calcification occurs in a coronal to apical direction with the chamber receding. In posterior teeth with bifurcations and trifurcations, secondary dentin is deposited preferentially on the floor of the chamber, decreasing the cervical to apical dimension of the chamber.[32,33] The mesiodistal and buccolingual dimensions remain relatively the same, as does the cusp to roof distance. Dystrophic calcifications related to caries, restorations, attrition abrasion, and erosion also can occur. In general, the pulp chamber is located at the cementoenamel junction (CEJ).[34,35] In young teeth, the pulp horns are at approximately the level of the height of contour.

The major objectives of the access openings include (1) removal of the chamber roof and all coronal pulp tissue, (2) locating all canals, 3) unimpeded straight-line access of the instruments in the canals to the apical one third or the first curve (if present), and (4) conservation of tooth structure. Prior to initiating treatment, the clinician should assess the existing coronal structure, restorations present, tooth angulation in the arch, and the position, size, depth, and shape of the pulp chamber. A parallel preoperative radiograph or digital image is essential. Additional angled radiographs or digital images may aid the identification of additional canals and roots. Bitewing radiographs and digital images offer the most accurate and distortion-free information on chamber anatomy in posterior teeth. Recent advances in cone beam computed tomography (CBCT) imaging allow three-dimensional viewing of the pulp chamber and radicular space.[36,37] Conservation of tooth structure is important for subsequent restorative treatment and the long-term prognosis.[38] Maintaining adequate structure in the cervical region is assured by not extending the access preparation beyond the natural external chamber walls. The distance from the surface of the clinical crown to the peripheral vertical wall of the pulp chamber is the same throughout the circumference of the tooth at the level of the CEJ and the orifices of the root canals are located at the angles in the floor-wall junction[39]

General Principles

The general principles for endodontic access are outline form, convenience form, caries removal, and toilet of the cavity.

Outline form is the recommended shape for access of a normal tooth with radiographic evidence of a pulp chamber and canal space. The outline form assures the correct shape and location and provides straight-line access to the apical portion of the canal or to the first curvature. The access preparation must remove tooth structure that would impede the cleaning and shaping of the canal or canals. The outline form is a projection of the internal tooth anatomy onto the external root structure. The form can change with time. As an example, in anterior teeth with mesial and distal pulp horns the access is triangular. In older individuals with chamber calcification, the pulp horns are absent, so the access is ovoid.

Convenience form allows modification of the ideal outline form to facilitate unstrained instrument placement and manipulation. As an example, the use of nickel-titanium rotary instruments requires straight-line access. An access might be modified to permit placement and manipulation of the nickel-titanium instruments. Another example is a premolar exhibiting three roots. The outline form might be made more triangular to facilitate canal location.

Caries removal is essential for several reasons. First, removing caries permits the development of an aseptic environment before entering the pulp chamber and radicular space. Second, it allows assessment of restorability before treatment. Third, caries removal provides sound tooth structure so that an adequate provisional restoration can be placed. Unsupported tooth structure is removed to ensure a coronal seal during and after treatment so that the reference point for length determination is not lost should fracture occur.

Toilet of the cavity involves preventing materials and objects from entering the chamber and canal space. A common error is entering the pulp chamber before the coronal structure or restorative materials have been adequately prepared. As a result, these materials enter the canal space and may block the apical portion of the canal.

Canal Morphologies

Five major canal morphologies have been identified (Fig. 15.7).[40] They include round, ribbon or figure eight, ovoid, bowling pin, kidney bean, and C-shape. With the exception of the round morphologic shape, each presents unique problems for adequate cleaning and shaping.

General Considerations

In difficult cases the access can be prepared without the rubber dam in place. This allows visualization of the tooth shape, orientation, and position in the dental arch. When the canal or chamber is located, the rubber dam is applied. *Caution:* Until the rubber dam is in place, broaches and files cannot be used (see Fig. 15.1).

Care must be taken to prevent tooth structure or restorative materials from entering the radicular portion of the root if additional expansion of the access is necessary after the chamber is exposed. When an access is to be enlarged or restorative materials removed after chamber exposure, the radicular space must be protected. The canal orifice and chamber floor can be blocked by placing gutta-percha temporary stopping. The material is heated and then compacted with a plugger. The temporary stopping is removed with heat (preferred) or solvents after completion of the access preparation.

Before beginning the access, the clinician should assess the preoperative radiographs to determine the degree of case difficulty. At this stage the estimated depth of access is calculated. This is a measurement from the midlingual surface of anterior teeth and the occlusal surface of posterior teeth to the coronal portion of the pulp chamber. Calculated in millimeters, this information is then transferred to the access bur and provides information on the depth necessary to expose the pulp. If the estimated depth of access is reached and the pulp has not been encountered, the access depth and orientation must be reevaluated. A parallel radiograph exposed with the rubber dam removed helps determine the depth and orientation so that perforations and unnecessary removal of tooth structure can be avoided (see Fig. 15.33).

The estimated depth of access for anterior teeth is similar in different tooth groups.[41] The maxillary central and lateral incisors average 5.5 mm for the central incisor and 5 mm for the lateral incisor. The mandibular central and lateral incisors average 4.5 mm for the central incisor and 5 mm for the lateral incisor. The maxillary canine averages 5.5 mm and the mandibular canine, with its longer clinical crown, averages 6 mm. In maxillary furcated premolars, the average distance from the cusp buccal cusp tip to the roof of the chamber is 7 mm.[42] For maxillary molars the distance is 6 mm, and for the mandibular molars it is 6.5 mm. With an average pulp chamber height of 2 mm, the access depth for most molars should not extend beyond 8 mm (the floor of the chamber).[35]

Access openings are best accomplished using fissure burs in the high-speed handpiece. A number of special burs are also available for access. No single bur type is superior. For the clinician with a knowledge of anatomy and morphology and the appropriate clinical skills and judgment, bur selection is a personal choice (Figs. 15.8 and 15.9). Regardless of the high-speed bur chosen, the bur is placed in the chamber and removed while rotating. High-speed burs are not used in the canals. Failure to follow these principles can result in breakage (Fig. 15.10).

Visualization of the internal anatomy is enhanced during access by using a fiberoptic handpiece and microscopy.[43]

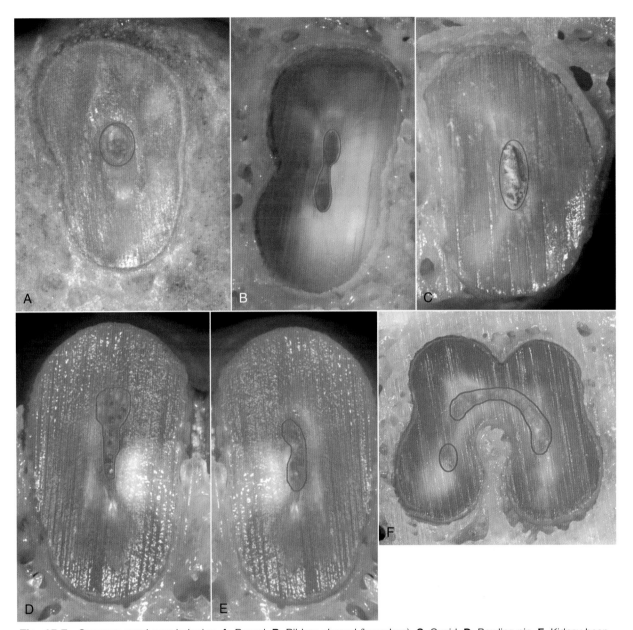

Fig. 15.7 Common canal morphologies. **A,** Round. **B,** Ribbon shaped (hourglass). **C,** Ovoid. **D,** Bowling pin. **E,** Kidney bean shaped. **F,** C-shaped.

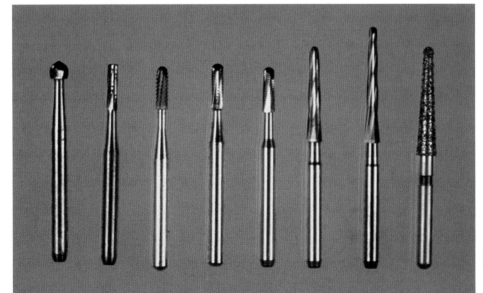

Fig. 15.8 Examples of access burs. *Left to right,* No. 4 round carbide, No. 557 carbide, Great White, Beaver bur, Transmetal, Multipurpose bur, Endo Z bur, and Endo Access bur.

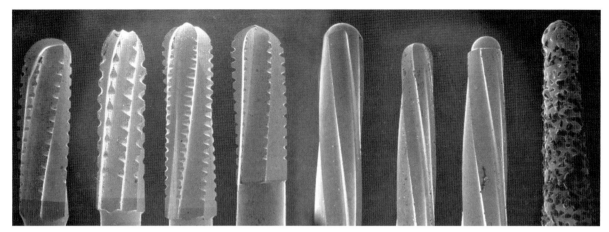

Fig. 15.9 *Left to right,* Magnified image of the Great White, Beaver bur, Transmetal, H34L, 269GK, Multipurpose bur, Endo Z bur, and Endo Access bur.

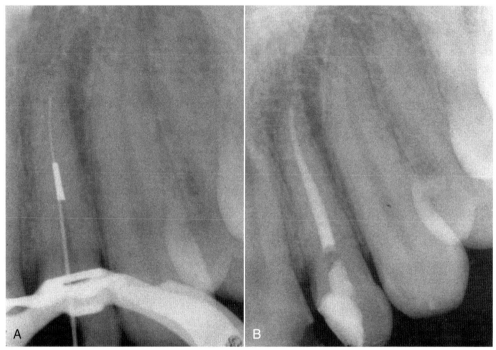

Fig. 15.10 **A,** Fractured fissure bur and working length file bypassing the obstruction. **B,** After the bur was removed with files and ultrasonics.

Illumination is the key. A sharp endodontic explorer is used to detect the canal orifice or to aggressively dislodge calcifications. When a canal is located, a small file or path-finding instrument (.06, .08, or .10 stainless steel file) is used to explore the canal and determine canal patency close to the apical foramen. Care should be exercised during this process to avoid forcing tissue apically, which might result in canal blockage (Fig. 15.11). This procedure is performed in the presence of irrigant or lubricant.

Often, in an attempt to preserve tooth structure, the access openings are constricted and underprepared. This creates problems with locating canals and gaining straight-line access. Removal of restorative materials during access is often indicated knowing that following treatment a new restoration will be placed. Removal enhances visibility and may reveal undetected canals, caries, or coronal fractures. When difficulties occur with calcifications or extensive restorations, the operator may become disoriented. The discovery of one canal can serve as a reference in locating the remaining canals. A file can be inserted and an angled radiograph exposed to reveal which canal has been located (see Chapter 13).

It is important not to violate marginal ridges during access preparation in any of the tooth groups.

Complex restorations, such as crowns and fixed partial dentures, may have changed the coronal landmarks used in canal location. A tipped tooth might be "uprighted" or a rotated tooth "realigned." Loss of orientation can result in incorrect identification of a canal, and searching for the other canals in the wrong direction results in excessive removal of tooth structure, perforation, or failure to locate and debride all canals.

Access through crowns with extensive foundations may make visibility difficult. Class V restorations may have induced coronal calcification or could have been placed

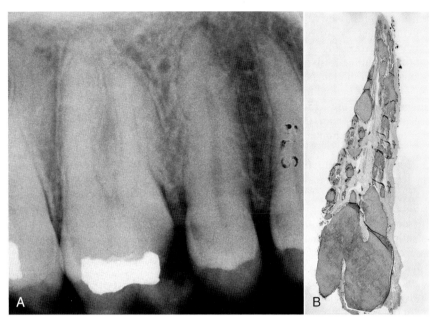

Fig. 15.11 **A,** Maxillary first molar shows extensive mesial caries. **B,** Histologic section of pulp tissue from the palatal canal reveals extensive calcification. Early canal exploration should be done with small files to avoid forcing the tissue and calcification apically and blocking the canal.

directly into the pulp space or the canals. In some instances, it may be best to remove restorative materials that interfere with visualization before initiating root canal treatment.

A modification of the armamentarium for teeth restored with crowns has been advocated for all-ceramic crowns. The initial outline and penetration through ceramic (porcelain) restorative material are made with a round diamond bur in the high-speed handpiece with water coolant. After penetration into dentin, a fissure bur is used. In teeth with porcelain-fused-to-metal restorations, a metal cutting bur is recommended. When possible, the access should remain in metal to reduce the potential for fracture in the porcelain. Evidence indicates that with a water coolant and careful instrumentation, diamond and carbide burs are equally effective.[44] The access is restored with amalgam after the root canal treatment.

In summary, aids in canal location include a knowledge of pulp anatomy and morphology; parallel straight-on and angled radiographs or digital images; a sharp endodontic explorer; interim radiographs or digital images; long-shanked, slow-speed burs (Fig. 15.12); ultrasonic instruments for troughing; dye staining; irrigation; transillumination; and enhanced vision with loupes or microscopy.[45]

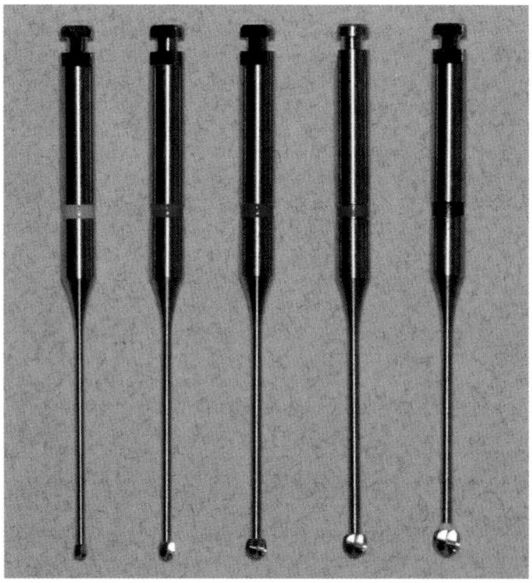

Fig. 15.12 Mueller burs have a round cutting head attached to a long shank. The long shank is not designed to drill deep into the root, but rather to extend the head of the slow-speed handpiece away from the tooth and permit better visibility.

ACCESS OPENINGS AND CANAL LOCATION*

Maxillary Central and Lateral Incisors

The maxillary central incisor has one root and one canal.[46] In young individuals, the prominent pulp horns require a triangular outline form to ensure that tissue and obturation materials, which otherwise might cause coronal discoloration, are removed (Fig. 15.13). Although the canal is centered in the

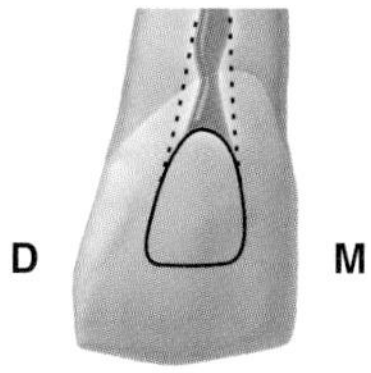

D   M

Fig. 15.13 A triangular outline form for access of the maxillary central incisor.

---

*See Appendix, Pulpal Anatomy and Access Preparations, for color illustrations showing the size, shape, and location of the pulp space in each tooth.

root at the CEJ and when the tooth is viewed from a mesial to distal orientation, it is evident that the crown is not directly in line with the long axis of the root (Fig. 15.14). For this reason, the establishment of the outline form and initial penetration into enamel are made with the bur perpendicular to the lingual surface of the tooth. This outline form is made in the middle third of the lingual surface (Figs. 15.15 and 15.16). After penetration to the depth of 2 to 3 mm, the bur is reoriented to coincide with the long axis and lingual orientation of the root.

After penetration to a depth of 2 to 3 mm, the bur is reoriented to coincide with the long axis and lingual orientation of the root. This reduces the risk of a lateral perforation through the facial surface. An additional common error is failure to remove the lingual shelf (see Fig. 15.15, *C*), which results in inadequate access to the entire canal. The canal is located by using a sharp endodontic explorer. When calcification has occurred, long-shanked burs in a slow-speed handpiece can be used (see Figs. 15.12 and 15.24, *D*). These burs move the head of the handpiece away from the tooth and enhance the ability to see exactly where the bur is placed in the tooth.

Access for the maxillary lateral incisor is similar to that for the central incisor. A triangular access is indicated in young patients with pulp horns (Fig. 15.17); as the pulp horns recede, the outline form becomes ovoid (Fig. 15.18).

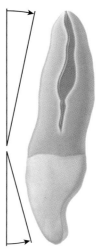

Fig. 15.14 Note the lingual inclination of the root in relation to the crown. In addition, the pattern of calcification occurs from the coronal portion of the pulp apically.

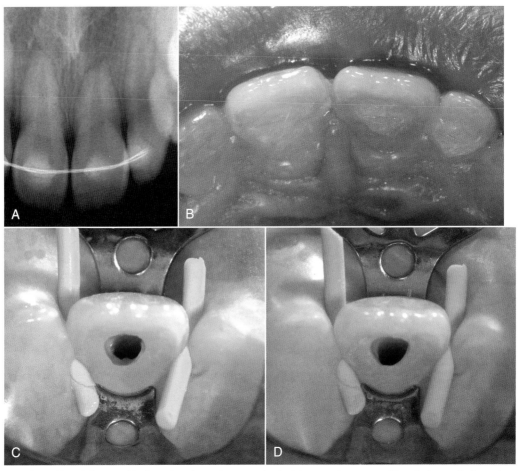

Fig. 15.15 A maxillary left central incisor showing pulp necrosis. **A,** A large pulp space with pulp horns that requires a triangular access outline. **B,** The lingual surface after removal of the orthodontic retaining wire. Note that tooth #9 is slightly discolored. **C,** The initial triangular access form exposing the chamber. Note that the lingual shelf has not been removed to expose the lingual wall. **D,** Removal of the lingual shelf, and completed access.

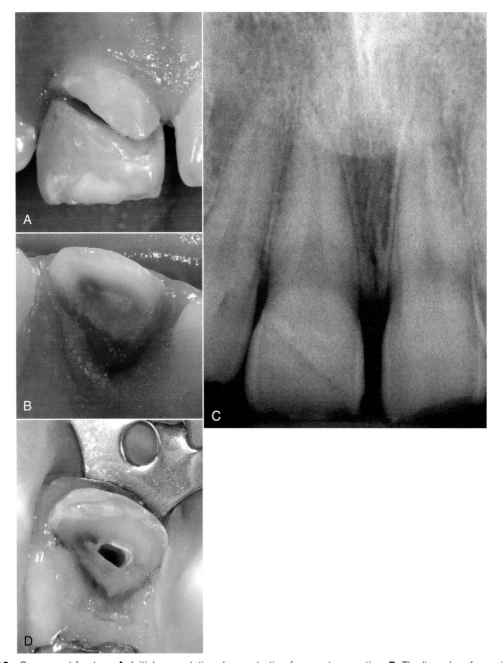

Fig. 15.16 Crown-root fracture. **A,** Initial presentation demonstrating fragment separation. **B,** The lingual surface with the segment removed. **C,** Preoperative radiograph. **D,** The extent of the fracture subgingivally requires a unique approach to isolation. Note that a premolar clamp is placed on the gingival tissues for isolation.

Fig. 15.17 Triangular outline form of the maxillary lateral incisor.

Dens invaginatus (or dens en dente) is a common developmental defect in the maxillary lateral incisor that results in pulp necrosis.[47,48] Additionally, a lingual groove may be found in maxillary lateral incisors, as evidenced by a narrow probing defect. These developmental defects complicate treatment and affect the prognosis.

Maxillary Canines

The maxillary canines have one canal in a single root. In general, pulp horns are absent, so the outline form is ovoid in the middle third of the lingual surface (Figs. 15.19 and 15.20). As attrition occurs, the chamber appears to move more incisally because of the loss of structure. In cross section the pulp

 15-2B

255

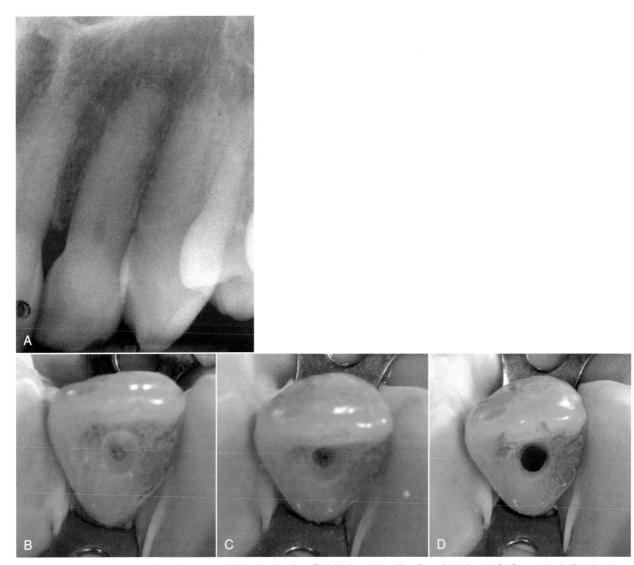

Fig. 15.18 **A,** Lateral incisor with a receded pulp chamber. **B,** Initial ovoid outline form is initiated. **C,** Coronal calcification is indicated by the color change. **D,** Completed access.

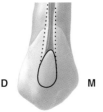

D   M

Fig. 15.19 Outline form for the maxillary canine.

is wide in a faciolingual direction compared to the mesiodistal dimension.

Maxillary Premolars

The maxillary first and second premolars have a similar coronal structure; therefore, the outline form is similar for these two teeth. It is centered in the crown and has an ovoid shape in the faciolingual direction (Figs. 15.21 and 15.22). An important anatomic consideration with these teeth is the mesial concavity at the CEJ. This is an area in which a lateral

perforation is likely to occur. When two canals are present, the canal orifices are located under the buccal and lingual cusp tips, equidistant from a line drawn through the center of the chamber in a mesial to distal direction. The cross-sectional morphology shows a kidney bean– or ribbon-shaped configuration. In rare instances when three canals are present, the outline form is triangular, with the base to the facial and the apex toward the lingual.

Maxillary Molars

The maxillary first and second molars have similar access outline forms. The outline form is triangular and located in the mesial half of the tooth, with the base to the facial and the apex toward the lingual (Figs. 15.23 and 15.24). The transverse or oblique ridge is left mostly intact. The external references for canal location serve as a guide in developing the outline form. The mesiobuccal canal orifice lies slightly distal to the mesiobuccal cusp tip. The distobuccal canal orifice lies distal and slightly lingual to the main mesiobuccal canal and is in line with the buccal groove. The lingual or palatal canal

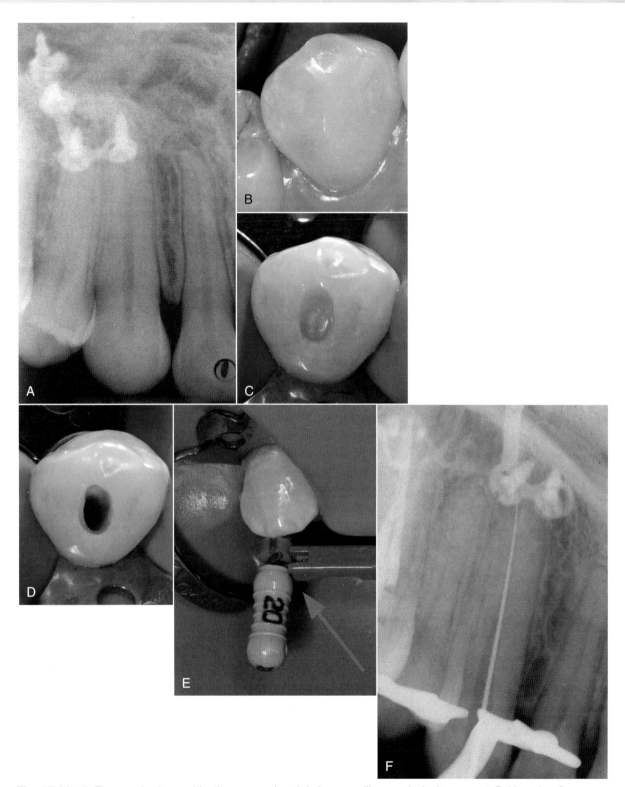

Fig. 15.20 **A,** The apex is obscured by the screws placed during a maxillary surgical advancement. **B,** Lingual surface. **C,** Initial access outline into dentin. **D,** Access is finalized. **E,** Apex locator *(arrow)*. **F,** Working length.

orifice generally exhibits the largest orifice and lies slightly distal to the mesiolingual cusp tip. The mesiobuccal root is very broad in a buccolingual direction, thus a small second canal is common.[49-53] The mesiolingual canal orifice (commonly referred to as the *MB2 canal*) is located 1 to 3 mm lingual to the main mesiobuccal canal (MB1 canal) and is slightly mesial to a line drawn from the mesiobuccal to the lingual or palatal canal. The initial movement of the canal from the chamber is often not toward the apex but laterally toward the mesial (Fig. 15.25). Removal of the coronal dentin (cornice) in this area permits exposure of the canal as it begins to move apically and facilitates negotiation (Figs. 15.26 and **257**

15.27; also see Figs. 15.24 and 15.25).[54] The operating microscope is a valuable aid.[29,38,43,52]

Mandibular Central and Lateral Incisors

15-2F The mandibular incisors are narrow in the mesiodistal dimension and broad faciolingually. There may be one canal with an ovoid or a ribbon-shaped configuration; often two canals are present. When there are two canals, the facial canal is easier to locate and is generally straighter than the lingual canal, which is often shielded by a lingual bulge. Because the tooth is often tipped facially, the lingual canal is difficult to locate; perforations primarily occur on the facial surface.

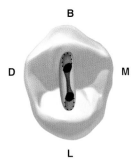

Fig. 15.21 Ovoid outline form for the maxillary premolars.

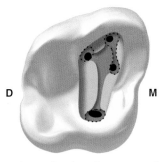

Fig. 15.23 Triangular outline form for access of the maxillary molar.

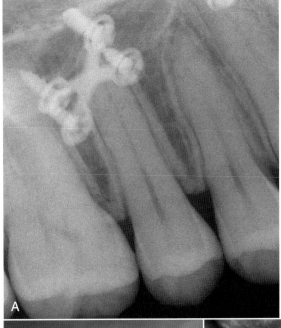

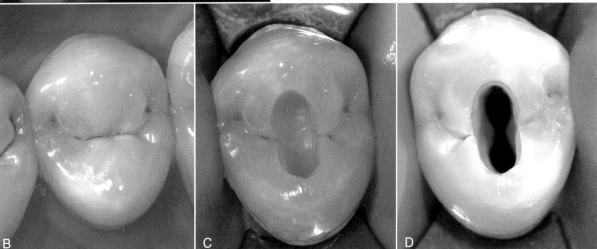

Fig. 15.22 **A,** Note the obstructed view of the apical region. **B,** Maxillary right second premolar. **C,** The initial outline form prepared into dentin. **D,** The chamber and canals are accessed.

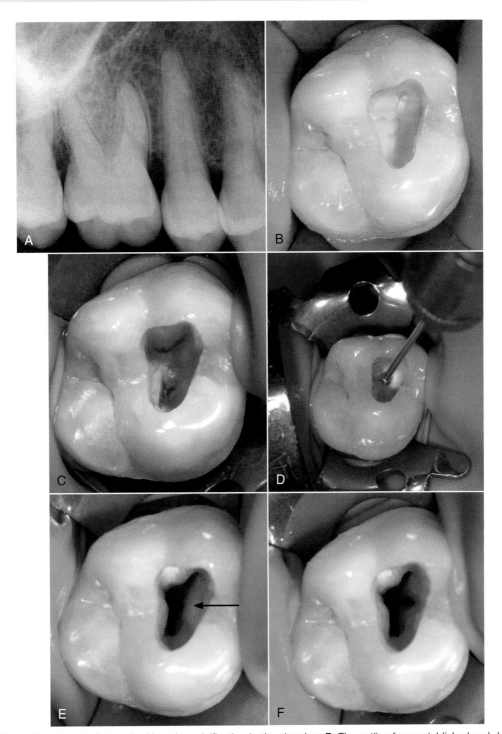

Fig. 15.24 **A,** Maxillary left first molar. Note the calcification in the chamber. **B,** The outline form established and dentin removed apically in layers. **C,** Exposure of the pulp horns. **D,** Use of a Mueller bur to completely unroof the chamber. Note the visibility and ability for precise removal of dentin. **E,** The completed access. The mesiobuccal canal is evident under the mesiobuccal cusp tip, the distobuccal canal is found opposite the buccal groove and slightly lingual to the main mesiobuccal canal, and the palatal canal is located under the mesiolingual cusp tip. Note the identification of the mesiolingual canal *(arrow).* **F,** Removal of the dentinal cornice that covers the mesiolingual canal to reveal the canal orifice. (See Appendix, Pulpal Anatomy and Access Preparations, for color illustrations showing the size, shape, and location of the pulp space within each tooth.)

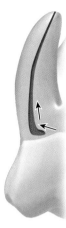

Fig. 15.25 The mesiolingual canal as it leaves the pulp chamber. Canals that are not negotiable but detected by an explorer may move laterally before proceeding apically.

The narrow mesiodistal dimension of these teeth makes access and canal location difficult. In young patients with mesiodistal pulp horns, the outline form is triangular with the base incisally and the apex gingivally. As the pulp recedes over time and the pulp horns disappear, the shape becomes more ovoid. The access is positioned in the middle third of the lingual surface (Figs. 15.28 and 15.29). Because of the small size of these teeth and the presence of mesiodistal concavities, access must be precisely positioned. The initial outline form is established into dentin with the bur perpendicular to the lingual surface. At a depth of 2 to 3 mm, the bur is reoriented along the long axis of the root. Because the percentage of teeth with two canals is reported to be 25% to 40%,[55,56] the lingual surface of the chamber and canal must be diligently explored with a small, precurved stainless steel file. A Gates-Glidden drill is used on the lingual to remove the dentin bulge.

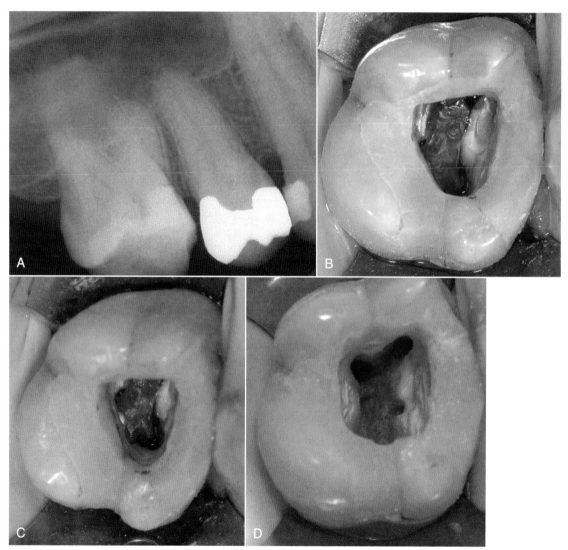

Fig. 15.26 **A,** Maxillary left first molar showing calcification. **B** and **C,** Initial access and identification of a pulp stone. Color and a thin line surrounding the periphery identify the hemorrhage. **D,** The pulp chamber with the stone removed. (See Appendix, Pulpal Anatomy and Access Preparations, for color illustrations showing the size, shape, and location of the pulp space within each tooth.)

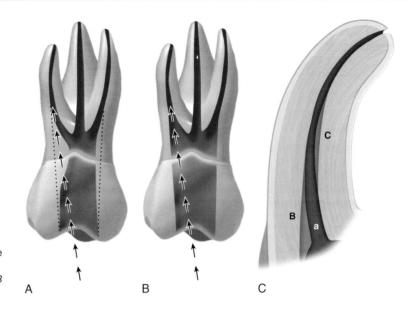

Fig. 15.27 **A,** The dashed lines show where dentin must be removed to achieve straight-line access. **B,** The access completed. **C,** The original canal *(a)* is modified using Gates-Glidden burs to remove tooth structure at *B* and *C.*

A   B   C

Fig. 15.28 Lingual outline form for the mandibular incisor.

In cases of attrition, the access moves toward the incisal surface. With the use of nickel-titanium rotary instruments, straight-line access is imperative. A more incisal approach on the lingual or facial surface is justified.[57] A modification of the access for the incisors is a facial approach.[58] This provides better visibility and can be used when there is crowding or when the canal is receded below the CEJ.

Mandibular Canines

The mandibular canines usually have a long, slender crown compared to the maxillary canine, which is shorter and wider in a mesiodistal direction. The tooth may have one or two roots. The root is broad in a faciolingual dimension and therefore may contain two canals.[49] The outline form is ovoid and positioned in the middle third of the crown on the lingual surface (Figs. 15.30 and 15.31). On access opening into the chamber, the lingual surface should be explored for the presence of a lingual canal. As attrition occurs, the access must be more incisal, and in severe cases it may actually include the incisal edge of the tooth.

Mandibular Premolars

The mandibular premolars appear to be easy to treat, but the anatomy may be complex. One, two, or three roots are possible, and canals often divide deep within the root in these complex morphologic configurations.[49,59] The crown of the first premolar has a prominent buccal cusp and a vestigial lingual cusp. In addition, there is a lingual constriction. Mesiodistal projections reveal that the chamber and canal orifice are positioned buccally. The access is therefore ovoid in a buccolingual dimension and positioned buccal to the

central groove (Figs. 15.32 and 15.33). It extends just short of the buccal cusp tip. The mandibular second premolar has a prominent buccal cusp, but the lingual cusp can be more prominent than with the first premolar. There is also a lingual constriction, so the outline form is ovoid from buccal to lingual and positioned centrally (Fig. 15.34).

Mandibular Molars

The mandibular molars are similar in anatomic configuration; however, there are subtle differences. The most common mandibular first molar configuration is two canals in the mesial root, although three have been reported,[60] and one canal in the distal root. A second canal is present in the distal root in 30% to 35% of cases (Fig. 15.35).[61,62] The roots often has a kidney bean shape in cross section with the concavity in the furcal region. The most common configuration for the mandibular second molar is two canals in the mesial root and one canal in the distal root. The incidence of four canals is low.[61]

The coronal reference points for canal location in the mandibular molar roots are influenced by the position of the crown on the root and by the lingual tipping of these teeth in the arch (Fig. 15.36). The mesiobuccal canal orifice is located slightly distal to the mesiobuccal cusp tip. The mesiolingual canal orifice is located in the area of the central groove area and slightly distal compared to the mesiobuccal canal. The distal canal is located near the intersection of the buccal, lingual, and central grooves. When a distobuccal canal is present, the orifice can be found buccal to the main distal canal and often is slightly more mesial. The mandibular first molar may even have a distinct separate extra distal root. Because of these anatomic relationships, the access outline form is rectangular or trapezoidal and positioned in the mesiobuccal portion of the crown (Fig. 15.37). An additional variation in mandibular molars is the presence of a middle mesial canal (Fig. 15.38).

During access preparation, the cervical bulge that overlies the canal orifices of the mesiobuccal and mesiolingual canals is removed (Fig. 15.39), permitting straight-line access to the first curve or apical portion of the root by reducing the emergence profile. This also enhances entry into the canals.

Text continued on p. 267 **261**

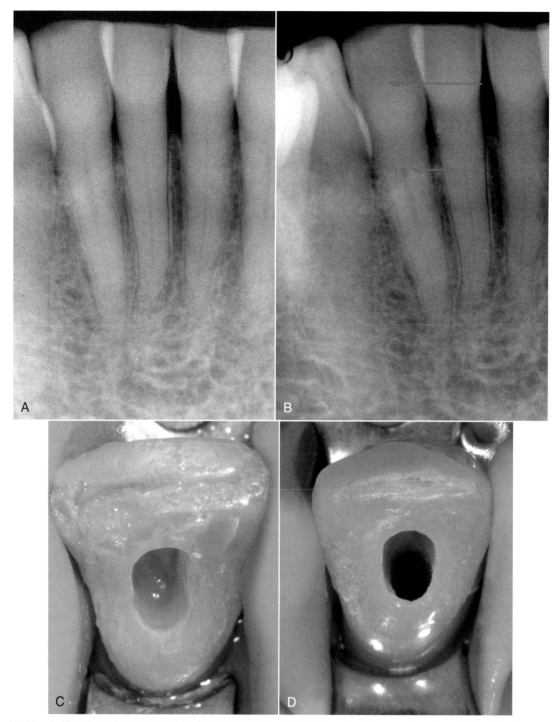

Fig. 15.29 **A,** Mandibular lateral incisor. **B,** Calculation of the estimated depth of access from the middle of the lingual surface to the coronal extent of the pulp. **C,** The initial outline form is more oval due to the receded chamber. **D,** Completed access.

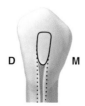

Fig. 15.30 Lingual ovoid outline form for the mandibular canine.

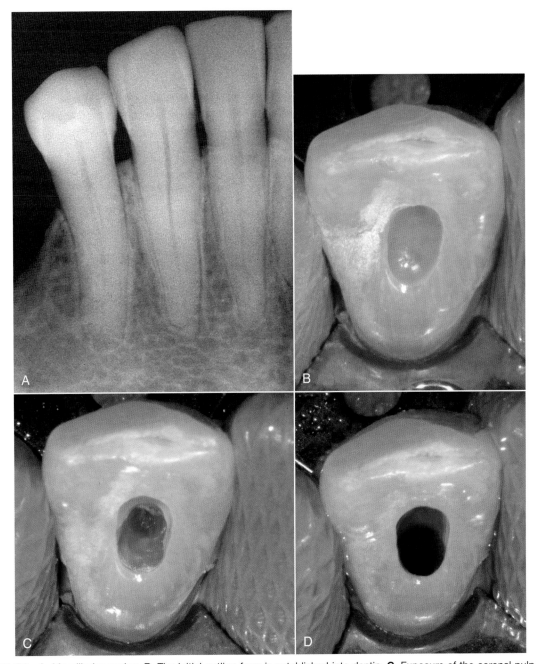

Fig. 15.31 **A,** Mandibular canine. **B,** The initial outline form is established into dentin. **C,** Exposure of the coronal pulp. **D,** The completed access opening.

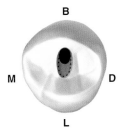

Fig. 15.32 Ovoid outline form for the mandibular first premolar. Note that the access is buccal to the central groove.

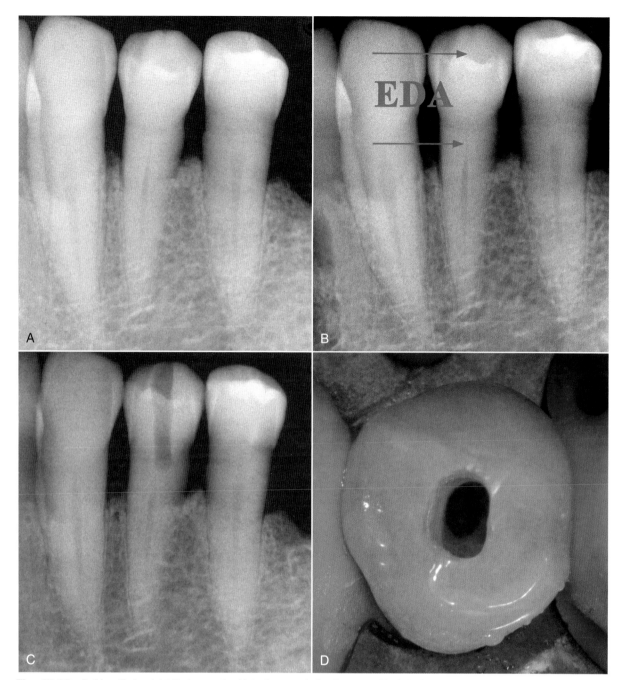

Fig. 15.33 **A,** Mandibular right first premolar. Note the receded pulp space. **B,** Calculation of the estimated depth of access. **C,** The estimated depth of access is reached, and the canal is not located. The rubber dam is removed and a straight-on parallel radiograph exposed. The film/digital image indicates that the canal is located mesial to the opening. **D,** The completed access.

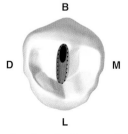

Fig. 15.34 Ovoid outline form for the mandibular second premolar.

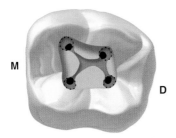

Fig. 15.35 Rectangular outline form for the mandibular first molar. Note that the mesiobuccal canal is located under the mesiobuccal cusp, and the mesiolingual canal lies centrally in relation to the crown and slightly to the distal of the mesiobuccal canal. The distolingual canal is located centrally, and the distobuccal canal lies more buccal and mesial to the main canal.

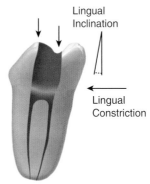

Fig. 15.36 Proximal view of a mandibular molar demonstrating the lingual inclination in the dental arch and a lingual constriction of the crown at the cementoenamel junction. Note that the mesiobuccal and mesiolingual canals are uniformly spaced within the root. However, with coronal access, the external reference points for the canal's location are the mesiobuccal cusp tip and the central groove as it crosses the mesial marginal ridge.

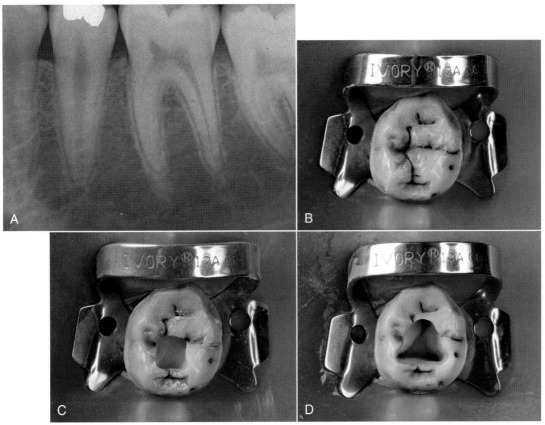

Fig. 15.37 **A,** The preoperative radiograph of a mandibular first molar. **B,** The preoperative occlusal anatomy. **C,** The initial access outline form. **D,** The completed access cavity demonstrating the two mesial canals and the single distal canal. (See Appendix, Pulpal Anatomy and Access Preparations, for color illustrations showing the size, shape, and location of the pulp space within each tooth.)

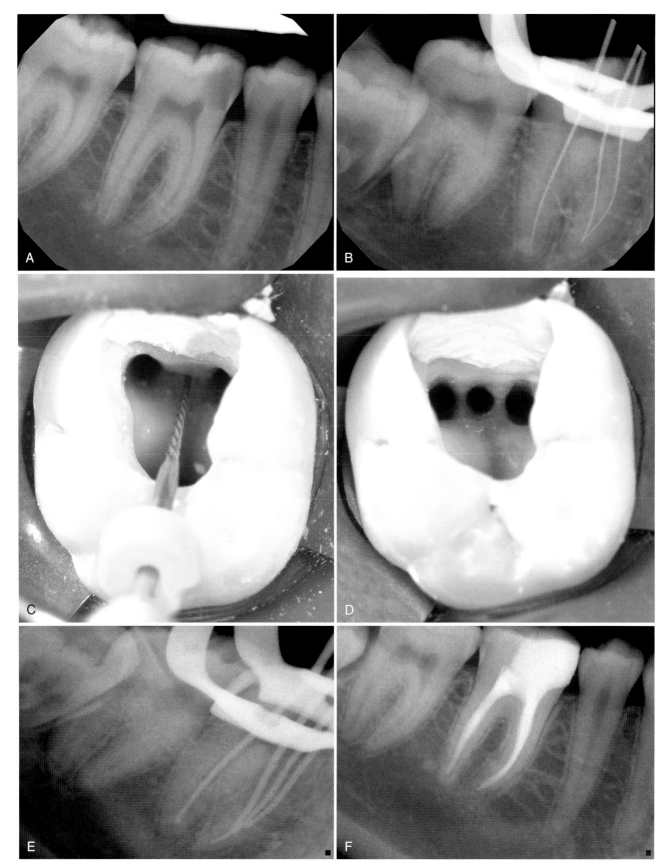

Fig. 15.38 **A,** Preoperative radiograph of a mandibular first molar with a middle mesial canal. **B,** Original working length radiographic image. **C,** Middle mesial canal located. **D,** Prepared canal. **E,** Master cone radiographic image. **F,** Postoperative radiographic image of tooth #30.

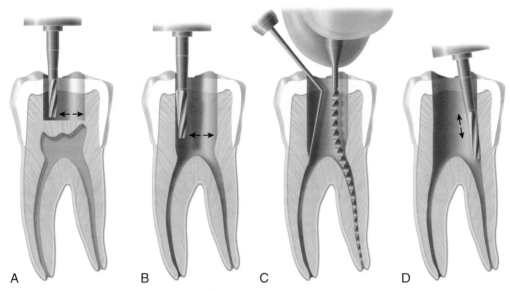

A   B   C   D

Fig. 15.39 Basic steps in access preparation. **A,** The access cavity is outlined deep into dentin and close to the estimated depth of access with the high-speed handpiece. **B,** Penetration and unroofing are achieved by fissure high-speed bur or slow-speed latch-type burs. Other bur configurations are acceptable. **C, D** Canal orifices are located and identified with an endodontic explorer. Small files are used to negotiate to the estimated working length. The dentin shelf that overlies and obscures the orifices is removed.

ERRORS IN ACCESS

Inadequate Preparation

Errors in access preparations are varied (Fig. 15.40). A common error is inadequate preparation, which has several significant consequences. Direct effects are decreased access and visibility, which prevent the clinician from locating the canals. The ability to remove the coronal pulp tissue and subsequent obturation materials is limited, and straight-line access cannot be achieved. Inadequate straight-line access can indirectly lead to errors during the cleaning and shaping. When files are deflected by coronal interferences, procedural errors, such as loss of working length, apical transportation, ledging, and apical perforation, are likely in curved canals. A No. 25 file or above has a straightening force that overcomes the confining resistance of the dentin wall. The file cuts on the outer surface apical to the curvature and the inner wall coronal to the curve. Adequate straight-line access decreases the canal curvature and reduces the coronal interferences, allowing the instrument to work more freely in the canal.[62]

Excessive Removal of Tooth Structure

The excessive removal of tooth structure has direct consequences and unlike inadequate preparation is irreversible and cannot be corrected. A minimum consequence is weakening of the tooth and subsequent coronal fracture. Evidence indicates that appropriate access and strategic removal of tooth structure that does not involve the marginal ridges do not significantly weaken the remaining coronal structure.[63] The marginal ridges provide the faciolingual strength to the crown[64]; access openings do not require removal of tooth structure in this area.[65]

The ultimate result of removing excessive tooth structure is perforation. Perforations in single-rooted teeth are located on the lateral surface. In multirooted teeth, perforations may be lateral or furcal (see Chapter 19).

LENGTH DETERMINATION

Radiographic Evaluation

The *working length* is defined as the distance from a predetermined coronal reference point (usually the incisal edge in anterior teeth and a cusp tip in posterior teeth) to the point where the cleaning and shaping and obturation should terminate. The reference point must be stable so that fracture does not occur between visits. Unsupported cusps that are weakened by caries or restorations should be reduced. The point of termination is empirical and based on anatomic studies; it should be 1 mm from the radiographic apex.[66,67] This accounts for the deviation of the foramen from the apex, and the distance from the major diameter of the foramen to the area where a dentinal matrix can be established apically. 15-3

Before access, an estimated working length is calculated by measuring the total length of the tooth on the diagnostic parallel radiograph or digital image. If the canal is curved, the canal length can be measured by placing a file that has been curved to duplicate the canal morphology against the film. The stop can be adjusted to coincide with the reference point, while the file tip is aligned with the radiographic apex. After adjustment of the stop, the file is straightened and the length measured. From a practical perspective, a calculation to the nearest 0.5 mm should be made. Then 2 mm are subtracted to account for the foramen distance (1 mm) and radiographic image distortion/magnification (1 mm).[68] This provides a safety factor so that instruments are not placed beyond the apex. Violation of the apex may result in inoculation of the periapical tissues with necrotic tissue, debris, and bacteria[69] and can lead to extrusion of materials during obturation[70,71] and a less favorable prognosis.[72]

After access preparation, a small file is used to explore the canal and establish patency to the estimated working length. The largest file to bind is then inserted to this estimated length; a file that is loose in the canal may be displaced during

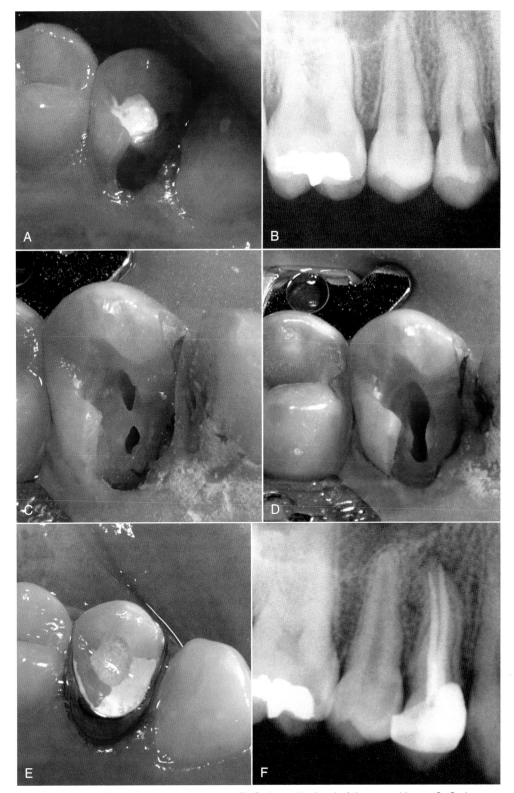

Fig. 15.40 **A,** Access made through gross mesial caries. **B,** Caries at the level of the crestal bone. **C,** Caries removal provides an aseptic operating field and allows assessment of restorability. Note that the previous access failed to deroof the chamber. **D,** Appropriate access reveals a ribbon-shaped pulp chamber. **E,** An orthodontic band placed to provide isolation. **F,** Postobturation.

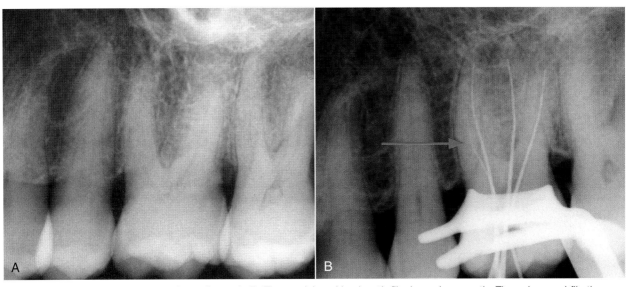

Fig. 15.41 **A,** Parallel preoperative radiograph. **B,** The mesial working length film is made correctly. The apices and file tips are clearly visible. Note the mesiolingual canal *(arrow)*.

film exposure or forced beyond the apex if the patient bites down inadvertently. Millimeter markings on the file shaft or rubber stops on the instrument shaft are used for length control. A sterile millimeter ruler or measuring device can be used to adjust the stops on the file. To ensure accurate measurement and length control during canal preparation, the stop must physically contact the coronal reference point. To obtain an accurate measurement, the minimum size of the working length should be a No. 20 file. With files smaller than No. 20, it is difficult to interpret the location of the file tip on the working length film or digital image. In multirooted teeth, files are placed in all canals before the film is exposed.

Angled films or digital images are necessary to separate superimposed files and structures (Fig. 15.41),[73] to provide an efficient method of determining the working length, and to reduce radiation to the patient. It is imperative that the rubber dam be left in place during working length determination to ensure an aseptic environment and to protect the patient from swallowing or aspirating instruments. The film/digital sensor can be held with a hemostat or a positioning device (Fig. 15.42).

A modified paralleling technique is used to position the film/digital sensor and the cone; this has been shown to be superior to the bisecting-angle technique.[74,75] With the modified paralleling technique, the film/digital sensor is positioned by using a hemostat approximately parallel to the long axis of the tooth. The cone is then positioned so that the central beam strikes the film at a 90-degree angle (Fig. 15.43). Although this technique is reliable, it is not foolproof.[76]

Other clinical factors should be considered in establishing the corrected working length. These include tactile sensation,[77] the patient's response, and hemorrhage. The use of tactile sensation may be valuable in large tapering canals; however, in small cylindrical canals, the rate of taper of the files may exceed the rate of taper of the canal and binding occurs coronally, giving the false sense of constriction. Preflaring the canal before length determination increases the tactile sensation significantly compared to unflared canals.[78]

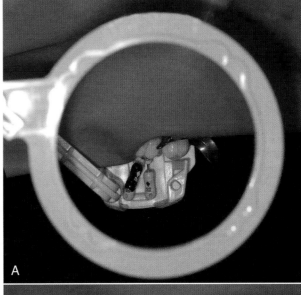

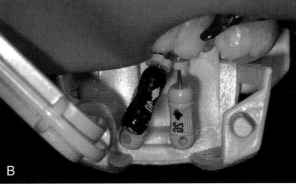

Fig. 15.42 **A,** Positioning device for holding working films. The ring assists in cone alignment. **B,** Close-up view of the device in position.

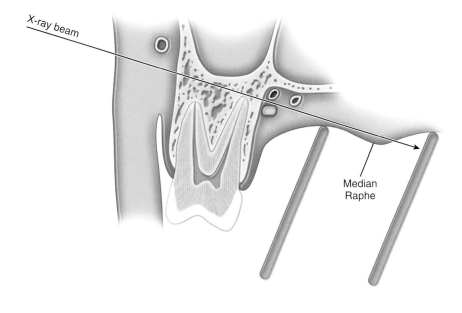

X-ray beam

Median
Raphe

Fig. 15.43 Proper positioning of the radiograph when making a working length radiograph. To capture the palatal root, the film should be placed on the opposite side of the midline.

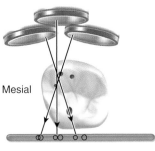

Mesial

Fig. 15.44 Separation of the mesiobuccal and mesiolingual canals achieved by varying the horizontal angle. With maxillary molars, maximum separation occurs with a mesial cone angulation because of the mesial location of the mesiolingual canal in relation to the mesiobuccal canal.

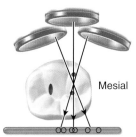

Mesial

Fig. 15.45 Separation of the mesiobuccal and mesiolingual canals achieved by varying the horizontal angle. With mandibular molars, maximum separation occurs with a distal orientation because of the mesial location of the mesiobuccal canal in relation to the mesiolingual canal.

After the film or sensor exposure, the corrected working length is calculated. The distance from the file tip to the radiographic apex is determined. If the distance is greater than 1 mm, a calculation is made (adding or subtracting length) so that the file tip is positioned 1 mm from the radiographic apex. If the correction is greater than 3 mm, a second working length radiograph or distal image should be made with the file placed at the adjusted length.

With angled radiographs or distal images, the canal determination is based on the buccal object or SLOB rule (same lingual, opposite buccal; see Chapter 12).[79,80] Because maxillary anterior teeth have only one canal, no angle is necessary. Mesial angles are recommended for premolars and maxillary molars (Fig. 15.44). Distal angulation is recommended for the mandibular incisors and molars (Fig. 15.45). For maxillary posterior teeth, the film should be placed on the opposite side of the midline to facilitate capture of the palatal roots on the film (see Fig. 15.43).

Electronic Apex Locators

Apex locators are also used in determining length.[81,82] Contemporary apex locators are based on the principle that the flow of higher frequencies of alternating current is facilitated in a biologic environment compared to lower frequencies. Passing two differing frequencies through the canal results in the higher frequency impeding the lower frequency (Fig. 15.46). The impedance values that change relative to each other are measured and converted to length information. At the apex, the impedance values are at their maximum differences. Unlike previous models, the impedance apex locator operates accurately in the presence of electrolytes.[83] Apex locators are helpful in length determination but must be confirmed with radiographs. Films or digital images help confirm the appropriate length and can identify missed canals. If the file is not centered in the root, a second canal is likely to be present.

An apex locator is very helpful in patients with structures or objects that obstruct visualization of the apex, patients who have a gag reflex and cannot tolerate films, and patients with medical problems that prohibit the holding of a film or sensor.

The use of apex locators and electric pulp testers in patients with cardiac pacemakers has been questioned.[84-89] In a recent study involving 27 patients with either implanted cardiac pacemakers or cardioverter/defibrillators, two impedance apex locators and one electric pulp tester did not interfere with the functioning of any of the cardiac devices.[90] However, it may be advisable not to use these devices in these patients; other means of length determination and pulp testing are available.

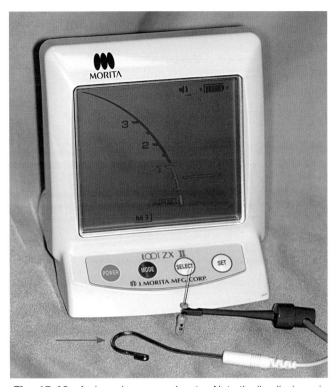

Fig. 15.46 An impedance apex locator. Note the lip clip *(arrow)*.

REFERENCES

1. Cohen S, Schwartz S: Endodontic complications and the law. *J Endod* 13:191-197, 1987.
2. Anabtawi MF, Gilbert GH, Bauer MR, et al: Rubber dam use during root canal treatment: findings from The Dental Practice-Based Research Network, *J Am Dent Assoc* 144:179-186, 2013.
3. Huggins DR: The rubber dam: an insurance policy against litigation, *J Indiana Dent Assoc* 65:23-24, 1986.
4. Taintor JF, Biesterfeld RC: A swallowed endodontic file: case report, *J Endod* 4:254-255, 1978.
5. Forrest WR, Perez RS: AIDS and hepatitis prevention: the role of the rubber dam, *Oper Dent* 11:159, 1986.
6. Cochran MA, Miller CH, Sheldrake MA: The efficacy of the rubber dam as a barrier to the spread of microorganisms during dental treatment, *J Am Dent Assoc* 119:141-144, 1989.
7. Samaranayake LP, Reid J, Evans D: The efficacy of rubber dam isolation in reducing atmospheric bacterial contamination, *ASDC J Dent Child* 56:442-444, 1989.
8. Miller RL, Micik RE: Air pollution and its control in the dental office, *Dent Clin North Am* 22:453-476, 1978.
9. Wong RC: The rubber dam as a means of infection control in an era of AIDS and hepatitis, *J Indiana Dent Assoc* 67:41-43, 1988.
10. de Andrade ED, Ranali J, Volpato MC, et al: Allergic reaction after rubber dam placement, *J Endod* 26:182-183, 2000.
11. Madison S, Jordan RD, Krell KV: The effects of rubber dam retainers on porcelain fused-to-metal restorations, *J Endod* 12:183-186, 1986.
12. Zerr M, Johnson WT, Walton RE: Effect of rubber-dam retainers on porcelain fused to metal. *Gen Dent* 44:132-134; quiz, 41-42; 1996.
13. Schwartz SF, Foster JK Jr: Roentgenographic interpretation of experimentally produced bony lesions. I, *Oral Surg Oral Med Oral Pathol* 32:606-612, 1971.
14. Jeffrey IW, Woolford MJ: An investigation of possible iatrogenic damage caused by metal rubber dam clamps, *Int Endod J* 22:85-91, 1989.
15. Weisman MI: A modification of the No. 3 rubber dam clamp, *J Endod* 9:30-31, 1983.
16. Liebenberg WH: Access and isolation problem solving in endodontics: anterior teeth, *J Can Dent Assoc* 59:663-667, 70-71, 1993.
17. Liebenberg WH: Access and isolation problem solving in endodontics: posterior teeth, *J Can Dent Assoc* 59:817-822, 1993.
18. Wakabayashi H, Ochi K, Tachibana H, et al: A clinical technique for the retention of a rubber dam clamp, *J Endod* 12:422-424, 1986.
19. Iglesias AM, Urrutia C: Solution for the isolation of the working field in a difficult case of root canal therapy, *J Endod* 21:394-395, 1995.
20. Kalkwarf KL, Krejci RF, Wentz FM, et al: Epithelial and connective tissue healing following electrosurgical incisions in human gingiva, *J Oral Maxillofac Surg* 41:80-85, 1983.
21. Garguilo AW, Wentz FM, Orban B: Dimensions of the dentogingival junction in humams, *J Periodontol* 32:261-267, 1961.
22. Kalkwarf KL, Krejci RF, Wentz FM: Healing of electrosurgical incisions in gingiva: early histologic observations in adult men, *J Prosthet Dent* 46:662-672, 1981.
23. Azzi R, Kenney EB, Tsao TF, et al: The effect of electrosurgery on alveolar bone, *J Periodontol* 54:96-100, 1983.
24. Johnson RH: Lengthening clinical crowns, *J Am Dent Assoc* 121:473-476, 1990.
25. Becker W, Ochsenbein C, Becker BE: Crown lengthening: the periodontal-restorative connection, *Compend Contin Educ Dent* 19:239-240; 42, 44-46, passim; quiz, 56; 1998.
26. Kaldahl WB, Becker CM, Wentz FM: Periodontal surgical preparation for specific problems in restorative dentistry, *J Prosthet Dent* 51:36-41, 1984.
27. Lovdahl PE, Gutmann JL: Periodontal and restorative considerations prior to endodontic therapy, *Gen Dent* 28:38-45, 1980.
28. Goto Y, Nicholls JI, Phillips KM, et al: Fatigue resistance of endodontically treated teeth restored with three dowel-and-core systems, *J Prosthet Dent* 93:45-50, 2005.
29. Libman WJ, Nicholls JI: Load fatigue of teeth restored with cast posts and cores and complete crowns, *Int J Prosthodont* 8:155-161, 1995.
30. Johnson GK, Sivers JE: Forced eruption in crown-lengthening procedures, *J Prosthet Dent* 56:424-427, 1986.
31. Hermsen KP, Ludlow MO: Disinfection of rubber dam and tooth surfaces before endodontic therapy, *Gen Dent* 35:355-356, 1987.
32. Tidmarsh BG: Micromorphology of pulp chambers in human molar teeth, *Int Endod J* 13:69-75, 1980.
33. Shaw L, Jones AD: Morphological considerations of the dental pulp chamber from radiographs of molar and premolar teeth, *J Dent* 12:139-145, 1984.
34. Patel S, Rhodes J: A practical guide to endodontic access cavity preparation in molar teeth, *Br Dent J* 203:133-140, 2007.
35. Deutsch AS, Musikant BL: Morphological measurements of anatomic landmarks in human maxillary and mandibular molar pulp chambers, *J Endod* 30:388-390, 2004.
36. Patel S, Dawood A, Ford TP, et al: The potential applications of cone beam computed tomography in the management of endodontic problems, *Int Endod J* 40:818-830, 2007.
37. Scarfe WC, Levin MD, Gane D, et al: Use of cone beam computed tomography in endodontics, *Int J Dent* 10:20-25, 2009..
38. Clark D, Khademi J: Modern molar endodontic access and directed dentin conservation, *Dent Clin North Am* 54:249-273, 2010.
39. Krasner P, Rankow HJ: Anatomy of the pulp-chamber floor, *J Endod* 30:5-16, 2004.
40. Weine FS: *Endodontic therapy*, ed 6, St Louis, 2004, Mosby.
41. Lee MM, Rasimick BJ, Turner AM, et al: Morphological measurements of anatomic landmarks in pulp chambers of human anterior teeth, *J Endod* 33:129-131, 2007.
42. Deutsch AS, Musikant BL, Gu S, et al: Morphological measurements of anatomic

landmarks in pulp chambers of human maxillary furcated bicuspids, *J Endod* 31:570-573, 2005.

43. Baldassari-Cruz LA, Lilly JP, Rivera EM: The influence of dental operating microscope in locating the mesiolingual canal orifice, *Oral Surg Oral Med Oral Pathol Oral Radiol Endod* 93:190-194, 2002.

44. Haselton DR, Lloyd PM, Johnson WT: A comparison of the effects of two burs on endodontic access in all-ceramic high lucite crowns, *Oral Surg Oral Med Oral Pathol Oral Radiol Endod* 89:486-492, 2000.

45. de Carvalho MC, Zuolo ML: Orifice locating with a microscope, *J Endod* 26:532-534, 2000.

46. Kasahara E, Yasuda E, Yamamoto A, et al: Root canal system of the maxillary central incisor, *J Endod* 16:158-161, 1990.

47. Dankner E, Harari D, Rotstein I: Dens evaginatus of anterior teeth: literature review and radiographic survey of 15,000 teeth, *Oral Surg Oral Med Oral Pathol Oral Radiol Endod* 81:472-475, 1996.

48. Gound TG: Dens invaginatus: a pathway to pulpal pathology—a literature review, *Pract Periodontics Aesthet Dent* 9:585-594; quiz, 96; 1997.

49. Green D: Double canals in single roots, *Oral Surg Oral Med Oral Pathol* 35:689-696, 1973.

50. Kulild JC, Peters DD: Incidence and configuration of canal systems in the mesiobuccal root of maxillary first and second molars, *J Endod* 16:311-317, 1990.

51. Pineda F: Roentgenographic investigation of the mesiobuccal root of the maxillary first molar, *Oral Surg Oral Med Oral Pathol* 36:253-260, 1973.

52. Stropko JJ: Canal morphology of maxillary molars: clinical observations of canal configurations, *J Endod* 25:446-450, 1999.

53. Weine FS, Healey HJ, Gerstein H, et al: Canal configuration in the mesiobuccal root of the maxillary first molar and its endodontic significance, *Oral Surg Oral Med Oral Pathol* 28:419-425, 1969.

54. Acosta Vigouroux SA, Trugeda Bosaans SA: Anatomy of the pulp chamber floor of the permanent maxillary first molar, *J Endod* 4:214-219, 1978.

55. Benjamin KA, Dowson J: Incidence of two root canals in human mandibular incisor teeth, *Oral Surg Oral Med Oral Pathol* 38:122-126, 1974.

56. Rankine-Wilson RW, Henry P: The bifurcated root canal in lower anterior teeth, *J Am Dent Assoc* 70:1162-1165, 1965.

57. Mauger MJ, Waite RM, Alexander JB, et al: Ideal endodontic access in mandibular incisors, *J Endod* 25:206-207, 1999.

58. Clements RE, Gilboe DB: Labial endodontic access opening for mandibular incisors: endodontic and restorative considerations, *J Can Dent Assoc* 57:587-589, 1991.

59. Vertucci FJ: Root canal morphology of mandibular premolars, *J Am Dent Assoc* 97:47-50, 1978.

60. Vertucci FJ: Root canal anatomy of the human permanent teeth, *Oral Surg Oral Med Oral Pathol* 58:589-599, 1984.

61. Hartwell G, Bellizzi R: Clinical investigation of in vivo endodontically treated mandibular and maxillary molars, *J Endod* 8:555-557, 1982.

62. Skidmore AE, Bjorndal AM: Root canal morphology of the human mandibular first molar, *Oral Surg Oral Med Oral Pathol* 32:778-784, 1971.

63. Reeh ES, Messer HH, Douglas WH: Reduction in tooth stiffness as a result of endodontic and restorative procedures, *J Endod* 15:512-516, 1989.

64. Sedgley CM, Messer HH: Are endodontically treated teeth more brittle? *J Endod* 18:332-335, 1992.

65. Wilcox LR, Walton RE: The shape and location of mandibular premolar access openings, *Int Endod J* 20:223-227, 1987.

66. Chapman CE: A microscopic study of the apical region of human anterior teeth, *J Br Endod Soc* 3:52-58, 1969.

67. Dummer PM, McGinn JH, Rees DG: The position and topography of the apical canal constriction and apical foramen, *Int Endod J* 17:192-198, 1984.

68. Vande Voorde H, Bjorndal AM: Estimating endodontic "working length" with paralleling radiographs, *Oral Surg Oral Med Oral Pathol* 27:106, 1969.

69. Ricucci D, Pascon EA, Ford TR, et al: Epithelium and bacteria in periapical lesions, *Oral Surg Oral Med Oral Pathol Oral Radiol Endod* 101:239-249, 2006.

70. Ricucci D, Langeland K: Apical limit of root canal instrumentation and obturation. Part 2. A histological study, *Int Endod J* 31:394-409, 1998.

71. Ricucci D: Apical limit of root canal instrumentation and obturation. Part 1. Literature review, *Int Endod J* 31:384-393, 1998.

72. Schaeffer MA, White RR, Walton RE: Determining the optimal obturation length: a meta-analysis of literature, *J Endod* 31:271-274, 2005.

73. Dummer PM, Lewis JM: An evaluation of the endometric probe in root canal length estimation, *Int Endod J* 20:25-29, 1987.

74. Forsberg J: A comparison of the paralleling and bisecting-angle radiographic techniques in endodontics, *Int Endod J* 20:177-182, 1987.

75. Forsberg J: Radiographic reproduction of endodontic "working length" comparing the paralleling and the bisecting-angle techniques, *Oral Surg Oral Med Oral Pathol* 64:353-360, 1987.

76. Olson AK, Goerig AC, Cavataio RE, et al: The ability of the radiograph to determine the location of the apical foramen, *Int Endod J* 24:28-35, 1991.

77. Seidberg BH, Alibrandi BV, Fine H, et al: Clinical investigation of measuring working lengths of root canals with an electronic device and with digital-tactile sense, *J Am Dent Assoc* 90:379-387, 1975.

78. Stabholz A, Rotstein I, Torabinejad M: Effect of preflaring on tactile detection of the apical constriction, *J Endod* 21:92-94, 1995.

79. Goerig AC, Neaverth EJ: A simplified look at the buccal object rule in endodontics, *J Endod* 13:570-572, 1987.

80. Richards AG: The buccal object rule, *Dent Radiogr Photogr* 53:37, 1980.

81. McDonald NJ: The electronic determination of working length, *Dent Clin North Am* 36:293-307, 1992.

82. Pratten DH, McDonald NJ: Comparison of radiographic and electronic working lengths, *J Endod* 22:173-176, 1996.

83. Fouad AF, Rivera EM, Krell KV: Accuracy of the Endex with variations in canal irrigants and foramen size, *J Endod* 19:63-67, 1993.

84. Beach CW, Bramwell JD, Hutter JW: Use of an electronic apex locator on a cardiac pacemaker patient, *J Endod* 22:182-184, 1996.

85. Garofalo RR, Ede EN, Dorn SO, et al: Effect of electronic apex locators on cardiac pacemaker function, *J Endod* 28:831-833, 2002.

86. Moshonov J, Slutzky-Goldberg I: Apex locators: update and prospects for the future, *Int J Comput Dent* 7:359-370, 2004.

87. Simon AB, Linde B, Bonnette GH, et al: The individual with a pacemaker in the dental environment, *J Am Dent Assoc* 91:1224-1229, 1975.

88. Woolley LH, Woodworth J, Dobbs JL: A preliminary evaluation of the effects of electrical pulp testers on dogs with artificial pacemakers, *J Am Dent Assoc* 89:1099-1101, 1974.

89. Gomez G, Duran-Sindreu F, Jara Clemente F, et al: The effects of six electronic apex locators on pacemaker function: an in vitro study, *Int Endod J*:46:399-405, 2013.

90. Wilson BL, Broberg C, Baumgartner JC, et al: Safety of electronic apex locators and pulp testers in patients with implanted cardiac pacemakers or cardioverter/defibrillators, *J Endod* 32:847-852, 2006.

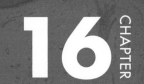

Cleaning and shaping

Ove A. Peters, W. Craig Noblett

CHAPTER OUTLINE

Principles of Cleaning
Principles of Shaping
Apical Canal Preparation
Pretreatment Evaluation
Principles of Cleaning and Shaping Techniques
Smear Layer Management
Irrigants

Lubricants
Preparation Errors
Preparation Techniques
Criteria for Evaluating Cleaning and Shaping
Intracanal Medicaments
Temporary Restorations

LEARNING OBJECTIVES

After reading this chapter, the student should be able to:

1. State reasons and describe strategies for enlarging the cervical portion of the canal to promote straight-line access.
2. Define how to determine the appropriate size of the master apical file.
3. Describe objectives for both cleaning and shaping and explain how to determine when these have been achieved.
4. Illustrate shapes of differently created preparations and draw these both in longitudinal and cross-sectional diagrams.
5. Illustrate probable actual shapes of preparations with iatrogenic errors created in curved canals.
6. Describe techniques for shaping canals that have irregular shapes, such as round, oval, hourglass, bowling pin, kidney bean, or ribbon.
7. Describe techniques for manual and engine-driven preparation of root canals.
8. Distinguish between apical stop, apical seat, and open apex and discuss how to manage obturation in each.
9. Describe appropriate techniques for removing the pulp.
10. Characterize the difficulties of preparation in the presence of anatomic aberrations that make complete debridement difficult.

11. List properties of suitable irrigants and identify which irrigant meets most of the criteria.
12. Describe the techniques that provide the maximal irrigant effect.
13. Discuss the properties and role of chelating and decalcifying agents.
14. Explain how to minimize preparation errors in small, curved canals.
15. Describe techniques for negotiating severely curved, "blocked," "ledged," or constricted canals.
16. Describe in general the principles of application of ultrasonic devices for enhanced root canal disinfection.
17. Evaluate in general alternative means of cleaning and shaping and list advantages and disadvantages of each.
18. Discuss nickel-titanium (NiTi) hand and rotary instruments and how the physical properties of this metal affect cleaning and shaping.
19. Discuss the properties and role of intracanal, interappointment medicaments.
20. List the principal temporary filling materials and describe techniques for their placement and removal.
21. Describe temporization of extensively damaged teeth.
22. Outline techniques and materials used for long-term temporization.

Successful root canal treatment is based on establishing an accurate diagnosis and developing an appropriate treatment plan; applying knowledge of tooth anatomy and morphology (shape); and performing the debridement, disinfection, and obturation of the entire root canal system. Historically, emphasis was on obturation and sealing the radicular space. However, no technique or material provides a seal that is completely impervious to moisture from either the apical or coronal aspect. Early studies on prognosis indicated that failures were attributable to incomplete obturation.[1] This proved fallacious, because obturation reflects only the adequacy of the cleaning and shaping. Canals that are poorly

273

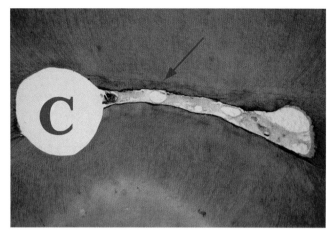

Fig. 16.1 Cross section through a root showing the main canal *(C)* and a fin *(arrow)* and associated cul-de-sac after cleaning and shaping using files and sodium hypochlorite. Note the tissue remnants in the fin.

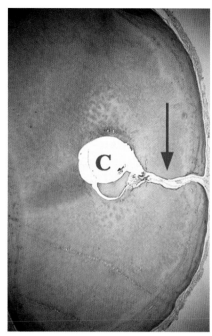

Fig. 16.2 The main canal *(C)* has a lateral canal *(arrow)* extending to the root surface. After cleaning and shaping with sodium hypochlorite irrigation, tissue remains in the lateral canal.

obturated may be incompletely cleaned and shaped. Adequate cleaning and shaping and establishing a coronal seal are the essential elements of successful treatment, and obturation is less important for short-term success.[2] Elimination (or significant reduction) of the inflamed or necrotic pulp tissue and microorganisms is the most critical factor. The role of obturation in long-term success has not been established; however, obturation may be significant in preventing recontamination either from the coronal or apical direction. Sealing the canal space after cleaning and shaping helps entomb any remaining organisms[3] and, with the coronal seal, prevents or at least delays recontamination of the canal and periradicular tissues. However, some bacterial species have been shown to survive entombment.[4]

PRINCIPLES OF CLEANING

Nonsurgical root canal treatment is a predictable method of retaining a tooth that otherwise would require extraction. Root canal treatment in a tooth with a vital pulp is more often successful than is root canal treatment of a tooth diagnosed with a necrotic pulp and periradicular pathosis.[5] The reason for this difference in outcome is the persistent presence of microorganisms and their metabolic byproducts. The most significant factors in the clinician's inability to completely remove intracanal microorganisms are tooth anatomy and morphology. Instruments are believed to *contact and plane the canal walls* to debride the canal (Figs. 16.1 to 16.4), aided by irrigating solutions. Morphologic factors include lateral canals (Fig. 16.2) and accessory canals, canal curvatures, canal wall irregularities, fins, cul-de-sacs (Fig. 16.1), and isthmuses. These aberrations make total debridement virtually impossible. Therefore, a practical objective of cleaning is to significantly reduce the irritants, not totally eliminate them.

Currently, there are no reliable clinical methods to assess cleaning efficacy. The presence of clean dentinal shavings, the color of the irrigant, and canal enlargement three file sizes beyond the first instrument to bind have been used to assess the adequacy of cleaning; however, these do not correlate well with debridement. Obtaining *glassy smooth walls* is

a suggested indicator,[6] but this property cannot be assessed beyond the coronal aspect of the root canal system.

PRINCIPLES OF SHAPING

The purpose of shaping is to facilitate cleaning and provide space for placing obturating materials. The main objective of shaping is to maintain or develop a continuously tapering funnel from the canal orifice to the apex. This reduces procedural errors during apical enlargement. The degree of enlargement is partly dictated by the method of obturation. For lateral compaction of gutta-percha, the canal should be enlarged sufficiently to permit placement of the spreader to within 1 to 2 mm of the working length. There is a correlation between the depth of spreader penetration and the quality of the apical seal.[7] For warm vertical compaction techniques, the coronal enlargement must permit the placement of pluggers to within 3 to 5 mm of the working length.[8]

As dentin is removed from the canal walls, the root becomes less resistant to fracture.[9] The degree of shaping is determined by preoperative root dimensions, the obturation technique, and the restorative treatment plan. Narrow, thin roots (e.g., those of the mandibular incisors) may not be enlarged to the same degree as more bulky roots (e.g., those of the maxillary central incisors).

APICAL CANAL PREPARATION

Termination of Cleaning and Shaping
Although the concept of cleaning and shaping the root canal space is simple, consensus has not been reached on some points. One example is the extent of the apical preparation. Early studies identified the dentinocemental junction as the

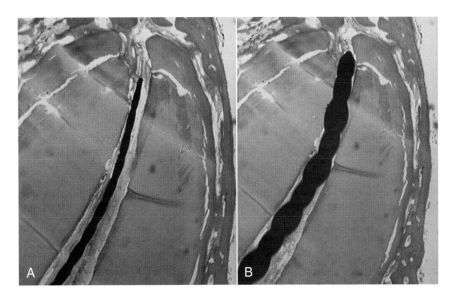

Fig. 16.3 **A,** A No. 15 file in the apical canal space. Note that this size file is inadequate for planing the walls. **B,** A No. 40 file more closely approximates the canal morphology. (Courtesy Dr. Randy Madsen.)

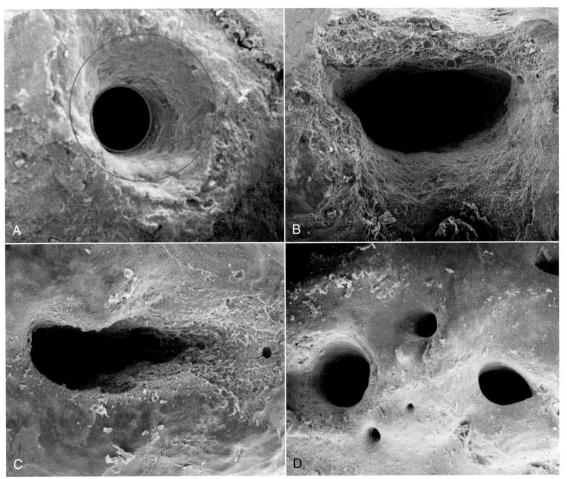

Fig. 16.4 **A,** The classic apical anatomy, consisting of the major diameter of the foramen and the minor diameter of the constriction. **B,** An irregular ovoid apical canal shape and external resorption. **C,** A bowling pin apical morphology and an accessory canal. **D,** Multiple apical foramina.

area where the pulp ends and the periodontal ligament begins. Unfortunately, this is a histologic landmark, and its position (which is irregular within the canal) cannot be determined clinically.

Traditionally, the apical point of termination, also known as the *working length* (WL), has been 1 mm from the radiographic apex. A classic study described the apical portion of the canal with the major diameter of the foramen and the minor diameter of the constriction (see Fig. 16.4).[10] The *apical constriction* is defined as the narrowest portion of the canal; the average distance from the foramen to the constriction was found to be 0.5 mm. Another study found the **275** classic apical constriction to be present in only 46% of the teeth studied. Also, when present, it varied in shape and in relationship to the apical foramen.[11] Variations from the classic appearance consist of the tapering constriction, multiple constrictions, and a parallel apical canal part.[11] To complicate the issue, the foramen is rarely located at the anatomic apex. Recently, micro-computed tomography data have provided a more realistic portrait of the apical canal morphology (Fig. 16.5).

Apical anatomy has also been shown to be quite variable (see Fig. 16.4, B, and Fig. 16.5). A study found no typical pattern for foraminal openings; it also found that no foramen coincided with the apex of the root.[12] The same group reported the foramen-to-apex distance to range from 0.2 to 3.8 mm.

It has also been noted that the foramen-to-constriction distance increases with age,[10] and root resorption may destroy the classic anatomic constriction.[13] Resorptive processes are common with pulp necrosis and apical bone resorption. Therefore root resorption is an additional factor to consider in length determination.

In a prospective study, significant adverse factors influencing success and failure were the presence of a perforation, preoperative periradicular disease, and incorrect length of the root canal filling.[14,15] The authors speculated that canals filled more than 2 mm short harbored necrotic tissue, bacteria, and irritants and that when retreated, these canals could be cleaned and sealed.[14] A meta-analysis evaluation of success and failure indicated a better success rate when the obturation was confined to the canal space.[16] A review of several studies on endodontic outcomes confirms that extrusion of materials decreases success.[5,17,18] In one study examining cases with pulp necrosis, better success was achieved when the procedures terminated at or within 2 mm of the radiographic apex. Obturation shorter than 2 mm from the apex or past the apex resulted in a decreased success rate. In teeth with vital inflamed pulp tissue, termination between 1 and 3 mm was acceptable.[17] Two larger studies confirmed that overfill was associated with inferior outcomes.[5,18]

The exact clinical point of apical termination of the preparation and obturation remains a matter of debate. Compacting

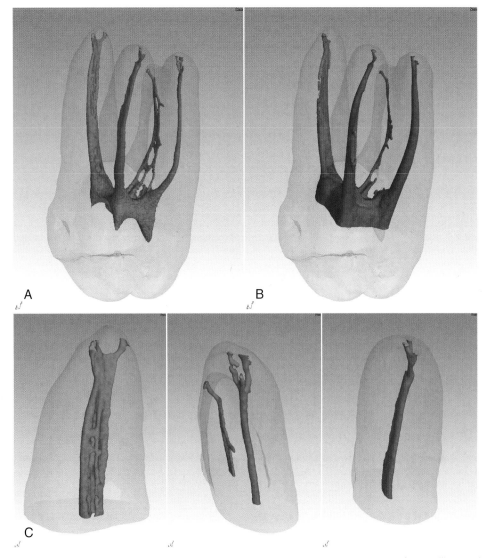

Fig. 16.5 **A,** Micro-computed tomography reconstruction of an unprepared root canal system of a maxillary molar.
B, Prepared canal system, enlarged to an apical size 30 in the palatal and 25 in the mesiobuccal and distobuccal canal.
C, Magnified view of the initial canal configuration for all three apices.

the gutta-percha and sealer against the apical dentin matrix (constriction of the canal) is important in creating a seal. The decision on where to terminate the preparation is based on a knowledge of apical anatomy, tactile sensation, radiographic interpretation, apex locators, apical bleeding, and the patient's response. To prevent extrusion, the cleaning and shaping procedures should be confined to the radicular space. Canals filled to the radiographic apex are actually slightly overextended.[12]

Degree of Apical Enlargement

Generalizations can be made regarding tooth anatomy and morphology, although each tooth is unique. The length of canal preparation is often emphasized, with little consideration given to important factors such as canal diameter and shape. Because morphology is variable, there is no standardized apical canal size. Traditionally, preparation techniques were determined by the desire to limit procedural errors and by the method of obturation. A small apical preparation reduces the incidence of preparation errors (discussed later) but may decrease the antimicrobial efficacy of cleaning procedures. It appears that with traditional hand instruments, apical transportation occurs in many curved canals enlarged beyond a No. 20 stainless steel file.[19]

The criteria for cleaning and shaping should be based on the ability to adequately deliver sufficient amounts of irrigant and not on a specific obturation technique. The ability of irrigants to reach the apical portion of the root canal depends on the canal's size and taper and the irrigation device used.[20-22]

Larger preparation sizes have been shown to provide adequate irrigation and debris removal and significantly decrease the number of microorganisms.[23-26] However, any removal of dentin has the potential to weaken radicular structure; therefore, the use of an irrigation adjunct designed to promote irrigation efficacy in smaller canals may be advantageous.[27,28]

In principle, there may to be a relationship between increasing the size of the apical preparation and canal cleanliness[29] and bacterial reduction.[30,31] Instrumentation techniques that advocate minimal apical preparation may be ineffective at achieving the goal of cleaning and disinfecting the root canal space.[29,31] However, this concept reaches its limits when too large a preparation leads to procedural errors[32,33] and when modifications created in the hard tissue block the very anatomy that was to be cleaned (Fig. 16.6).[34]

A variety of microbial species can penetrate deep into dentinal tubules.[35] These intratubular organisms are sheltered from endodontic instruments, the action of irrigants, and intracanal medicaments. Dentin removal appears to be the primary method for decreasing their numbers. However, it may not be possible to remove bacteria that are deep in the tubules, regardless of the technique. There is a correlation between the number of organisms present and the depth of tubular

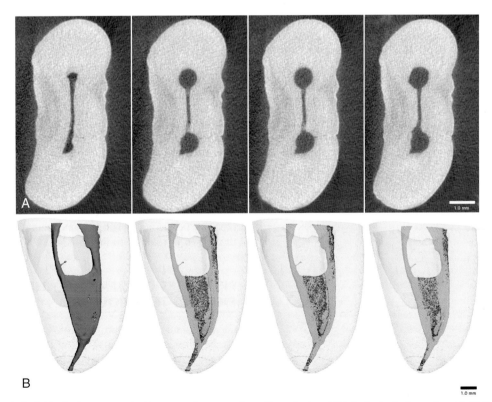

Fig. 16.6 **A,** Individual micro-computed tomography scans from the apical root third of a typical specimen before and after root canal preparation and irrigation with sodium hypochlorite (NaOCl), subsequent irrigation with ethylenediaminetetraacetic acid (EDTA), and final passive ultrasonic irrigation using again NaOCl (from left to right). **B,** The corresponding three-dimensional reconstructions of the whole canal system are depicted in the bottom panel. (Modified from Paqué F, Boessler C, Zehnder M: Accumulated hard tissue debris levels in mesial roots of mandibular molars after sequential irrigation steps, *Int Endod J* 44[2]:148, 2011.)

penetration[36]; in teeth with apical periodontitis, bacteria may penetrate the tubules to the periphery of the root.[37,38]

Elimination of Etiology

The development of nickel-titanium instruments has dramatically changed the techniques of cleaning and shaping; these instruments have been rapidly adopted by clinicians in many countries.[39-41] The primary advantage of these flexible instruments is seen in shaping, specifically a significant reduction in the incidence of preparation errors.[32]

Neither hand instruments nor rotary files have been shown to completely debride the canal.[24,42,43] Mechanical enlargement of the canal space dramatically reduces the number of microorganisms present in the canal,[44] but it cannot render the canal sterile.[24] Therefore, the use of antimicrobial irrigants has been recommended, in addition to mechanical preparation techniques.[45] There is currently no consensus on the most appropriate irrigant or concentration of solution, although sodium hypochlorite (NaOCl) is the most widely used irrigant.

Unfortunately, solutions such as NaOCl that are designed to kill bacteria[45-47] are often toxic to the host cells[48-51]; therefore, extrusion beyond the canal space is to be avoided.[52,53] A major factor in the effectiveness of irrigants is the volume of irrigant used during the procedure. Increasing the volume produces cleaner preparations.[54]

Apical Patency

In the apical patency technique, small hand files are repeatedly placed to or slightly beyond the apical foramen during canal preparation (Fig. 16.7). A benefit of this technique during cleaning and shaping procedures is that it ensures that the working length is not lost and that the apical portion of the root is not packed with tissue, dentin debris, and bacteria

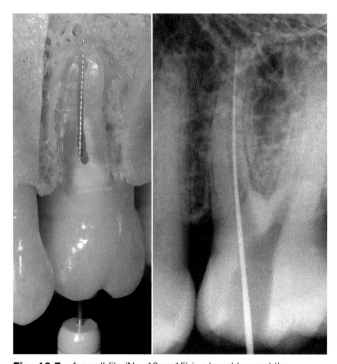

Fig. 16.7 A small file (No. 10 or 15) is placed beyond the radiographic apex to maintain patency of the foramen. Note that the tip extends beyond the apical foramen.

(see Fig. 16.6, *A*). This technique has raised some concerns about extrusion of dentinal debris, bacteria, and irrigants.[55] However, in a recent large, retrospective study, the apical patency technique was identified as a factor possibly associated with higher success rates.[5] Moreover, at least in vitro, microorganisms do not appear to be transported beyond the confines of the canal by patency filing.[56] Small files are not directly effective in debridement (see Fig. 16.3), but achieving patency may be helpful in enhancing irrigation efficacy[57] and in electronic length determination.

Studies evaluating treatment failure have noted the presence of bacteria outside the radicular space,[58] in addition to several other factors, and in some cases bacteria have been shown to exist as plaques or biofilms on the external root structure.[59]

PRETREATMENT EVALUATION

Before treatment, each case should be evaluated for its degree of difficulty. Normal anatomy and anatomic variations are determined, as are variations in canal morphology.[60]

One or more preoperative radiographs of diagnostic quality are assessed. The longer a root, the more difficult it is to treat. Apically, a narrow, curved root is susceptible to perforation; in multirooted teeth, a narrow area midroot could result in a stripping perforation toward the root concavity. The degree and location of curvature are determined. Canals are seldom straight, and curvatures in a faciolingual direction are normally not visible on the radiograph. Sharp curvatures or dilacerations are more difficult to manage than is a continuous, gentle curve. Roots with an S-shape or bayonet configuration are very difficult to treat. Intracanal mineralization also complicates treatment. Such mineralization generally occurs in a coronal to apical direction (see Fig. 14-14); therefore, a large, tapering canal may become more cylindrical with irritation or age.

The presence of resorption also complicates treatment. With internal resorption, it is difficult to pass instruments through the coronal portion of the canal and the resorptive defect and into the apical portion. Also, files do not remove tissue, necrotic debris, and bacteria from the resorptive defect. External resorption may perforate the canal space and present problems with hemostasis and isolation. Restorations may obstruct access and visibility and change the orientation of the crown in relation to the root.

PRINCIPLES OF CLEANING AND SHAPING TECHNIQUES

Cleaning and shaping are separate and distinct concepts but are performed concurrently. The criteria of canal preparation include developing a continuously tapered funnel, maintaining the original shape of the canal, maintaining the apical foramen in its original position, keeping the apical opening as small as possible, and developing glassy-smooth walls.[8] The cleaning and shaping procedures are designed to maintain an apical matrix for compacting the obturating material, regardless of the obturation technique.[8]

The clinician must be knowledgeable about a variety of techniques and instruments involved in the treatment of the myriad variations in canal anatomy. There is no consensus or clinical evidence on which technique or instrument design or type is clinically superior.[33,61]

Nickel-titanium files have been incorporated into endodontics because of their flexibility and resistance to cyclic fatigue.[62] The resistance to cyclic fatigue permits these instruments to be used in a rotary handpiece, which gives them an advantage over stainless steel files. Nickel-titanium (NiTi) files are manufactured in both hand and rotary versions and have been demonstrated to produce superior shaping compared to stainless steel hand instruments.[32,61,63]

NiTi instruments are available in a variety of designs, many with increased taper compared to the .02 mm standardized stainless steel files. Common tapers are .04 and .06, and the tip diameters may or may not conform to the traditional manufacturing specifications. The file systems can vary the taper while maintaining the same tip diameter, or they can use varied tapers with International Organization for Standardization (ISO) standardized tip diameters; some NiTi instruments have multiple tapers along their cutting portions.

A useful procedure for root canal preparation using current instruments unfolds in stages. Stage 1 is a defined preflaring, performed before bringing any hand file to the apical third of the canal. Depending on the expected canal difficulty, instruments may reach working length during stage 2 (e.g., if there is only one curvature). If preoperative assessments have indicated that an S-shape or multiple curvatures are present, it may be useful to introduce a stage 3, in which the estimated WL is finally reached; in such cases, stage 2 is used to create additional enlargement into the secondary curvature.[64]

In general, the use of nickel-titanium rotary instruments should be preceded by a manual exploration of the canal to the desired preparation length, also known as *glide path verification*. This step is performed with one or more small K-files that are not precurved. If it is possible to predictably reach working length without precurving, rotary instruments may be used to the desired length. However, caution should be used in S-shaped canals, canals that join within a single root (type II configuration), and canals with severe dilacerations. Canals in which ledge formation is present and very large canals in which instruments fail to contact the canal walls do not lend themselves to rotary preparation. In general, for rotary root canal preparation, straight-line access to the canal is essential.

Instrument fracture can occur as a result of torsional forces or cyclic fatigue.[33] Torsional forces develop because of frictional resistance; therefore, as the surface area increases along the flutes, the greater the friction and the more potential for fracture. Torsional stress can be reduced by limiting file contact and using a crown-down preparation technique, in addition to liquid irrigants (e.g., NaOCl), during the procedure.

Cyclic fatigue occurs as a file rotates in a curved canal.[65] At the point of curvature, the outer surface of the file is under tension and the inner surface of the instrument is compressed. As the instrument rotates, the areas of tension and compression alternate, and crack initiation begins, ultimately leading to fracture. There is often no visible evidence that fracture is imminent; therefore, the frequency with which a nickel-titanium instrument is used should be monitored.[66] In difficult, calcified, or severely curved canals, the instruments should be used only once.[61]

SMEAR LAYER MANAGEMENT

During cleaning and shaping, organic pulpal materials and inorganic dentinal debris accumulate. Not only are these pressed into accessory canals, fins, and isthmuses (see Fig. 16.6), they also are deposited on the radicular canal wall, producing an amorphous, irregular smear layer (Fig. 16.8).[67] With pulp necrosis, the smear layer may be contaminated with bacteria and their metabolic byproducts. The smear layer is superficial, having a thickness of 1 to 5 μm, and debris can be packed into the dentinal tubules to varying distances.[68]

There is no consensus on removal of the smear layer before obturation.[67,69,70] The advantages and disadvantages of smear layer removal remain controversial; however, evidence generally supports removal of the smear layer prior to obturation.[67,71] The organic debris present in the smear layer might constitute a substrate for bacterial growth, and it has been suggested that the smear layer prevents sealer contact with the canal wall, permitting leakage. In addition, viable

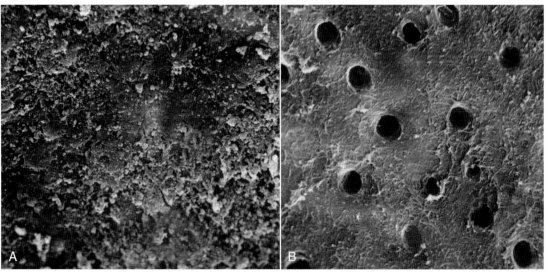

Fig. 16.8 **A,** A canal wall with the smear layer present. **B,** The smear layer removed with 17% EDTA.

Box 16.1 Properties of an Ideal Irrigant

Organic tissue solvent
Inorganic tissue solvent
Antimicrobial action
Nontoxic
Low surface tension
Lubricant

microorganisms in the dentinal tubules may use the smear layer as a substrate for sustained growth. If the smear layer is not removed, it may slowly disintegrate with leaking obturation materials, or it may be removed by acids and enzymes that are produced by viable bacteria left in the tubules or that enter via coronal leakage.[3] The presence of a smear layer may also interfere with the action and effectiveness of root canal irrigants and interappointment disinfectants.[47]

With smear layer removal, filling materials adapt better to the canal wall.[72,73] Also, removal of the smear layer enhances the adhesion of sealers to dentin and tubular penetration[69,72-74] and permits the penetration of all sealers to varying depths.[75] Removal of the smear layer reduces both coronal and apical leakage.[71,76]

IRRIGANTS

The ideal properties for an endodontic irrigant are listed in Box 16.1.[67] Currently, no solution meets all the requirements outlined. In fact, no techniques appear able to completely clean the root canal space.[34,77-79] Frequent irrigation is necessary to flush and remove the debris generated by the mechanical action of the instruments. At the same time, preparation of the radicular wall creates hard tissue debris that is typically pushed into the accessory anatomy, blocking access for subsequent irrigation.[34] Therefore, coordinated use of mechanical shaping and irrigation is imperative to maximize the antibacterial efficacy of endodontic procedures.

Sodium Hypochlorite

As mentioned, the most common irrigant is NaOCl, also known as household bleach. The advantages of an NaOCl solution include mechanical flushing of debris from the canal, the ability to dissolve vital[80] and necrotic tissue,[81] antimicrobial action,[42] and lubricating action.[82] In addition, NaOCl is inexpensive and readily available.[83]

Free chlorine in NaOCl dissolves necrotic tissue by breaking down proteins into amino acids. There is no proven appropriate concentration of NaOCl, but concentrations ranging from 0.5% to 5.25% have been recommended. A common concentration is 2.5%, a concentration at which the potential for toxicity is reduced, yet some tissue dissolving and antimicrobial activity is maintained.[84,85] Because the action of the irrigant is related to the amount of free chlorine, an increase in volume can compensate for a decrease in concentration. Warming the solution can also increase its effectiveness.[86,87] However, NaOCl is limited in its ability to dissolve canal content because of limited contact with tissues in all areas of the root canal system.

Because of toxicity, extrusion is to be avoided.[49,53,88] The irrigating needle must be placed *loosely* in the canal

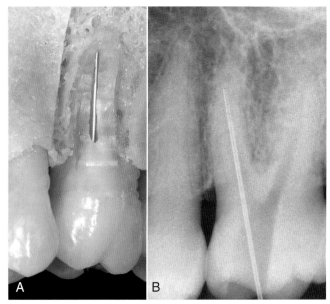

Fig. 16.9 For effective irrigation, the needle must be placed in the apical one third of the root and must not bind.

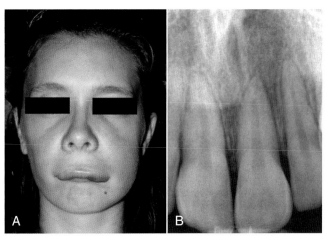

Fig. 16.10 A sodium hypochlorite accident during treatment of the maxillary left central incisor. Extensive edema occurred in the upper lip and was accompanied by severe pain.

(Fig. 16.9). Insertion to binding and slight withdrawal minimizes the potential for extrusion and a sodium hypochlorite accident (Fig. 16.10). Special care should be taken when irrigating a canal with an open apex. To control the depth of insertion, the needle is bent slightly at the appropriate length or a rubber stopper is placed on the needle.

The irrigant does not move apically more than 1 mm beyond the irrigation tip, so deep placement with small-gauge needles enhances irrigation (see Fig. 16.9).[89] During rinsing, the needle is moved up and down constantly to produce agitation and prevent binding or wedging of the needle.

EDTA

Ethylenediaminetetraacetic acid (EDTA)[90] is another frequently used irrigant; its activity is directed toward removal of the smear layer. Irrigation with 17% EDTA for 1 minute, followed by a final rinse with NaOCl,[91] is a recommended method. Chelators such as EDTA remove the inorganic components and leave the organic tissue elements intact. NaOCl is then necessary for removal of the remaining organic components; however, the use of NaOCl after chelating agents may lead to excessive demineralization of radicular wall dentin.[92] Demineralization results in removal of the smear layer and plugs and enlargement of the tubules.[93,94] The action is most effective in the coronal and middle thirds of the canal and is diminished in the apical third.[90,95]

Reduced efficacy may be a reflection of canal size[96] or anatomic variations such as irregular or sclerotic tubules.[97,98] The variable structure of the apical dentin presents a challenge during endodontic obturation with adhesive materials.

The recommended time for removal of the smear layer with EDTA is 1 minute.[90,99,100] The small particles of the smear layer are primarily inorganic and have a high surface-to-mass ratio, which facilitates removal by acids and chelators. EDTA exposure over 10 minutes causes excessive removal of both peritubular and intratubular dentin.[100] Citric acid has also been shown to be an effective means of removing the smear layer.[101,102]

Chlorhexidine

Chlorhexidine has a broad spectrum of antimicrobial activity, provides a sustained action,[88,103] and has little toxicity.[104-107] Two percent chlorhexidine has an antimicrobial action similar to that of 5.25% NaOCl,[104] and it is more effective against *Enterococcus faecalis*.[88] NaOCl and chlorhexidine are synergistic in their ability to eliminate microorganisms.[105] A disadvantage of chlorhexidine is its inability to dissolve necrotic tissue and remove the smear layer. Moreover, clinical studies do not confirm that the use of chlorhexidine is associated with better outcomes.[5]

MTAD

An alternative method for disinfecting while at the same time removing the smear layer uses a mixture composed of a tetracycline isomer, an acid, and a detergent (MTAD) as a final rinse to remove the smear layer.[108] The effectiveness of MTAD in completely removing the smear layer is enhanced when low concentrations of NaOCl are used as an intracanal irrigant before the use of MTAD.[109] A 1.3% NaOCl concentration was recommended; MTAD may be superior to NaOCl in antimicrobial action.[110,111] MTAD has been shown to be effective in killing *E. faecalis,* an organism commonly found in failing treatments, and it may prove beneficial during retreatment. It is biocompatible,[112] does not alter the physical properties of the dentin,[112] and enhances bond strength.[113] Although there is encouraging in vitro data, MTAD has not been shown to be clinically beneficial at this point.[114]

QMix

Use of a recently introduced irrigant, marketed as QMix,[115] follows an underlying strategy similar to that for MTAD; in addition, QMix has the potential not only to remove the smear layer, but also to provide antibiofilm activity. QMix consists of a proprietary mix of chlorhexidine, EDTA, and a surface-active agent. Although this is a new material and nothing is known about its contribution to clinical outcomes, it appears that smear layer removal is similar to that seen with 17% EDTA,[116] and antimicrobial effects are adequate.[117,118] However, tissue dissolution with prior canal shaping and use of NaOCl are still required.[119]

Ultrasonics

Ultrasonic activation is used to enhance irrigation and to remove materials from the canal, including posts and silver cones. Ultrasonically powered instruments may also be used for thermoplastic obturation and root-end preparation during surgery; however, shaping curved root canals with ultrasonic instruments has been shown to create preparation errors and is no longer recommended.[120-122]

The main mechanism of adjunctive cleaning with ultrasonics is acoustic microstreaming,[123] which is described as complex, steady-state streaming patterns in vortex-like motions or eddy flows that are formed close to the instrument. Agitation of the irrigant with an ultrasonically activated instrument after completion of cleaning and shaping has the benefit of increasing the effectiveness of the solution.[96,124-126]

LUBRICANTS

Lubricants facilitate manipulation of hand files during cleaning and shaping. They are an aid in initial canal negotiation, especially in small and constricted canals without taper.

Glycerin is a mild alcohol that is inexpensive, nontoxic, aseptic, and somewhat soluble. A small amount can be placed along the shaft of the file or deposited in the canal orifice. Counterclockwise rotation of the file carries the material apically. The file can then be worked to length using a watch-winding motion.

Paste lubricants can incorporate chelators. One advantage to paste lubricants is that they can suspend dentinal debris and prevent apical compaction. One proprietary product consists of glycol, urea peroxide, and EDTA in a special water-soluble base. It has been demonstrated to exert antimicrobial action.[127] Another type is composed of 19% EDTA in a water-soluble, viscous solution. A disadvantage of these EDTA compounds appears to be the deactivation of NaOCl by reducing the available chlorine[128] and potential toxicity.[129] The addition of EDTA to the lubricants has not proved effective.[130] In general, files remove dentin faster than the chelators can soften the canal walls. When nickel-titanium rotary techniques are used, aqueous solutions (e.g., NaOCl), rather than paste lubricants, should always be present in the root canal to reduce torque.[82]

PREPARATION ERRORS

Regardless of the technique used in root canal preparation, procedural errors can occur. These include loss of working length, apical transportation, apical perforation, instrument fracture, and stripping perforations.

Loss of working length has several causes, including failure to have an adequate reference point from which the working length is determined, packing of tissue and debris in the apical portion of the canal, ledge formation, and inaccurate measurement of files.

Apical transportation and zipping occur when relatively inflexible files are used to prepare curved canals. The restoring force of the file (the tendency to return to the original straight shape of the file) exceeds the threshold for cutting dentin in a curved canal (Figs. 16.11 and 16.12).[131] When this apical transportation continues with larger and larger files, a teardrop shape develops, and *apical perforation* can occur on the lateral root surface (Fig. 16.11). Transportation in curved canals already begins with a No. 25 file.[19] Enlargement of curved canals at the working length beyond a No. 25 file can be done only when an adequate coronal flare is developed.

As stated before, *instrument fracture* occurs with torsional and cyclic fatigue. Locking the flutes of a file in the canal wall while continuing to rotate the coronal portion of the instrument is an example of torsional fatigue (Fig. 16.13). Cyclic fatigue results when strain develops in the metal. File fracture occurs more frequently with rotaries but may also involve hand instruments such as K-type and Hedstrom files.[132]

Stripping perforations occur in the furcal region of curved roots and frequently in the mesial roots of maxillary and mandibular molars (Figs. 16.14 and 16.15). The canal in this

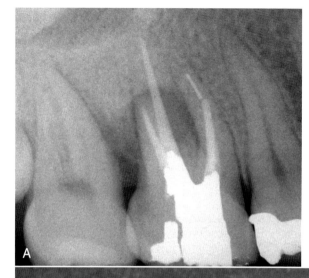

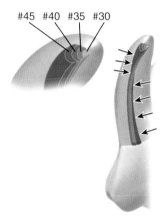

Fig. 16.11 Procedural errors of canal transportation, zipping and strip perforation, occur during standardized preparation when files remove dentin from the outer canal wall apical to the curve and from the inner wall coronal to the curve. This is related to the restoring force (stiffness) of the files. Note that in the apical portion, the transportation takes the shape of a teardrop as the larger files are used.

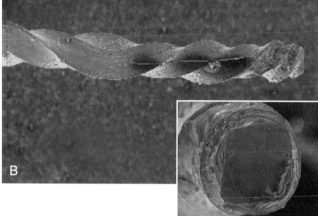

Fig. 16.13 **A,** No. 35 file fractured in the mesiobuccal canal. **B,** Scanning electron microscope examination reveals torsional failure at the point of fracture. Note the tightening of the flutes near the fracture and the unwinding of the flutes along the shaft.

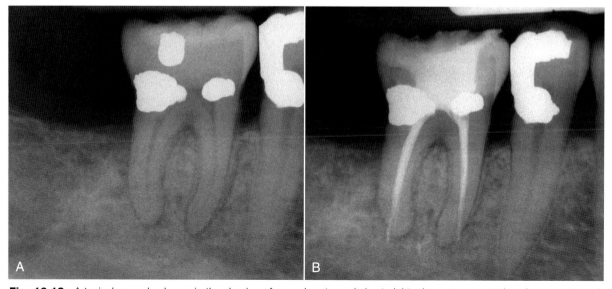

Fig. 16.12 A typical procedural error in the shaping of curved root canals is straightening or transportation. A comparison of preoperative *(left)* and postoperative *(right)* radiographs in this case reveals that mesial and distal canals have been transported, and there are apical perforations.

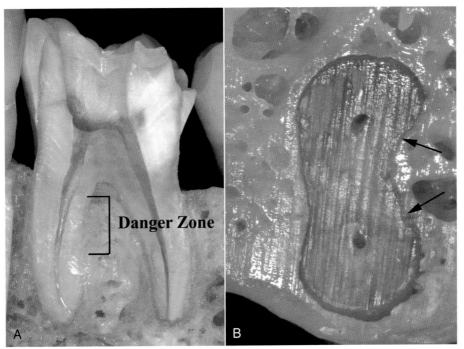

Fig. 16.14 **A,** The furcal region of molars at the level of the curvature (danger zone) is a common site of stripping perforation. **B,** Note the concavity *(arrows)* in the furcation area of this mandibular molar.

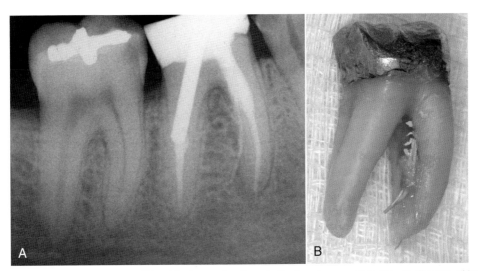

Fig. 16.15 Straight-line access can result in stripping perforations in the furcal areas of molars. **A,** The use of large Gates-Glidden drills and overpreparation have resulted in the stripping perforation. **B,** Note that the perforation is in the concavity of the furcation.

area of the root is not always centered in cross sections; before preparation, the average distance to the furcal wall (danger zone) is less than the distance to the bulky outer wall (safety zone). An additional complicating factor is the furcal concavity of the root.[133]

PREPARATION TECHNIQUES

Working Length Determination

A major step in clinical endodontics, regardless of the instruments used, is the determination of the apical termination of cleaning and shaping, in addition to obturation procedures.

Using diagnostic radiographs, an estimate of the working length can be obtained. With a staged preparation sequence (as detailed previously), during the first stage files are not placed in the root canal to the WL; rather, their use is restricted to the coronal and middle thirds of the canal. However, during all shaping stages, care should be taken not to inadvertently overextend the instruments. As soon as a small file appears to reach the estimated termination point, the use of an electronic apex locator is recommended. These units typically provide an accurate assessment of the location of the narrowest canal diameter and can detect the position of the test file relative to the periodontal ligament. Exposing a radiograph with the test file in place then verifies the measurement.

283

Based on this information, clinicians may note the working length for the canal as the distance between a coronal reference point and the apical termination point. Based on clinical evidence[5,18] and classic studies,[134] the working length should terminate just short of the electronically measured canal length. During canal preparation, working lengths tend to shorten because the enlarged canal provides a straighter path to the apical termination point; however this effect is minimized with coronal flaring. Nevertheless, the clinician should check the working length periodically and correct it if needed.

Hand Instrumentation
Watch Winding
Watch winding is reciprocating, back-and-forth (clockwise/counterclockwise) rotation of the instrument in an arch and is used to negotiate canals and to work files to place. The first file that reaches tentative working length and slightly binds is called the *initial apical file* (IAF). Light apical pressure is applied to move the file deeper into the canal.

Reaming
Reaming is defined as the clockwise cutting rotation of the file. In general, the instruments are placed into the canal until binding is encountered. The instrument is then rotated clockwise 180 to 360 degrees to plane the walls and enlarge the canal space.

Filing
Filing is defined as placing the file into the canal and pressing it laterally while withdrawing it along the path of insertion to scrape (plane) the wall. A modification is the quarter turn–pull technique. This involves placing the file to the point of binding, rotating the instrument 90 degrees, and then pulling the instrument along the canal wall. Any filing technique has a tendency to straighten curved canals.

Circumferential Filing
Circumferential filing is used for canals that are larger and/or not round. The file is placed into the canal and withdrawn in a directional manner sequentially against the mesial, distal, buccal, and lingual walls. Circumferential filing is not very effective beyond the coronal third of a root canal.[135,136]

Standardized Preparation
After 1961, instruments were manufactured with a standard formula. Clinicians used a preparation technique of sequentially enlarging the canal space with smaller to larger instruments at the working length (Box 16.2).[137] In theory, this created a standardized preparation of uniform taper. Unfortunately, in cylindrical and small, curved canals, procedural errors were identified with this technique.[138]

Step-Back Technique
The step-back technique reduces procedural errors and improves debridement.[138,139] After coronal flaring, the apical canal diameter is determined with the initial apical file (the first file that binds at the WL). Subsequent preparation to the WL, up to the master apical file (MAF), creates the apical preparation size (e.g., size No. 35); the succeeding larger files are shortened by 0.5- or 1-mm increments from the previous file length (Figs. 16.16 and 16.17) up to the final file (e.g.,

Box 16.2 Descriptors for Files Used During Root Canal Preparation

Working length (WL)
Initial apical file (IAF)
Master apical file (MAF)
Final file (FF)
Final apical file (FAF)

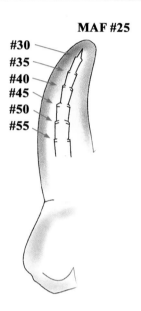

MAF #25

#30
#35
#40
#45
#50
#55

Fig. 16.16 The step-back technique is designed to provide a tapering preparation. The process begins with one file size larger than the master apical file, with incremental shortening of either 0.5 or 1 mm.

size No. 60). This step-back process creates a flared, tapering preparation while reducing procedural errors. The last file used in the step-back sequence becomes the final file (FF). This type of preparation is superior to standardized serial filing and reaming techniques in debridement and maintaining the canal shape.[139]

Step-Down Technique
The step-down technique is advocated for cleaning and shaping procedures because it removes coronal interferences and provides coronal taper. Originally advocated for hand file preparation,[140] the step-down technique also has been incorporated into techniques using nickel-titanium files. With the pulp chamber filled with irrigant or lubricant, the canal is explored with a small instrument to assess the morphology (curvature). The working length can be established at this time. The coronal one third of the canal is then flared with Gates-Glidden drills or NiTi orifice shapers. A large file (e.g., No. 60) is then placed in the canal, and a watch-winding motion is used until resistance is encountered.[140] The process is repeated with sequentially smaller files until the apical portion of the canal is reached. The working length and the initial apical file (the first file that binds at working length) can be determined if this was not accomplished initially. The apical portion of the canal can now be prepared by enlarging the canal to the master apical file at the working length. Apical taper is accomplished using a step-back technique.

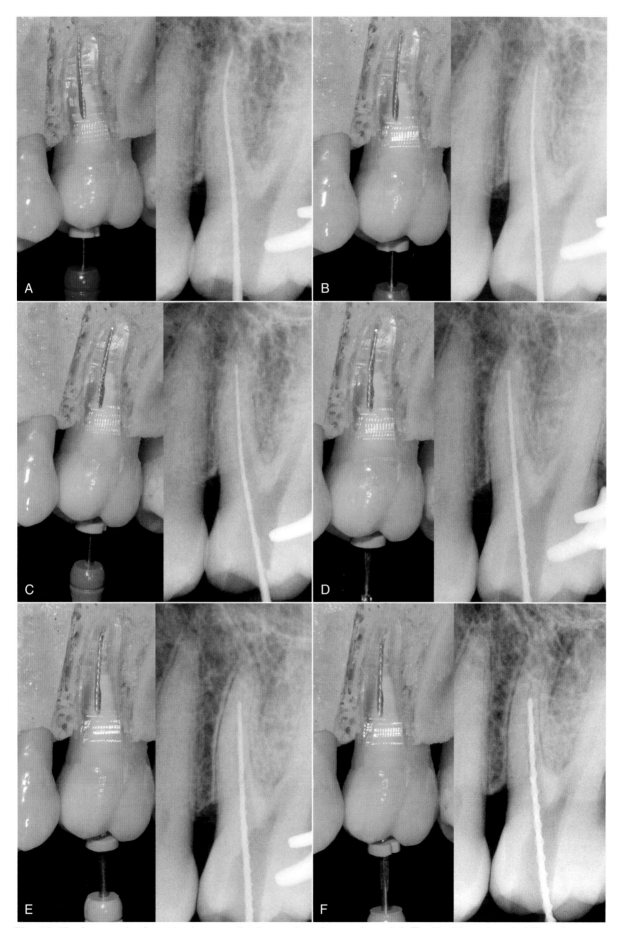

Fig. 16.17 An example of step-back preparation in a moderately curved canal. **A,** The No. 25 master apical file at the corrected working length of 21 mm. **B,** The step-back process begins with the No. 30 file at 20.5 mm. **C,** No. 35 file at 20 mm. **D,** No. 40 file at 19.5 mm. **E,** No. 45 file at 19 mm. **F,** No. 50 file at 18.5 mm.

285

Continued

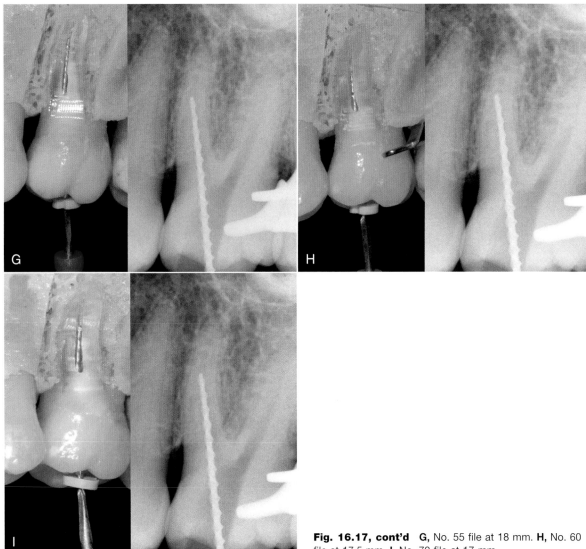

Fig. 16.17, cont'd **G,** No. 55 file at 18 mm. **H,** No. 60 file at 17.5 mm. **I,** No. 70 file at 17 mm.

Passive Step-Back Technique

The passive step-back technique is a modification of the incremental step-back technique.[8,141] After the apical diameter of the canal has been determined, the next higher instrument is inserted until it *first* makes contact (binding point). It is then rotated one-half turn and removed (Fig. 16.18). The process is repeated, with larger and larger instruments placed to their binding point. This entire instrument sequence is then repeated. With each sequence, the instruments drop deeper into the canal, creating a tapered preparation. Advantages to the technique include a knowledge of canal morphology, removal of debris and minor canal obstructions, and a gradual passive, slight enlargement of the canal in an apical to coronal direction.

Anticurvature Filing

Anticurvature filing is advocated during coronal flaring procedures to preserve the furcal wall in the treatment of molars (Fig. 16.19). As stated before, canals are often not centered in mesial roots of maxillary and mandibular molars; instead, they are located closer to the furcation. Stripping perforations occur primarily during use of the Gates-Glidden drills, but also can happen with overzealous use of hand instruments. To

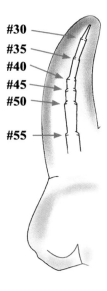

Fig. 16.18 Passive step-back. Smaller to larger files are inserted to their initial point of binding and then rotated 180 to 360 degrees and withdrawn. This process creates slight taper and coronal space and permits larger instruments to reach the apical one third.

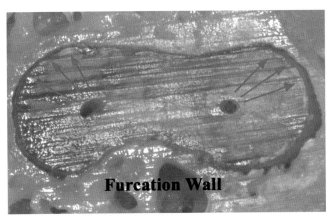

Furcation Wall

Fig. 16.19 The anticurvature filing technique. Instruments are directed away from the furcal "danger zone" toward the line angles (safety zone) where the bulk of dentin is greater.

prevent this procedural error, the Gates-Glidden drills should be confined to the canal space coronal to the root curvature and used in a step-back or step-down manner (Figs. 16.20 and 16.21). Gates-Glidden drills and laterally cutting NiTi orifice shapers can also be used directionally in an anticurvature fashion to selectively remove dentin from the bulky wall (safety zone) toward the line angle, protecting the inner or furcal wall (danger zone) coronal to the curve (Fig. 16.19).

Balanced Force Technique

The balanced force technique recognizes the fact that instruments are guided by the canal walls when rotated.[142] Because files with a symmetric cross section cut in both a clockwise and counterclockwise rotation, the balanced force approach to instrumentation involves placing the file to length and then using a clockwise rotation (less than 180 degrees) to engage the dentin. This is followed by a counterclockwise rotation (at

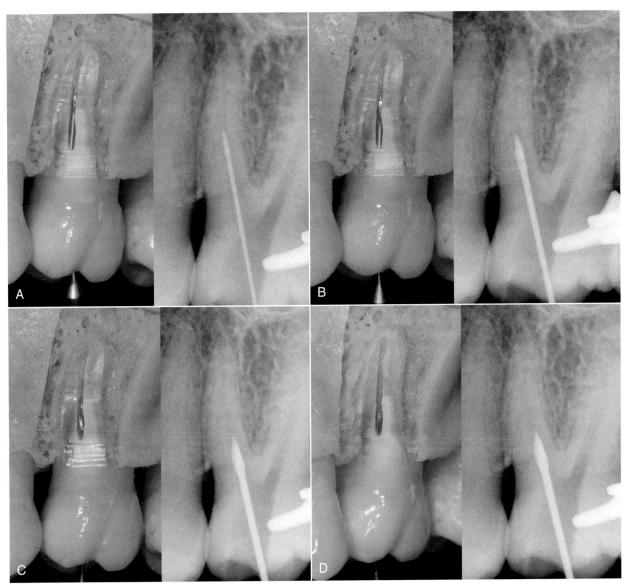

Fig. 16.20 Straight-line access in a maxillary left first molar with Gates-Glidden drills used in a slow-speed handpiece for a step-back technique. The No. 1 Gates is used until resistance **(A)**, followed by the No. 2, which should not go past the first curvature **(B)**. The No. 3 Gates is used 3 to 4 mm into the canal **(C)**, followed by the No. 4 instrument **(D)**.

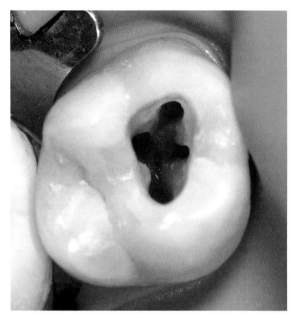

Fig. 16.21 A maxillary first molar after straight-line access with the Gates-Glidden drills.

least 120 degrees) with apical pressure to cut and enlarge the canal. The degree of apical pressure varies from light pressure with small instruments to heavy pressure with large instruments. The clockwise rotation pulls the instrument into the canal in an apical direction. The counterclockwise cutting rotation forces the file in a coronal direction while cutting circumferentially. After the cutting rotation, the file is repositioned and the process is repeated until the working length is reached. At this point, a final clockwise rotation is used to evacuate the debris. The balanced force method is considered the most effective hand instrumentation technique.[63,77]

Recapitulation

Recapitulation is important regardless of the technique selected (Fig. 16.22) and is accomplished by taking a small file to the working length to loosen accumulated debris and then flushing it with 1 to 2 mL of irrigant. Recapitulation is performed between each successive enlarging instrument, regardless of the cleaning and shaping technique.

Shaping Modifications

The apical configuration in a given case may be recognized as an apical stop, apical seat, or open apex. In addition to assessing a diagnostic radiograph, the clinician detects these configurations by placing the MAF to the corrected working length after shaping is completed. If the MAF easily extends past the WL, the apical configuration is open. If the MAF stops at the WL, a file one or two sizes smaller is placed to the same depth. If this file also stops, the apical configuration is called an *apical stop*. When the smaller file goes past the corrected working length, the apical configuration is a *seat*.

In a small, curved canal, enlargement should be restricted to three sizes larger than the initial apical file to decrease the potential for transportation. In a straight canal, it may be larger without producing a procedural error. Because a properly prepared canal exhibits taper, the small files at the corrected working length can be used to enlarge the canal without transportation. Additional apical enlargement is performed

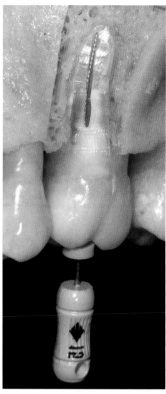

Fig. 16.22 Recapitulation is accomplished between each instrument by reaming with the master apical file or a smaller instrument, minimizing packing of debris and loss of length.

with an irrigant in the canal and employs a reaming action at the corrected working length. The last file used becomes the so-called final apical file (FAF). Because this file contacts only the apical portion of the canal, the technique may result in a less irregular apical preparation. The canal is then irrigated, the smear layer is removed with a decalcifying agent, and the canal is dried with paper points.

Engine-Driven Instruments
Gates-Glidden Drills

Gates-Glidden drills are suited for straight-line access modification (see Figs. 16.20 and 16.21). A No. 2 Gates (approximately size No. 70) is often used first, followed by the No. 3 (approximately size No. 90) and perhaps the No. 4 (approximately size No. 110). In very narrow canals, a No. 1 Gates (approximately size No. 50) may be needed. It is important to remember the size of the Gates-Glidden drills. If the canal orifice cannot accommodate a No. 50 file, careful hand instrumentation should be performed to provide adequate initial coronal space; alternatively, a tapered NiTi orifice shaper may be used in such a case. To prevent stripping perforations, Gates-Glidden drills should not be placed apical to canal curvatures.

Nickel-Titanium Rotary Instruments

Nickel-titanium rotary preparation is typically performed in a staged approach using coronal flaring; however, the specific technique is based on the instrument system selected. One instrument sequence uses nickel-titanium files in a crown-down approach with a constant taper and variable ISO tip sizes (Fig. 16.23). With this technique, a .06 taper is selected.

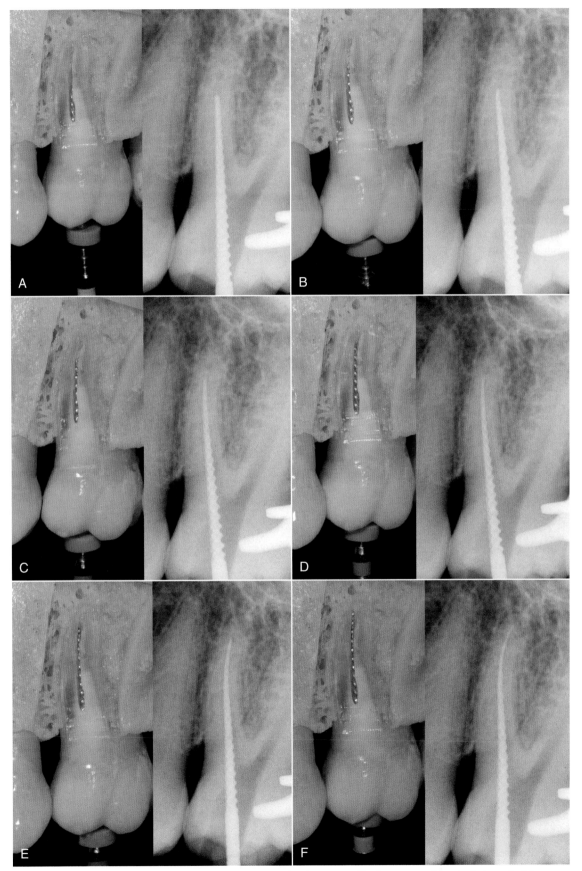

Fig. 16.23 The mesiobuccal canal is prepared using nickel-titanium rotary files in a crown-down technique. In this sequence, each instrument has the same .06 taper with varied ISO standardized tip diameters. Instruments were used to resistance. The process begins with a .06/45 file to resistance at 16 mm **(A),** followed by a .06/40 instrument at 17 mm **(B). C,** The .06/35 file is used to 18 mm. **D,** The .06/30 at 19 mm. **E,** The .06/25 at 20 mm. **F,** The .06/20 file is used to the corrected working length of 21 mm.

Initially, a size .06/45 file is used until resistance, followed by the .06/40, .06/35, .06/30, .06/25, and .06/20. In another technique, nickel-titanium files with a constant tip diameter are used also in a crown-down sequence. The initial file is a .10/20 instrument, the second a .08/20, the third a .06/20, and the fourth a .04/20 (Fig. 16.24). Many variations of these basic approaches have been recommended for different file designs. More recently introduced systems try to limit the number of file sizes, up to the point of using only one size for the majority of canals. Obviously, one size does not fit all canals shapes, and modifications frequently must be made when such a system is used.

A critical point with all rotaries is the handling of these files. In addition to the manufacturer's guidelines for individual files, several general principles should be followed.[61,143] For example, instrument insertions should follow an in-and-out pattern; each instrumentation step should consist of three

to five movements and should not exceed 10 to 15 seconds. Apically directed force should typically not exceed the force required to bend the rotary when placed on a tabletop. Most NiTi files are made of austenitic alloy and work best with a lower rather than higher rotational speed (e.g., 250 rpm). However, martensitic rotaries work better with higher speeds, (e.g., 500 rpm).[144]

In the currently marketed electric motors, the torque setting is already programmed. These settings are a reasonable protection against instrument breakage due to torsional loading but are less effective with greater tapers (e.g., .06 and .08).[33] All rotaries work best in irrigated canals and not in the presence of a gel-type lubricant, such as RC Prep.[82]

Nickel-titanium rotaries should not be placed into an unexplored canal, but rather should follow hand instruments, which establish a glide path that then can be followed by rotaries.[145] It is important to note that hand files for glide path

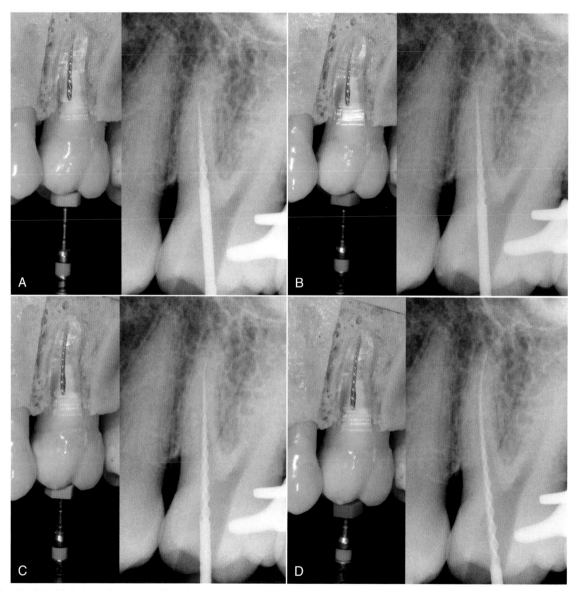

Fig. 16.24 Nickel-titanium rotary files with a standardized ISO tip diameter and variable tapered files can be used in canal preparation. In this sequence, the instruments have a standardized tip diameter of 0.20 mm. Initially, a .10/20 file is used **(A)**, followed by a .08/20 file **(B). C,** The third instrument is a .06/20 file. **D,** The final instrument, a .04/20 file, is used to the corrected working length of 21 mm.

preparation should not be precurved; only then can rotaries predictably follow.

Frequently NiTi rotaries are combined with hand files or other rotary instruments. One such combination technique uses the following steps: coronal flaring, nickel-titanium rotary preparation to the WL, and additional apical enlargement (Box 16.3). After access, the irrigated canal is explored with a No. 10 or No. 15 K-file into the midroot area. Sometimes a canal is already naturally flared and wide (e.g., a maxillary central incisor or canine in a younger patient). In such cases a No. 10 file may immediately be placed to the estimated working length and a working length radiograph can be obtained. For more constricted canals, Gates-Glidden drills or better NiTi orifice shapers can be used to accomplish early coronal flaring. This step facilitates irrigation and removes coronal interferences, which in turn permits easier access to the apical portion of the root canal and more accurate determination of the apical constriction location[146] and size.[147]

In the presence of irrigant or gel-based lubricant, the canal is negotiated to full length with hand files used in a watch-winding motion. If an impediment is felt, the negotiation files need to be precurved. However, to secure a glide path for subsequent rotary use, the clinician must confirm that a straight No. 15 K-file can reach the corrected working length. The tightness of fit of the negotiation file at the WL gives an estimate of the canal size; however, coronal interferences do not permit a more accurate assessment at this point.

The middle and apical portions of the canal then are prepared using nickel-titanium rotary instruments (see Figs. 16.23 and 16.24). Rotary files are used with a crown-down approach to reach the corrected working length. Using this approach with continuously tapered rotaries creates coronal taper and reduces the contact area of the file, so torsional forces are reduced.[148] Differently designed NiTi rotaries may follow a single-length principle, according to the manufacturer's recommendations.

Emphasis traditionally has been placed on determining the canal length, with comparatively little consideration given to the canal diameter in the apical portion of the root. Because every canal is unique in its morphology, apical canal diameters must be assessed. After initial preparation to length, the size of the apical portion of the canal is determined by placing successively larger instruments to the corrected WL until slight binding is encountered (Fig. 16.25). Often, the next larger instrument will not go to the corrected working length. If it does go to length, a subjective estimation of the apical diameter must be made according to the degree of binding. This file is the MAF (initial file to bind). It is defined as the largest file to bind slightly at the corrected working length after straight-line access. This provides an estimate of the canal diameter

before cleaning and shaping and is the point where the step-back preparation begins. Unfortunately this technique often underestimates actual constriction diameters[149]; therefore, additional apical enlargement may be performed.

When the body of the canal has been shaped, the apical portion may be additionally prepared using hand or rotary files (Fig. 16.26). The first instrument selected for this portion of the shaping process is one size larger than the MAF (estimated canal diameter at the WL). Recent clinical evidence has suggested that such an enlargement may be beneficial to the outcome.[150]

CRITERIA FOR EVALUATING CLEANING AND SHAPING

After cleaning and shaping procedures, the canal should exhibit "glassy smooth" walls, and there should be no evidence of dentin filings, debris, or irrigant in the canal. This can be directly determined in the coronal root canal portion when an operating microscope is used to visualize endodontic procedures; it can only be indirectly determined in the more apical portion of the root canal by tactile feedback during instrumentation.

Shaping is evaluated by assessing the canal taper and identifying the apical configuration in size and shape. For obturation with lateral compaction, a small finger spreader ideally should go to within 1 mm of the corrected working length without binding. For warm vertical compaction, the plugger should reach to within 5 mm of the corrected working length (Fig. 16.27).

The following principles and concepts should be applied, regardless of the instruments or technique selected.

1. Initial canal exploration is always performed with smaller hand files to gauge the canal's size, shape, and configuration.
2. Copious irrigation must be provided between instruments in the canal.
3. Coronal preflaring facilitates the placement of larger files (either hand or rotary) to working length and reduces procedural errors, such as loss of working length and canal transportation.
4. Apical canal enlargement proceeds gradually, using sequentially larger files, regardless of the flaring technique.
5. Debris is loosened and dentin is removed from all walls on the outstroke or with a rotating action at or close to the working length.
6. Instrument binding or dentin removal on insertion should be avoided. Files are teased to length using a watch-winding action. This is a back-and-forth rotating motion of the file between the thumb and forefinger, continually working the file apically. Careful file manipulation in an irrigant-filled canal helps prevent apical packing of debris and minimizes extrusion of debris into the periradicular tissues.
7. Circumferential filing is used for canals with cross-sectional shapes that are not round. The file is placed into the canal and withdrawn in a directional manner against the mesial, distal, buccal, and lingual walls.
8. After each insertion the file is removed and the flutes are cleaned of debris; the file can then be reinserted into the **291**

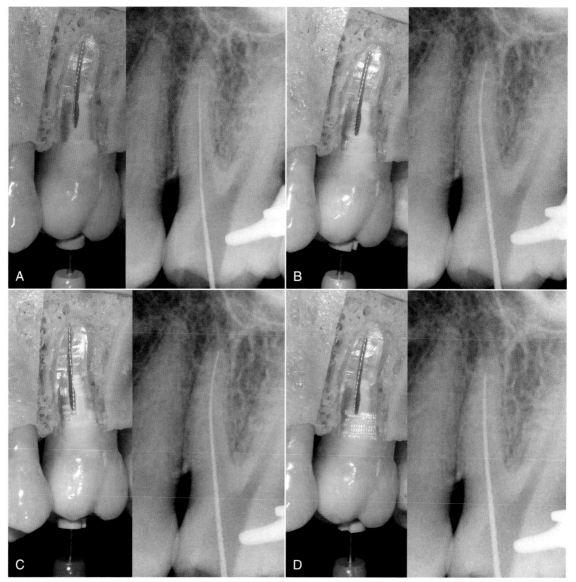

Fig. 16.25 After straight-line access in this maxillary molar, the actual constriction size is determined by successively placing small to larger files to the corrected working length. **A,** A No. 15 stainless steel file is placed to 21 mm without resistance. **B,** A No. 20 file is placed to 21 mm without resistance. **C,** The No. 25 file reaches 21 mm with slight binding. **D,** A No. 30 file is then placed and does not go the corrected working length, indicating that the initial canal size in the apical portion of the canal is No. 25.

canal to plane the next wall. Debris is removed from the file by wiping it with an alcohol-soaked gauze or a cotton roll.[151]

9. Recapitulation is done to loosen debris by placing a small file to the corrected working length, followed by irrigation to mechanically remove the material. During recapitulation the canal walls are not planed and the canal is not enlarged.

10. Small, long, curved canals are the most difficult and tedious to enlarge. They require extra caution during preparation because they are the most prone to loss of length and transportation.

11. Overenlargement of curved canals by files attempting to straighten themselves leads to procedural errors (see Fig. 16.11).

12. Overpreparation of canal walls toward the furcation may result in a stripping perforation in the danger zone, where root dentin is thinner (see Fig. 16.12).

13. Instruments, irrigants, debris, and obturating materials should be contained within the canal. These are all known physical or chemical irritants that can induce periradicular inflammation and may delay or compromise healing.

14. Creation of an apical stop may be impossible if the apical foramen is already very large. An apical taper (seat) is attempted but with care. Overusing large files aggravates the problem by creating an even larger apical opening.

15. Forcing or locking (binding) files into dentin produces unwanted torsional force. This tends to untwist the file, which in turn stresses the instrument possibly to the point of fracture.

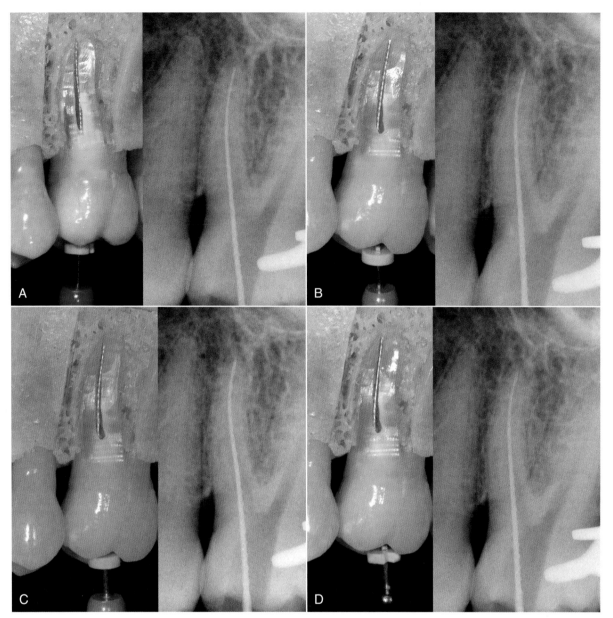

Fig. 16.26 Final apical enlargement **A,** The master apical file (No. 25) at the corrected working length of 21 mm. **B,** Enlargement with a No. 30 file to the corrected working length of 21 mm. **C,** Further enlargement with a No. 35 file. **D,** Final enlargement to a No. 40 file. The final instrument used becomes the final apical file (FAF).

INTRACANAL MEDICAMENTS

Intracanal medicaments have a long history of use as interim appointment dressings (Box 16.4). They have been used for the following three purposes: (1) to reduce interappointment pain, (2) to decrease the bacterial count and prevent regrowth, and (3) to render the canal contents inert.

Clinical evidence of the effectiveness of these agents is mixed; this has led to increased interest in the efficacy of so-called single-visit endodontic therapy. Only a few prospective studies have directly compared single and multiple visit strategies, and a meta-analysis favored single-visit treatment.[152] Two well-done clinical studies[153,154] showed microorganisms in the accessory anatomy and isthmuses, and also in the main canal, after single-visit treatment and in the majority of the cases with calcium hydroxide placement.

Box 16.4 Groupings of Commonly Used Intracanal Medicaments

Calcium hydroxide
Phenolics
Aldehydes
Halides
Steroids
Antibiotics
Combinations

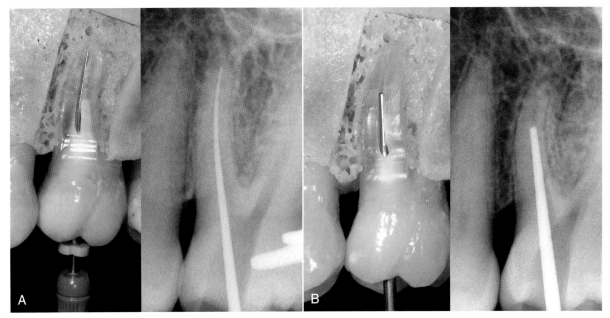

Fig. 16.27 The coronal taper is assessed using the spreader or plugger depth of penetration. **A,** With lateral compaction, a finger spreader should fit loosely 1 mm from the corrected working length with space adjacent to the spreader. **B,** For warm vertical compaction, the plugger should go to within 5 mm of the corrected working length.

Calcium Hydroxide

One intracanal agent that is effective in inhibiting microbial growth in canals is calcium hydroxide.[155] The antimicrobial activity of calcium hydroxide is a result of the alkaline pH, and this agent may aid in dissolving necrotic tissue remnants and bacteria and their byproducts.[156-158] Interappointment use of calcium hydroxide in the canal demonstrates no pain-reduction effects.[159] Calcium hydroxide has been recommended for use in teeth with necrotic pulp tissue and bacterial contamination. It probably has little benefit in teeth with vital pulps. Calcium hydroxide should be placed as a powder mixed with a liquid (e.g., local anesthetic solution, saline, or sterile water) to form a slurry; or it can be introduced into the canal as a proprietary paste supplied in a syringe (Fig. 16.28). A Lentulo spiral is effective and efficient for placement.[160-162] Spinning the paste into the canal by rotating a file counterclockwise and using an injection technique is not as effective. It is important to place the material deeply and densely for maximum effectiveness. To accomplish this, straight-line access should be performed, and the apical portion of the canal should be prepared to a No. 25 file or greater. Removal after placement is difficult,[163] especially in the apical portion of the root.

Phenols and Aldehydes

The majority of the phenols and aldehydes have nonspecific action and can destroy host tissues in addition to microbes.[164-166] Historically it was thought that these agents were effective, although their use was based on opinion and empiricism. The phenols and aldehydes are toxic, and the aldehydes are fixative agents.[167,168] When placed in the radicular space, they have access to the periradicular tissues and the systemic circulation.[169,170] Research has demonstrated that their clinical use is not justified.[171-175] Clinical studies assessing the ability of these agents to prevent or control interappointment pain indicate that they are not effective.[176-179]

Corticosteroids

Corticosteroids are antiinflammatory agents that have been advocated for reducing postoperative pain by suppressing inflammation. The use of corticosteroids as intracanal medicaments may diminish lower level postoperative pain in certain situations[180]; however, evidence also suggests that they may be ineffective, particularly with higher pain levels.[179] Irreversible pulpitis and acute apical periodontitis are examples of conditions in which steroid use might be beneficial.[180-182]

Chlorhexidine

Chlorhexidine has recently been advocated as an intracanal medicament.[183,184] A 2% gel is recommended, which can be used alone or mixed with calcium hydroxide. The combination of chlorhexidine and calcium hydroxide has greater antimicrobial activity than calcium hydroxide mixed with saline,[185] and periradicular healing in animal models appears to be enhanced.[186] However, a recent randomized clinical trial did not show that the combination of calcium hydroxide and 2% chlorhexidine was advantageous, compared to single-appointment treatment in cases with periapical lesions, after 1 year of observation.[187]

TEMPORARY RESTORATIONS*

As stated before, root canal treatment may involve more than one visit. Also, unless it is limited to a routine access cavity, the final restoration is usually not completed in the same appointment as the root canal treatment, and a temporary restoration is then required. In special situations, when definitive restoration has to be deferred, the temporary must last several months.

---

*Courtesy of Dr. Harold Messer.

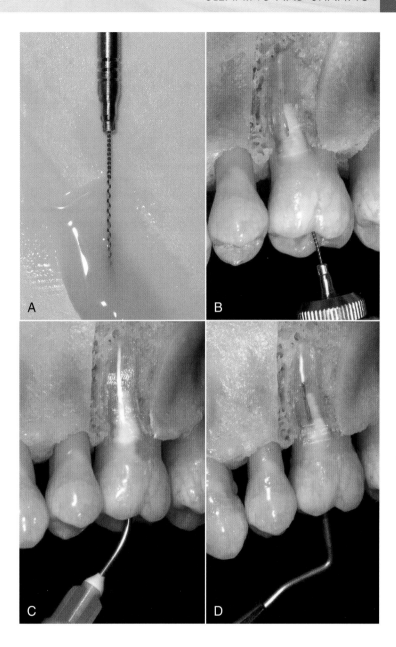

Fig. 16.28 Calcium hydroxide placement. **A,** Calcium hydroxide mixed with glycerin to form a thick paste. **B,** Placement with a Lentulo spiral. **C,** Injection of a proprietary paste. **D,** Compaction of calcium hydroxide powder with a plugger.

Objectives of Temporization

The temporary restoration must do the following:

1. Seal coronally, preventing ingress of oral fluids and bacteria and egress of intracanal medicaments.
2. Enhance isolation during treatment procedures.
3. Protect tooth structure until the final restoration is placed.
4. Allow ease of placement and removal.
5. Satisfy esthetics, but always as a secondary consideration to providing a seal.

These objectives depend on the intended duration of use. Therefore, different materials are required, depending on time, occlusal load and wear, complexity of access, and loss of tooth structure.

Routine Access Cavities

Many access cavities involve only one surface and are surrounded by dentin walls or by porcelain or metal (if the restoration is retained). The temporary must last several days to

several weeks. Numerous types are available, including premixed cements that set on contact with moisture (Cavit); reinforced zinc oxide–eugenol cements, such as intermediate restorative material (IRM); glass ionomer cements (GICs), such as Fuji IX; and specially formulated light-polymerized composite materials, such as temporary endodontic restorative material (TERM).[188] Ease of use and good sealing ability make Cavit an excellent routine material for smaller cavities, but low strength and rapid occlusal wear limit its use to short-term sealing. IRM and TERM provide improved wear resistance, although their sealing ability is probably marginally less than that of Cavit.[189,190] More durable restorative materials, especially glass ionomer cements, tend to provide the best seal. A double seal of Fuji IX over Cavit provides a durable and effective barrier to microbial leakage. It is not known whether experimental leakage differences based on bacterial leakage or dye penetration are significant clinically, especially since thermocycling and occlusal loading are often not part of the testing procedure.[191] Clinically, 4 mm of Cavit provided

Cotton Pellet

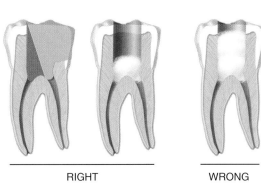

RIGHT   WRONG

Fig. 16.29 Techniques for temporization. *Left,* These two techniques are correct. Either minimal space is occupied by cotton, or no cotton pellet is used, particularly if the proximal is to be restored. *Right,* This technique is incorrect. Most of the chamber is packed with cotton, which leaves inadequate space and strength for the material (3 to 4 mm are required), and cotton fibers may promote bacterial leakage. (Courtesy Dr. L. Wilcox and Dr. H. Messer.)

an effective seal against bacterial penetration for 3 weeks.[192] Most critical are the thickness and placement of the material and the cavity size.

Techniques of Placement

The quality of the coronal seal depends on the thickness of the material, how it is compacted into the cavity, and the extent of contact with sound tooth structure or restoration. A minimum depth of 3 to 4 mm is required around the periphery, preferably 4 mm or more to allow for wear. In anterior teeth, the access is oblique to the tooth surface; care must be taken to ensure that the material is at least 3 mm thick in the cingulum area.

Cavit (or a similar material) is placed as follows. The chamber and cavity walls should be dry. Cavit can be placed directly over the obturated canal orifices; more commonly, a thin layer of cotton or a small section of a sterile sponge is placed over the canal orifices to prevent canal blockage[193] (Fig. 16.29). Care must be taken not to incorporate cotton fibers into the restorative material because they can promote rapid leakage.[194] Cavit is packed into the access opening with a plastic instrument in increments from the bottom up and pressed against the cavity walls and into undercuts (Fig. 16.30). Excess is removed, and the surface is smoothed with moist cotton. The patient should avoid chewing on the tooth for at least an hour.

Subsequent removal using a high-speed bur requires care to avoid damage to the access opening. Alternatively, an ultrasonic tip can be used.

Extensive Coronal Breakdown

Extensive mesial/occlusal/distal (MOD) cavities and teeth without marginal ridges or with undermined cusps require a stronger filling material (high-strength GIC), and care must be taken to ensure an adequate thickness and good marginal adaptation proximally. The temporary filling material should extend well into the pulp chamber, deep to the proximal margin, to ensure a marginal seal. Reducing the height of

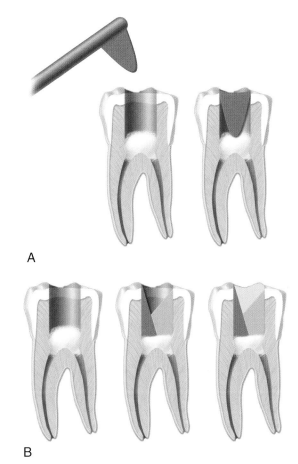

A

B

Fig. 16.30 Techniques for placing temporary material. **A,** A single large "blob" placed in the access opening will not seal the walls. **B,** The incremental technique is correct; successive layers are added, and each layer is pressed against the chamber walls before the next is applied. (Courtesy Dr. L. Wilcox and Dr. H. Messer.)

undermined cusps well out of occlusion reduces the risk of fracture. For severely broken-down teeth, a cusp-onlay amalgam or a well-fitting orthodontic band cemented onto the tooth (restored with glass ionomer cement) provides a durable temporary restoration and strengthens the tooth against fracture.[195] At the next appointment, access is prepared through the restoration.

Provisional Post Crowns

The use of a provisional crown with an incorporated resin post may be required, particularly when a cast post and core is being fabricated for a visible tooth with little remaining coronal tooth structure. However, the use of such a provisional crown retained with a temporary post has inherent problems. Using the canal space for a provisional post precludes use of an intracanal medicament, and the coronal seal depends entirely on the cement. The coronal seal is generally inadequate, with a loosely fitting and mobile provisional post and crown.[196] However, in spite of these potential difficulties, such provisional restorations may be required while cast posts and cores are being fabricated. Because of the potential problems, it is prudent to cement the definitive post as soon as possible.

When such a provisional crown-post combination is being used, the post should fit the canal snugly (not binding) and extend apically 4 to 5 mm short of working length and coronally to within 2 to 3 mm of the incisal edge. A polycarbonate shell is trimmed to a good fit; autopolymerizing material then is added to the inside of the shell to mold to the root face and attach to the post. After contouring and occlusal adjustment, provisional luting cement (Temp Bond or similar cement) is placed on the coronal 3 to 4 mm of the post and root face, and the unit is cemented into place. A provisional removable partial overdenture is a useful alternative; access remains excellent, and there is little chance of disturbing the coronal seal between appointments.

Long-Term Temporary Restorations

Few indications exist to justify delaying the final restoration, and endodontic procedures (other than trauma management) rarely require prolonged treatment. If a temporary restoration has to last more than a few weeks, a durable material should be used, such as amalgam, GIC, or acid-etch composite. A double seal with a liner of glass ionomer or flowable composite is placed over the coronal aspect of the root canal filling. The pulp chamber is filled with a layer of Cavit, allowing for sufficient thickness of the restorative material to ensure strength and wear resistance. Subsequent access to the canal space is readily achieved without damage to remaining tooth structure because the layer of Cavit can be easily removed.

REFERENCES

1. Ingle JI: *Endodontics*, ed 5, London, Ontario, 2002, BC Decker.
2. Sabeti MA, Nekofar M, Motahhary P, et al: Healing of apical periodontitis after endodontic treatment with and without obturation in dogs, *J Endod* 32(7):628, 2006.
3. Delivanis PD, Mattison GD, Mendel RW: The survivability of F43 strain of *Streptococcus sanguis* in root canals filled with gutta-percha and Procosol cement, *J Endod* 9(10):407, 1983.
4. Sedgley CM, Lennan SL, Applebe OK: Survival of *Enterococcus faecalis* in root canals ex vivo, *Int Endod J* 38(10):735, 2005.
5. Ng YL, Mann V, Gulabivala K: A prospective study of the factors affecting outcomes of nonsurgical root canal treatment. Part 1. Periapical health, *Int Endod J* 44(7):583, 2011.
6. Walton RE: Current concepts of canal preparation, *Dent Clin North Am* 36(2):309, 1992.
7. Allison DA, Weber CR, Walton RE: The influence of the method of canal preparation on the quality of apical and coronal obturation, *J Endod* 5(10):298, 1979.
8. Schilder H: Cleaning and shaping the root canal, *Dent Clin North Am* 18(2):269, 1974.
9. Wilcox LR, Roskelley C, Sutton T: The relationship of root canal enlargement to finger spreader–induced vertical root fracture, *J Endod* 23(8):533, 1997.
10. Kuttler Y: Microscopic investigation of root apexes, *J Am Dent Assoc* 50(5):544, 1955.
11. Dummer PMH, McGinn JH, Rees DG: The position and topography of the apical canal constriction and apical foramen, *Int Endod J* 17(4):192, 1984.
12. Gutierrez JH, Aguayo P: Apical foraminal openings in human teeth, *Oral Surg Oral Med Oral Pathol Oral Radiol Endod* 79(6):769, 1995.
13. Malueg LA, Wilcox LR, Johnson W: Examination of external apical root resorption with scanning electron microscopy, *Oral Surg Oral Med Oral Pathol Oral Radiol Endod* 82(1):89, 1996.
14. Farzaneh M, Abitbol S, Friedman S: Treatment outcome in endodontics—the Toronto study, phases I and II: orthograde retreatment, *J Endod* 30(9):627, 2004.
15. de Chevigny C, Dao TT, Basrani BR, et al: Treatment outcome in endodontics—the Toronto study, phase 4: initial treatment, *J Endod* 34(3):258, 2008.
16. Schaeffer MA, White RR, Walton RA: Determining the optimal obturation length: a meta-analysis of literature, *J Endod* 31(4):271, 2005.
17. Wu MK, Wesselink PR, Walton RE: Apical terminus location of root canal treatment procedures, *Oral Surg Oral Med Oral Pathol Oral Radiol Endod* 89(1):99, 2000.
18. Ricucci D, Russo J, Rutberg M, et al: A prospective cohort study of endodontic treatments of 1,369 root canals: results after 5 years, *Oral Surg Oral Med Oral Pathol Oral Radiol Endod* 112(6):825, 2011.
19. Eldeeb ME, Boraas JC: The effect of different files on the preparation shape of severely curved canals, *Int Endod J* 18(1):1, 1985.
20. Chow TW: Mechanical effectiveness of root canal irrigation, *J Endod* 9(11):475, 1983.
21. Ram Z: Effectiveness of root canal irrigation, *Oral Surg Oral Med Oral Pathol* 44(2):306, 1977.
22. Salzgeber RM, Brilliant JD: An in vivo evaluation of the penetration of an irrigating solution in root canals, *J Endod* 3(10):394, 1977.
23. Ørstavik D, Kerekes K, Molven O: Effects of extensive apical reaming and calcium hydroxide dressing on bacterial infection during treatment of apical periodontitis: a pilot study, *Int Endod J* 24(1):1, 1991.
24. Dalton BC, Ørstavik D, Phillips C, et al: Bacterial reduction with nickel-titanium rotary instrumentation, *J Endod* 24(11):763, 1998.
25. Sjögren U, Figdor D, Spångberg L, et al: The antimicrobial effect of calcium hydroxide as a short-term intracanal dressing, *Int Endod J* 24(3):119, 1991.
26. Wu YN, Shi JN, Huang LZ, et al: Variables affecting electronic root canal measurement, *Int Endod J* 25(2):88, 1992.
27. Haapasalo M, Shen Y, Qian W, et al: Irrigation in endodontics, *Dent Clin North Am* 54(2):291, 2010.
28. vd Sluis LW, Versluis M, Wesselink PR: Passive ultrasonic irrigation of the root canal: a review of the literature, *Int Endod J* 40(6):415, 2007.
29. Usman N, Baumgartner JC, Marshall JG: Influence of instrument size on root canal débridement, *J Endod* 30(2):110, 2004.
30. Rollison S, Barnett F, Stevens RH: Efficacy of bacterial removal from instrumented root canals in vitro related to instrumentation technique and size, *Oral Surg Oral Med Oral Pathol Oral Radiol Endod* 94(3):366, 2002.
31. Card SJ, Sigurdsson A, Ørstavik D, et al: The effectiveness of increased apical enlargement in reducing intracanal bacteria, *J Endod* 28(11):779, 2002.
32. Pettiette MT, Delano EO, Trope M: Evaluation of success rate of endodontic treatment performed by students with stainless-steel K-files and nickel-titanium hand files, *J Endod* 27(2):124, 2001.
33. Peters OA: Current challenges and concepts in the preparation of root canal systems: a review, *J Endod* 30(8):559, 2004.
34. Paqué F, Boessler C, Zehnder M: Accumulated hard tissue debris levels in mesial roots of mandibular molars after sequential irrigation steps, *Int Endod J* 44(2):148, 2011.
35. Love RM, Jenkinson HF: Invasion of dentinal tubules by oral bacteria, *Crit Rev Oral Biol Med* 13(2):171, 2002.
36. Akpata ES: Effect of endodontic procedures on the population of viable microorganisms in the infected root canal, *J Endod* 2(12):369, 1976.
37. Matsuo T, Shirakami T, Ozaki K, et al: An immunohistological study of the localization of bacteria invading root pulpal walls of teeth with periapical lesions, *J Endod* 29(3):194, 2003.
38. Peters LB, Wesselink PR, Buijs JF, et al: Viable bacteria in root dentinal tubules of teeth with apical periodontitis, *J Endod* 27(2):76, 2001.
39. Bird DC, Chambers D, Peters OA: Usage parameters of nickel-titanium rotary instruments: a survey of endodontists in the United States, *J Endod* 35(9):1193, 2009.
40. Parashos P, Messer HH: Uptake of rotary NiTi technology within Australia, *Aust Dent J* 50(4):251, 2005.
41. Bjørndal L, Reit C: The adoption of new endodontic technology amongst Danish general dental practitioners, *Int Endod J* 38(1):52, 2005.
42. Waltimo T, Trope M, Haapasalo M, et al: Clinical efficacy of treatment procedures in endodontic infection control and one year follow-up of periapical healing, *J Endod* 31(12):863, 2005.
43. Shuping GB, Ørstavik D, Sigurdsson A, et al: Reduction of intracanal bacteria using nickel-titanium rotary instrumentation and various medications, *J Endod* 26(12):751, 2000.
44. Siqueira JF Jr, Lima KC, Magalhaes FAC, et al: Mechanical reduction of the bacterial population in the root canal by three instrumentation techniques, *J Endod* 25(5):332, 1999.
45. Siqueira JF Jr, Rocas IN, Santos SR, et al: Efficacy of instrumentation techniques and irrigation regimens in reducing the bacterial population within root canals, *J Endod* 28(3):181, 2002.
46. Tanomaru Filho M, Leonardo MR, da Silva LA: Effect of irrigating solution and calcium hydroxide root canal dressing on the repair of apical and periapical tissues of teeth with periapical lesion, *J Endod* 28(4):295, 2002.
47. Ørstavik D, Haapasalo M: Disinfection by endodontic irrigants and dressings of experimentally infected dentinal tubules, *Endod Dent Traumatol* 6(4):142, 1990.
48. Gernhardt CR, Eppendorf K, Kozlowski A, et al: Toxicity of concentrated sodium hypochlorite used as an endodontic irrigant, *Int Endod J* 37(4):272, 2004.
49. Pashley EL, Birdsong NL, Bowman K, et al: Cytotoxic effects of NaOCl on vital tissue, *J Endod* 11(12):525, 1985.
50. Reeh ES, Messer HH: Long-term paresthesia following inadvertent forcing of sodium hypochlorite through perforation in maxillary incisor, *Endod Dent Traumatol* 5(4):200, 1989.
51. Witton R, Brennan PA: Severe tissue damage and neurological deficit following extravasation of sodium hypochlorite solution during routine endodontic treatment, *Br Dent J* 198(12):749, 2005.

52. Brown DC, Moore BK, Brown CE Jr, et al: An in vitro study of apical extrusion of sodium hypochlorite during endodontic canal preparation, *J Endod* 21(12):587, 1995.

53. Hülsmann M, Hahn W: Complications during root canal irrigation: literature review and case reports, *Int Endod J* 33(3):186, 2000.

54. Yamada RS, Armas A, Goldman M, et al: A scanning electron microscopic comparison of a high volume final flush with several irrigating solutions. Part 3, *J Endod* 9(4):137, 1983.

55. Lambrianidis T, Tosounidou E, Tzoanopoulou M: The effect of maintaining apical patency on periapical extrusion, *J Endod* 27(11):696, 2001.

56. Izu KH, Thomas SJ, Zhang P, et al: Effectiveness of sodium hypochlorite in preventing inoculation of periapical tissue with contaminated patency files, *J Endod* 30(2):92, 2004.

57. Vera J, Arias A, Romero M: Dynamic movement of intracanal gas bubbles during cleaning and shaping procedures: the effect of maintaining apical patency on their presence in the middle and cervical thirds of human root canals-an in vivo study, *J Endod* 38(2):200, 2012.

58. Nair PN: On the causes of persistent apical periodontitis: a review, *Int Endod J* 39(4):249, 2006.

59. Carr GB, Schwartz RS, Schaudinn C, et al: Ultrastructural examination of failed molar retreatment with secondary apical periodontitis: an examination of endodontic biofilms in an endodontic retreatment failure, *J Endod* 35(9):1303, 2009.

60. AAE Endodontic Case Difficulty Assessment Form and Guidelines. American Association of Endodontists, Chicago, 2010.

61. Peters OA, Paqué F: Current developments in rotary root canal instrument technology and clinical use: a review, *Quintessence Int* 41(6):479, 2010.

62. Walia H, Brantley WA, Gerstein H: An initial investigation of the bending and torsional properties of Nitinol root canal files, *J Endod* 14(7):346, 1988.

63. Peters OA, Schönenberger K, Laib A: Effects of four NiTi preparation techniques on root canal geometry assessed by micro-computed tomography, *Int Endod J* 34(3):221, 2001.

64. McSpadden JT, Bonaccorso A, Tocchio C, et al: The zone technique, *Endo-Endodontic Practice Today (UK)* 2(1):33, 2008.

65. Pruett JP, Clement DJ, Carnes DL: Cyclic fatigue testing of nickel-titanium endodontic instruments, *J Endod* 23(2):77, 1997.

66. Zuolo ML, Walton RE: Instrument deterioration with usage: nickel-titanium versus stainless steel, *Quintessence Int* 28(6):397, 1997.

67. Torabinejad M, Handysides R, Khademi AA, et al: Clinical implications of the smear layer in endodontics: a review, *Oral Surg Oral Med Oral Pathol Oral Radiol Endod* 94(6):658, 2002.

68. McComb D, Smith DC: A preliminary scanning electron microscopic study of root canals after endodontic procedures, *J Endod* 1(7):238, 1975.

69. Sen BH, Piskin B, Baran N: The effect of tubular penetration of root canal sealers on dye microleakage, *Int Endod J* 29(1):23, 1996.

70. Chailertvanitkul P, Saunders WP, MacKenzie D: The effect of smear layer on microbial coronal leakage of gutta-percha root fillings, *Int Endod J* 29(4):242, 1996.

71. Clark-Holke D, Drake D, Walton R, et al: Bacterial penetration through canals of endodontically treated teeth in the presence or absence of the smear layer, *J Dent* 31(4):275, 2003.

72. Oksan T, Aktener BO, Sen BH, et al: The penetration of root canal sealers into dentinal tubules: a scanning electron microscopic study, *Int Endod J* 26(5):301, 1993.

73. Wennberg A, Ørstavik D: Adhesion of root canal sealers to bovine dentine and gutta-percha, *Int Endod J* 23(1):13, 1990.

74. Leonard JE, Gutmann JL, Guo IY: Apical and coronal seal of roots obturated with a dentine

bonding agent and resin, *Int Endod J* 29(2):76, 1996.

75. Kokkas AB, Boutsioukis A, Vassiliades LP, et al: The influence of the smear layer on dentinal tubule penetration depth by three different root canal sealers: an in vitro study, *J Endod* 30(2):100, 2004.

76. Cobankara FK, Adanr N, Belli S: Evaluation of the influence of smear layer on the apical and coronal sealing ability of two sealers, *J Endod* 30(6):406, 2004.

77. Siqueira JF Jr, Araujo MC, Garcia PF, et al: Histological evaluation of the effectiveness of five instrumentation techniques for cleaning the apical third of root canals, *J Endod* 23(8):499, 1997.

78. Wu MK, Wesselink PR: Efficacy of three techniques in cleaning the apical portion of curved root canals, *Oral Surg Oral Med Oral Pathol Oral Radiol Endod* 79(4):492, 1995.

79. Tan BT, Messer HH: The quality of apical canal preparation using hand and rotary instruments with specific criteria for enlargement based on initial apical file size, *J Endod* 28(9):658, 2002.

80. Rosenfeld EF, James GA, Burch BS: Vital pulp tissue response to sodium hypochlorite, *J Endod* 4(5):140, 1978.

81. Svec TA, Harrison JW: Chemomechanical removal of pulpal and dentinal debris with sodium hypochlorite and hydrogen peroxide vs normal saline solution, *J Endod* 3(2):49, 1977.

82. Peters OA, Boessler C, Zehnder M: Effect of liquid and paste-type lubricants on torque values during simulated rotary root canal instrumentation, *Int Endod J* 38(1):223, 2005.

83. Jungbluth H, Peters C, Peters OA, et al: Physicochemical and pulp tissue dissolution properties of some household bleach brands compared with a dental sodium hypochlorite solution, *J Endod* 38(3):372, 2012.

84. Zehnder M: Root canal irrigants, *J Endod* 32(5):389, 2006.

85. Zehnder M, Kosicki D, Luder H, et al: Tissue-dissolving capacity and antibacterial effect of buffered and unbuffered hypochlorite solutions, *Oral Surg Oral Med Oral Pathol Oral Radiol Endod* 94(6):756, 2002.

86. Berutti E, Marini R: A scanning electron microscopic evaluation of the débridement capability of sodium hypochlorite at different temperatures, *J Endod* 22(9):467, 1996.

87. Gambarini G, De Luca M, Gerosa R: Chemical stability of heated sodium hypochlorite endodontic irrigants, *J Endod* 24(6):432, 1998.

88. Oncag O, Hosgor M, Hilmioglu S, et al: Comparison of antibacterial and toxic effects of various root canal irrigants, *Int Endod J* 36(6):423, 2003.

89. Abou-Rass M, Piccinino MV: The effectiveness of four clinical irrigation methods on the removal of root canal debris, *Oral Surg Oral Med Oral Pathol* 54(3):323, 1982.

90. Hülsmann M, Heckendorff M, Lennon A: Chelating agents in root canal treatment: mode of action and indications for their use, *Int Endod J* 36(12):810, 2003.

91. Baumgartner JC, Mader CL: A scanning electron microscope evaluation of four root canal irrigation regimes, *J Endod* 13(4):147, 1987.

92. Mai S, Kim YK, Arola DD, et al: Differential aggressiveness of ethylenediamine tetraacetic acid in causing canal wall erosion in the presence of sodium hypochlorite, *J Dent* 38(3):201, 2010.

93. Guignes P, Faure J, Maurette A: Relationship between endodontic preparations and human dentin permeability measured in situ, *J Endod* 22(2):60, 1996.

94. Hottel TL, El-Rafai NY, Jones JJ: A comparison of the effects of three chelating agents on the root canals of extracted human teeth, *J Endod* 25(11):716, 1999.

95. Lim TS, Wee TY, Choi MY, et al: Light and scanning electron microscopic evaluation of Glyde File Prep in smear layer removal, *Int Endod J* 36(5):336, 2003.

96. Krell KV, Johnson RJ: Irrigation patterns of ultrasonic endodontic files. II. Diamond coated files, *J Endod* 14(2):535, 1988.

97. Mjør IA, Smith MR, Ferrari M, et al: The structure of dentine in the apical region of human teeth, *Int Endod J* 34(5):346, 2001.

98. Paqué F, Luder HU, Sener B, et al: Tubular sclerosis rather than the smear layer impedes dye penetration into the dentine of endodontically instrumented root canals, *Int Endod J* 39(1):18, 2006.

99. Scelza MF, Teixeira AM, Scelza P: Decalcifying effect of EDTA-T, 10% citric acid, and 17% EDTA on root canal dentin, *Oral Surg Oral Med Oral Pathol Oral Radiol Endod* 95(2):234, 2003.

100. Calt S, Serper A: Smear layer removal by EGTA, *J Endod* 26(8):459, 2000.

101. Haznedaroglu F: Efficacy of various concentrations of citric acid at different pH values for smear layer removal, *Oral Surg Oral Med Oral Pathol Oral Radiol Endod* 96(3):340, 2003.

102. Baumgartner JC, Brown CM, Mader CL, et al: A scanning electron microscopic evaluation of root canal débridement using saline, sodium hypochlorite, and citric acid, *J Endod* 10(11):525, 1984.

103. Rosenthal S, Spångberg L, Safavi K: Chlorhexidine substantivity in root canal dentin, *Oral Surg Oral Med Oral Pathol Oral Radiol Endod* 98(4):488, 2004.

104. Jeansonne MJ, White RR: A comparison of 2.0% chlorhexidine gluconate and 5.25% sodium hypochlorite as antimicrobial endodontic irrigants, *J Endod* 20(6):276, 1994.

105. Kuruvilla JR, Kamath MP: Antimicrobial activity of 2.5% sodium hypochlorite and 0.2% chlorhexidine gluconate separately and combined, as endodontic irrigants, *J Endod* 24(7):472, 1998.

106. Vahdaty A, Pitt Ford TR, Wilson RF: Efficacy of chlorhexidine in disinfecting dentinal tubules in vitro, *Endod Dent Traumatol* 9(6):243, 1993.

107. White RR, Hays GL, Janer LR: Residual antimicrobial activity after canal irrigation with chlorhexidine, *J Endod* 23(4):229, 1997.

108. Torabinejad M, Khademi AA, Babagoli J, et al: A new solution for the removal of the smear layer, *J Endod* 29(3):170, 2003.

109. Torabinejad M, Cho Y, Khademi AA, et al: The effect of various concentrations of sodium hypochlorite on the ability of MTAD to remove the smear layer, *J Endod* 29(4):233, 2003.

110. Shabahang S, Pouresmail M, Torabinejad M: In vitro antimicrobial efficacy of MTAD and sodium hypochlorite, *J Endod* 29(7):450, 2003.

111. Shabahang S, Torabinejad M: Effect of MTAD on *Enterococcus faecalis*–contaminated root canals of extracted human teeth, *J Endod* 29(9):576, 2003.

112. Zhang B, Alysandratos KD, Angelidou A, et al: Human mast cell degranulation and preformed TNF secretion require mitochondrial translocation to exocytosis sites: relevance to atopic dermatitis, *J Allergy Clin Immunol* 127(6):1522, 2011.

113. Machnick TK, Torabinejad M, Munoz CA, et al: Effect of MTAD on the bond strength to enamel and dentin, *J Endod* 29(12):818, 2003.

114. Malkhassian G, Manzur AJ, Legner M, et al: Antibacterial efficacy of MTAD final rinse and two percent chlorhexidine gel medication in teeth with apical periodontitis: a randomized double-blinded clinical trial, *J Endod* 35(11):1483, 2009.

115. Stojic S, Shen Y, Qian W, et al: Antibacterial and smear layer removal ability of a novel irrigant, QMiX, *J Endod* 45(4):1365, 2012.

116. Dai L, Khechen K, Khan S, et al: The effect of QMix, an experimental antibacterial root canal irrigant, on removal of canal wall smear layer and debris, *J Endod* 37(1):80, 2011.

117. Wang Z, Shen Y, Haapasalo M: Effectiveness of endodontic disinfecting solutions against young and old *Enterococcus faecalis* biofilms in dentin canals, *J Endod* 38(10):1376, 2012.

118. Morgental RD, Singh A, Sappal H, et al: Dentin inhibits the antibacterial effect of new and conventional endodontic irrigants, *J Endod* 39(3):406, 2013.

119. Ordinola-Zapata R, Bramante CM, Brandao Garcia R, et al: The antimicrobial effect of new and conventional endodontic irrigants on intraorally infected dentin, *Acta Odont Scand* 71(3-4): 424, 2013.

120. Cymerman JJ, Jerome LA, Moodnik RM: A scanning electron microscope study comparing the efficacy of hand instrumentation with ultrasonic instrumentation of the root canal, *J Endod* 9(8):327, 1983.

121. Schulz-Bongert U, Weine FS, Schulz-Bongert J: Preparation of curved canals using a combined hand-filing, ultrasonic technique, *Comp Cont Educ Dent* 16(3):270, 1995.

122. Chenail BL, Teplitsky PE: Endosonics in curved root canals. II, *J Endod* 14(5):214, 1988.

123. Ahmad M, Pitt Ford TJ, Crum LA: Ultrasonic débridement of root canals: acoustic streaming and its possible role, *J Endod* 13(10):490, 1987.

124. Cameron JA: The use of ultrasonics in the removal of the smear layer: a scanning electron microscope study, *J Endod* 9(7):289, 1983.

125. Archer R, Reader A, Nist R, et al: An in vivo evaluation of the efficacy of ultrasound after step-back preparation in mandibular molars, *J Endod* 18(11):549, 1992.

126. Weller RN, Brady JM, Bernier WE: Efficacy of ultrasonic cleaning, *J Endod* 6(9):740, 1980.

127. Steinberg D, Abid-el-Raziq D, Heling I: In vitro antibacterial effect of RC-Prep components on *Streptococcus sobrinus*, *Endod Dent Traumatol* 15(4):171, 1999.

128. Zehnder M, Schmidlin PR, Sener B, et al: Chelation in root canal therapy reconsidered, *J Endod* 31(11):817, 2005.

129. Cehreli ZC, Onur MA, Tasman F, et al: Effects of current and potential dental etchants on nerve compound action potentials, *J Endod* 28(3):149, 2002.

130. Goldberg F, Abramovich A: Analysis of the effect of EDTAC on the dentinal walls of the root canal, *J Endod* 3(3):101, 1977.

131. Powell SE, Wong PD, Simon JH: A comparison of the effect of modified and nonmodified instrument tips on apical canal configuration. II, *J Endod* 14(5):224, 1988.

132. Parashos P, Messer HH: Rotary NiTi instrument fracture and its consequences, *J Endod* 32(11):1031, 2006.

133. Degerness RA, Bowles WR: Dimension, anatomy and morphology of the mesiobuccal root canal system in maxillary molars, *J Endod* 36(6):985, 2010.

134. Sjögren U, Hagglund B, Sundqvist G, et al: Factors affecting the long-term results of endodontic treatment, *J Endod* 16(10):498, 1990.

135. Wu MK, vd Sluis LW, Wesselink PR: The capability of two hand instrumentation techniques to remove the inner layer of dentine in oval canals, *Int Endod J* 36(3):218, 2003.

136. Paqué F, Balmer M, Attin T, et al: Preparation of oval-shaped root canals in mandibular molars using nickel-titanium rotary instruments: a micro-computed tomography study, *J Endod* 36(4):703, 2010.

137. Ingle JI: A standardized endodontic technique using newly development instruments and filling materials, *Oral Surg Oral Med Oral Pathol* 14(1):83, 1961.

138. Weine FS, Kelly RF, Lio PJ: The effect of preparation procedures on original canal shape and on apical foramen shape, *J Endod* 1(8):255, 1975.

139. Walton RE: Histologic evaluation of different methods of enlarging the pulp canal space, *J Endod* 2(10):304, 1976.

140. Morgan LF, Montgomery S: An evaluation of the crown-down pressureless technique, *J Endod* 10(10):491, 1984.

141. Torabinejad M: Passive step-back technique, *Oral Surg Oral Med Oral Pathol* 77(4):398, 1994.

142. Roane JB, Sabala CL, Duncanson MG Jr: The "balanced force" concept for instrumentation of curved canals, *J Endod* 11(5):203, 1985.

143. Rotary Instrumentation: an Endodontic Perspective. American Association of Endontists, Chicago, 2008.

144. Bardsley S, Peters CI, Peters OA: The effect of three rotational speed settings on torque and apical force with vortex rotary instruments in vitro, *J Endod* 37(6):860, 2011.

145. Patino PV, Biedma BM, Liebana CR, et al: The influence of a manual glide path on the separation rate of NiTi rotary instruments, *J Endod* 31(2):114, 2005.

146. Stabholz A, Rotstein I, Torabinejad M: Effect of preflaring on tactile detection of the apical constriction, *J Endod* 21(2):92, 1995.

147. Pecora JD, Capelli A, Guersoli A, et al: Influence of cervical preflaring on apical file size determination, *Int Endod J* 38(7):430, 2005.

148. Schrader C, Peters OA: Analysis of torque and force with differently tapered rotary endodontic instruments in vitro, *J Endod* 31(2):120, 2005.

149. Paqué F, Zehnder M, Marending M: Apical fit of initial K-files in maxillary molars assessed by micro-computed tomography, *Int Endod J* 43(4):328, 2010.

150. Saini HR, Tewari S, Sangwan P, et al: Effect of different apical preparation sizes on outcome of primary endodontic treatment: a randomized controlled trial, *J Endod* 38(10):1309, 2012.

151. Ferreira Murgel CA, Walton RE, Rittman B, et al: A comparison of techniques for cleaning endodontic files after usage: a quantitative scanning electron microscopic study, *J Endod* 16(5):214, 1990.

152. Sathorn C, Parashos P, Messer HH: Effectiveness of single- versus multiple-visit endodontic treatment of teeth with apical periodontitis: a systematic review and meta-analysis, *Int Endod J* 38(6):347, 2005.

153. Nair PN, Henry S, Cano V, et al: Microbial status of apical root canal system of human mandibular first molars with primary apical periodontitis after "one-visit" endodontic treatment, *Oral Surg Oral Med Oral Pathol Oral Radiol Endod* 99(2) 2005.

154. Vera J, Siqueira JF, Ricucci D, et al: One- versus two-visit endodontic treatment of teeth with apical periodontitis: a histobacteriologic study, *J Endod* 38(8):1040, 2012.

155. Law A, Messer H: An evidence-based analysis of the antibacterial effectiveness of intracanal medicaments, *J Endod* 30(10):689, 2004.

156. Yang SF, Rivera EM, Baumgardner KR, et al: Anaerobic tissue-dissolving abilities of calcium hydroxide and sodium hypochlorite, *J Endod* 21(12):613, 1995.

157. Safavi KE, Nichols FC: Effect of calcium hydroxide on bacterial lipopolysaccharide, *J Endod* 19(2):76, 1993.

158. Safavi KE, Nichols FC: Alteration of biological properties of bacterial lipopolysaccharide by calcium hydroxide treatment, *J Endod* 20(3):127, 1994.

159. Walton RE, Holton IFJ, Michelich R: Calcium hydroxide as an intracanal medication: effect on posttreatment pain, *J Endod* 29(10):627, 2003.

160. Rivera EM, Williams K: Placement of calcium hydroxide in simulated canals: comparison of glycerin versus water, *J Endod* 20(9):445, 1994.

161. Sigurdsson A, Stancill R, Madison S: Intracanal placement of Ca(OH)₂: a comparison of techniques, *J Endod* 18(8):367, 1992.

162. Torres CP, Apicella MJ, Yancich PP, et al: Intracanal placement of calcium hydroxide: a comparison of techniques, revisited, *J Endod* 30(4):225, 2004.

163. Lambrianidis T, Kosti E, Boutsioukis C, et al: Removal efficacy of various calcium hydroxide/chlorhexidine medicaments from the root canal, *Int Endod J* 39(1):55, 2006.

164. Chang YC, Tai KW, Chou LS, et al: Effects of camphorated parachlorophenol on human periodontal ligament cells in vitro, *J Endod* 25(12):779, 1999.

165. Spångberg L: Cellular reaction to intracanal medicaments, *Trans Int Conf Endod* 5(0):108, 1973.

166. Spångberg L, Rutberg M, Rydinge E: Biologic effects of endodontic antimicrobial agents, *J Endod* 5(6):166, 1979.

167. Harrison JW, Bellizzi R, Osetek EM: The clinical toxicity of endodontic medicaments, *J Endod* 5(2):42, 1979.

168. Thoden van Velzen SK, Feltkamp-Vroom TM: Immunologic consequences of formaldehyde fixation of autologous tissue implants, *J Endod* 3(5):179, 1977.

169. Walton RE, Langeland K: Migration of materials in the dental pulp of monkeys, *J Endod* 4(6):167, 1978.

170. Myers DR, Shoaf HK, Dirksen TR, et al: Distribution of 14C-formaldehyde after pulpotomy with formocresol, *J Am Dent Assoc* 96(5):805, 1978.

171. Doran MG, Radtke PK: A review of endodontic medicaments, *Gen Dent* 46(5):484, 1998.

172. Harrison JW, Baumgartner JC, Svec TA: Incidence of pain associated with clinical factors during and after root canal therapy. Part 1. Interappointment pain, *J Endod* 9(9):384, 1983.

173. Byström A, Claesson R, Sundqvist G: The antibacterial effect of camphorated paramonochlorophenol, camphorated phenol and calcium hydroxide in the treatment of infected root canals, *Endod Dent Traumatol* 1(5):170, 1985.

174. Walton RE: Intracanal medicaments, *Dent Clin North Am* 28(4):783, 1984.

175. Harrison JW, Baumgartner CJ, Zielke DR: Analysis of interappointment pain associated with the combined use of endodontic irrigants and medicaments, *J Endod* 7(6):272, 1981.

176. Maddox DL, Walton RE, Davis CO: Incidence of post-treatment endodontic pain related to medicaments and other factors, *J Endod* 3(12):447, 1977.

177. Kleier DJ, Mullaney TP: Effects of formocresol on posttreatment pain of endodontic origin in vital molars, *J Endod* 6(5):566, 1980.

178. Torabinejad M, Kettering JD, McGraw JC, et al: Factors associated with endodontic interappointment emergencies of teeth with necrotic pulps, *J Endod* 14(5):261, 1988.

179. Trope M: Relationship of intracanal medicaments to endodontic flare-ups, *Endod Dent Traumatol* 6(5):226, 1990.

180. Ehrmann EH, Messer HH, Adams GG: The relationship of intracanal medicaments to postoperative pain in endodontics, *Int Endod J* 36(12):868, 2003.

181. Chance K, Lin L, Shovlin FE, et al: Clinical trial of intracanal corticosteroid in root canal therapy, *J Endod* 13(9):466, 1987.

182. Chance KB, Lin L, Skribner JE: Corticosteroid use in acute apical periodontitis: a review with clinical implications, *Clin Prev Dent* 10(1):7, 1988.

183. Dametto FR, Ferraz CCR, Paula B, et al: In vitro assessment of the immediate and prolonged antimicrobial action of chlorhexidine gel as an endodontic irrigant against *Enterococcus faecalis*, *Oral Surg Oral Med Oral Pathol Oral Radiol Endod* 99(6):768, 2005.

184. Dammaschke T, Schneider U, Stratmann U, et al: Effect of root canal dressings on the regeneration of inflamed periapical tissue, *Acta Odont Scand* 63(3):143, 2005.

185. Gomes BPFD, Vianna ME, Sena NT, et al: In vitro evaluation of the antimicrobial activity of calcium hydroxide combined with chlorhexidine gel used as intracanal medicament, *Oral Surg Oral Med Oral Pathol Oral Radiol Endod* 102(4):544, 2006.

186. De Rossi A, Silva LAB, Leonardo MR, et al: Effect of rotary or manual instrumentation, with or without a calcium hydroxide/1% chlorhexidine intracanal dressing, on the healing of experimentally induced chronic periapical lesions, *Oral Surg Oral Med Oral Pathol Oral Radiol Endod* 99(5):628, 2005.

187. Penesis VA, Fitzgerald PI, Fayad MI, et al: Outcome of one-visit and two-visit endodontic treatment of necrotic teeth with apical periodontitis: a randomized controlled trial with one-year evaluation, *J Endod* 34(3):251-257, 2008.

188. Naoum HJ, Chandler NP: Temporization for endodontics, *Int Endod J* 35(12):964, 2002.

189. Barthel CR, Zimmer S, Wussogk R, et al: Long-term bacterial leakage along obturated roots restored with temporary and adhesive fillings, *J Endod* 27(9):559, 2001.

190. Zmener O, Banegas G, Pameijer CH: Coronal microleakage of three temporary restorative materials: an in vitro study, *J Endod* 30(8):582, 2004.

191. Mayer T, Eickholz P: Microleakage of temporary restorations after thermocycling and mechanical loading, *J Endod* 23(5):320, 1997.

192. Beach CW, Calhoun JC, Bramwell JD, et al: Clinical evaluation of bacterial leakage of endodontic temporary filling materials, *J Endod* 22(9):459, 1996.

193. Vail MM, Steffel CL: Preference of temporary restorations and spacers: a survey of diplomates of the American Board of Endodontists, *J Endod* 32(6):513, 2006.

194. Newcomb BE, Clark SJ, Eleazer PD: Degradation of the sealing properties of a zinc oxide–calcium sulfate–based temporary filling material by entrapped cotton fibers, *J Endod* 27(12):789, 2001.

195. Pane ES, Palamara JE, Messer HH: Stainless steel bands in endodontics: effects on cuspal flexure and fracture resistance, *Int Endod J* 35(5):467, 2002.

196. Gutmann JL: The dentin-root complex: anatomic and biologic considerations in restoring endodontically treated teeth, *J Prosthet Dent* 67(4):458, 1992.

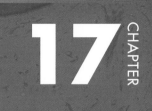

Preparation for restoration

Harold H. Messer, Charles J. Goodacre

CHAPTER OUTLINE

Risks to Survival of Root-Filled Teeth
Structural and Esthetic Considerations
Coronal Seal
Restoration Timing

Restoration Design
Preparation of Tooth and Canal Space for Post and Core
Post Type, Retention, and Core Systems
Restoring Access Through an Existing Restoration

LEARNING OBJECTIVES

After reading this chapter, the student should be able to:

1. Describe the main factors involved in the survival of root-filled teeth.
2. Summarize factors contributing to loss of tooth strength and describe the structural importance of remaining tooth tissue.
3. Explain the importance of a coronal seal and how it is achieved.
4. Describe the requirements of an adequate restoration.
5. Outline postoperative risks to the unrestored tooth.
6. Discuss the rationale for immediate restoration.

7. Identify restorative options before root canal treatment is started.
8. Discuss the advantages and disadvantages of direct and indirect restorations.
9. Outline indications for post placement in anterior and posterior teeth.
10. Describe common post systems and the advantages and disadvantages of each.
11. Describe core materials and their placement.
12. Describe techniques for restoring an access opening through an existing restoration.

Prompt restoration is required to minimize the risk of tooth fracture and coronal leakage. Restorability should be confirmed before root canal treatment begins. All caries and any existing restorations should be removed, both to reduce the risk of marginal leakage during treatment[1] and to reveal the extent of residual tooth structure.[2] Options for restoration, based on the amount of remaining tooth structure and functional demands, are also considered at this stage.[2,3] In most cases, restoration is straightforward, but the choice must be based on sound principles if the tooth is to be retained long term as a functional unit. This chapter considers principles of restoration rather than detailed techniques, which are beyond the scope of this textbook.

RISKS TO SURVIVAL OF ROOT-FILLED TEETH

Although root-filled teeth are at greater risk of extraction than vital teeth,[4] their long-term survival rate is very high. Numerous studies investigating the survival of root-filled teeth have documented that at most 1% to 2% are lost per year,[5-8] and one very large study of almost 1.5 million cases reported that

only 2.9% of teeth were lost after 8 years.[7] A recent meta-analysis showed a mean survival of 87% after 8 to 10 years.[5] The restoration is the key to survival.

The major risks to root filled teeth are as follows:

1. *Caries and periodontal disease.* Caries and periodontal disease are responsible for up to half of all extractions of root-filled teeth.[9-11] Emerging evidence suggests that root-filled teeth may be more susceptible to caries than vital teeth, though the biologic reasons for increased susceptibility are unknown.[12,13]
2. *Lack of definitive restoration.* A surprisingly high percentage of teeth are not appropriately restored after root canal treatment.[6,10,14] In one study of U.S. insurance data,[6] almost 30% of teeth had not been restored 2 years after root canal treatment, and 11% of these teeth were extracted.
3. *Inadequate restoration.* Lack of coronal coverage is the major restorative factor in tooth loss after root canal treatment.[5-7,15] Of the extracted teeth in the study mentioned previously involving 1.5 million teeth, 85% did not have coronal coverage.[7] The lack of cuspal protection predisposes the tooth to unrestorable cusp or crown

301

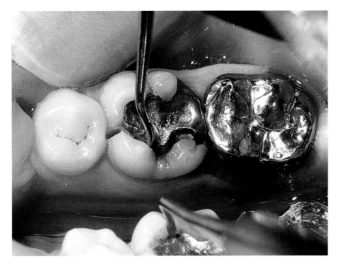

Fig. 17.1 Crown-root fracture (split tooth) of a root canal–treated tooth restored with amalgam but lacking protection of undermined, weakened cusps. (Courtesy Dr. H. Colman.)

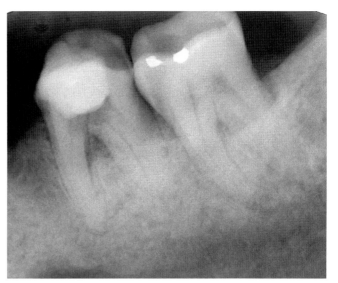

Fig. 17.2 Teeth requiring root canal treatment have commonly been structurally compromised by caries and restorative procedures.

fracture. Direct restoration does not provide adequate protection unless the access opening is confined to the occlusal surface.

4. *Occlusal stresses.* Teeth serving as abutments for fixed or removable prostheses are at significantly increased risk of loss, as are teeth lacking mesial and distal proximal support from adjacent teeth.[5,6,16]

5. *Endodontic factors.* Typically only about 10% of extractions result from an endodontic cause, including persistent pain.[9-11,17] Endodontic problems (development or persistence of a periapical lesion) are generally amenable to further management rather than extraction. Procedural problems (e.g., perforations) may also lead to extraction.[17]

STRUCTURAL AND ESTHETIC CONSIDERATIONS

Teeth function in a challenging environment, with heavy occlusal forces and repeated loading at a frequency of more than 1 million cycles per year over many decades of clinical life. Caries, restorative procedures, and occlusal stresses add to the risk of serious damage to teeth during normal function, and root-filled teeth are at greater risk than intact teeth. As noted previously, unrestorable crown fracture is a common sequel to inadequately protected root-filled teeth (Fig. 17.1).[15,18] It is important to understand the basis for this fracture susceptibility when planning the restoration.

Structural Changes in Dentin

It is now generally recognized that many mechanical properties of the dentin of root-filled teeth differ only to a minor extent from those of the dentin of vital teeth (strength, hardness, modulus of elasticity).[19,20] Similarly, the moisture content of dentin is unaffected by loss of pulp vitality.[21] Despite the seemingly minor differences, other biomechanical factors may result in substantial differences between vital and root-filled teeth.[22] The fracture toughness of dentin is probably a very important property in relation to fracture susceptibility, but it has not been widely investigated in relation to the dentin of the root-filled tooth. The loss of dentinal fluid, which may

play a role in stress distribution and stress relief, could also contribute to changes in the response of root-filled teeth to occlusal stresses.[23]

Loss of Tooth Structure

Most teeth requiring root canal treatment are already structurally compromised by caries and subsequent restorative procedures. Every step of root canal treatment and restoration removes additional dentin. Teeth are measurably weakened even by occlusal cavity preparation; greater loss of tooth structure further compromises strength. Loss of one or both marginal ridges is the major contributor to reduced cuspal stiffness (strength) (Fig. 17.2).[24,25] Endodontic access has only a minor effect on decreasing cuspal strength when the access cavity is surrounded by solid walls of dentin.[24] In a tooth already seriously compromised by caries, trauma, or large restorations, the access cavity is more significant, particularly if the adjacent marginal ridges have been lost.[26] Excessive coronal flaring also results in greater susceptibility to cusp fractures.[27]

Biomechanical Factors

The occlusal loads to which teeth are subjected during normal function generate large stresses in teeth that are capable of causing cusp fracture and even vertical root fracture in intact vital teeth.[28] Cuspal flexure (movement under loading) weakens the premolars and molars over time.[25] As cavity preparations become larger and deeper, unsupported cusps become weaker and show more deflection under occlusal loads.[24-26] Greater cuspal flexure leads to cyclic opening of the margins between the tooth and the restorative material. The alteration of the internal canal morphology resulting from endodontic and restorative procedures may also contribute to loss of rigidity. The distribution of stresses in the restored root-filled tooth subjected to occlusal load is markedly changed from those in the intact, vital tooth.[22] Fatigue is also a factor; cusps become progressively weaker with repetitive flexing. Hence, the restoration must be designed to minimize cuspal flexure to protect against fracture and marginal leakage.

Esthetic Factors

Increasingly, patients wish to enhance the esthetic appearance of restorations, and for root-filled teeth this often involves metal-ceramic or all-ceramic crowns. It is necessary to allow adequate thickness of the ceramic to provide a more natural appearance. Removal of tooth structure during preparation for metal-ceramic and all-ceramic crowns is greater than for a cusp overlay cast restoration or an all-metal crown.[29-31] Residual coronal tooth structure may be further weakened as a result.

Requirements for an Adequate Restoration

Based on the concepts discussed, the definitive restoration should (1) preserve remaining tooth structure, although not at the expense of appropriate restoration; (2) protect remaining tooth structure and in particular minimize cuspal flexure; (3) provide a coronal seal; and (4) satisfy function and esthetics. Care must be taken to ensure that esthetic demands do not lead to the weakening of teeth by excessive removal of remaining tooth structure.

CORONAL SEAL

Coronal leakage is a major cause of endodontic failure.[32,33] Even a well-obturated canal does not provide an enduring barrier to bacterial penetration,[34] and we rely on the restoration for long-term integrity of the coronal seal. The restoration may provide the coronal seal either as a separate step (e.g., placing a barrier over canal orifices)[35,36] or, more commonly, as an integral part of the restoration. For direct restoration of a simple access cavity, a bonded restoration provides the most reliable seal.[37] Experimental leakage studies consistently demonstrate that leakage occurs around a post, regardless of the type of post or luting cement.[38] However, a crown with an adequate ferrule, plus a post and core foundation, provides an effective barrier against coronal leakage.[39,40]

A frequently asked question with regard to lost or leaking restorations is, "How long can a root filling be exposed to oral fluids before it should be retreated?" The question has no clear answer. Experimental studies suggest that complete leakage along the length of the root filling occurs rapidly, within days or weeks.[41,42] A recent review, however, concluded that coronal leakage may be clinically less significant than is suggested by experimental laboratory leakage studies.[43] Clinically, periapical lesions may not develop even several years after the coronal seal is lost, and bacterial invasion is often limited to the coronal third of the canal.[44,45] The commonly accepted guideline is that the root filling should be replaced if it is exposed to oral fluids for more than 2 to 3 months.[32] However, if the root filling has been performed to a high technical standard and periapical pathology is absent, it may be sufficient to replace the lost or leaking restoration rather than the entire root filling.[43]

RESTORATION TIMING

Unless there are specific reasons for delay, definitive restoration is completed as soon as practical.[32,37,46] Most provisional restorative materials used to seal the endodontic access opening have low wear and fracture resistance; substantial occlusal wear and loss of the coronal seal may occur within

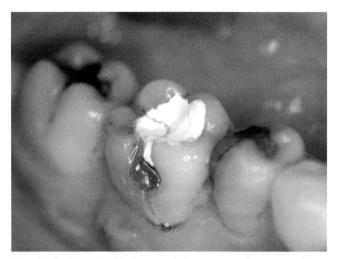

Fig. 17.3 Unrestorable fracture during root canal treatment. The lack of cuspal protection combined with deep anatomic grooves led to fracture within days of endodontic access.

weeks. The tooth is at its weakest after access and remains so until it has been appropriately restored. The provisional restoration does not provide complete protection against occlusal forces, even when the tooth is out of occlusion. Unrestorable fracture during or soon after treatment is all too common (Fig. 17.3). Protection can be provided in the form of an orthodontic band cemented around the tooth.

For most teeth, it is unnecessary to wait for radiographic evidence of healing before the definitive restoration is placed. Prompt restoration may improve the prognosis because it provides better protection against fracture and loss of the coronal seal. With a guarded prognosis, the rationale for postponing definitive restoration is based on the nature of further management if failure occurs. Orthograde retreatment is usually possible through the restoration (addressed later in this chapter) unless a post is placed in the canal. If correction requires surgery, there is no reason to delay restoration. The only reason for delay is a questionable prognosis, as when failure would lead to extraction.

When definitive restoration of the tooth is delayed, the provisional restoration must be durable and must protect, seal, and meet functional and esthetic demands. Provisional materials such as Cavit are inadequate.[47] For posterior teeth, some form of cuspal protection is desirable, even with provisional restorations.[48] A good long-term posterior provisional restoration is an amalgam core that covers weakened cusps, thus providing functional and sealing protection. The definitive crown preparation can be completed later without removing the core (Fig. 17.4). Comparable anterior restorations are more challenging owing to esthetic demands and difficulties with the coronal seal.[37] A one-piece provisional post-crown is at risk of dislodgment, thereby compromising an adequate seal.[49] It is preferable to place a definitive post and core immediately when a provisional crown is indicated.[46,50]

RESTORATION DESIGN

Principles and Concepts

Three practical principles are important in ensuring function and durability.

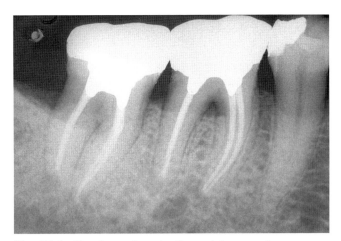

Fig. 17.4 Chamber and canal orifices retain an amalgam core, taking advantage of natural undercuts. The teeth can be prepared for crowns without removing the amalcore, or the amalgams may be definitive restorations if the cusps are adequately protected. (Courtesy D.P. Parashos.)

1. *Conservation of tooth structure.* Some anterior root canal–treated teeth are intact or minimally restored, and there is evidence supporting restoration of only the coronal access opening rather than a crown or a crown combined with a post and core,[51,52] requiring little if any additional tooth structure removal. Some data even indicate that molars that are intact (except for small endodontic access openings) can be restored using only composite resin.[53] However, most root canal–treated posterior teeth and some anterior teeth are structurally compromised, and crown placement is required so that the cusps and remaining tooth structure can be encompassed, which minimizes the potential for tooth fracture and enhances tooth longevity.[15,18] The process used by some practitioners of routinely decoronating an endodontically treated tooth and then rebuilding it is neither desirable nor in keeping with contemporary science.
2. *Retention.* The definitive coronal restoration of a root canal–treated tooth may consist only of a restoration filling the endodontic access opening that is retained by surrounding tooth structure. When the tooth is structurally compromised and a crown is needed, it is retained by remaining dentin and a restorative material core that replaces missing tooth structure. If the core cannot be adequately retained by the remaining coronal tooth structure, a post can be placed into the pulp chamber and root canal to provide retention for the core. Because posts weaken teeth[54-58] and may produce root fracture or lead to root perforation during preparation of the root canal,[59] they should be used only when the core cannot be retained by some other means, such as mechanical and chemical bonding of a restorative material.[60,61]
3. *Protection of remaining tooth structure.* In posterior teeth, this applies to protecting weakened cusps by minimizing their flexure and fracture. The restoration is designed to encompass the cusps and minimize the chance of tooth fracture and also to transmit functional loads through the tooth to the suspensory apparatus.

Planning the Definitive Restoration
The choice of definitive restoration is straightforward when the root canal–treated tooth is intact or only minimally

restored with an appropriate restoration. The preferred treatment is removal of the provisional restoration in the endodontic access opening and also any other material (e.g., cotton pellets). The root canal filling material should be visible; amalgam or composite resin then is used to restore the area, depending on esthetic requirements.

When the tooth requires a crown, the type of definitive treatment can be determined only after the existing restoration (or restorations) have been removed, to ensure that there is no caries present and to expose the remaining sound tooth structure. Visualizing the restorative preparation in advance ensures that structural requirements for retention of the core are preserved. Increasingly, esthetic demands dictate the use of all-ceramic or metal-ceramic crowns for definitive tooth restoration. These materials usually function satisfactorily, but they have less favorable physical properties than all-metal restorations, particularly in mouths where occlusal forces are heavy, as evidenced by wear facets and parafunctional habits such as bruxism.

Anterior Teeth
Whenever possible, direct restoration of the endodontic access opening (e.g., etched and bonded composite resin) is used; this is sufficient for teeth that are otherwise largely intact. For more extensively damaged anterior teeth (trauma, large proximal restorations), complete coronal coverage using a metal-ceramic or all-ceramic crown supported by a post and core is indicated. The choices for premolars and molars are more varied.

Posterior Teeth
Direct Restorations
Restorations placed directly into the endodontic access opening (amalgam or composite resin) are conservative, but their use must be carefully considered. The restoration must protect against coronal fracture. Indications for restoration of only the coronal access opening include the following:
1. Minimal tooth structure is lost before and during root canal treatment; a conservative access preparation is present with intact marginal ridges, and the tooth can be restored without further preparation.
2. The long-term prognosis of the tooth is uncertain, but a durable restoration is needed during the observation period.

Posterior teeth with substantial tooth structure loss may be restored with amalgam if it is esthetically acceptable and if unsupported cusps are adequately protected by the amalgam.[62] Some cuspal coverage amalgams have lasted for many years (Fig. 17.5), whereas others have fractured due to the presence of heavy occlusal forces. Assessment of occlusal forces and functional activity helps determine whether a cuspal coverage amalgam is a suitable restoration. A conventional Class II amalgam without cuspal coverage does not provide cuspal protection and ordinarily should not be used.[63] At a minimum, cusps adjacent to a lost marginal ridge should be onlayed with sufficient thickness of amalgam (at least 2 mm)[64] to resist occlusal forces (Fig. 17.5). The amalgam should extend into the pulp chamber and canal orifices to aid retention. The amalgam may subsequently serve as a core for an indirect cast restoration if indicated (Fig. 17.6). Bonded amalgams have also been used, but their clinical performance in root-filled teeth has not been well documented, and bond failure is likely

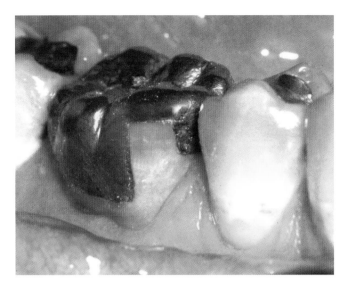

Fig. 17.5 Cuspal coverage amalgam replaced distobuccal and distal cusps while also protecting mesiobuccal and lingual cusps with 2 mm of amalgam. It functioned well for more than 10 years, at which point the patient requested a crown on the tooth.

to be catastrophic in the presence of weakened, unprotected cusps.

There are esthetic deficits when amalgam is used in visible teeth, and the need for a tooth-colored restoration warrants the use of bonded composite resin restorations. The use of bonding continues to escalate as materials and techniques improve, and good results have been reported in a long-term prospective clinical study of composite resin restorations.[65] Proximal leakage and recurrent proximal caries remains a concern, particularly when the restorations have subgingival margins and were placed without the use of a rubber dam.

Indirect Restorations
All-metal cast restorations (onlays and three-quarter and complete crowns) provide excellent occlusal protection and are optimal when the loss of tooth structure requires a crown. The attractiveness of onlays is that the tooth preparation design is more conservative than complete coverage preparations, yet provides good cuspal coverage (Fig. 17.7). The strength of gold allows conservative tooth reduction, with a reverse bevel providing effective cuspal coverage. Complete coverage all-metal crowns are used when there is insufficient coronal tooth structure present for a more conservative restoration or if functional or parafunctional stresses require the protective effect of complete coronal coverage.

When a tooth is prepared for a crown, the coronal access opening should be restored and sealed with an amalgam or a bonded composite resin as part of the core foundation for the crown. Glass ionomer can also be used to restore the access opening, as long as its purpose is to seal the opening and it is not forming a substantial portion of the axial walls that will be used for retention of the crown.

The esthetic requirements of many patients prevent the use of all-metal crowns. Metal-ceramic or all-ceramic crowns have become the most frequently used materials for root canal–treated posterior teeth. These types of complete crowns provide a reliable, strong restoration that protects against root

fracture (Fig. 17.8).[61,66,67] However, root canal treatment may have required substantial tooth structure removal and that, coupled with the reduction needed for a crown, can necessitate placement of a core restoration and sometimes a post to retain the core. To plan the core shape there must be complete exposure of the tooth's perimeter. Gingival retraction cord and sometimes soft tissue removal via electrosurgery or use of a laser are beneficial methods that help prevent undersized cores being made because of incomplete viewing of the finish line. When a core is used as a foundation for the crown without the use of a post, the material must be well retained into remaining tooth structure and must be of sufficient thickness so that the material will not fracture during function, resulting in crown failure (Fig. 17.9).

PREPARATION OF TOOTH AND CANAL SPACE FOR POST AND CORE

Coronal Tooth Preparation
The first procedure when restoring a tooth that requires a post and core and crown is to prepare the coronal tooth structure for the type of crown to be used. Even when substantial coronal tooth structure is missing, the remaining portion should be prepared first so structural integrity can be assessed. Any thin, friable coronal tooth structure that remains after tooth preparation should be removed and replaced as part of the core, rather than have it fracture when subjected to force during removal of the provisional restoration at the crown cementation appointment or fracture during occlusal functioning after cementation of the definitive crown.

Post Selection
A post is used to retain the core. The need for a post is dictated by the amount of remaining coronal tooth structure available to retain the core. A major disadvantage of posts is that they do not reinforce the tooth, but rather further weaken it by additional removal of dentin and by creating stresses that predispose to root fracture.[60,61,68-70] Therefore, posts are only used when the core cannot be retained in the tooth by other means.

A post system should be selected that fits the requirements of the tooth and restoration. The tooth should not be prepared and adapted to the post system; rather, the post system and preparation design should be selected as appropriate to the tooth and its morphology. Therefore, custom-cast posts and cores are preferred for roots that have very tapered root canals. Also, roots with substantial developmental depressions are best served by using cast posts and cores made to fit the existing morphology after root canal treatment rather than removing tooth structure to make the root fit the form of a prefabricated post. Mandibular incisors, maxillary first premolars, and mandibular molars are examples of teeth that are best restored using cast posts and cores. Additionally, some teeth have oval root canals that are wide faciolingually but narrow mesiodistally, and they are best restored with cast posts and cores (Fig. 17.10). Prefabricated round posts are well-suited for use in teeth that have somewhat more rounded roots and root canals because removal of some root structure to adapt the tooth to the post usually does not result in substantive weakening as long as the diameter of the post is not excessive.

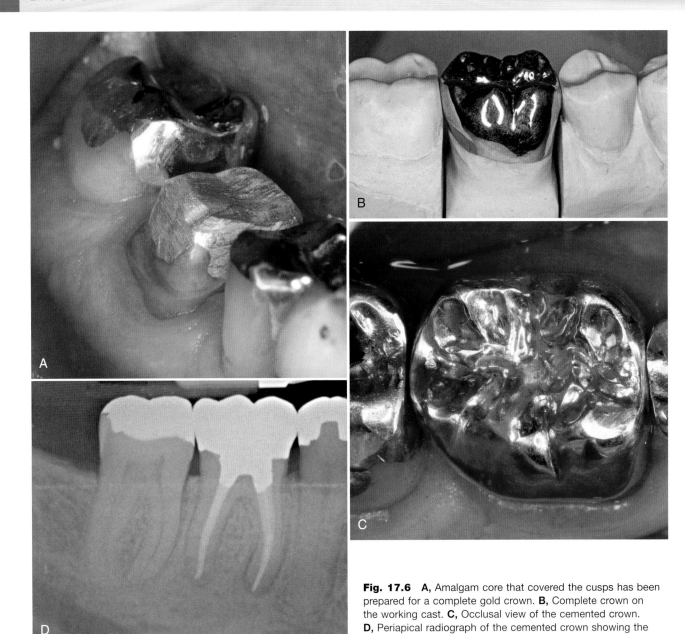

Fig. 17.6 **A,** Amalgam core that covered the cusps has been prepared for a complete gold crown. **B,** Complete crown on the working cast. **C,** Occlusal view of the cemented crown. **D,** Periapical radiograph of the cemented crown showing the amalgam core extended into the pulp chamber.

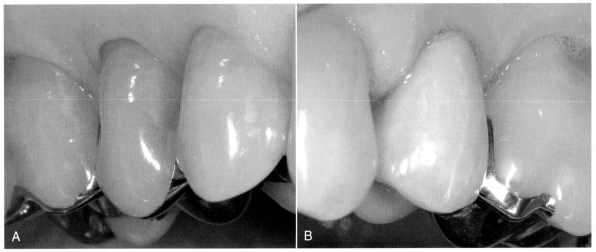

Fig. 17.7 Cast gold onlay on second premolar incorporating buccal reverse bevel for protection against cuspal flexure. This technique may not satisfy the esthetic requirements of many patients.

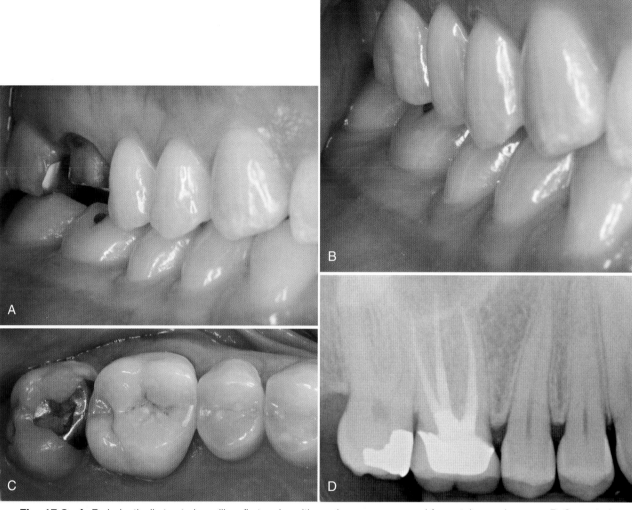

Fig. 17.8   A, Endodontically treated maxillary first molar with amalgam core prepared for metal-ceramic crown. **B,** Cemented crown. **C,** Occlusal view of the crown. **D,** Periapical radiograph showing the cemented crown and amalgam core.

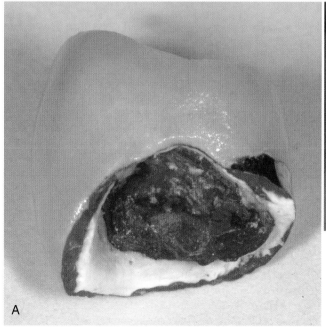

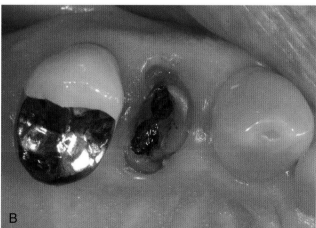

Fig. 17.9   A, The patient presented with crown failure due to fracture of the amalgam core. **B,** The amalgam core had no mechanical retention into the remaining tooth structure, and the mesiodistal dimension did not provide sufficient strength because of the narrow morphology of the first premolar. (Courtesy Dr. N. Baba.)

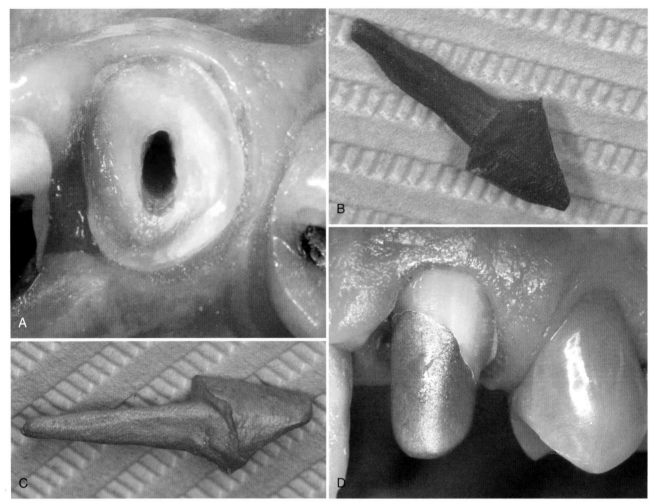

Fig. 17.10 **A,** Maxillary canine with oval root canal. This tooth is not morphologically suited for a prefabricated post because the post would contact only a small portion of the mesial and distal walls, or the tooth would have to be extensively prepared to a round form, weakening the tooth or possibly perforating it where the proximal root depressions are present. **B,** A resin pattern was made directly in the tooth. **C,** The pattern was invested and cast. **D,** The cast post and core are cemented, and the tooth is ready for final preparation. (Courtesy Dr. J. Kan.)

There has been a debate regarding how the post should interact with the tooth under load and whether the post material should be similar in stiffness to root dentin (carbon fiber, quartz fiber), somewhat stiffer (titanium and gold), or much stiffer (stainless steel and cobalt-chromium alloys).[71] Stiff posts have been successfully used for decades, but they may lead to tooth fracture, whereas the more flexible posts deform with the tooth and tend to fail without fracturing the tooth.[72] Bonding between the post and the tooth may allow the restored tooth to deform more with loading, compared with the conventional approach of using an indirect restoration much more rigid than the tooth. Long-term clinical trials will determine how posts should interact with teeth and what degree of stiffness functions best.

Tooth-colored post and core materials are needed beneath all-ceramic crowns to prevent gingival discoloration and to allow some light transmission through the crown and tooth; this situation has created increased interest in fiber posts (Fig. 17.11). The desire to have posts flex in concert with tooth structure has also raised interest in fiber posts. Carbon fiber and quartz fiber posts appear to be advantageous with regard to root fracture potential because fewer root fractures were recorded in laboratory studies in these posts compared to metal posts.[73,74] Several clinical studies have reported no root fractures,[75-84] and other clinical studies have reported a small number of root fractures.[85-88] However, these types of posts were less retentive than metal posts in laboratory tests,[89] indicating the need for optimal post length. Clinical results with fiber posts have been mixed; many studies have reported high levels of success, but other, longer term studies[79,87,88] have reported higher failure rates (11[86,88] to 28%[79]). Post loosening, post fracture, and even root fracture has been reported. As a result, it is proposed that fiber posts be used cautiously when post length is less than optimal (Fig. 17.12), when peripheral walls are missing (Fig. 17.13),[90] or when heavy occlusal forces or parafunctional habits are present.[91]

It has been determined in the laboratory that threaded posts create stress in the root of a tooth.[70,92] Additionally, a meta-analysis of clinical studies indicates that the survival rate for threaded posts is 81%, whereas it is 91% for cemented posts.[93] Therefore, threaded posts are not recommended.

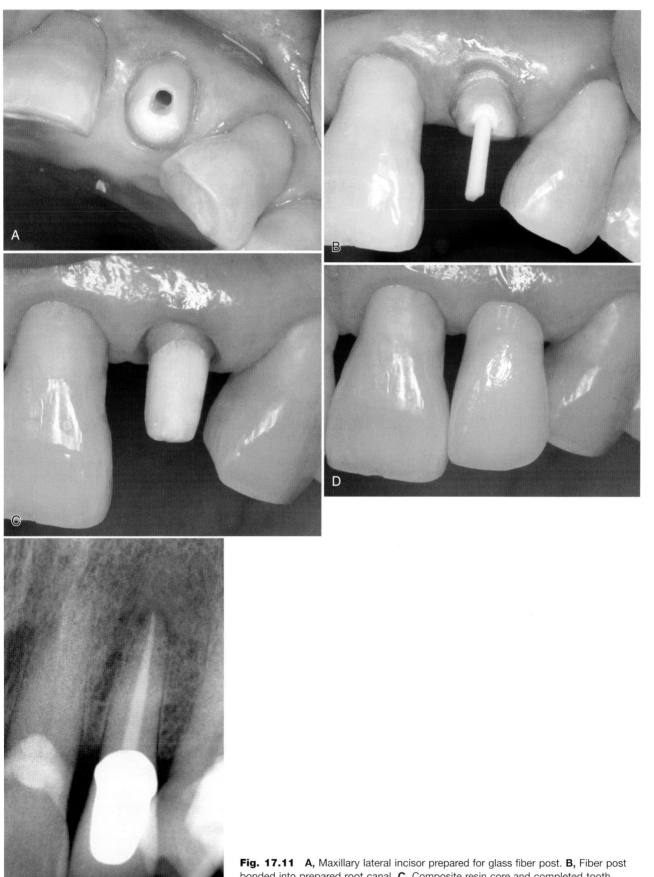

Fig. 17.11 **A,** Maxillary lateral incisor prepared for glass fiber post. **B,** Fiber post bonded into prepared root canal. **C,** Composite resin core and completed tooth preparation. **D,** Cemented crown. **E,** Radiograph showing the zirconia core with porcelain veneer and slightly radiopaque fiber post.

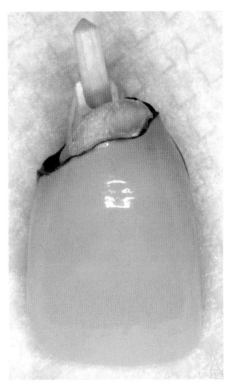

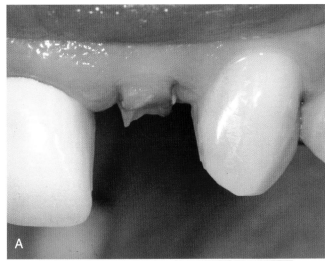

Fig. 17.12 Excessively short fiber post that rapidly failed and resulted in fracture of the remaining facial tooth structure, visible inside the crown. (Courtesy Dr. N. Baba.)

Post Space Preparation

When a post is required for core retention, the minimum post space (length, diameter, and taper) should be prepared consistent with that need. Preparation consists of removing gutta-percha to the required length, followed by the least amount of enlargement and shaping needed to receive the post (Fig. 17.14). Caution is required because excessive removal of gutta-percha results in a defective apical seal.[94,95] Because there is evidence that longer posts are more retentive[95,96] and have less potential to cause root fracture than do short posts,[96-100] optimizing post length is appropriate as long as the apical seal is not compromised. Therefore, rather than using proportional guidelines for determining post length (e.g., one half the root length or equal to the crown height), the amount of apical gutta-percha required to maintain an apical seal should be used as a guide to length. For all teeth but molars, it is recommended that 5 mm of apical gutta-percha be retained and the post extended to that level (Fig. 17.14). For molars, the length is determined by the potential for root thinning or perforation.[101] Based on this molar data, posts should be extended only 5 mm into the root canal and only in the primary molar roots (mesial root of the mandibular molars and palatal root of the maxillary molars) (Fig. 17.15).

Excessive dentin removal seriously weakens the root, which may predispose it to root fracture. Additionally, a perforation may occur if the cutting instrument deviates from the canal or if the preparation is too large or extends beyond the straight portion of the canal. Radiographs may be deceptive as a guide to root curvature and diameter by disguising root concavities and faciolingual curves.[102] As a general rule, the post diameter should be minimal, particularly apically, and not more than one third the root diameter (Fig. 17.15).[103] Tapered post preparations minimize the amount of tooth

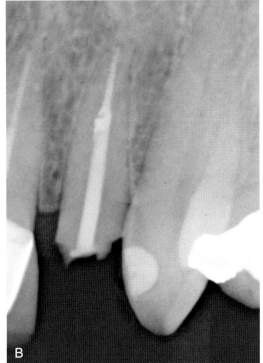

Fig. 17.13 **A,** Fiber post that fractured. Note the lack of peripheral walls to help support the post. **B,** Radiograph showing the fractured fiber post. (Courtesy Dr. N. Baba.)

structure removed apically and thereby reduce the amount of tooth structure removed.

Removal of Gutta-Percha

Whenever possible, gutta-percha is removed immediately after obturation to ensure the most predictable apical seal.[104] At this stage, the dentist is most familiar with the canal features, including shape, length, size, and curvature. Depending on the obturation technique, the canal may be filled only to the desired length, or gutta-percha may be removed to the desired length using a hot instrument. The remaining gutta-percha is then vertically condensed in the apical canal before the sealer has set. The obturation radiograph confirms that sufficient gutta-percha remains (5 mm). Studies have shown that canal leakage occurs when only 2 or 3 mm

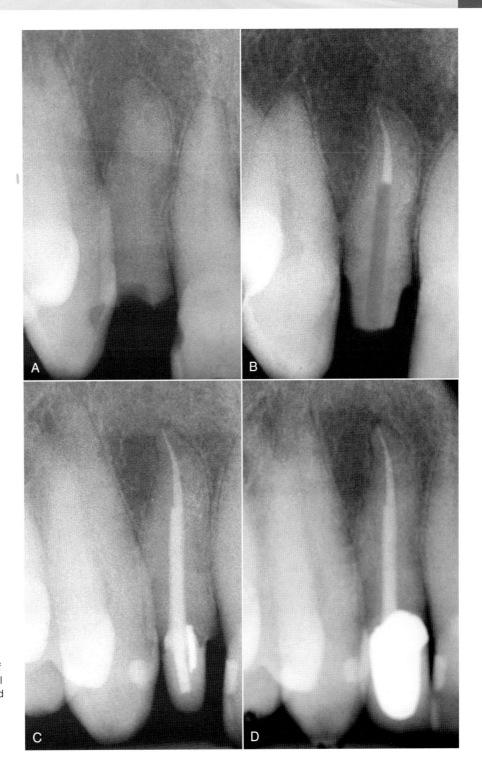

Fig. 17.14 **A** and **B**, Post space preparation showing adequate retention of gutta-percha to provide an enduring apical seal. **C,** The post (here a Parapost) is fitted so that no gap occurs between the post and remaining gutta-percha, and a resin composite core is built up. **D,** Crown in place.

of gutta-percha is retained apically; however, little or no leakage occurs with 4 mm or more.[104,105] Therefore, 4 mm of gutta-percha provides an appropriate apical seal. However, because of variation in the angulation of clinical radiographs, it is proposed that at least 5 mm of radiographic gutta-percha be retained.

Gutta-percha removal at a subsequent appointment is satisfactory.[104-106] A safe procedure is the use of a heated instrument. Gutta-percha is removed in increments to the desired length using a heat carrier or heated plugger. Any instrument that penetrates to the desired depth can be used, as long as it has sufficient heat capacity. Alternative means of

removal include solvents and mechanical techniques. Problems with solvents (e.g., chloroform, xylene, or eucalyptol) include messiness and an unpredictable depth of penetration. Rotary instruments, such as Peeso reamers and Gates-Glidden drills, have been safely used for decades, but their use requires caution because they can remove dentin quickly. Additionally, they can create a channel that does not follow the root canal, causing root thinning or, worse yet, perforation. They may also "grab" and displace the apical gutta-percha. Nickel-titanium rotary instruments specially designed for preparing post spaces are available; these have a noncutting tip and a noncutting lateral surface. It has been determined that they can be effective[107] and that they pose minimal risk of ledging or canal transportation.[108,109]

Finishing the Post Space

After the post length and diameter have been established, the post space may need further refinement to eliminate small undercuts. If gutta-percha has been adequately removed, rotary instruments can be used for final canal shaping; however, as stated previously, they should be used carefully to avoid excessive tooth removal that weakens the root or causes a perforation. Final shaping can also be performed using hand manipulation of the rotary instruments because only small amounts of tooth need to be removed in most situations.

Ferrule

The use of a cervical ferrule (circumferential band of metal) that encompasses the tooth structure is a key method of preventing tooth fracture (Fig. 17.16). Ferrules formed by the crown that extend cervically to engage the tooth structure apical to the core help teeth resist fracture, whereas ferrules

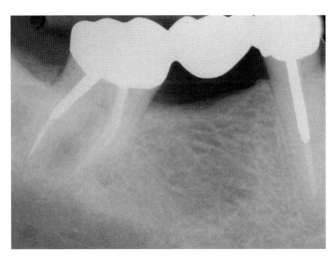

Fig. 17.15 Molar abutment for fixed partial denture has a post in the distal root that extends 5 mm beyond the base of the pulp chamber into the root canal. The post was prepared with a tapered form to minimize tooth reduction. In the premolar abutment, a parallel-wall post was used because of the more favorable root morphology and dimensions.

created by the core engaging the coronal tooth structure are generally not effective.[110-113] Crown ferrules that encompass more than 1 mm of tooth structure are the most effective in helping teeth resist fracture.[111] Ferrules that encompass 2 mm of tooth structure around the entire circumference of a tooth produce greater fracture resistance than ferrules that engage only part of the tooth circumference (Fig. 17.17).[112,113]

POST TYPE, RETENTION, AND CORE SYSTEMS

Anterior Teeth

Either a prefabricated post with direct core buildup (see Fig. 17.16) or a cast post and core (see Fig. 17.10) can be used for anterior teeth. Prefabricated posts should passively fit the root prior to cementation to minimize wedging forces. Screw-retained posts are contraindicated; they predispose to vertical root fracture and are difficult to remove.

A cast metal post and core is fabricated as a single unit. The post portion provides unit strength and retention, and the core cannot separate from the post. Custom fitting of the post and core to the existing root morphology permits minimal dentin removal both from the canal space and coronally, plus maximum ferrule effect without crown lengthening.[112,113] The core shape should conform to the remaining coronal tooth structure.

Anterior root canal–treated teeth must withstand lateral forces from mandibular excursive movements which, if transmitted excessively via a post, can fracture the root. Consideration should be given to the occlusal scheme. Where possible, the excursive load should be limited, with more force being borne by adjacent, more structurally sound teeth.

Posterior Teeth

Premolars with substantial loss of coronal structure, particularly maxillary premolars, are best restored with a cast post and core (Fig. 17.18). Narrow mesiodistal root width and substantial developmental root depressions, coupled with tapered roots, may result in excessive removal of root structure when the tooth is prepared for a prefabricated post. Additionally, the mesiodistal thinness of the tooth may not permit adequate core thickness in association with a prefabricated post. Minimal enlargement during post space preparation is essential to preserve sufficient dentin thickness.[103] In

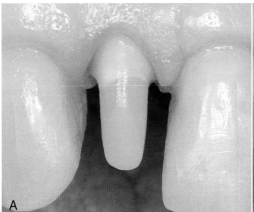

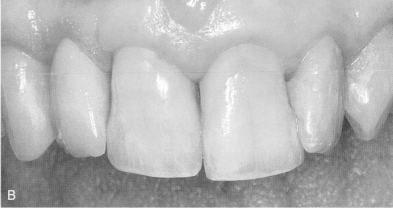

Fig. 17.16 **A,** Composite resin core buildup, with a ferrule incorporated into the preparation so that the crown can grasp the tooth structure cervical to the core. **B,** The metal-ceramic crown as the definitive restoration.

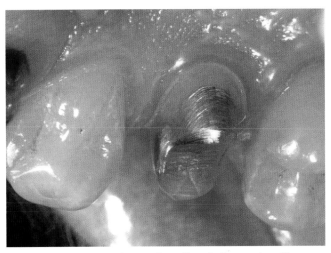

Fig. 17.17 Root canal–treated maxillary first premolar with a ferrule extending 2 mm beyond the core for optimal resistance to tooth fracture.

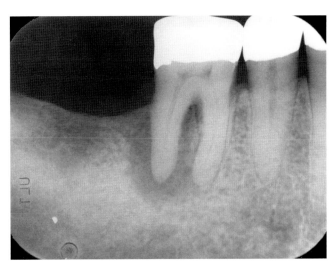

Fig. 17.19 Pulp necrosis several years after preparation and placement of a full-coverage restoration. Root canal treatment is now required through the crown, with the attendant risks of perforation or loss of retention.

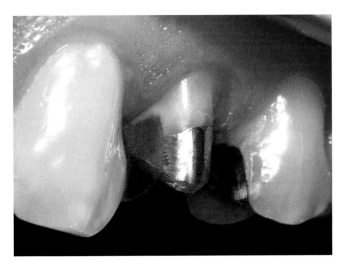

Fig. 17.18 A cast post and core provides the best foundation for restoring maxillary premolars.

maxillary premolars with two roots, the palatal canal should be used for the post because the facial root can frequently have a concavity on the furcal aspect of the root.[103,114] A small, short (2 to 3 mm) post in the buccal canal can be used to provide some retention and antirotation.

Molars, which have larger pulp chambers, permit direct core options; the volume of the core is greater and the chamber shape provides retention. Most molars can be restored with a direct core only, without a post (see Fig. 17.6). However, with minimal remaining coronal tooth structure and a small pulp chamber, a post may be needed to provide retention for the core.

The longest and straightest canal is preferred for the post, typically the palatal canal of maxillary molars and the distal canal of mandibular molars.[102] These roots are known as the "primary roots" for post placement. Other canals are narrower and more curved and are in weaker roots with surface concavities. These should be used only (and cautiously) if other factors preclude placement in the larger canals. Additional core retention, when needed, is supplemented by extending the core material 1 to 2 mm into the remaining canal orifices.

A wide variety of passively seated prefabricated posts is available. Parallel-sided posts provide greater retention than tapered posts. However, they require more post space preparation than cast posts and cores; matching post size to canal size is important to minimize dentin removal. The post should have close approximation to the root canal walls without binding, but it need not contact dentin throughout its entire length to achieve adequate retention. Threaded screw posts should not be used.

Tooth preparation for a molar core requires little removal of tooth structure; the core is retained by the morphology of the pulp chamber and natural undercuts in the chamber. A coronoradicular core of amalgam (Amalcore) condensed into the chamber and slightly into canal orifices provides a passive, strong core (see Figs. 17.4 and 17.6).[115] With fast-setting amalgam, the tooth may be prepared for the crown at the same visit, although preparation is easier when the material has fully hardened. A widely used alternative to amalgam is composite resin, which has a fracture resistance comparable to that of amalgam and produces more favorable tooth fracture patterns if failure occurs.[69,116] Composite resin has the advantage of allowing immediate crown preparation.[69] Glass ionomer cements do not have sufficient shear strength for use as a core material.

Pins

Practitioners have used pins safely for many years, but some have determined that there is no need for retentive pins.[64] Those who do not use pins cite the stresses and microfractures generated in dentin and the risk of perforation. They also suggest that the antirotation benefit of the pin is best achieved by other means, such as a slightly out-of-round preparation.

RESTORING ACCESS THROUGH AN EXISTING RESTORATION

Occasionally, pulps undergo irreversible pulpitis or necrosis after placement of a crown, requiring root canal treatment (Fig. 17.19).[59,68,117] Access through the restoration, with **313** subsequent definitive repair of the opening, is preferable to making a new crown.

For the restoration to remain functional, three conditions must be met: (1) the interface between the restoration and the repair material must provide a good coronal seal; (2) retention of the crown must not be compromised; and (3) the final core structure must support the restoration against functional or minor traumatic stresses. Access, particularly if overextended, may leave only a thin shell of axial dentin, especially in anterior teeth and premolars. Retention then depends almost entirely on the repair material. Fortunately, the chamber and canal are available to create a core that provides adequate retention and support in many instances. Compared to restorative material alone, placement of a post through an access opening and through an existing crown into the root canal adds little additional support and retention and is rarely indicated.

The repair material should have high compressive and shear strength. Amalgam is an excellent material that maintains (and even improves) its seal with time and is easily condensed into the entire chamber and access opening as a single unit. Composite resins are usually the material of choice in tooth-colored crowns.[69] Glass ionomer and other cements do not have the requisite shear strength.

REFERENCES

1. Abbott PV: Assessing restored teeth with pulp and periapical diseases for the presence of cracks, caries and marginal breakdown, *Aust Dent J* 49:33, 2004.
2. McDonald AV, Setchell D: Developing a tooth restorability index, *Dent Update* 32:343, 2005.
3. Bandlish RB, McDonald AV, Setchell DJ: Assessment of the amount of remaining coronal dentine in root-treated teeth, *J Dent* 34:699, 2006.
4. Caplan DJ, Cai J, Yin G, et al: Root canal filled versus non-root canal filled teeth: a retrospective comparison of survival times, *J Public Health Dent* 65:90, 2005.
5. Ng Y-L, Mann V, Gulabivala K: Tooth survival following non-surgical root canal treatment: a systematic review of the literature, *Int Endod J* 43:171, 2010.
6. Lazarski MP, Walker WA, Flores CM, et al: Epidemiological evaluation of the outcomes of nonsurgical root canal treatment in a large cohort of insured dental patients, *J Endod* 27:791, 2001.
7. Salehrabi R, Rotstein I: Endodontic treatment outcomes in a large patient population in the USA: an epidemiological study, *J Endod* 30:846, 2004.
8. Chen SC, Chueh LH, Hsaio CK, et al: An epidemiological study of tooth retention after non-surgical endodontic treatment in a large population in Taiwan, *J Endod* 33:226, 2007.
9. Chen SC, Chueh LH, Hsaio CK, et al: First untoward events and reasons for tooth extraction after non-surgical endodontic treatment in Taiwan, *J Endod* 34:671, 2008.
10. Zadik Y, Sandler V, Bechor R, et al: Analysis of factors related to tooth extraction of endodontically treated teeth, *Oral Surg Oral Med Oral Pathol Oral Radiol Endod* 106:e31, 2008.
11. Touré B, Faye B, Kane AW, et al: Analysis of reasons for extraction of endodontically treated teeth: a prospective study, *J Endod* 37:1512, 2011.
12. Merdad K, Sonbul H, Bukhary S, et al: Caries susceptibility of endodontically versus nonendodontically treated teeth, *J Endod* 37:139, 2011.
13. Frisk F, Merdad K, Reit C, et al: Root-filled teeth and recurrent caries: a study of three repeated cross-sectional samples from the city of Jönköping, Sweden, *Acta Odontol Scand* 69:401, 2011.
14. Lynch CD, Burke FM, Ni Riordáin R, et al: The influence of coronal restoration type on the survival of endodontically treated teeth, *Eur J Prosthodont Restor Dent* 12:171, 2004.
15. Aquilino SA, Caplan DJ: Relationship between crown placement and the survival of endodontically treated teeth, *J Prosthet Dent* 87:256, 2002.
16. Alley BS, Kitchens GG, Alley LW, et al: A comparison of survival of teeth following endodontic treatment performed by general dentists or by specialists, *Oral Surg Oral Med Oral Pathol Oral Radiol Endod* 98:115, 2004.
17. Ng Y-L, Mann V, Gulabivala K: A prospective study of the factors affecting outcomes of non-surgical root canal treatment. Part 2. Tooth survival, *Int Endod J* 44:610, 2011.
18. Vire DE: Failure of endodontically treated teeth: classification and evaluation, *J Endod* 17:338, 1991.
19. Huang T-JG, Schilder H, Nathanson D: Effects of moisture content and endodontic treatment on some mechanical properties of human dentin, *J Endod* 18:209, 1992.
20. Sedgley CM, Messer HH: Are endodontically treated teeth more brittle? *J Endod* 18:332, 1992.
21. Papa J, Cain C, Messer HH: Moisture content of endodontically treated vs vital teeth, *Endod Dent Traumatol* 10:91, 1994.
22. Kishen A: Mechanisms and risk factors for fracture predilection in endodontically treated teeth. *Endod Topics* 13:57, 2006.
23. Kahler B, Swain MV, Moule A: Fracture toughening mechanisms responsible for differences in work to fracture of hydrated and dehydrated dentine, *J Biomech* 36:229, 2003.
24. Reeh ES, Messer HH, Douglas WH: Reduction in tooth stiffness as a result of endodontic and restorative procedures, *J Endod* 15:512, 1989.
25. Hood JAA: Biomechanics of the intact, prepared and restored tooth: some clinical implications, *Int Dent J* 41:25, 1991.
26. Panitvisai P, Messer HH: Cuspal deflection in molars in relation to endodontic and restorative procedures, *J Endod* 21:57, 1995.
27. Hansen EK, Asmussen E: Cusp fracture of endodontically treated posterior teeth restored with amalgam: teeth restored in Denmark before 1975 versus after 1979, *Acta Odontol Scand* 51:73, 1993.
28. Chan CP, Lin CP, Tseng SC, et al: Vertical root fracture in endodontically versus non-endodontically treated teeth: a survey of 315 cases in Chinese patients, *Oral Surg Oral Med Oral Pathol Oral Radiol Endod* 87:504, 1999.
29. Edelhoff D, Sorensen JA: Tooth structure removal associated with various preparation designs for anterior teeth, *J Prosthet Dent* 87:503, 2002.
30. Seow LL, Toh CG, Wilson NH: Remaining tooth structure associated with various preparation designs for anterior teeth, *Eur J Prosthodont Restor Dent* 13:57, 2005.
31. Hussain SKF, McDonald A, Moles DR: In vitro study investigating the mass of tooth structure removed following endodontic and restorative procedures, *J Prosthet Dent* 98:260, 2007.
32. Slutzky-Goldberg I, Slutzky H, Gorfil C, et al: Restoration of endodontically treated teeth: review and treatment recommendations, *Int J Dent* 2009;2009:150251. doi: 10.1155/2009/150251. Epub 2010 Jan 26.
33. Nair PNR: On the causes of persistent apical periodontitis: a review, *Int Endod J* 39:249, 2006.
34. Gillen BM, Looney SW, Gu L-S, et al: Impact of the quality of coronal restoration versus the quality of root canal fillings on success of root canal treatment: a systematic review and meta-analysis, *J Endod* 37:895, 2011.
35. Guerra JA, Skribner JE, Lin LM: Influence of base on coronal microleakage of post-prepared teeth, *J Endod* 20:589. 1994.
36. Jenkins S, Kulild J, Williams K, et al: Sealing ability of three materials in the orifices of root canal systems obturated with gutta-percha, *J Endod* 32:225, 2006.
37. Schwartz RS, Fransman R: Adhesive dentistry and endodontics: materials, clinical strategies and procedures for restoration of access cavities: a review, *J Endod* 31:151, 2005.
38. Wu MK, Pehlivan Y, Kontakiotis EG, et al: Microleakage along apical root fillings and cemented posts, *J Prosthet Dent* 79:264, 1998.
39. Nissan J, Rosner O, Gross O, et al: Coronal leakage in endodontically treated teeth restored with posts and complete crowns using different luting agent combinations, *Quintessence Int* 42:317, 2011.
40. Schmid-Schwap M, Graf A, Preinerstorfer A, et al: Microleakage after thermocycling of cemented crowns: a meta-analysis, *Dent Mater* 27:8555, 2011.
41. Magura ME, Kafrawy AH, Brown CE Jr, et al: Human saliva coronal microleakage in obturated root canals: an in vitro study, *J Endod* 17:324, 1991.
42. Khayat A, Lee SJ, Torabinejad M: Human saliva penetration of coronally unsealed obturated root canals, *J Endod* 19:458, 1993.
43. Kainan D, Moshonov J, Smidt A: Is endodontic re-treatment mandatory for every relatively old temporary restoration? A narrative review, *J Am Dent Assoc* 142:391, 2011.
44. Ricucci D, Gröndahl K, Bergenholtz G: Periapical status of root-filled teeth exposed to the oral environment by loss of restoration or caries, *Oral Surg Oral Med Oral Pathol Oral Radiol Endod* 90:354, 2000.
45. Ricucci D, Bergenholtz G: Bacterial status in root-filled teeth exposed to the oral environment by loss of restoration and fracture or caries: a histopathological study of treated cases, *Int Endod J* 36:787, 2003.
46. Tang W, Wu Y, Smales RJ: Identifying and reducing risks for potential fractures in endodontically treated teeth, *J Endod* 36:609, 2010.
47. Friedman S, Shani J, Stabholz A, et al: Comparative sealing ability of temporary filling materials evaluated by leakage of radiosodium, *Int Endod J* 19:187, 1986.
48. Pane ES, Palamara JE, Messer HH: Stainless steel bands in endodontics: effects on cuspal flexure and fracture resistance, *Int Endod J* 35:467, 2002.
49. Fox K, Gutteridge DL: An in vitro study of coronal microleakage in root canal–treated teeth restored by the post and core technique, *Int Endod J* 30:361, 1997.
50. Demarchi MGA, Sato EFL: Leakage of interim post and cores used during laboratory fabrication of custom posts, *J Endod* 28:328, 2002.
51. Gluskin AH, Radke RA, Frost SL, et al: The mandibular incisor: rethinking guidelines for post and core design, *J Endod* 21:33, 1995.
52. Pontius O, Hutter JW: Survival rate and fracture strength of incisors restored with different post and

core systems and endodontically treated incisors without coronoradicular reinforcement, *J Endod* 28:710, 2002.

53. Nagasiri R, Chitmongkolsuk S: Long-term survival of endodontically treated molars without crown coverage: a retrospective cohort study, *J Prosthet Dent* 93:164, 2005.

54. Lovdahl PE, Nicholls JI: Pin-retained amalgam cores vs cast-gold dowel-cores, *J Prosthet Dent* 38:507, 1977.

55. Guzy GE, Nicholls JI: In vitro comparison of intact endodontically treated teeth with and without endo-post reinforcement, *J Prosthet Dent* 42:39, 1979.

56. Leary JM, Aquilino SA, Svare CW: An evaluation of post length within the elastic limits of dentin, *J Prosthet Dent* 57:277, 1987.

57. Trope M, Maltz DO, Tronstad L: Resistance to fracture of restored endodontically treated teeth, *Endod Dent Traumatol* 1:108, 1985.

58. McDonald AV, King PA, Setchell DJ: In vitro study to compare impact fracture resistance of intact root-treated teeth, *Int Endod J* 23:304, 1990.

59. Goodacre CJ, Bernal G, Rungcharassaeng K, et al: Clinical complications in fixed prosthodontics, *J Prosthet Dent* 90:31, 2003.

60. Gutmann JL: The dentin-root complex: anatomic and biologic considerations in restoring endodontically treated teeth, *J Prosthet Dent* 67:458, 1992.

61. Assif D, Nissan J, Gafni Y, et al: Assessment of the resistance to fracture of endodontically treated molars restored with amalgam, *J Prosthet Dent* 89:462, 2003.

62. Plasmans PJ, Creugers NH, Mulder J: Long-term survival of extensive amalgam restorations, *J Dent Res* 77:453, 1998.

63. Linn J, Messer HH: Effect of restorative procedures on the strength of endodontically treated molars, *J Endod* 20:479, 1994.

64. Summit JB, Burgess JO, Berry TG, et al: The performance of bonded vs pin-retained complex amalgam restorations, *J Am Dent Assoc* 132:923, 2001.

65. Mannocci F, Qualtrough AJ, Worthington HV, et al: Randomized clinical comparison of endodontically treated teeth restored with amalgam or with fiber posts and resin composite: five-year results, *Oper Dent* 30:9, 2005.

66. Sorensen JA, Martinoff JT: Intracoronal reinforcement and coronal coverage: a study of endodontically treated teeth, *J Prosthet Dent* 51:780, 1984.

67. Valderhaug J, Jokstad A, Ambjornsen E, et al: Assessment of the periapical and clinical status of crowned teeth over 25 years, *J Dent* 25:97, 1997.

68. Goodacre CJ, Spolnik KJ: The prosthodontic management of endodontically treated teeth: a literature review. I. Success and failure data, treatment concepts, *J Prosthodont* 3:243, 1994.

69. Schwartz RS, Robbins JW: Post placement and restoration of endodontically treated teeth: a literature review, *J Endod* 30:289, 2004.

70. Obermayr G, Walton RE, Leary JM, et al: Vertical root fracture and relative deformation during obturation and post cementation, *J Prosthet Dent* 66:181, 1991.

71. Asmussen E, Peutzfeldt A, Sahafi A: Finite element analysis of stresses in endodontically treated, dowel-restored teeth, *J Prosthet Dent* 94:321, 2005.

72. Sirimai S, Riis DN, Morgano SM: An in vitro study of the fracture resistance and the incidence of vertical root fracture of pulpless teeth restored with six post-and-core systems, *J Prosthet Dent* 81:262, 1999.

73. Akkayan B, Gulmez T: Resistance to fracture of endodontically treated teeth restored with different post systems, *J Prosthet Dent* 87:431, 2002.

74. Newman MP, Yaman P, Dennison J, et al: Fracture resistance of endodontically treated teeth restored with composite posts, *J Prosthet Dent* 89:360, 2003.

75. Fredriksson M, Astback J, Pamenius M, et al: A retrospective study of 236 patients with teeth restored by carbon fiber–reinforced epoxy resin posts, *J Prosthet Dent* 80:151, 1998.

76. Glazer B: Restoration of endodontically treated teeth with carbon fiber posts: a prospective study, *J Can Dent Assoc* 66:613, 2000.

77. Malferrari S, Monaco C, Scotti R: Clinical evaluation of teeth restored with quartz fiber–reinforced epoxy resin posts, *Int J Prosthodont* 16:39, 2003.

78. Monticelli F, Grandini S, Goracci C, et al: Clinical behavior of translucent-fiber posts: a 2-year prospective study, *Int J Prosthodont* 16:593, 2003.

79. King PA, Setchell DJ, Rees JS: Clinical evaluation of a carbon fiber reinforced endodontic post, *J Oral Rehabil* 30:785, 2003.

80. Tidehag P, Lundström J, Larsson B, et al: A 7-year retrospective study of Composipost root canal posts (abstract 4080), *J Dent Res* 83(Special Issue A), 2004.

81. Grandini S, Goracci C, Tay FR, et al: Clinical evaluation of the use of fiber posts and direct resin restorations for endodontically treated teeth, *Int J Prosthodont* 18:399, 2005.

82. Mannocci F, Qualtrough AJ, Worthington HV, et al: Randomized clinical comparison of endodontically treated teeth restored with amalgam or with fiber posts and resin composite: five-year results, *Oper Dent* 30:9, 2005.

83. Cagidiaco MC, Radovic I, Simonetti M, et al: Clinical performance of fiber post restorations in endodontically treated teeth: 2-year results, *Int J Prosthodont* 20:293, 2007.

84. Turker SB, Alkumru HN, Evren B: Prospective clinical trial of polyethelene fiber ribbon–reinforced, resin composite build-up restorations, *Int J Prosthodont* 20:55, 2007.

85. Wennström J: The C-Post system, *Compend Contin Educ Dent* 20(Suppl):S80, 1996.

86. Naumann M, Blankenstein F, Dietrich T: Survival of glass fiber–reinforced composite post restorations after 2 years: an observational clinical study, *J Dent* 33:305, 2005.

87. Segerstrom S, Astback J, Ekstrand KD: A retrospective long term study of teeth restored with prefabricated carbon fiber reinforced epoxy resin posts, *Swed Dent J* 30:1, 2006.

88. Ferrari M, Cagidiaco MC, Goracci C, et al: Long-term retrospective study of the clinical performance of fiber posts, *Am J Dent* 20:287, 2007.

89. Gallo JR, Miller T, Xu X, et al: In vitro evaluation of the retention of composite fiber and stainless steel posts, *J Prosthodont* 11:25, 2002.

90. Signore A, Kaitsas V, Ravera G, et al: Clinical evaluation of an oval-shaped prefabricated glass fiber post in endodontically treated premolars presenting an oval canal cross-section: a retrospective cohort study, *Int J Prosthodont* 24:255, 2011.

91. Mehta SB, Millar BJ: A comparison of the survival of fibre posts cemented with two different composite resin systems, *Br Dent J* 205:600, 2008 (Online: E23.DOI:10.1038/sj.bdj.2008.1036).

92. Henry PJ: Photoelastic analysis of post core restorations, *Aust Dent J* 22:157, 1977.

93. Creugers NH, Mentink AG, Kayser AF: An analysis of durability data on post and core restorations, *J Dent* 21:281, 1993.

94. Kvist T, Rydin E, Reit C: The relative frequency of periapical lesions in teeth with root canal–retained posts, *J Endod* 15:578, 1989.

95. Pappen AF, Bravo M, Gonzalez-Lopez S, et al: An in vitro study of coronal leakage after intraradicular preparation of cast-dowel space, *J Prosthet Dent* 94:214, 2005.

96. Colley IT, Hampson EL, Lehman ML: Retention of post crowns: an assessment of the relative efficiency of posts of different shapes and sizes, *Br Dent J* 124:63, 1968.

97. Johnson JK, Sakumura JS: Dowel form and tensile form, *J Prosthet Dent* 40:645, 1978.

98. Standlee JP, Caputo AA, Collard EW, et al: Analysis of stress distribution by endodontic posts, *Oral Surg Oral Med Oral Pathol Oral Radiol Endod* 33:952, 1972.

99. Trabert KC, Caputo AA, Abou-Rass M: Tooth fracture: a comparison of endodontic and restorative treatments, *J Endod* 4:341, 1978.

100. Hunter AJ, Feiglin B, Williams JF: Effects of post placement on endodontically treated teeth, *J Prosthet Dent* 62:166, 1989.

101. Abou-Rass M, Jann JM, Jobe D, et al: Preparation of space for posting: effect of thickness of canal walls and incidence of perforation in molars, *J Am Dent Assoc* 104:834, 1982.

102. Perez E, Zillich R, Yaman P: Root curvature localizations as indicators of post length in various tooth groups, *Endod Dent Traumatol* 2:58, 1986.

103. Raiden G, Costa L, Koss S, et al: Residual thickness of root in first maxillary premolars with post space preparation, *J Endod* 25:502, 1999.

104. Fan B, Wu MK, Wesselink PR: Coronal leakage along apical root fillings after immediate and delayed post space preparation, *Endod Dent Traumatol* 15:124, 1999.

105. Goodacre CJ, Spolnik KJ: The prosthodontic management of endodontically treated teeth: a literature review. II. Maintaining the apical seal, *J Prosthodont* 4:51, 1995.

106. Abramovitz I, Tagger M, Tamse A, et al: The effect of immediate vs delayed post space preparation on the apical seal of a root canal filling: a study in an increased-sensitivity pressure-driven system, *J Endod* 26:435, 2000.

107. Coniglio I, Magni E, Goracci C, et al: Post space cleaning using a new nickel titanium endodontic drill combined with different cleaning regimens, *J Endod* 34:83, 2008.

108. Rödig T, Hülsmann M, Kahlmeier C: Comparison of root canal preparation with two rotary NiTi instruments: ProFile .04 and GT Rotary, *Int Endo J* 40:553, 2007.

109. Cheung GS, Liu CS: A retrospective study of endodontic treatment outcome between nickel-titanium rotary and stainless steel hand filing techniques, *J Endod* 35:938, 2009.

110. Sorensen JA, Engelman MJ: Ferrule design and fracture resistance of endodontically treated teeth, *J Prosthet Dent* 63:529, 1990.

111. Libman WJ, Nicholls JI: Load fatigue of teeth restored with cast posts and cores and complete crowns, *Int J Prosthodont* 8:155, 1995.

112. Tan PL, Aquilino SA, Gratton DG, et al: In vitro fracture resistance of endodontically treated central incisors with varying ferrule heights and configurations, *J Prosthet Dent* 93:331, 2005.

113. Ng CC, Dumbrigue HB, Al-Bayat MI, et al: Influence of remaining coronal tooth structure location on the fracture resistance of restored endodontically treated anterior teeth, *J Prosthet Dent* 95:290, 2006.

114. Tamse A, Katz A, Pilo R: Furcation groove of buccal root of maxillary first premolars: a morphometric study, *J Endod* 26:359, 2000.

115. Nayyar A, Walton RE, Leonard LA: An amalgam coronal-radicular dowel and core technique for endodontically treated posterior teeth, *J Prosthet Dent* 43:511, 1980.

116. Pilo R, Cardash HS, Levin E, et al: Effect of core stiffness on the in vitro fracture of crowned, endodontically treated teeth, *J Prosthet Dent* 88:302, 2002.

117. Cheung GS, Lai SC, Ng RP: Fate of vital pulps beneath a metal-ceramic crown or a bridge retainer, *Int Endod J* 38:521, 2005.

Obturation

James C. Kulild, Bekir Karabucak

LEARNING OBJECTIVES

After reading this chapter, the student should be able to:

1. Recognize the clinical criteria that determine when to obturate.
2. List the criteria for the ideal obturating material.
3. Describe the purpose of obturation and the reasons inadequate obturation may result in treatment failure.
4. Identify the core obturating materials most commonly used and list their constituents and physical properties.
5. Describe the advantages and disadvantages of each core material.
6. Discuss the indications and contraindications for obturation with each core material.
7. Differentiate between standardized, nonstandardized, and tapered sizes of gutta-percha (GP) cones and discuss when each is indicated.
8. Define and differentiate between lateral and vertical compaction and suggest where each is indicated.
9. Describe the lateral compaction technique.
10. Discuss the significance of depth of spreader penetration during lateral compaction.
11. Describe the vertical compaction technique.
12. Describe briefly other techniques used for obturation, including thermoplasticization, thermocompaction, paste injection, core carrier systems, and sectional obturation.
13. Describe the custom cone (chloroform-softened) technique and discuss when it is indicated.
14. Describe the preparation of the canal for obturation.
15. Review the techniques for final drying and apical clearing.
16. Discuss the technique for fitting the master cones.
17. List criteria for the ideal sealer.
18. Describe a technique for mixing and placing a sealer.
19. Discuss the technique for removing excess sealer and obturating material from the chamber and explain why this process is necessary.
20. Discuss the clinical and radiographic criteria for evaluating the quality of obturation.

OBJECTIVES OF "OBTURATION"

Historically, obturation has been considered one of the critical steps of root canal treatment and, when not properly performed, a potential cause of treatment failure. An early and often quoted report[1] stated that most treatment failures could be attributed to inadequate obturation. Healing was evaluated radiographically at various times after root canal treatment.[1] Such retrospective surveys, however, have major limitations; the outcome may demonstrate clearly a correlation between the observed failures and poorly obturated root canal systems (RCSs), but just because two events are associated does not prove cause and effect. In other words, although RCSs in these failed treatments may not have demonstrated radiographically dense obturations, other factors may have caused irritation of the periapical tissues and failure, such as (1) loss of or an inadequate coronal seal, (2) inadequate debridement and disinfection, (3) missed and untreated RCSs, (4) vertical root fractures, (5) significant periodontal disease, (6) coronal fractures, (7) poor aseptic technique, and (8) procedural errors (e.g., incorrect length, ledging, zipping, and perforations).

Significantly, a periapical lesion may heal temporarily after debridement without obturation.[2] Although this is not an acceptable treatment option, it does demonstrate an important concept: *what is removed from the RCS is more important than what is inserted into it.* The goal is to create a watertight seal to maintain a clean and disinfected RCS environment and to provide an optimum state for the health of the periapical tissues.

The objective of obturation is to create a watertight seal along the length of the RCS from the coronal opening to the apical termination. Traditionally the importance of establishing and maintaining a *coronal* seal has been overlooked; the quality of the coronal seal wasn't deemed important. However, it is now known to be as important as the apical seal to a long-term favorable outcome.[3] A watertight coronal seal can prevent residual microbes in the RCS from gaining access to the periodontal ligament, causing disease. It also minimizes the entry of new microbes into the RCS from the apical foramen, lateral or accessory canals, coronal opening, or odontoblastic tubule dead tracts.

POTENTIAL CAUSES OF FAILURE

Most treatment failures related to deficiencies in obturation are long-term failures. A low volume of irritant or the slow release of irritant into periapical tissues causes damage that is not apparent in the short term. *The persistence or development of periapical pathosis may not be evident for months or even years after treatment.* Therefore, recall evaluation to assess healing is important. Obturation-related failures may occur in different ways as described in the following sections.

Apical Seal
Leaving Debris in the RCS
Bacteria, tissue debris, and other irritants are usually not totally removed during cleaning and shaping (see Chapter 16). These constitute a potential source of irritation to periapical tissues that may not allow healing. Sealing these irritants in the RCS during obturation may prevent (or limit) their escape into the surrounding tissues. This seal must remain intact indefinitely because this reservoir of irritants may persist and cause disease years later. Interestingly, some bacteria sealed in the canal may lose viability, probably because of lack of substrate.[4] Other bacteria may remain dormant, waiting for the introduction of substrate to proliferate and cause disease. Even dead bacteria or their remnants can be irritating or antigenic and cause inflammation and negative immunologic consequences.[5]

Traditionally the apical foramen has been viewed as the main point of entry of microbes into the RCS. Later investigations have reported that, in fact, coronal microleakage often is the primary means of microbial entry.[6]

Coronal Seal
Irritants from the Oral Cavity
A coronal seal is extremely important because if the myriad of irritants present in the oral cavity gain access to the RCS and subsequently to the periapical tissues, they may cause inflammation and prevent healing. Irritants include microorganisms, food, chemicals, or other agents that pass through the mouth.

If a properly obturated RCS is exposed to saliva, a dissolution of sealer (with subsequent leakage over a relatively short period) may occur.[7-9] This results in leakage of bacteria, toxins, and chemicals into, and around, the gutta-percha (GP).[10] The consequences of sealer loss are obvious; communication between the oral cavity and the periodontal ligament (PDL) eventually becomes complete via accessory canals, dead tracts, or the apical foramen.

It is not possible to determine clinically whether the passage of irritants from the oral cavity to the periapex has occurred.

Therefore, it is unwise to restore a tooth in which an RCS has been exposed to saliva, bacteria, food debris, or other irritants from the oral cavity. Coronal exposure of the obturating material for longer than a short period, through loss of restoration, recurrent caries, or defective margins, requires retreatment. The duration of exposure that indicates retreatment depends on various factors, such as the quality of the obturation, the length of the RCS, and/or the surface area of exposure.

Restoration
Proper material selection and a superlative placement technique are critical. This aspect of the overall treatment is an integral part of obturation. The restoration acts as a protector of tooth structure and is the primary coronal seal, whether temporary or definitive. These factors are discussed in detail in Chapter 17.

Lateral Seal
The lateral seal is not as critical as the apical and coronal seals. Lateral/accessory canals are normally subcrestal and do not communicate with the oral cavity. However, establishment of a seal in the middle third of the RCS is also important. Lateral canals are often found in these regions; they constitute a potential channel for irritants from the RCS to the PDL (Fig. 18.1).[11]

Length of Obturation
The extent of the obturation mass relative to the apical foramen is also important. Ideally, obturating materials should remain within the RCS.

Overextension (Overfill)
Overextensions are undesirable. Prognostic studies report that failures increase with time when the primary obturating material has been extruded beyond the apical foramen.[12,13] Histological examination of periapical tissues after overextension (overfill) typically demonstrates increased inflammation and delayed or impaired healing.[14] Patients also experience more postobturation discomfort. Two other problems with overextension are irritation from the material itself and an inadequate apical seal.

Obturating Materials
Whether the obturation material is core or sealer, both are irritants, to a greater or lesser degree, when in contact with host tissues.[15] The GP core can cause mild tissue irritation initially. Sealers are toxic and invoke a foreign body response and inflammation when they are in contact with tissues.[16,17] The irritation from the sealer continues until the sealer sets. A small amount of sealer passing out of the foramen into PDL may not be a significant problem. However, when there is gross overextension of the primary obturating material and the sealer, persistent inflammation[14] and failure can result (Fig. 18.2).

Lack of Apical Seal Secondary to Overextension
Lack of an adequate apical seal may be even more important than irritation from the materials. GP, like amalgam, requires a matrix to compact against. An analogy is trying to compact and form amalgam into a Class II preparation without a metal matrix. The same is true of GP and sealer. Absence of an apical matrix or barrier may prevent sufficient lateral and

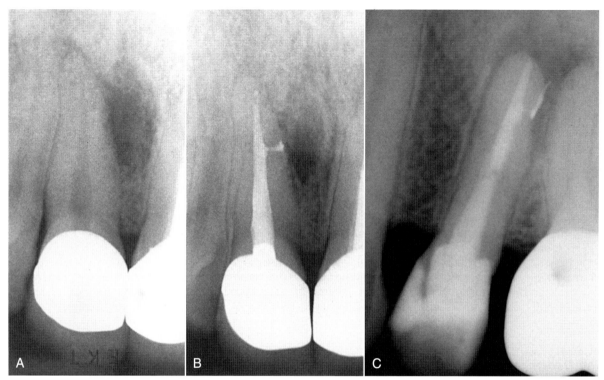

Fig. 18.1 **A,** Pulp necrosis with apical and lateral radiolucent lesions. **B,** On obturation, a lateral canal was detected communicating with the periodontium. This lesion should heal after removal of necrotic pulp tissue in the main canal and then obturation. **C,** Completed obturation showing lateral canal with extrusion of sealer along the periodontium. The lesion should heal within 6 months to 1 year. (**C** courtesy Dr. J. Fransen.)

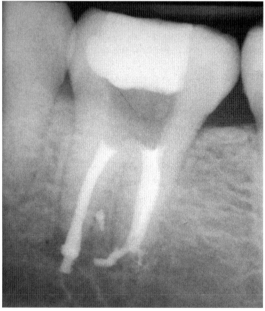

Fig. 18.2 Overfill of both mesial and distal canals. Lack of apical resistance and retention form (no apical matrix) permitted the extrusion of the gutta-percha/sealer mass.

vertical compaction, resulting in an inadequate seal. A tapered apical preparation helps form an adequate matrix for GP compaction and facilitates an adequate apical seal, with or without a small amount of sealer passing through the foramen into the PDL.

Obturation Short of the Apical Construction (Underfill)

An underfill results when both the preparation and the obturation mass are short of the desired working length (WL) or when the obturation does not extend to the WL. Either of these circumstances, or failure to treat a canal, may contribute to lack of healing, particularly long term (Fig. 18.3).

The "optimal" preparation/obturation length for a properly prepared RCS is slightly short of the apical foramen. Preparation or obturation excessively short of these lengths (more than 3 mm) may leave existing or potential irritants in the RCS. Periapical inflammation may then develop over an extended period, depending on the volume of irritants or the balance established between irritants and the immune system.

Compared with overfill, underfill is less of a problem, as indicated by outcome assessment and histologic studies.[18] Therefore, it is preferable to err on the short side to confine everything to the interior of the RCS.

Lateral Canals

The role of lateral and/or accessory canals in root canal treatment has been a subject of debate. These canals connect the RCS to the PDL. Irritants in the RCS, such as bacteria and necrotic debris, may gain access to the lateral PDL and initiate inflammation (see Fig. 18.1). Histological examination of roots after debridement has demonstrated that lateral canals are rarely, if ever, debrided.[19] However, certain techniques tend to move core material and/or sealer (primarily) into a lateral or accessory canal.[20] When the main RCS has been adequately cleaned, shaped, and obturated, radiolucencies adjacent to lateral canals heal as readily as periapical lesions.

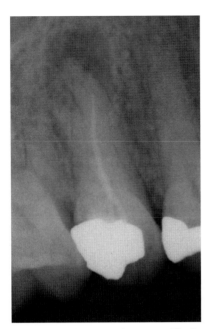

Fig. 18.3 Failure caused by operative errors. The buccal canal is underprepared (inadequate debridement) and incompletely obturated (short fill); the palatal canal is neither instrumented nor filled.

This typically occurs whether the obturating material has or has not been expressed into a lateral or accessory canal. In general, the obturation of lateral canals is inconsequential to the outcome of most root canal treatments, despite the claims that certain techniques fill lateral canals.[21]

Vertical Root Fractures

A vertical root fracture (VRF) is a devastating occurrence that usually requires removal of the tooth or the fractured root through a root amputation or hemisection. Signs and symptoms, in addition to radiographic findings, demonstrate that bone loss and soft tissue lesions are common.[22] Lateral forces exerted during obturation or post placement are major etiologic factors in VRFs, owing to their wedging action.[23-27] However, many crown/root fractures are idiopathic. The pathogenesis, findings, and prevention of vertical fractures are discussed further in Chapter 8.

TIMING OF OBTURATION

When questions arise, such as, "When is treatment to be completed?" or "Is it time to obturate?" the following factors must be considered: signs and symptoms, pulp and periapical status, and difficulty of the procedure. Combinations of these factors affect the decisions made about the number of appointments and the timing of obturation.

Patient's Symptoms

In general, if the patient presents with severe symptoms and the diagnosis is symptomatic (acute) apical periodontitis or abscess, obturation is contraindicated. These are emergency situations; therefore, it is preferable to manage the immediate problem and delay definitive treatment. Acute apical abscesses have been treated in a single appointment,[28] although this is generally not recommended.

Painful irreversible pulpitis is a different situation. Because the inflamed pulp (the source of the pain) is removed, obturation may be completed at the same appointment, time permitting.

Pulp and Periapical Status
Vital Pulp

If time and the situation permit, the procedure may be completed in a single visit, regardless of the inflammatory status of the pulp.

Necrotic Pulp

Without significant periapical discomfort, obturation may be completed during the same appointment as RCS preparation. Pulp necrosis with asymptomatic apical periodontitis or chronic apical abscess, or condensing osteitis *alone,* is not necessarily a contraindication to single-appointment treatment.

There may be advantages to multiple appointments. Placement of an intracanal antimicrobial dressing (e.g., calcium hydroxide) reduces bacteria. Calcium hydroxide in the RCS for 7 days reduces the bacterial load.[29] A comparison of single-visit to multiple-visit intracanal calcium hydroxide treatment did not demonstrate differences in the long-term prognosis.[30] However, the presence of bacteria in the RCS at the time of obturation may have a significant impact on the long-term prognosis.[31] At present, there are no definitive conclusions about when single- or multiple-visit procedures are indicated in which situations. The decision for obturation should be based on thorough canal disinfection procedures.

One situation that contraindicates single-visit care is the persistence of exudation into the RCS during preparation. The potential for post-treatment exacerbation is increased if the periapical lesion is productive and generates continual drainage. If the canal is sealed, pressure and corresponding tissue destruction may proceed rapidly. In these cases, cleaning and shaping are completed, followed by calcium hydroxide placement. In general, exudation is diminished and controllable at a subsequent appointment, and obturation may then be completed.

Degree of Difficulty

Complex cases are time-consuming and may be better managed in multiple appointments. If the treatment period would exceed 2 hours and/or the clinician believes that he or she may be better prepared to treat the case at subsequent appointments, obturation should be delayed.

Culture Results

Obtaining cultures is a procedure in use many years ago. The principle was to obtain negative cultures prior to obturation. However, there was no substantive documentation that the technique or the outcomes were valid.[32] Thus, this technique is no longer used universally.

Number of Appointments

The decision on the number of appointments needed usually is made during initial treatment planning. The decision to schedule another appointment, when made *during* an appointment, reflects a change of circumstances. For example, the

Box 18.1   Desirable Properties of Obturating Materials

Grossman suggested that the ideal obturant would do the following[34]:

- Be easily introduced into the canal
- Seal the canal laterally and apically
- Not shrink after insertion.
- Be impervious to moisture
- Be bactericidal or at least discourage bacterial growth
- Be radiopaque
- Not stain the tooth structure
- Not irritate periapical tissues or affect the tooth structure
- Be sterile or easily sterilized
- Be easily removed from the root canal

Currently, no material or combination of materials satisfies all these criteria.

patient or dentist becomes tired or has lost patience, or the RCS continues to drain.

CORE OBTURATING MATERIALS

Primary obturating materials are usually solid or semisolid (paste or softened form). These comprise the bulk of material that will fill the RCS and may or may not be used with a sealer. A sealer is essential with all solid obturating materials, although sealers behave differently with different obturating materials and techniques.[33]

Obturating materials may be introduced into the canals in different forms and may be manipulated by different means once inside. These materials and methodologies are discussed in some detail; alternatives also are discussed, but in less detail. Whatever the material, there are desirable properties that must be considered (Box 18.1).[34]

Solid Materials

Solids have major advantages over semisolids (pastes). Although various materials have been used, the only one universally accepted as the primary material is gutta-percha. It has withstood the test of time and research and is by far the most commonly used.[35] Synthetic resin–based core materials are also available (these are discussed later in the chapter).

Major advantages of solid cores over semisolid paste types is the clinician's ability to better control length and also a reasonable ability of the solid material to adapt itself to irregularities and create an adequate seal throughout the root canal system (RCS).

Gutta-Percha
Composition
The primary bulk ingredient of a GP cone is zinc oxide (±75%). GP, which is a congener of rubber, accounts for approximately 20% and gives the cone its unique properties (e.g., plasticity). The remaining ingredients are binders, opaquers, and coloring agents.

Shapes
GP cones are available in two basic shapes, standard and nonstandard (or conventional). In general, standardized sizes

conform to the requirements of either the International Organization of Standardization (ISO) or the American Dental Association/American National Standards Institute (ADA/ANSI). Nonstandard materials and equipment do not conform to those requirements. Standardized cones are designed to have the same size and taper as the corresponding endodontic instruments used to prepare the RCS; that is, a No. 40 cone with an 0.04 taper should correspond to a No. 40 nickel-titanium (NiTi) rotary instrument with an 0.04 taper.

Clinical observations and studies indicate that commercially available so-called standardized cones show wide variations in size and taper.[36] This lack of uniformity is not critical; however, canal shape after preparation is also variable.

GP master cones (MCs) with varying tapers tend to be selected according to the method of canal preparation or to match the master apical file tip size and corresponding taper.

Advantages
GP was introduced as an obturating material more than 160 years ago.[30] Due to its usefulness and popularity, it has become the standard to which other obturating materials are compared.

GP has a number of advantages. *First,* because of its plasticity, it adapts with compaction to irregularities in prepared canals, especially when thermoplasticized. *Second,* it is relatively easy to manage and manipulate, even with complex obturation techniques. *Third,* GP is relatively easy to remove from the RCS, either partially to allow post placement or totally for retreatment. *Fourth,* GP is relatively biocompatible, being nearly inert over time when in contact with connective tissue.[15] If a cone becomes contaminated, it can be effectively sterilized by immersion in sodium hypochlorite (1% concentration or greater) for 1 minute.[37]

Sealability
Studies show that, regardless of the technique, the use of GP without a sealer does not result in an adequate seal.[38,39] Disadvantages of GP include lack of chemical adhesion to each other and, more important, to dentin. When heat is applied or GP is mixed with solvents (e.g., chloroform or eucalyptol), it shrinks markedly during cooling or with evaporation of the solvent,[40] leaving space between the core and dentinal walls.[41] A sealer is used because it fills the spaces between the GP cones and between the GP and the RCS wall. However, it has been reported that the sealer does not predictably fill all of these spaces and coat the walls.[42]

Methods of Obturation
As stated earlier, obturation methods are varied and imaginative. Enterprising dentists and manufacturers have devised (and sell) a variety of devices (with special techniques) in an attempt to enable the clinician to obturate more quickly and effectively.

The most popular obturation method is lateral compaction, followed by warm vertical compaction. Other techniques involve either chemical or physical alteration of the GP in an attempt to render the material more plastic, which assists in adaption to either additional GP or the RCS walls.

Another variation is a system that includes a solid core (carrier) surrounded by a coating of GP. The carrier may be stainless steel or titanium but is more typically plastic. After RCS preparation, the carrier and GP are warmed in a heater specifically designed for this purpose and placed in the canal as a unit.

Other technologies have been introduced that involve warming, plasticizing, and injecting GP. All are discussed in more detail later in this chapter.

Resin

Synthetic polyester resin–based polymers have been advocated as an obturation material (Fig. 18.4).[43,44] The core material, composed of polycaprolactone with fillers of bioactive glass and other components, is used with a dual-cured Bis-GMA resin sealer and self-etching primer.[44] This combination is an attempt to form a single entity, or so-called monoblock, in the RCS; it involves a chemical bond between the sealer and dentin and the sealer and core material. The material has been reported to be noncytotoxic, biocompatible, and nonmutagenic and has been approved for use by the U.S. Food and Drug Administration (FDA). Early research reported that this material was more resistant to leakage than GP.[44] More recent evidence indicates no difference in leakage compared to more standard techniques.[45,46] The resin cores, available in nonstandard and standard sizes, have handling properties similar to those of GP and can be removed by solvents and heat if retreatment is indicated. Pellets are also available for use in thermoplastic injection techniques. As yet there are no controlled clinical trials with long-term evaluation to demonstrate how this system compares to GP as an obturating material.

Silver Points

Silver points were designed to correspond to the last file size used in preparation and presumably to fill the RCS precisely

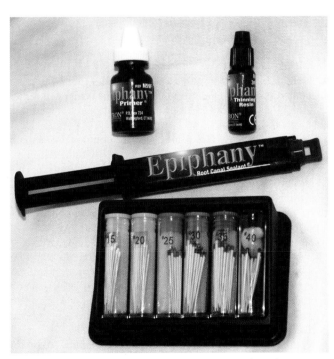

Fig. 18.4 A resin-based obturation system contains primer, sealer, and cones. The cones resemble gutta-percha and can be placed using lateral or warm vertical compaction; pellets are available for thermoplastic injection. (Courtesy Axis/SybronEndo, Orange, CA.)

in all dimensions. This would be ideal if the preparation were round, a shape that is rarely achieved. It is impossible to predictably prepare an RCS to a uniformly round shape.[47] It was thought that silver points had oligodynamic properties, but later evidence indicated that they did not.

Although the short-term sealability success of silver points seemed comparable to that of GP, silver points are a poor long-term choice as a routine obturating material.[48,49] Their major disadvantages are lack of adaptability (Fig. 18.5) and possible toxicity to periapical tissues from corrosion.[50] Also, because of their tight frictional fit, silver cones are difficult to remove, either totally during retreatment or partially during post space preparation.[51]

Silver cones are not recommended.

Pastes (Semisolids)

It seemed like a great idea: why not develop a paste or cement with bioactive ingredients? This material could be mixed in a liquid or putty form and injected to the WL, obturating the entire RCS, and then allowed to set. The process would be faster, the paste would fill the entire canal space, and obturation would be much simpler.

Although the concept is appealing, there are significant practical difficulties. The major disadvantages with the use of paste materials are lack of predictable length control, shrinkage, toxicity of ingredients, preclinical difficulties in introduction of the material without voids, and resorbability of the materials.

Paste filling is not recommended.

Types
Zinc Oxide–Eugenol (ZnOE)

ZnOE may be used in its pure state in primary teeth because it is resorbable as the tooth is exfoliated. However, it is generally not advocated in permanent teeth. Other formulations combine ZnOE with various additives. The types known as N2 and RC2B are most common. These are derivations of Sargenti's formula and contain opaquers, metallic oxides (lead) or chlorides (mercuric), steroids (at times), plasticizers, paraformaldehyde, and various other ingredients. Claims of antimicrobial properties, biologic therapeutic activity, and superiority are made for these paste formulations. However, no scientific evidence exists verifying that they contribute any beneficial aspects to healing. In fact, most of these additives are very toxic.[52] In 1998 the American Association of Endodontists issued a position statement on the use of paraformaldehyde-containing endodontic filling materials.

Use of these materials is below the standard of care and therefore not recommended.[53]

Plastics

It has been suggested that a resin-based sealer, such as AH26 or Diaket, be used as the sole obturating material. *These sealers have the same disadvantages as other pastes and are therefore not recommended.*

Techniques of Placement

Various methodologies have been advocated for insertion of pastes and/or sealers. Two popular methods are injection and placement with a Lentulo spiral.

Injection is accomplished using a syringe-type device with a barrel and special needles.[54] The paste is mixed and placed **321**

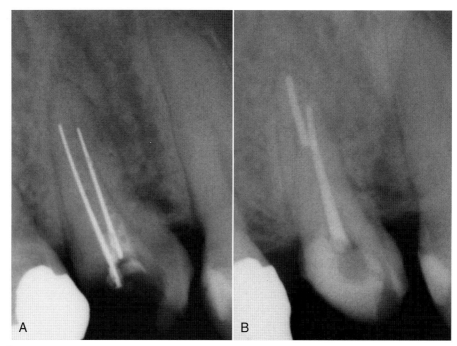

Fig. 18.5 **A,** Obturation with silver points. Retreatment is necessary due to loss of coronal restoration, short obturation, and inadequate debridement. **B,** Retreatment and obturation using vertical compaction of gutta-percha and sealer. Post space was provided for the final restoration. (Courtesy Dr. T. Remmers.)

in the barrel, a screw handle is inserted and twisted, and the paste is extruded through the needle. The needles are placed deep in the canal, and the paste is expressed as the needles are slowly backed out of the canal. Advocates claim that this method completely fills the canal from the apical portion to the canal orifice. However, it is not unusual for voids to develop, resulting in a short or overextended obturation.

Paste placement is assisted using Lentulo spiral drills. The paste is mixed and placed into the chamber, and the Lentulo drill is spun into the RCS. The RCS is filled with paste, and the drill is slowly withdrawn, as with the syringe device. The reverse spiral on the Lentulo is what carries the paste into the RCS.

Both techniques are more attractive in theory than in fact. Neither technique has demonstrated an ability to seal effectively over time or to completely obturate the RCS.

Moreover, because of a lack of predictable length control, both injection and placement by Lentulo spiral drill have major deficiencies and are not recommended.

Advantages and Disadvantages of Pastes

The advantages of pastes are speed, relative ease of use, and use of a single material. The equipment needed, at least with the Lentulo spiral technique, is relatively simple, comprising only a limited assortment of special drills.

The disadvantages are lack of predictability and lack of consistent length control. Also, it is difficult to avoid overextension or underfill (Fig. 18.6). Another major disadvantage is inconsistent sealability.[55] This may be related to three factors: (1) large voids or discrepancies within the material or adjacent to the walls; (2) shrinkage of ZnOE on setting, which leaves space for microleakage; and (3) solubility of pastes in tissue or oral fluids.

SEALERS

Sealer, as an adjunct, accomplishes the objective of creating a watertight seal.[56] Sealer must be used in conjunction with the primary obturating material, regardless of the technique or material used. This makes the physical properties and placement of the sealer important.

Desirable Properties

Grossman outlined the criteria for an ideal sealer, which are presented in the following list.[56] None of the sealers currently available has all these ideal properties, but some have more than others.

- *Tissue tolerance.* The sealer and its components should cause neither tissue destruction nor cell death. All commonly used sealers show some degree of toxicity.[15] This toxicity is greatest when the sealer is unset but tends to diminish after setting and with time.[57]
- *No shrinkage with setting.* The sealer should remain dimensionally stable or even expand slightly on setting.
- *Slow setting time.* The sealer should provide adequate working time for placement and manipulation of obturating material, then set reasonably soon after obturation is complete. It is desirable to have sealer unset if post space is made immediately.
- *Adhesiveness.* A truly adhesive material forms a tight bond between the core material and dentin.
- *Radiopacity.* Sealer should be readily visible on radiographs so the operator knows where it is located both within the RCS and in the periapex when overextended. However, sealer should not be more radiopaque then core material because it would mask voids and obturation imperfections.

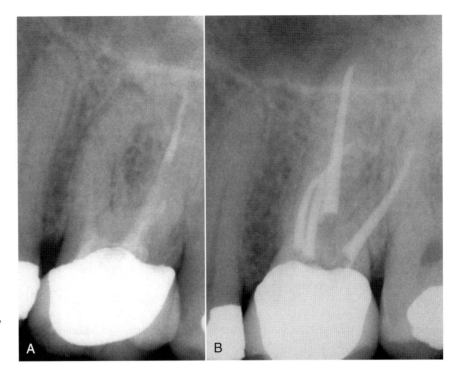

Fig. 18.6 A, Inadequate preparation, paste fills, and evidence of periapical disease. **B,** The tooth was retreated. A second mesiobuccal canal was located, instrumented, and obturated. All canals were obturated using warm vertical compaction with a resin core and sealer.

- *Absence of staining.* Remnants should not stain dentin or enamel. Currently, all tested sealers, particularly ZnOE-based sealers or those containing heavy metals, stain dentin to a greater or lesser degree.[58,59]
- *Solubility in solvent.* Occasionally, creation of post space or retreatment may be necessary days, months, or years after obturation. The sealer should be soluble in a solvent. Different sealers have different degrees of solubility in different solvents and with varying mechanical techniques.[60]
- *Insolubility to oral and tissue fluids.* Sealer should not resorb when in contact with tissue fluids. However, all sealers are soluble to a greater or lesser extent when in contact with oral fluids.[8]
- *Bacteriostatic properties.* Although a bactericidal sealer would seem to be desirable, a substance that kills bacteria could also be toxic to host tissues. At minimum, the sealer should not encourage bacterial growth.[61]
- *Ability to create a seal.* This is obviously an important physical property. The material must create and maintain a watertight seal apically, laterally, and coronally.

Types

In general, the four major types of sealers are ZnOE-based, plastics, glass ionomer, and those containing calcium hydroxide. Other variations and compounds have been proposed or are marketed as sealers; these should be considered experimental.

Certainly, the standard sealer with which all others are compared is the Grossman formulation, which has withstood the test of time and use, although some plastics (resins) are now widely used and have many desirable properties. Calcium hydroxide and glass ionomer types are newer and have interesting properties but also significant drawbacks.

ZnOE-Based Sealers

The major advantage of ZnOE-based sealers is their long history of successful use. Obviously, their positive qualities outweigh their negative aspects (staining, a *very* slow setting time,[62] nonadhesion, and solubility).

Grossman's Formulation

Grossman's formula is as follows:

Powder: Zinc oxide (body), 42 parts; staybelite resin (setting time and consistency), 27 parts; bismuth subcarbonate, 15 parts; barium sulfate (radiopacity), 15 parts; sodium borate, 1 part.

Liquid: Eugenol

Most ZnOE sealers in use today are variations of this original formula. Three problems with this formulation are its *very* slow setting time,[62] toxic effects on host tissue, and lack of adhesiveness.

Epoxy Resin

Epoxy has traditionally been available in a powder-liquid formula (AH26, AH Plus, and ThermaSeal Plus). Its advantages include antimicrobial action, adhesion, a long working time, ease of mixing, and very good sealability. Its disadvantages are staining, relative insolubility in solvents, some toxicity when unset, and some solubility to oral fluids. There are newer formulations without hexamine tetramine, which has been implicated in postobturation sensitivity.[63] This formulation is also easier to mix because it is composed of two pastes mixed equally.

Other Plastics

Other plastics are primarily of the methylmethacrylate type and are not commonly used.

Calcium Hydroxide

Calcium hydroxide sealers have been introduced in which the calcium hydroxide is incorporated into a ZnOE or plastic base. These sealers reportedly have biologic properties that stimulate a calcific barrier at the apex; however, these **323** properties have not been conclusively demonstrated in clinical or experimental use. Calcium hydroxide sealers show antimicrobial properties and adequate short-term sealability.[64] Questions have been raised about their long-term stability (greater solubility) and tissue toxicity.[65] Until further experimental and clinical data are available, these sealers have no demonstrated advantages.[65]

Glass Ionomer

Endodontic formulations of glass ionomer have been introduced recently. This material has the advantage of bonding to dentin, seems to provide an adequate apical and coronal seal, and is biocompatible.[66] However, its hardness and insolubility make retreatment and post space preparation more difficult, and it is difficult to treat the dentin properly to accept the material.[67] (Glass ionomer–impregnated GP used with a glass ionomer sealer is discussed later in the chapter.)

Ceramic-Based Sealer

Ceramic-based sealer is a recently introduced root canal sealer. It is based on a bioceramic composition with zirconium oxide, calcium silicates, calcium phosphate, and calcium hydroxide as its main constituents, besides fillers and thickening agents. The sealer has been reported as insoluble, radiopaque, and nonshrinking; it requires moisture to harden. Studies have shown that bioceramic sealer has minor cytotoxicity. However, further studies are necessary to determine the long-term effect of this sealer on the success of the treatment.[68]

Others

Various luting agents and basing and restorative materials have been tried and tested as endodontic sealers.[69] Examples are zinc phosphate cement, composite, and polycarboxylate cement. These materials have not proved satisfactory.

Mixing

ZnOE sealer types should be mixed to a thick consistency. They should string approximately 2 to 3 inches. The thicker the mix, the better the properties of the sealer, particularly in regard to stability, superiority of seal, and diminished toxicity.[70] Epoxy resins are mixed to a much thinner consistency.

Placement

Various techniques have been advocated for placement of a sealer, which is done before insertion of the core material. The sealer may be placed with paper points, files, ultrasonic activation of files, or special drills (Lentulo); as a coating on the primary cone; or by injection with special syringes. Although different methods have shown varying degrees of effectiveness in sealer application, no technique has proved superior.[71-73] In fact, sealers may not completely cover the interface between GP and the canal wall after obturation.[42]

A simple and effective technique is to coat the walls by picking up sealer on the final apical file or a one-size-smaller file (Fig. 18.7). The file is placed to length and slowly spun counterclockwise, which has the effect of carrying the sealer apically and coating the walls. A sterile file should be used at this step to prevent contamination and the mixing in of dentinal chips left on the file. Flooding the canal with sealer is neither necessary nor desirable because it may lead to overextension.

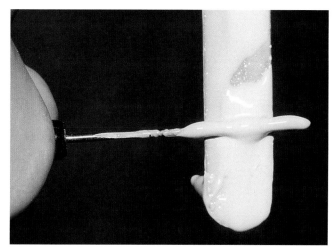

Fig. 18.7 An easy, effective method of sealer application. The file covered with sealer is inserted and spun counterclockwise to coat the canal walls.

Sealer is not placed in all canals at once unless it has a long working time. Removing sealer that has set is difficult. The Grossman formulations and epoxy resins are slow setting and may be placed in all canals.[61]

OBTURATION TECHNIQUES WITH GUTTA-PERCHA

Different approaches to obturation with GP can be used, depending on the size of the prepared canal, the final shape of the preparation, and irregularities within the canal. The overriding factor is clinician preference; no technique has been shown to be superior with regard to long-term outcomes.

Selection of Technique

The two traditional techniques are lateral and warm vertical compaction of GP. Sealability is similar for both.[74] As mentioned, the choice is dictated primarily by the clinician's preference and by custom, although there may be special situations indicating a particular use of each technique. Both must be used with a sealer.

More recent approaches have been introduced that depend on warming and softening formulations of GP with special devices and instruments and then placing the GP incrementally. Most of these techniques and devices are heavily marketed and promoted; they are discussed later in the chapter.

Other methods are also used, most involving alteration of the entire GP cone with a solvent such as chloroform or eucalyptol. These are technique sensitive and therefore are not widely used or taught.

Lateral Compaction

Lateral compaction is the most popular obturation technique, both in practice and as taught in most institutions.[75] A variation of lateral compaction is the solvent-softened (or custom-fitted tip) technique (outlined later in this chapter).

Indications

Lateral compaction of GP may be used in most clinical situations. Exceptions are severely curved or abnormally shaped canals and those with gross irregularities, such as internal resorption. However, lateral compaction may be combined with other obturation approaches.[76] In general, if the situation is not amenable to lateral compaction (or vertical compaction, if that is the usual approach) or is too difficult for the general practitioner, the patient should be referred to an endodontist.

Advantages

Lateral compaction is relatively uncomplicated, requires a relatively simple armamentarium, and seals and obturates as well as any other technique in conventional situations.[77] A major advantage of lateral compaction over most other techniques is length control. With establishment of a definitive apical stop and careful use of the spreader, the length of the GP filling can be predictably placed to the WL without concern for overextension. Additional advantages include relative predictability of retreatment, adaptation to the walls of the RCS, positive dimensional stability, and the ability to prepare post space.[78]

Disadvantages

The resultant obturation is not a homogeneous mass. The MC and accessory cones are compacted against each other, and the areas between all the cones are at least partially filled in by the sealer.[33] There are no other major disadvantages to lateral compaction, other than difficulties in obturating severely curved canals, an open apex, and canals with internal resorptive defects.

Technique of Lateral Compaction

Although there are variations, a workable and acceptable technique of lateral compaction is presented here.

Spreader or Plugger Selection

Selection and try-in of the spreader or plugger should be performed during the cleaning and shaping of the canal.

Finger spreaders or pluggers are preferred over standard (long-handled) spreaders because they afford better tactile sensation, an improved apical seal, better instrument control (Fig. 18.8), and reduced dentin stress during obturation.[24,78] Use of these finger instruments likely reduces the incidence of vertical root fractures during obturation. Stainless steel finger spreaders or pluggers are more flexible and can be inserted deeper than standard hand spreaders (Fig. 18.9).

Nickel-titanium finger spreaders have even more flexibility; these spreaders seem to produce less wedging force while penetrating deeper.[79] This advantage may result in less of a tendency to produce vertical root fractures. These spreaders do behave differently because of their flexibility and require practice for efficient use.

Master Cone Selection

Either a standard or nonstandard GP cone may be adapted as a master cone. An MC with the same tip size and taper as the

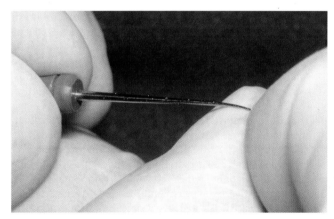

Fig. 18.8 Finger spreaders may be precurved to improve negotiation in curved canals.

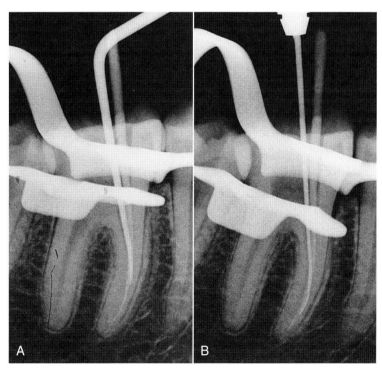

Fig. 18.9 Comparison of hand spreader with finger pluggers or spreaders. **A,** The stiff, more tapered hand spreader will not negotiate the curve. **B,** The smaller, more flexible finger spreader permits deeper penetration and produces a superior apical seal.

master apical file is selected and placed in the RCS. The MC should butt up against the apical stop with a solid feeling of obstructing further movement of the MC past the stop. In an apical preparation that is very irregular in shape and has no apical stop, the MC should be customized with a solvent-softened or heat-softened cone technique or the apical stop improved.

Fitting the MC

After final irrigation, the following steps are performed.

1. Because the MC fits only in the apical portion of the apically cleared, flared RCS, the amount of resistance to removal is slight (Fig. 18.10). A slight frictional fit at the apical portion is acceptable, and so-called tug-back is unnecessary.[80] However, there should be a definite stop when the cone fits into place. This prevents overextension of the obturation mass into the PDL. The cone is fitted to the WL.
2. A cone may be too small, as indicated by a buckling in the apical few millimeters (Fig. 18.11, *A*). A larger apical end can be created by cutting 1-mm increments off the tip of the MC until the proper fit is obtained (Fig. 18.11, *B*). Deep spreader penetration, to within 1 mm of the WL, should be accomplished with a prefitted spreader.[81] If the MC is too small for the preparation, the tip is trimmed (special trimmers are available) to increase the GP point size (Fig. 18.12), regardless of the taper.
3. The MC is removed by grasping it at the reference point, and the length is verified by measuring it on a ruler.
4. The length of the MC then is evaluated radiographically. The traditional close radiographic fit of the MC in the apical third is unrelated to the quality of the final seal.[80]
5. A GP cone that extends beyond the apical foramen demonstrates lack of a satisfactory apical stop and a poorly fitted master GP cone. This requires revalidation of the WL and establishment of an apical stop by progressing to larger file sizes slightly short of the working length until an acceptable stop is achieved. This step improves length control and the obturation.

Steps in Obturation

Although there are many combinations of obturating instruments and different types of GP, the method presented here is an effective and accepted technique. A suggested approach for

routine situations is matching the size of the finger spreader with the size of the accessory cone (Fig. 18.13). There is no precise correlation between accessory point size and the size of the finger spreader.

The following are the specific steps for lateral compaction (Figs. 18.14 to 18.16).

1. Sealer is placed on the apical 3 mm of the MC.
2. The MC is inserted slowly to allow excess cement to escape coronally; it is slowly moved apically and coronally three times to coat the walls of the RCS.
3. Before the spreader is inserted and removed, an accessory cone is picked up with locking pliers at the measured length, ready to be inserted.
4. The measured spreader is inserted between the MC and the walls to within 1 to 2 mm of the WL. The spreader taper is the mechanical force that laterally and vertically compacts the GP, creating a space for an additional accessory cone.
5. The spreader is freed for removal by back-and-forth rotation around its axis. The spreader is removed, and the measured fine accessory GP cone is immediately inserted into the space created.

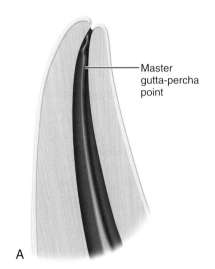

Master gutta-percha point

A

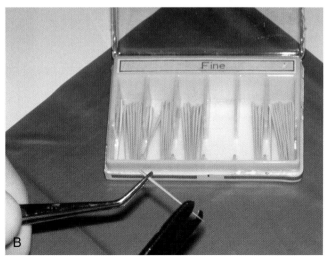

B

Fig. 18.11 **A,** A cone that appears buckled on the radiograph or on removal is much too small. **B,** A larger cone should be selected or clipped to form a larger size at the tip.

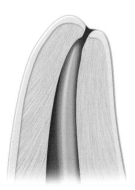

Fig. 18.10 The master cone needs only a slight frictional fit in the very apical region. This permits deep spreader penetration between the gutta-percha and the canal wall.

6. (Optional): A radiograph may be exposed after one or two cones have been placed before searing off the tops. If there are length problems, the cones can be easily retrieved. A new MC is fitted at a corrected length and the process repeated.

7. This procedure is repeated until the spreader can no longer be inserted beyond the apical third of the canal. Obturation may be evaluated with a radiograph at any time.

8. Excess GP is seared off with a hot instrument at the RCS orifice (Fig. 18.17).

9. The cervical portion of the warm GP is vertically compacted using the Glick No. 1, a No. 5-7 heater-plugger, or other appropriately sized, prefitted plugger.

10. It is generally advisable to place an orifice barrier over each orifice to a depth of at least 1 mm to help minimize leakage if the temporary restoration allows leakage from the oral cavity. An unfilled, tinted resin is useful for this purpose, so that if post space is required in the future, the orifice barrier can be easily seen and removed.

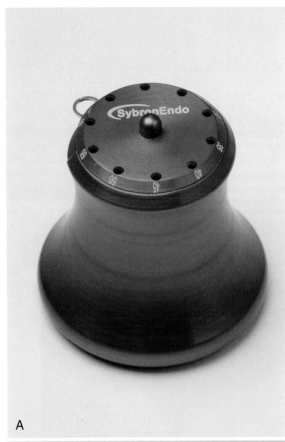

A

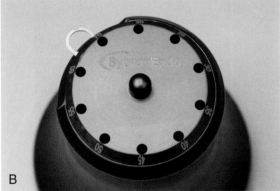

B

Fig. 18.12 **A,** Device capable of accurately clipping the tips of greater taper gutta-percha. **B,** Closer view of the tip sizes available

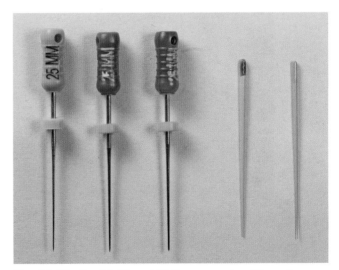

Fig. 18.13 Size 20, 25, and 30 finger spreaders, 25 mm long with associated rubber stopper, along with size 20 and 25 standardized gutta-percha accessory points.

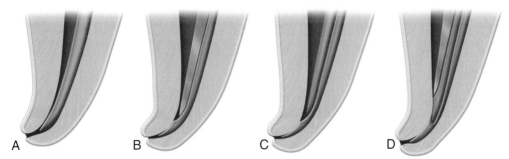

A B C D

Fig. 18.14 The steps of lateral compaction. **A,** The master cone is fitted. **B,** A finger spreader or plugger is inserted, ideally to 1 to 2 mm of the prepared length. **C,** The spreader is rotated and removed, and an accessory cone is placed in the space created. **D,** The process is repeated.

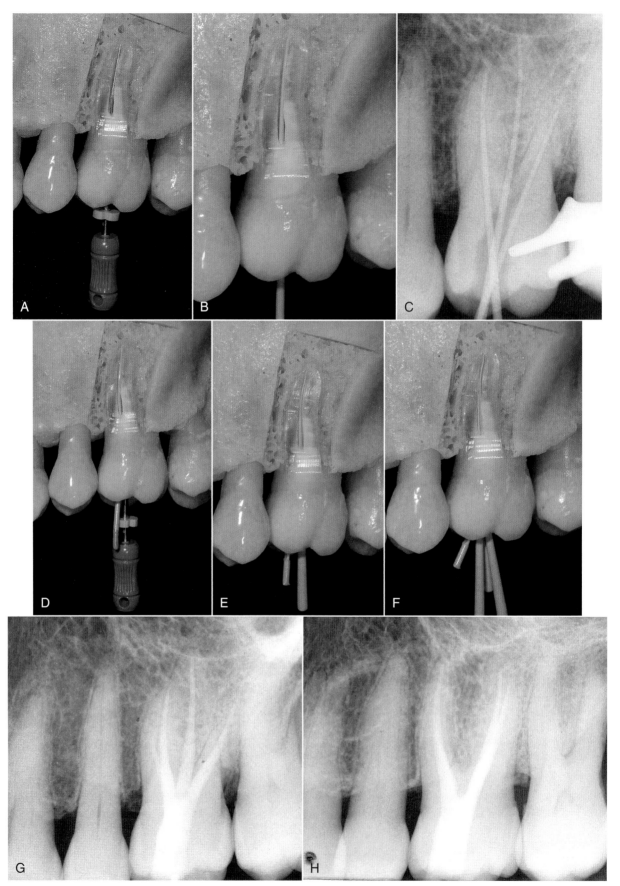

Fig. 18.15 Lateral compaction. **A,** An endodontic file is first inserted to check for proper depth of penetration. **B,** Standardized gutta-percha points are placed. **C,** Placement is verified radiographically. **D,** Once the sealer has been placed and the cone is to length, the spreader is inserted along the side of the cemented cone (here, in the mesiobuccal canal). **E,** An accessory cone is placed in the space created by the spreader. **F,** The process is repeated (i.e., reinsertion of the spreader, followed by placement of another accessory cone) until the spreader does not penetrate beyond the middle third of the canal. The cones are removed at the orifice with heat, and the coronal mass then is vertically compacted. **G,** The remaining canals are obturated in the same manner. **H,** The final radiograph demonstrates four canals properly obturated. (Courtesy Dr. W. Johnson.)

Ultrasonic Compaction

An alternative method involves lateral compaction with ultrasonic activation of the spreader, which heats the ultrasonic tip and subsequently the GP. The ultrasonic spreader is placed next to the MC and activated without water coolant. Apical pressure is exerted, and the spreader is inserted to within 1 mm of the WL. The advantages of this method are that the ultrasonic action may spread the sealer; the friction of the spreader thermoplasticizes the GP; and less force is required to place the spreader, which helps minimize the risk of a vertical root fracture.[82]

Finishing Procedure

The following are the steps for finishing the obturation procedure.

1. The chamber is cleaned thoroughly with cotton pellets moistened in alcohol or chlorhexidine followed by a dry cotton pellet. Remnants of GP or sealer may cause future discoloration (Fig. 18.18).
2. A temporary or definitive restoration is placed (see Chapter 17).
3. A radiograph is exposed with the restoration in place and the clamp removed to evaluate the quality of the completed obturation. An occlusal check is then performed.

Correcting Obturation Problems

Occasionally, voids or length problems are apparent radiographically. These should be corrected *immediately,* before the sealer has set.

For voids, GP is removed with hot pluggers until the spreader can be reinserted just beyond the void or discrepancy. Sealer is then reapplied, and lateral compaction is performed as described previously.

An advantage of exposing a radiograph before the excess GP is seared off is that the entire mass can usually be removed by grasping the cones with fingers or cotton pliers and removing the entire mass. Fitting of a new MC and reobturation can then be performed to achieve a satisfactory result.

If the excess GP has been seared off, an overextension can sometimes be corrected before the sealer sets by removing all the GP. When extruded beyond the apex, the overfilled GP is difficult to recover, particularly after the sealer sets. Extruded sealer can only be retrieved surgically (usually not necessary).

Obturating materials extruded beyond the apex are irritants and can affect healing, but generally they do not completely prevent resolution unless there is gross overfill of core material. ZnOE-based sealers often resorb from periapical tissues

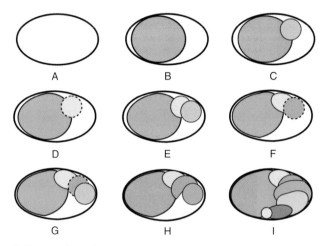

A. Prepared canal
B. Master cone inserted
C. Spreader placed
D. Placement of accessory cone (shown as dashed circle)
E-H. Continuation of lateral compaction
I. Completion of obturation

Fig. 18.16 Schematic of the steps of lateral compaction. Each insertion of the spreader to its most apical extent laterally compacts the gutta-percha cone toward the opposing wall. At the completion of the compaction, the canal is obturated with a series of cones that have been cold-welded together with sealer. (Courtesy Dr. J. Schweitzer.)

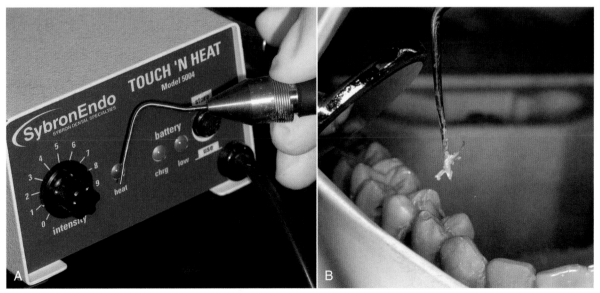

Fig. 18.17 **A,** A convenient, battery-powered heating device holds an assortment of tips. **B,** The tip is rapidly heated for removal of excess gutta-percha from the chamber or from the canal when creating a post space.

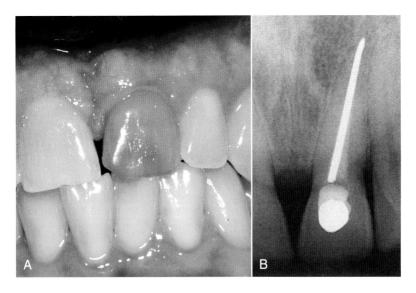

Fig. 18.18 Often discoloration is caused by improper technique and is preventable. **A,** A too-frequent unfortunate occurrence: gradual discoloration after root canal treatment. **B,** Causes include sealer remnants and a silver point extending into the chamber and amalgam restoring the lingual access. This tooth will be difficult to bleach because the stains are from metallic ions.

over time.[83] These situations should not be treated surgically unless failure to heal is evident on follow-up examination. If an abundance of sealer is overextended, consultation with an oral and maxillofacial surgeon is recommended, especially if the material is in the vicinity of, or extends into, the inferior alveolar canal.

Solvent-Softened Custom Cones

Chloroform and halothane have proven to be effective solvents. However, concerns about toxicity have been expressed. Concerns about chloroform are unfounded because recent evaluations show that, if used judiciously, chloroform is safe for retreatment and for the formation of custom cones.[84,85] The technique described here uses chloroform.

An impression of the apical 3 or 4 mm of the canal is made in the master cone. The objective is to fit the cone closely into the apical portion to try to create a better seal, but primarily to prevent extrusion of GP beyond the apex.[86,87]

Indications

Solvent-softened custom cones are indicated if (1) an apical stop is not present or (2) a stop is present but the apical portion of the canal is very large or irregular.

Technique

1. The MC selected is a larger standard or nonstandard cone that, when inserted, stops 2 to 4 mm short of the WL.
2. The apical 3 to 4 mm of the MC is softened by dipping it in chloroform for 1 to 2 seconds (Fig. 18.19). Halothane dipping is done for 3 to 4 seconds.
3. The cone is placed to the WL or to resistance Then, the cone is grasped at the reference point, removed, and measured. The process is repeated until the cone goes to the WL.
4. The cone is removed and the solvent allowed to evaporate. The cone tip should show an impression of the apical preparation (Fig. 18.20).
5. The cone is replaced in the same position and a confirmatory radiograph is made.
6. Sealer is applied to the apical 3 to 4 mm of the MC, which is moved up and down three times before placing to length.

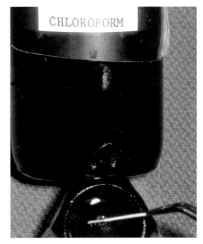

Fig. 18.19 The softened custom cone technique. The apical portion (3 to 4 mm) is dipped in chloroform for 1 to 2 seconds and then tamped in the canal.

7. The standard lateral compaction procedure follows, with spreader insertion, rotation, removal, and accessory cone placement until the spreader cannot be placed into the apical one third. More sealer is added by coating each accessory cone before placement.
8. A radiograph may be exposed to evaluate the obturation before searing off the excess coronally. The mass can easily be pulled out at this point and reobturation performed, if necessary.
9. Post space may be prepared immediately after obturation (Fig. 18.21).

Vertical Compaction

Vertical compaction is also an effective but more complex technique; its sealability is comparable to that of lateral compaction.[88] With the introduction of new devices, the warm vertical compaction technique has become somewhat more user friendly and also less time-consuming.

Indications

In general, vertical compaction can be used in the same situations as lateral compaction. It is preferred in a few circumstances, such as with internal resorption or other situations involving internal morphologic complexities.

Advantages and Disadvantages

The principal advantage of vertical compaction over lateral compaction is the ability to adapt the warmed and softened GP to the irregular surface architecture of the RCS.[89,90] Disadvantages include increased difficulty of length control, a more complicated procedure, and a larger assortment of required instruments.[88] Also, a somewhat larger canal preparation is necessary to allow insertion of the instruments to the required depths.

Technique

The warm vertical compaction technique requires a heat source and pluggers of various sizes for compaction of the thermoplasticized GP. Schilder pluggers begin at 0.4 mm in diameter (equal to ISO size No. 40) and increase by 0.1 mm for each successive instrument; the largest instrument is 1.1 mm in diameter (equal to ISO size No. 110).

The technique consists of fitting a GP cone with a taper similar to that of the instrumented RCS short of the apex and applying heat using a plugger. The GP is softened by the heat and becomes plastic. Pluggers are then placed in the canal with apical pressure to produce a hydraulic force that moves the GP apically, against the canal walls, and into RCS irregularities. such as accessory and lateral canals. GP is then added in small increments, and each increment of GP is heated and softened and packed vertically until the entire canal is filled. Detailed descriptions of the technique appear elsewhere.[91]

Other Warm Vertical Approaches

A recent modification of the warm vertical compaction technique is termed the *continuous wave of compaction*. Prerequisites for this technique are a tapering canal preparation, a constricted apical preparation, and an accurate cone fit. The technique is often used after preparation with nickel-titanium rotary files of greater taper. The heat source is an electrical device that supplies heat to a plugger on demand (Fig. 18.22). Pluggers are available in nonstandardized sizes that match the nonstandardized GP cones or in standardized sizes that match files of greater taper (Fig. 18.22). In addition, two hand

 18-1

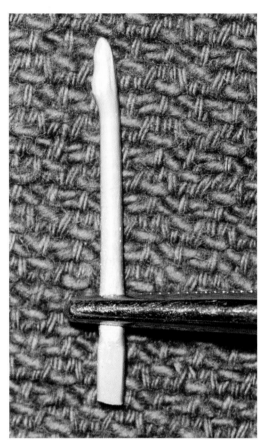

Fig. 18.20 After the softened cone has been tamped into the canal and then removed, it should show an impression of the apical region.

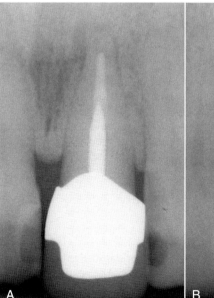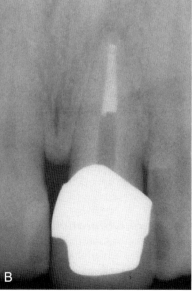

Fig. 18.21 **A,** Retreatment is required in this tooth due to persistent apical periodontitis. **B,** After post and gutta-percha removal and canal instrumentation, the apical 3 mm of the canal was impressed and obturated using a custom-formed gutta-percha cone. This was due to the irregular, resorptive nature of the apical portion of the canal. Post space was prepared after obturation. (Courtesy Dr. T. Remmers.)

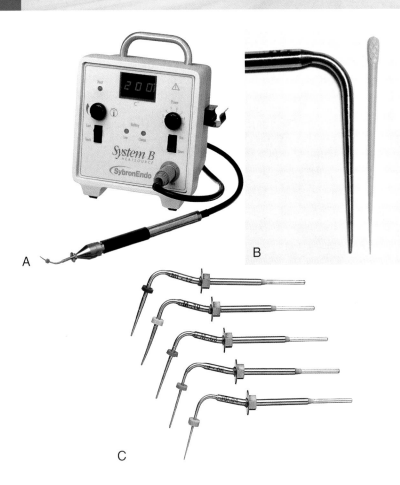

A

B

C

Fig. 18.22 A specialized heating device. **A,** Controlled current causes rapid heating of the plugger, which softens a prefit gutta-percha cone in the canal. **B,** "Continuous wave of condensation" plugger is designed to size-match the rotary file used to prepare the canal. Pluggers are also approximately matched to nonstandardized gutta-percha in an attempt to obturate the apical portion of a canal with a single cone. **C,** Pluggers are available in a variety of sizes and tapers. (Courtesy SybronEndo, Orange, Calif.)

pluggers of differing diameters are used to sustain and compact the GP apically.

Heat is applied at a prescribed temperature (200°C) for a short period, as determined by the clinician. Applying a constant source of heat to a prefitted GP cone allows hydraulic pressure to be applied in one continuous motion. As the plugger moves apically, the fit becomes more precise and the hydraulic pressure is increased, forcing the GP into canal irregularities. Details of the continuous wave of condensation technique are available in other publications.[92]

The continuous wave of compaction technique has not demonstrated advantages in long-term outcome, and there are inherent risks. When thermoplasticization is used, or any technique that physically alters GP, there is the potential for over-extension into the periapical tissues (Fig. 18.23) and for damage to the periodontal ligament and supporting alveolar bone from heat. An increase of 10°C above body temperature appears to be a critical threshold for permanent damage to osseous tissues at the surface of the root. Flame-heated carriers reach high temperatures and pose the greatest threat of damage to the periodontal structures.[93,94] When used properly, the injectable GP technique and the continuous wave compaction technique appear to produce temperature changes below the critical threshold.[95,96]

Sectional Obturation

A recent innovation is a technique that uses special devices and involves a two-phase sectional approach (Fig. 18.24). A small apical segment of GP is placed (down-packed), followed by back-filling of GP.[97,98] This technique seems

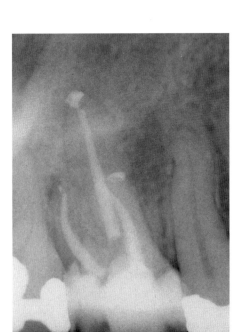

Fig. 18.23 Completed obturation using continuous wave of condensation with gutta-percha and sealer. This technique, as with any warm obturation method, tends to apically extrude sealer. The sealer usually absorbs with time. (Courtesy Dr. A. Hsiao.)

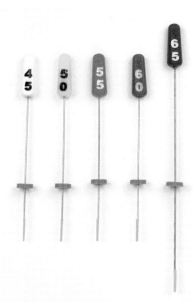

Fig. 18.24 Carriers with apical plugs of gutta-percha attached. Once inserted into a canal prepared with specially designed rotary files, the carrier is rotated in a counterclockwise direction to separate the gutta-percha from the carrier. The canal is then back-filled using lateral or warm compaction. Carriers are also available with resin plugs. (Courtesy Lightspeed Technology, San Antonio, Texas.)

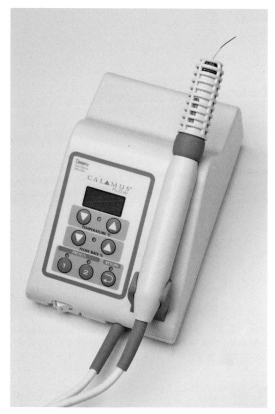

Fig. 18.26 A thermoplasticized injection device with 360-degree push-button technology and preloaded cartridges; this provides better tactile sensation for the injection of gutta-percha.

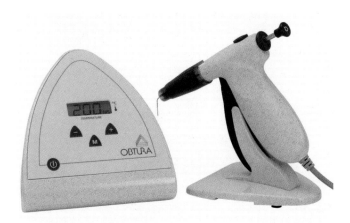

Fig. 18.25 A thermoplasticizing device. A high-heat gun softens gutta-percha into an injectable plastic mass. (Courtesy Obtura Spartan, Fenton, Mo.)

relatively fast and may prove useful but requires more investigation.[92] Details of the technique appear elsewhere.[93]

Thermoplasticized Injection
For thermoplasticization injection, specially formulated GP is warmed in injection devices (Fig. 18.25) and then injected in much the same manner as a caulking gun. Other devices are available that incorporate a 360 degree push-button technology and preloaded cartridges, allowing for better tactile sensation for the injection of GP (Fig. 18.26). When used in conjunction with a sealer, thermoplasticized injection provides an adequate seal.[99] This technique is useful in special situations (Fig. 18.27). However, lack of length control and shrinkage on cooling are potential disadvantages. This is a technique-sensitive methodology.

Solvent
Solvent techniques involve the total or partial dissolution of GP in solvents, primarily chloroform or eucalyptol. These techniques have names such as chloropercha, eucapercha, diffusion technique, or chloroform resin. Often these techniques are not used in conjunction with a standard sealer, but rather depend on softened GP to closely adapt to the wall of the RCS. The problem is that GP shrinks away from the walls as the solvents evaporate. Extensive leakage is generally seen with these techniques,[40] resulting in a poorer long-term prognosis.[100]

Solvent techniques are not recommended.

Carrier-Based Systems
Carrier-based systems typically use a plastic central carrier coated with GP. The carrier is flexible yet provides rigidity for the overlying GP. The obturators are tapered and standardized so that the carriers correspond to the size of instruments used in the prepared RCS. After preparation, the canal is dried and lightly coated with sealer. The appropriate-sized obturator is heated in a special oven and firmly placed to the WL. The carrier is then sectioned 1 to 2 mm above the orifice to the canal. These carrier/GP systems are equivalent to conventional GP obturation with apical sealing but may not consistently create a coronal seal (Fig. 18.28).[101-103] Special systems (devices) have been developed that use cross-linked GP as the carrier, allowing for easier placement and retreatment than can be done with traditional plastic or metal carriers (Fig. 18.29).

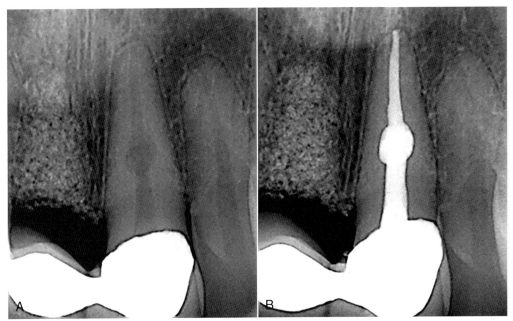

Fig. 18.27 Internal resorption. **A,** Lateral compaction is not the recommended technique for filling this defect once the canal has been cleaned and shaped. **B,** Thermoplastic injection of resin core obturating material was vertically compacted into the resorptive defect.

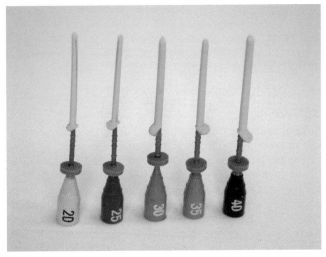

Fig. 18.28 A plastic carrier coated with gutta-percha is softened in a specially designed oven. Prior to obturation, the size verifier (without gutta-percha) is used to confirm the canal size. The tapered carrier both laterally and vertically compacts the gutta-percha as it is inserted into the sealer-lined canal. Once the gutta-percha has cooled, the handle is twisted off. (Courtesy Soft Core Axis Dental, Coppell, Texas.)

An advantage of the technique is the potential for the plasticized GP to effectively flow into RCS irregularities.[101] Disadvantages include a tendency for extrusion of the material periapically and difficulty removing the carrier and GP during retreatment.[102]

Newer Techniques and Materials

A new flowable GP obturation system was recently introduced (Fig. 18.30).[104] It is composed of a mixture of finely ground GP, silicone-based sealer, and silver particles. After trituration, the material is injected into a canal before the placement of a GP master cone. No compaction is necessary, and the

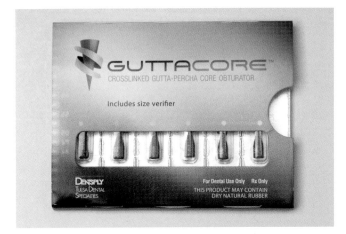

Fig. 18.29 Special systems (devices) have been developed that use cross-linked gutta-percha as the carrier; these allow easier placement and retreatment than do traditional plastic or metal carriers.

material reportedly self-cures in 30 minutes and expands slightly on setting. No heating is required with this system, and retreatment can be performed using conventional techniques. Clinically validated research on this material has been minimal and inconclusive.

Another recent development is glass ionomer–impregnated GP (Fig. 18.31).[105] The chemical bond between glass ionomers and dentin has been established.[106] However, the lack of an adequate bond to the core obturation material has been a major drawback for previous glass ionomer–based sealers. The current material apparently addresses this by incorporating glass ionomer particles into the GP cone, to which is applied a 2-µm glass ionomer coating. It is claimed (but has not been conclusively demonstrated) that these glass ionomer particles encourage the formation of a true bond between the glass ionomer–based sealer and the obturation cone. As with

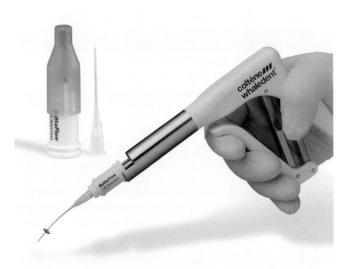

Fig. 18.30 GuttaFlow is a cold flowable injection system that combines a silicone-based matrix with finely ground gutta-percha. It is used with a master gutta-percha point, without the need for compaction. (Courtesy Coltene/Whaledent, Cuyahoga Falls, Ohio.)

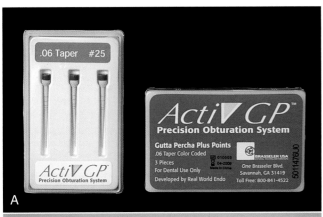

A

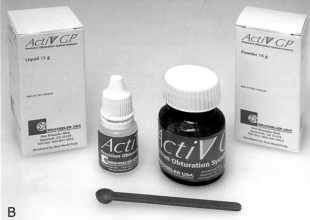

B

Fig. 18.31 Glass ionomer–coated gutta-percha points **(A)** are used with a glass ionomer sealer **(B)** to attempt to create a monoblock within the canal system. (Courtesy of Brasseler USA, Savannah, Ga.)

the polyester resin–based systems discussed previously, this bonding of the sealer to the dentin wall and obturation core is referred to as a *monoblock.* Because the working time of the glass ionomer–based sealer is insufficient, only a single-cone obturation technique is recommended. It is very difficult,

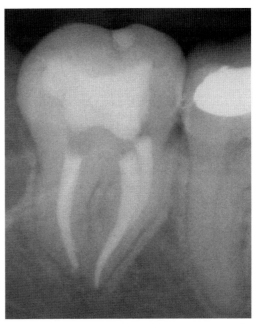

Fig. 18.32 Bayonet-shaped canals. Obturation was performed with a combination of techniques and materials. The result is good quality: no voids, uniform density, and the obturation reflects the taper created during canal preparation. Resin core and sealer were vertically compacted using the continuous wave technique, followed by back-filling with injectable thermoplasticized resin. (Courtesy Dr. T. Remmers.)

if not impossible, to adequately treat all the walls of the RCS with preparatory liquids. Research evaluating the efficacy of this system is not yet available.

Mineral trioxide aggregate (MTA) can be used as an alternative to GP for filling material.

 18-2

These new obturation systems are interesting and have potential. However, research verification of their clinical effectiveness is lacking.

EVALUATION OF OBTURATION

Surprisingly, evaluation of the completed obturation is difficult. The only means of immediate assessment is radiographic evaluation, which is imprecise at best. However, radiographic evaluation has been the standard and at least provides some criteria by which to judge the quality of the obturation .

Symptoms
The presence of symptoms for a few days after obturation is common and probably unrelated to the obturation itself. It reflects a different phenomenon, probably tissue irritation from the procedure.

Radiographic Criteria
A watertight seal cannot be evaluated on a radiograph. Only fairly gross discrepancies are visible, and these voids or deficiencies may or may not relate to lack of a seal and result in long-term failure.[107] The following are the radiologic evaluation criteria (Fig. 18.32).
- *Radiolucencies.* Voids in the body or at the interface of the obturating material and dentin wall indicate incomplete obturation.

- *Density.* The obturation mass should be of uniform density from the coronal to the apical aspect. The coronal region is more radiopaque than the apical region because of the greater thickness of the obturated mass in this area. The margins of GP should be distinct, with no fuzziness, indicating close adaptation to the walls of the RCS.
- *Length.* The material should extend to the prepared length and coronally be removed apically to a level apical to the orifice in posterior teeth and apical to the gingival margin in anterior teeth.
- *Taper.* The GP should reflect the prepared RCS. The taper need not be uniform but should be consistent.

Restoration

Whether definitive or temporary, the restoration should contact enough dentin surface to ensure a quality coronal seal.

Placement of the definitive buildup or restoration should be accomplished as soon as possible after obturation to help preclude leakage and contamination of the obturation and to protect weakened tooth structure. The restoration should also be placed under the rubber dam to maximize success.

THE FUTURE

Even though the materials and methodologies used today have resulted in high rates of healing, there is no question that better materials and methodologies remain undiscovered and await quality research and development that will open the doors to even better obturation, with resultant improvement in healing rates.

REFERENCES

1. Ingle JL, Beveridge E, Glick D, et al: The Washington study. In Ingle JI, Bakland LK, editors: *Endodontics*, ed 4, Baltimore, 1994, Williams & Wilkins.
2. Klevant FJH, Eggink CO: The effect of canal preparation on periapical disease, *Int Endod J* 16:68, 1983.
3. Ray H, Trope M, Buxt P, et al: Influence of various factors on the periapical status of endodontically treated teeth, *Int Endod J* 28:12, 1995.
4. Delivanis PD, Mattison GD, Mendel RW: The survivability of F43 strain of *Streptococcus sanguis* in root canals filled with gutta-percha and ProcoSol cement, *J Endod* 9:407, 1983.
5. Vianna ME, Horz HP, Conrads G, et al: Effect of root canal procedures on endotoxins and endodontic pathogens, *Oral Microbiol Imunol* 22:411, 2007.
6. Madison S, Swanson K, Chiles SA: An evaluation of coronal microleakage in endodontically treated teeth. II. Sealer types, *J Endod* 13:109, 1987.
7. Swanson KS, Madison S: An evaluation of coronal microleakage in endodontically treated teeth. I. Time periods, *J Endod* 13:56, 1987.
8. Khayat A, Lee SJ, Torabinejad M: Human saliva penetration of coronally unsealed obturated root canals, *J Endod* 19:458, 1993.
9. Magura ME, Kafrawy AH, Brown CE Jr, et al: Human saliva coronal microleakage in obturated root canals: an in vitro study, *J Endod* 17:324, 1991.
10. De-Deus G, Audi C, Murad C, et al: Sealing ability of oval-shaped canals filled using System B heat source with either gutta-percha or Resilon: an ex-vivo study using a polymicrobial leakage model, *Oral Surg Med Oral Pathol Oral Radiol Endod* 104:114, 2007.
11. Haapasalo M, Shen Y, Ricucci D: Reasons for persistent and emerging post-treatment endodontic disease, *Endod Topics* 18:31, 2011.
12. Strindberg LZ: The difference in the results of pulp therapy on certain factors, *Acta Odontol Scand Suppl* 14:21, 1956.
13. Smith C, Setchell D, Harty F: Factors influencing the success of conventional root canal therapy: a five-year retrospective study, *Int Endod J* 26:321, 1993.
14. Seltzer S, Soltanoff W, Smith J: Periapical tissue reactions to root canal instrumentation beyond the apex and root canal fillings short of and beyond the apex, *Oral Surg Oral Med Oral Pathol* 36:725, 1973.
15. Rappaport HM, Lilly GE, Kapsimalis P: Toxicity of endodontic filling materials, *Oral Surg Oral Med Oral Pathol* 18:785, 1964.
16. Olsson B, Sliwkowski A, Langeland K: Subcutaneous implantation for the biologic

evaluation of endodontic materials, *J Endod* 7:355, 1981.
17. Wu M, Wesselink P, Walton R: Apical terminus location of root canal treatment procedures, *Oral Surg Oral Med Oral Pathol* 89:99, 2000.
18. Sjogren U, Hagglund B, Sunqvist G, et al: Factors affecting the long-term results of endodontic treatment, *J Endod* 16:498, 1990.
19. Walton R: Histologic evaluation and comparison of different methods of pulp canal enlargement, *J Endod* 2:304, 1976.
20. Karabucak B, Kim A, Chen V, et al: The comparison of gutta-percha and Resilon penetration into lateral canals with different thermoplastic delivery systems, *J Endod* 34:847, 2008.
21. Ricucci D, Siqueira J: Fate of the tissue in lateral canals and apical ramifications in response to pathological conditions and treatment procedures, *J Endod* 36:1, 2010.
22. Walton RE, Michelich RJ, Smith GN: The histopathogenesis of vertical root fractures, *J Endod* 10:48, 1984.
23. Holcomb J, Pitts D, Nicholls J: Further investigation of spreader loads required to cause vertical root fracture during lateral condensation, *J Endod* 13:277, 1987.
24. Dang DA, Walton RE: Vertical root fracture and root distortion: effect of spreader design, *J Endod* 15:294, 1989.
25. Murgel CA, Walton RE: Vertical root fracture and dentin deformation in curved roots: the influence of spreader design, *Endod Dent Traumatol* 6:273, 1990.
26. Obermayr G, Walton RE, Leary JM, et al: Vertical root fracture and relative deformation during obturation and post cementation, *J Prosthet Dent* 66:181, 1991.
27. Barreto MS, Morales R, Breu de Rosa R, et al: Vertical root fractures and dentin defects: effects of root canal preparation, filling and mechanical cycling, *J Endod* 38:1135, 2012.
28. Saini HR, Tewari S, Sangwan P, et al: Effect of different apical preparation size on outcome of primary endodontic treatment: a randomized controlled trial, *J Endod* 38:1309, 2012.
29. Sjögren U, Figdor D, Spangberg L, et al: The antimicrobial effect of calcium hydroxide as a short-term intracanal dressing, *Int Endod J* 4:119, 1991.
30. Weiger R, Rosendahl R, Lost C: Influence of calcium hydroxide intracanal dressings on the prognosis of teeth with endodontically induced periapical lesions, *Int Endod J* 33:219, 2000.
31. Sjögren U, Figdor, Persson S, et al: Influence of infection at the time of root filling on the outcome

of endodontic treatment of teeth with apical periodontitis, *Int Endod J* 30:297, 1997.
32. Engstrom B, Segerstad L, Ramstrom G, et al: Correlation of positive cultures with the prognosis for root canal treatment, *Odontol Rev* 15:257, 1964.
33. Hugh C, Walton R, Facer R: Evaluation of intracanal sealer distribution with five different obturation techniques, *Quintessence Int* 36:721, 2005.
34. Grossman L: *Endodontic practice*, ed 11, p 242, Philadelphia, 1988, Lea & Febiger.
35. Marlin J, Schilder H: Physical properties of gutta percha, *Oral Surg Oral Med Oral Pathol* 32:260, 1971.
36. Cunningham KP, Walker MP, Kulild JC, et al: Variability of the diameter and taper of size #30, .04 gutta-percha cones, *J Endod* 32:1081, 2006.
37. Cardoso C, Kotaka C, Redmerski R, et al: Rapid decontamination of gutta-percha cones with sodium hypochlorite, *J Endod* 25:498, 1999.
38. Skinner RL, Himel VT: The sealing ability of injection-molded thermoplasticized gutta-percha with and without the use of sealers, *J Endod* 13:315, 1987.
39. Ravindranath M, Neelakantan P, Karpagavinayagam K, et al: The influence of obturation technique on sealer thickness and depth of sealer penetration into dentinal tubules evaluated by computer-aided digital analysis, *Gen Dent* 59:376, 2011.
40. Zakariasen KL, Stadem PS: Microleakage associated with modified eucapercha and chloropercha root canal filling techniques, *Int Endod J* 15:67, 1982.
41. Schilder H, Goodman A, Aldrich W: The thermomechanical properties of gutta-percha. V. Volume changes in bulk gutta-percha as a function of temperature and its relationship to molecular phase transformation, *Oral Surg Oral Med Oral Pathol* 59:285, 1985.
42. Facer R, Walton R: Intracanal distribution patterns of sealer after lateral condensation, *J Endod* 29:832, 2003.
43. Texeira FB, Texeira ECN, Thompson JY, et al: Fracture resistance of endodontically treated roots using a new type of resin filling material, *J Am Dent Assoc* 135:646, 2004.
44. Shipper G, Orstavik D, Texeira FB, et al: An evaluation of microbial leakage in roots filled with a thermoplastic synthetic polymer-based root canal filling material (Resinol), *J Endod* 30:342, 2004.
45. Biggs S, Knowles K, Ibarrola J, et al: In vitro assessment of the sealing ability of Resilon/Epiphany using fluid filtration, *J Endod* 32:759, 2006.

46. Baumgartner G, Zehnder M, Paque F: *Enterococcus faecalis* type strain leakage through root canals filled with gutta-percha/AH Plus or Resilon/Epiphany, *J Endod* 33:45, 2007.

47. Paque F, Balmer M, Attin T, et al: Preparation of oval-shaped root canals in the mandibular molars using nickel-titanium rotary instruments: a micro-computed tomography study, *J Endod* 36:703, 2010.

48. Johnson WT, Zakariasen KL: Spectrophotometric analysis of micro-leakage in the fine curved canals found in the mesial roots of mandibular molars, *Oral Surg Oral Med Oral Pathol* 56:305, 1983.

49. Timpawat S, Jensen J, Feigal RJ, et al: An in vitro study of the comparative effectiveness of obturating curved root canals with gutta-percha cones, silver cones, and stainless steel files, *Oral Surg Oral Med Oral Pathol* 55:180, 1983.

50. Zielke DR, Brady JM, del Rio CE: Corrosion of silver cones in bone: a scanning electron microprobe analysis, *J Endod* 1:11, 1975.

51. Krell K, Fuller M, Scott G: The conservative retrieval of silver cones in difficult cases, *J Endod* 10:269, 1984.

52. Serper A, Ucer O, Onur R, et al: Comparative neurotoxic effects of root canal filling materials on rat sciatic nerve, *J Endod* 24:592, 1998.

53. Concerning paraformaldehyde-containing endodontic filling materials and sealers American Association of Endodontics Position Statement, www.aae.org/guidelines/. October 13, 2013

54. Krakow A, Berk H: Efficient endodontic procedures with the use of the pressure syringe, *Dent Clin North Am* 9:387, 1965.

55. Fogel B: A comparative study of five materials for use in filling root canal spaces, *Oral Surg Oral Med Oral Pathol* 43:284, 1977.

56. Grossman L: *Endodontic practice*, ed 11, p 255, Philadelphia, 1988, Lea & Febiger.

57. Karapinar-Kazandag M, Bayrak OF, Yalvac ME, et al: Cytotoxicity of five endodontic sealers on L929 cell line and human pulp cells, *Int Endod J* 44:626, 2011.

58. van der Burgt T, Mullaney TP: Tooth discoloration induced by endodontic sealers, *Oral Surg Oral Med Oral Pathol* 61:84, 1986.

59. Parsons J, Walton R, Ricks-Williamson L: In vitro longitudinal assessment of coronal discoloration from endodontic sealers, *J Endod* 27:699, 2001.

60. Grossman LI: Solubility of root canal cements, *J Dent Res* 57:927, 1978.

61. Ørstavik D: Antibacterial properties of root canal sealers, cements and pastes, *Int Endod J* 14:27, 1981.

62. Allan N, Walton R, Schaffer M: Setting times for endodontic sealers under clinical usage and in vitro conditions, *J Endod* 27:421, 2000.

63. Leonardo M, Bezerra da Silva L, Filho M, et al: Release of formaldehyde by four endodontic sealers, *Oral Surg Oral Med Oral Pathol Oral Radiol Endod* 88:221, 1999.

64. Barnett F, Trope M, Rooney J, et al: In vivo sealing ability of calcium hydroxide–containing root canal sealers, *Endod Dent Traumatol* 5:23, 1989.

65. Desai S, Chandler N: Calcium hydroxide–based root canal sealers: a review, *J Endod* 35:475, 2009.

66. Pameijer C, Zmener O: Resin materials for root canal obturation, *Dent Clin North Am* 54:325, 2010.

67. Moshonov J, Trope M, Friedman S: Retreatment efficacy 3 months after obturation using glass ionomer cement, zinc oxide–eugenol, and epoxy resin sealers, *J Endod* 20:90, 1994.

68. Zhang W, Li Z, Peng B: Ex vivo cytotoxicity of a new calcium silicate–based canal filling material, *Int Endod J* 43:769, 2010.

69. Moradi S, Ghoddusi J, Forghani M: Evaluation of dentinal tubule penetration after the use of dentin bonding agent as a root canal sealer, *J Endod* 35:1563, 2009.

70. Benatti O, Stolf WL, Ruhnke LA: Verification of the consistency, setting time, and dimensional changes of root canal filling materials, *Oral Surg Oral Med Oral Pathol* 46:107, 1978.

71. Kahn F, Rosenberg P, Schertzer L, et al: An in-vitro evaluation of sealer placement methods, *Int Endod J* 30:181, 1997.

72. Wiemann AH, Wilcox LR: In vitro evaluation of four methods of sealer placement, *J Endod* 17:444, 1991.

73. Aguirre A, El Deeb M, Aguirre R: The effect of ultrasonics on sealer distribution and sealing of root canals, *J Endod* 23:759, 1997.

74. Director RC, Rabinowitz JL, Miline RS: The short-term sealing properties of lateral condensation, vertical condensation and Hydron using ^{14}C human serum albumin, *J Endod* 8:149, 1982.

75. Lee M, Winkler J, Hartwell G, et al: Current trends in endodontic practice: emergency treatments and technological armamentarium, *J Endod* 35:35, 2009.

76. Sakkal S, Weine FS, Lemian L: Lateral condensation: inside view, *Compendium* 12:796, 1991.

77. Amditis C, Blackler S, Bryant R, et al: The adaptation achieved by four root canal filling techniques as assessed by three methods, *Aust Dent J* 37:439, 1992.

78. Simons J, Ibanez B, Friedman S, et al: Leakage after lateral condensation with finger spreaders and D-11-T spreaders, *J Endod* 17:101, 1991.

79. Schmidt K, Walker T, Johnson J, et al: Comparison of nickel-titanium and stainless-steel spreader penetration and accessory cone fit in curved canals, *J Endod* 26:42, 2000.

80. Allison DA, Michelich RJ, Walton RE: The influence of MC adaptation on the quality of the apical seal, *J Endod* 11:166, 1981.

81. Yared GM, Bou Dagher FE: Elongation and movement of the gutta-percha MC during initial lateral condensation, *J Endod* 19:395, 1993.

82. Baumgardner K, Krell K: Ultrasonic condensation of gutta-percha: an in vitro dye penetration and scanning electron microscopic study, *J Endod* 16:253, 1990.

83. Augsberger RA, Peters DD: Radiographic evaluation of extruded obturation materials, *J Endod* 16:492, 1990.

84. McDonald MN, Vire DE: Chloroform in the endodontic operatory, *J Endod* 18:301, 1992.

85. Allard N, Andersson L: Exposure of dental personnel to chloroform in root-filling procedures, *Endod Dent Traumatol* 8:155, 1992.

86. Keane KM, Harrington GW: The use of chloroform softened gutta-percha MC and its effects on the apical seal, *J Endod* 10:57, 1984.

87. Yancich PP, Hartwell GR, Portell FR: A comparison of apical seal: chloroform versus eucalyptol-dipped gutta-percha obturation, *J Endod* 15:257, 1989.

88. Peng L, Ling Y, Tan H, et al: Outcome of root canal obturation by warm gutta-percha versus cold lateral condensation: a meta-analysis, *J Endod* 33:106, 2007.

89. Wolcott J, Himel V, Powell W: Effect of two obturation techniques on the filling of lateral canals and the main canal, *J Endod* 23:632, 1997.

90. DuLac K, Nielsen C, Tomazic T, et al: Comparison of the obturation of lateral canals by six techniques, *J Endod* 25:376, 1999.

91. Schilder H: Vertical compaction of warm gutta-percha. In Gerstein H, editor: *Techniques in clinical endodontics*, Philadelphia, 1983, Saunders.

92. Buchanan S: Continuous wave of condensation technique, *Endod Pract* 2:7, 1998.

93. Hand R, Hugel E, Tsaknis P: Effects of a warm gutta percha technique on the lateral periodontium, *Oral Surg Oral Med Oral Pathol* 36:872, 1983.

94. Lee F, VanCura J, BeGole E: A comparison of root surface temperatures using different obturation heat sources, *J Endod* 24:617, 1998.

95. Weller RN, Koch K: In vitro radicular temperatures produced by injectable thermoplasticized gutta-percha, *Int Endod J* 25:593, 1999.

96. Floren J, Weller RN, Pashly D, et al: Changes in root surface temperatures with in vitro use of the System B HeatSource, *J Endod* 25:593, 1999.

97. Santos M, Walker W, Carnes D: Evaluation of apical seal in straight canals after obturation using the Lightspeed sectional method, *J Endod* 25:609, 1999.

98. Senia S: Canal diameter: the forgotten dimension, *Endod Pract* 3:34, 2000.

99. Evans JT, Simon JHS: Evaluation of the apical seal produced by injected thermoplasticized gutta-percha in the absence of smear layer and root canal sealer, *J Endod* 12:101, 1986.

100. Ørstavik D, Kerekes K, Eriksen HM: Clinical performance of three endodontic sealers, *Endod Dent Traumatol* 3:178, 1987.

101. Chu CH, Lo ECM, Cheung GSP: Outcome of root canal treatment using Thermafil and cold lateral condensation filling techniques, *Int Endod J* 38:179, 2005.

102. Baumgardner K, Taylor J, Walton R: Canal adaptation and coronal leakage: lateral condensation compared to Thermafil, *J Am Dent Assoc* 126:351, 1995.

103. Ordinalo-Zapata R, Bramante M, Bernardineli N, et al: A preliminary study of the percentage of sealer penetration in roots obturated with the Thermafil and RealSeal-1 obturation techniques in mesial root canals of mandibular molars, *Oral Surg Oral Med Oral Pathol* 108:961, 2009.

104. Elayouti A, Achleithner C, Lost C, et al: Homogeneity and adaptation of a new gutta-percha paste to root canal walls, *J Endod* 31:687, 2005.

105. Koch K, Brave D: Endodontic synchronicity, *Compend Contin Educ Dent* 26:218, 2005.

106. De Bruyne MA, De Moor RJ: The use of glass ionomer cements in both conventional and surgical endodontics, *Int Endod J* 37:91, 2004.

107. Youngson C, Nattress B, Manogue M, et al: In vitro radiographic representation of the extent of voids within obturated root canals, *Int Endod J* 28:77, 1995.

Procedural accidents

Mahmoud Torabinejad, James D. Johnson

CHAPTER OUTLINE

Perforations During Access Preparation
Accidents During Cleaning and Shaping

Accidents During Obturation
Accidents During Post Space Preparation

LEARNING OBJECTIVES

After reading this chapter, the student should be able to:
1. Recognize procedural accidents and describe the causes, prevention, and treatment of the following:
   a. Pulp chamber perforation during access preparation
   b. Ledging
   c. Obstruction of the canal with dental materials or dentin shavings

d. Coronal or radicular perforation
e. Separated instrument
f. Obturation short of the prepared working length
g. Expression of obturation materials beyond the apex
h. Incomplete obturation
i. Vertical root fracture
j. Post space preparation mishaps

A s can other complex disciplines of dentistry, root canal therapy can present unwanted or unforeseen challenges that can affect the prognosis. These mishaps are collectively termed *procedural accidents*. However, fear of procedural accidents should not deter a practitioner from performing root canal treatment if proper case selection and competency issues are observed.

Knowledge of the etiologic factors involved in procedural accidents is essential for prevention. In addition, methods of recognition and treatment and the effects of such accidents on the prognosis must be learned. Most problems can be avoided by adhering to the basic principles of diagnosis, case selection, treatment planning, access preparation, cleaning and shaping, obturation, and post space preparation.

Examples of procedural accidents include swallowed or aspirated endodontic instruments, crown or root perforation, ledge formation, separated instruments, underfilled or overfilled canals, and vertically fractured roots. A good practitioner uses knowledge, dexterity, intuition, patience, and awareness of personal limitations to minimize these accidents. When an accident occurs during root canal treatment, the patient should be informed about (1) the incident, (2) procedures necessary for correction, (3) alternative treatment modalities, and (4) the effect of this accident on the prognosis. Proper medical-legal documentation is mandatory. A successful practitioner learns from past experiences and applies them to future challenges. In addition, the practitioner who knows her or his own limitations is able to recognize potentially difficult cases and refers the patient to an endodontist. The beneficiary is the patient, who thus receives the best care.

This chapter discusses the causes, prevention, and treatment of various types of procedural accidents that may occur at different phases of root canal treatment. The effects of these accidents on the short-term and long-term prognoses also are described.

PERFORATIONS DURING ACCESS PREPARATION

The prime objective of an access cavity is to provide an unobstructed or straight-line pathway to the apical foramen (Fig. 19.1). Accidents such as excess removal of tooth structure or perforation may occur during attempts to locate canals. Failure to achieve straight-line access is often the main etiologic factor for other types of intracanal accidents.

Causes

Despite anatomic variations in the configuration of various teeth, the pulp chamber in most cases is located in the *center* of the anatomic crown. The pulp system is located in the long axis of the tooth. Lack of attention to the degree of axial inclination of a tooth in relation to adjacent teeth and to alveolar bone may result in either gouging or perforation of the crown or the root at various levels (Fig. 19.2). After the proper access outline form has been established, failure to direct the bur parallel to the long axis of a tooth causes gouging or perforation of the root. This problem often occurs when the dentist must use the reflected image from an intraoral mirror to make the access preparation. In these situations, the natural

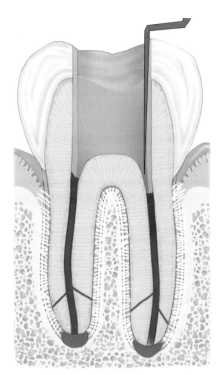

Fig. 19.1 Making an unobstructed and straight-line pathway to the apical foramen of root canals prevents accidental procedures.

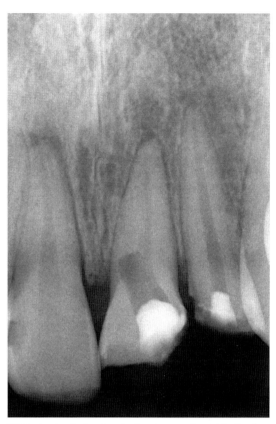

Fig. 19.2 Lack of attention to the degree of axial inclination of the central incisor in relation to adjacent teeth and to alveolar bone resulted in severe gouging and near perforation in an otherwise simple access preparation.

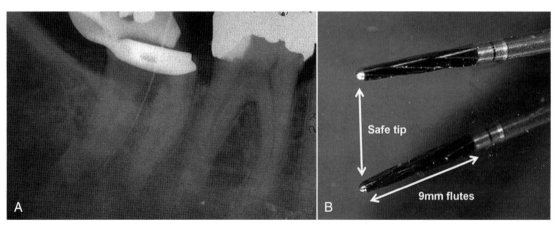

Fig. 19.3 **A,** Failure to recognize when the bur passes through the roof of the pulp chamber in a calcified pulp chamber may result in gouging or perforation of the furcation. The use of apex locators and angled radiographs is necessary for early perforation detection. Early detection reduces damage and improves repair. **B,** Use of a "safe-ended" access bur prevents perforation of the chamber floor.

tendency is to direct the bur away from the long axis of the root to improve vision through the mirror. Failure to check the orientation of the access opening during preparation may result in a perforation. The dentist should stop periodically to review the bur-tooth relationship. Aids for evaluating progress include transillumination, magnification, and radiographs.

Searching for the pulp chamber or orifices of canals through an underprepared access cavity may also result in accidents.

Failure to recognize when the bur passes through a small or flattened (disklike) pulp chamber in a multirooted tooth may also result in gouging or perforation of the furcation (Fig. 19.3, *A*). Use of a "safe-ended" access bur (Fig. 19.3, *B*) can prevent perforation of the chamber floor.

A cast crown often is not aligned in the long axis of the tooth; directing the bur along the misaligned casting may result in a coronal or radicular perforation.

Prevention
Clinical Examination

Thorough knowledge of tooth morphology, including both the surface and internal anatomies and their relationship, is mandatory to prevent pulp chamber perforations. Next, the location and angulation of the tooth must be related to adjacent teeth and alveolar bone to avoid a misaligned access preparation. In addition, radiographs of teeth from different angles provide information about the size and extent of the pulp chamber and the presence of internal changes such as calcification or resorption. *The radiograph is a two-dimensional projection of a three-dimensional object.* Varying the horizontal exposure angle provides at least a distorted view of the third dimension and may be helpful in supplying additional anatomic information. Cone beam computed tomography (CBCT) can also provide invaluable information in cases involving severe calcification or unusual canal anatomy. In complex cases, referral to an endodontist may be indicated.

Operative Procedures

Use of a rubber dam (Fig. 19.4) during root canal treatment is usually indicated.[1-3] However, when problems in locating pulp chambers are anticipated (e.g., tilted teeth, misoriented castings, or calcified chambers), initiating access without a rubber dam is preferred because it allows better crown-root alignment.[4] When access is made without rubber dam placement, no intracanal instruments, such as files, reamers, or broaches, should be used unless they are secured by a piece of floss[4] and a throat pack has been placed. Constricted chambers or canals must be sought patiently, with small amounts of dentin removed at a time.

Failure to recognize when the bur passes through the roof of the pulp chamber, if the chamber is calcified, may result in gouging or perforation of the furcation. As mentioned previously, after penetration of the roof of the chamber, use of a "safe-ended" access bur, such as the Endo Z (Dentsply/Maillefer, Tulsa, Oklahoma) or a pulp shaper bur (Dentsply/Tulsa Dental, Tulsa, Oklahoma), can prevent perforation of the chamber floor.

The use of electronic apex locators and angled radiographs is necessary for early perforation detection. Early detection reduces damage caused by continued treatment (irrigation, cleaning, and shaping) and improves the prognosis for nonsurgical repair.

Another useful method of providing isolation and also visualizing the crown-root alignment is the use of a "split" dam. This dam can be applied in the anterior region without a rubber dam clamp (see Chapter 15) or in posterior regions by quadrant isolation if a distal tooth can be clamped. Also, elimination of the metal clamp from the field of operation allows radiographic orientation of a coronal access preparation.

To orient the access, a bur may be placed in the preparation hole (secured with cotton pellets) and then radiographed (Fig. 19.5). This provides information about the depth of access in relation to the canal's location. Remember, a single canal is located in the center of the root. A direct facial radiograph shows the mesiodistal relationship; a mesial- or distal-angled film shows the faciolingual location. This procedure is helpful for locating small canals.

Use of a fiberoptic light during access preparation may assist in locating canals. This strong light illuminates the cavity when the beam is directed through the access opening (reflected light) and illuminates the pulp chamber floor (transmitted light). In the latter case, a canal orifice appears as a dark spot. Using magnifying glasses or an operative microscope[5-7] also aids in locating a small orifice. Magnification loupes (2.5 or greater) are helpful, especially when used with transillumination. The ultimate aid in canal location is the operating microscope. Patients with problems requiring significant magnification for canal location should be referred to an endodontist who has this specialized equipment.

Recognition and Treatment

Perforation into the periodontal ligament (PDL) or bone usually (but not always) results in immediate and continuous hemorrhage. The canal or chamber is difficult to dry, and placement of a paper point or cotton pellet may increase or renew the bleeding. Bone is relatively avascular compared with soft tissue. Mechanical perforation may initially produce only hemorrhage equal to that of pulp tissue.

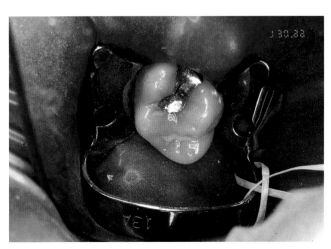

Fig. 19.4 A rubber dam must be applied in the anterior and posterior teeth. It provides isolation of the target tooth and prevents procedural accidents.

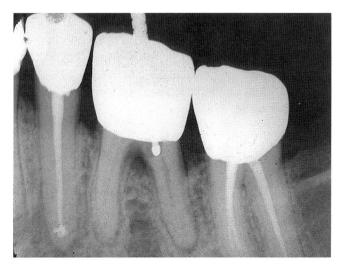

Fig. 19.5 A small bur is placed during access preparation when orientation is a problem. This provides information about angulation and depth of bur penetration.

Perforations must be recognized early to avoid subsequent damage to the periodontal tissues with intracanal instruments and irrigants. Early signs of perforation may include one or more of the following: (1) sudden pain during the working length determination when local anesthesia was adequate during access preparation; (2) the sudden appearance of hemorrhage; (3) burning pain or a bad taste during irrigation with sodium hypochlorite; and (4) other signs, including a radiographically malpositioned file or a PDL reading from an apex locator that is short of the working length on an initial file entry.

Unusually severe postoperative pain may result from cleaning and shaping procedures performed through an undetected perforation. At a subsequent appointment the perforation site will be hemorrhagic because of inflammation of the surrounding tissues. The overall prognosis of the tooth must be evaluated with respect to the strategic value of the tooth, the location and size of the defect, and the potential for repair.

Perforation into the PDL at any location has a negative effect on the long-term prognosis. The dentist must inform the patient of the questionable prognosis[1] and closely monitor the long-term periodontal response to any treatment. In addition, the patient must know what signs or symptoms indicate failure and, if failure occurs, what the subsequent treatment will be.

Perforations during access cavity preparation present a variety of problems. When a perforation occurs or is strongly suspected, the patient should be considered for referral to an endodontist. In general, a specialist is better equipped to manage these patients (Fig. 19.6). Also, after long-term evaluation, other procedures, such as surgery, may be necessary if future failure occurs.

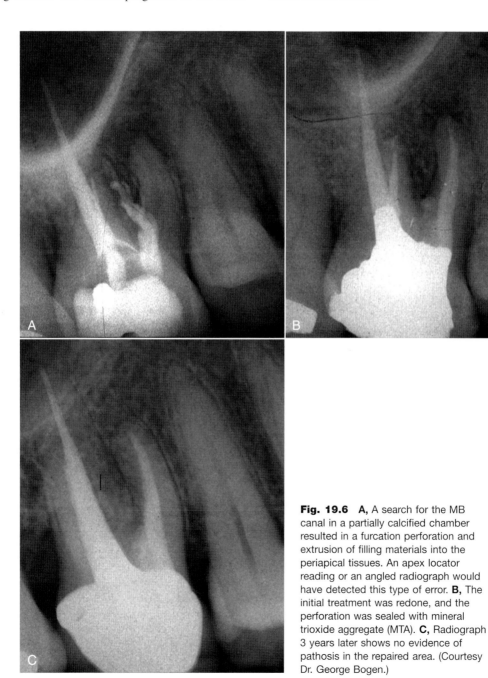

Fig. 19.6 **A,** A search for the MB canal in a partially calcified chamber resulted in a furcation perforation and extrusion of filling materials into the periapical tissues. An apex locator reading or an angled radiograph would have detected this type of error. **B,** The initial treatment was redone, and the perforation was sealed with mineral trioxide aggregate (MTA). **C,** Radiograph 3 years later shows no evidence of pathosis in the repaired area. (Courtesy Dr. George Bogen.)

Lateral Root Perforation

The location and size of the perforation during access are important factors in a lateral perforation. If the defect is located at or above the height of crestal bone, the prognosis for perforation repair is favorable.[8,9] These defects can be easily "exteriorized" and repaired with a standard restorative material, such as amalgam, glass ionomer, or composite. Periodontal curettage or a flap procedure is occasionally required to place, remove, or smooth excess repair material. In some cases, the best repair is placement of a full crown with the margin extended apically to cover the defect.

Teeth with perforations below the crestal bone in the coronal third of the root generally have the poorest prognosis. Attachment often recedes, and a periodontal pocket forms, with attachment loss extending apically to at least the depth of the defect. The treatment goal is to position the apical portion of the defect above the crestal bone. Orthodontic root extrusion is generally the procedure of choice for teeth in the esthetic zone.[10-12] Surgical crown lengthening may be considered when the esthetic result will not be compromised or when adjacent teeth require surgical periodontal therapy. Internal repair of these perforations with mineral trioxide aggregate (MTA) has been shown to provide an excellent seal compared to other materials.[13]

Furcation Perforation

A perforation of the furcation is generally one of two types: the "direct" or the "stripping" type. Each is created and managed differently, and the prognoses vary. A *direct perforation* usually occurs during a search for a canal orifice. It is more of a "punched-out" defect into the furcation with a bur and is usually accessible, may be small, and may have walls. This type of perforation should be immediately (if possible) repaired with MTA (Fig. 19.7). If proper conditions exist (dryness), glass ionomer or composite can be used to seal the defect. The prognosis is usually good if the defect is sealed immediately.

A *stripping perforation* involves the furcation side of the coronal root surface and results from excessive flaring with files or drills. Whereas direct perforations are usually accessible and therefore can be repaired nonsurgically, stripping perforations are generally inaccessible, requiring more elaborate approaches. The usual consequences of untreated stripping perforations are inflammation and subsequent development of a periodontal pocket. Long-term failure results from leakage of the repair material, which produces periodontal breakdown with attachment loss. Skillful use of MTA has significantly improved the prognosis of nonsurgical repair of stripping perforations compared with other repair materials (Fig. 19.8).

Nonsurgical Treatment

If feasible, nonsurgical repair (Fig. 19.9) of furcation perforations is preferred over surgical intervention.[4] Traditionally, materials such as amalgam, gutta-percha, zinc oxide–eugenol, Cavit, calcium hydroxide, freeze-dried bone, and indium foil have been used clinically and experimentally to seal these defects.[14-23] Repair is difficult because of potential problems with visibility, hemorrhage control, and management and sealing ability of the repair materials. In general, perforations occurring during access preparation should be sealed immediately, but the patency of the canals must be protected. Immediate repair of the perforations with MTA offers the best results for perforation repair.[22-27]

Surgical Treatment

Surgery requires more complex restorative procedures and more demanding oral hygiene from the patient.[9] Surgical alternatives include repair of the perforation with MTA if accessible by a surgical approach. If the perforation is not repairable or accessible by a surgical approach, hemisection, bicuspidization, root amputation, or intentional replantation should be considered. Teeth with divergent roots and bone levels that allow preparation of adequate crown margins are suitable for either hemisection or bicuspidization. Intentional replantation (Fig. 19.10) is indicated when the defect is inaccessible or when multiple problems exist, such as a perforation combined with a separated instrument, or when the prognosis for other surgical procedures is poor. Dentist and patient must recognize that the prognosis for treatment of surgically altered teeth is guarded because of the increased technical difficulty associated with restorative procedures and the demanding oral hygiene requirements. The remaining roots are prone to caries, periodontal disease, and vertical root fracture. Treatment planning options, including extraction, should be discussed with the patient when the prognosis is poor.

Prognosis

Factors affecting the long-term prognosis of teeth after perforation repair include the location of the defect in relation to the crestal bone, length of the root trunk, accessibility for repair, size of the defect, presence or absence of a periodontal communication to the defect, time lapse between perforation and repair, sealing ability of the restorative material, and subjective factors, such as the technical competence of the dentist and the attitude and oral hygiene practices of the patient.[4] Early recognition and repair improve the prognosis by minimizing damage to the periodontal tissues from bacteria, files, and irrigants. Additionally, a small perforation (less than 1 mm) causes less tissue destruction and is more amenable to repair than a larger perforation. Electronic apex locators or angled radiographs with files in place aid in early detection.

An unrecognized or untreated perforation in the furcation usually results in a periodontal defect that communicates through the gingival sulcus within weeks or sometimes days.

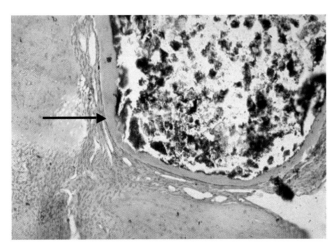

Fig. 19.7 Immediate repair of a perforation in the furcation of a dog premolar with MTA results in the formation of cementum *(arrow)* adjacent to the material.

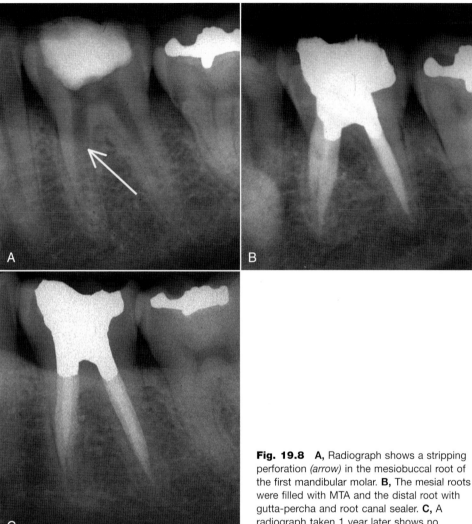

Fig. 19.8 **A,** Radiograph shows a stripping perforation *(arrow)* in the mesiobuccal root of the first mandibular molar. **B,** The mesial roots were filled with MTA and the distal root with gutta-percha and root canal sealer. **C,** A radiograph taken 1 year later shows no periradicular pathosis.

A preexisting periodontal communication caused by perforation worsens the prognosis; the time between perforation and repair should be as short as possible.[22,28] Immediate sealing of the defect reduces the incidence of periodontal breakdown. To best determine the long-term prognosis, the dentist must monitor the patient's symptoms, any radiographic changes and, most important, the periodontal status. Radiographs and periodontal probing during recall examination are the best measures of success or failure of the repair procedure.

ACCIDENTS DURING CLEANING AND SHAPING

The most common procedural accidents during cleaning and shaping of the root canal system are ledge formation, artificial canal creation, root perforation, instrument separation, and extrusion of irrigating solution periapically. Correction of these accidents is usually difficult, and the patient should be referred to an endodontist.

Ledge Formation
By definition, a ledge has been created when the working length can no longer be negotiated and the original patency of the canal is lost. The major causes of ledge formation include (1) inadequate straight-line access into the canal, (2) inadequate irrigation or lubrication, (3) excessive enlargement of a curved canal with files, and (4) packing of debris in the apical portion of the canal.

Prevention of a Ledge
Preoperative Evaluation
Prevention of ledging begins with examination of the preoperative radiograph of the canal for curvatures, length, and initial size.

Curvatures
Most important is the coronal third of the root canal. Severe coronal curvature predisposes the apical canal to ledging. Straight-line access to the orifice of the canal can be achieved during access preparation, but accessibility to the apical third of the canal is achieved only with coronal flaring. Severe apical curvatures require a proper sequence of cleaning and shaping procedures to maintain patency (see Chapter 16).

Length
Longer canals are more prone to ledging than shorter canals. Careful attention to maintaining patency is required to prevent ledging.

343

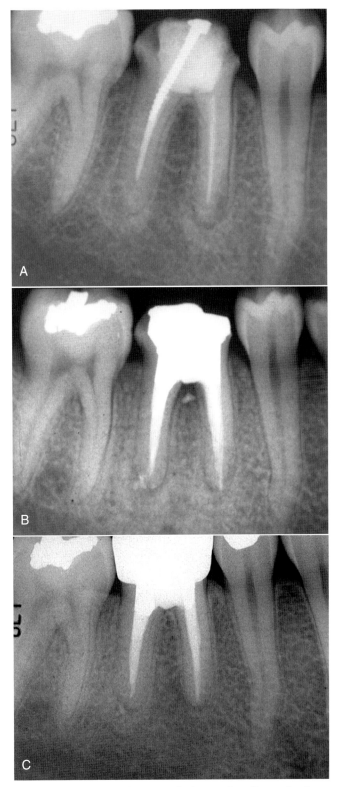

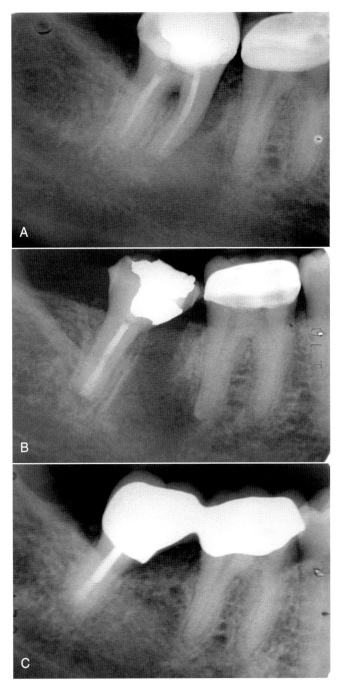

Fig. 19.9 **A,** Periapical radiograph shows a furcation perforation in the first mandibular molar. **B,** The root canal was retreated, and the perforation was repaired with MTA. **C,** Radiograph taken 26 months later shows no evidence of furcal pathosis.

Fig. 19.10 **A,** Postoperative radiograph from a 58-year-old female after endodontic treatment. The patient is percussion sensitive, and periapical lesions are present. A 7-mm periodontal pocket exists on the mesiobuccal aspect of the mesial root of the second molar. A fracture is suspected, and extract-replant was performed for diagnostic reasons. The tooth was extracted, and a fracture was noted on the mesial root. **B,** The mesial root was resected, and the tooth was replanted after retrofilling of the distal root with MTA. **C,** Radiograph 1 year later shows osseous repair and restoration of this tooth. The periodontal pocket healed.

Initial Size

Smaller diameter canals are more easily ledged than larger diameter canals.

In summary, *the canals most prone to ledging are small, curved, and long.* Radiographs are two dimensional and cannot provide accurate information about the actual shape and curvature of the root canal system. All root canals have some degree of curvature, including faciolingual curves, which may not be apparent on straight facial exposures.

Technical Procedures

Determination of working length in the cleaning and shaping process is a continuation of the access preparation. Optimum straight-line access to the apical third is not achieved until cleaning and shaping have been completed. An accurate working length measurement is a requirement because cleaning and shaping short of the ideal length become a prelude to ledge formation. Frequent recapitulation and irrigation, along with the use of lubricants, are mandatory. Sodium hypochlorite may be used initially for hemorrhage control and removal of debris. However, this agent alone may not be adequate to provide maximum lubrication.

Silicone, glycerin, and wax-based lubricants are commercially available for canal lubrication. Because these materials are viscous, they are carried into the apical regions of the canal with the file. Enhanced lubrication permits easier file insertion, reduces stress to the file, and assists with the removal of debris. The lubricant is easily removed with sodium hypochlorite irrigation. Flexible files (nickel-titanium) with noncutting tips reduce the chances of ledge formation.

With hand files, a one-eighth to one-fourth reaming motion should be used in the apical third. A filing motion directed away from the furcation is used to form the funnel shape of the canal and reduce the coronal curvature. Each file must be worked until it is loose before a larger size is used.

Canals with a severe coronal curvature require a passive step-back cleaning and shaping technique (see Chapter 16). A No. 15 file is used at working length. With maximum irrigation or lubrication, the canal is passively and progressively flared in a step-back fashion. The No. 15 file is recapitulated many times to maintain patency. This preflaring technique reduces the coronal curvature and enlarges the canal. Better control of the files is gained for enlarging and cleaning the apical third of the canal as the last step (see the section Apical Canal Preparation in Chapter 16). Using this technique, the chances of ledge formation are reduced. Rotary files with increased taper blend and join the shape into a tapering funnel.

Management of a Ledge

Once created, a ledge is difficult to correct. An initial attempt should be made to bypass the ledge with a No. 10 steel file to regain working length. The file tip (2 to 3 mm) is sharply bent and worked in the canal in the direction of the canal curvature. Lubricants are helpful. A "picking" motion is used to attempt to feel the catch of the original canal space, which is slightly short of the apical extent of the ledge. If the original canal is located, the file is then worked with a reaming motion and a repeated, short, up-and-down movement to maintain the space and remove debris (Fig. 19.11), although this may be only partially successful. Once a ledge has been created, even if it is initially bypassed, instruments and obturating materials tend to be continually directed into the ledge.

If the original canal cannot be located by this method, cleaning and shaping of the existing canal space is completed at the new working length. At times, flaring of the canal may allow the ledge to be bypassed by providing improved access to the apical canal. Small, curved files are used in the manner previously described in a final attempt to bypass the ledge. If this is successful, the apical canal space must be sequentially cleaned and flared to an appropriate size. Complete removal or reduction of the ledge facilitates obturation.

Prognosis

Failure of root canal treatment associated with ledging depends on the amount of debris left in the uninstrumented and unfilled portion of the canal. The amount depends on when ledge formation occurred during the cleaning and shaping process. In general, short and cleaned apical ledges have a good prognosis. Teeth with vital pulp tissue apical to a ledge generally have a better prognosis than teeth with necrotic, infected tissue, apical to a ledge, that had not been cleaned out before the formation of the ledge. The patient must be informed of the prognosis, the importance of the recall examination, and signs that indicate failure. Future appearance of clinical symptoms or radiographic evidence of failure may require referral for apical surgery or retreatment.

Artificial Canal Creation
Cause and Prevention

Deviation from the original pathway of the root canal system and creation of an artificial canal cause an exaggerated ledge. This situation arises from the factors that cause ledge formation; therefore, the recommendations for preventing ledge formation should be followed to avoid creation of artificial canals. The unfortunate sequence is as follows: A ledge is created, and the proper working length is lost. The operator, eager to regain that length, "bores" apically with each file, creating an artificial canal. Used persistently, the file eventually perforates the root surface. Aggressive use of stainless steel files is the most common cause of this problem.

Management

Negotiating the original canal with the exaggerated ledge is normally very difficult. Rarely can the original canal be located, renegotiated, and prepared. To obturate, the dentist should determine whether a perforation exists. Methods include apex locator readings, hemorrhage on paper points while drying, and radiographs with a file in position. If a perforation is confirmed, the working length is adjusted to create an apical stop within sound tooth structure at the adjusted length with larger files, and obturation is begun. If there is no perforation, the canal is obturated with a warm or softened gutta-percha technique in conjunction with a root canal sealer. If there is a perforation, the defect should be repaired internally or surgically (see the section Root Perforations in this chapter). The formation of an apical barrier with MTA permits obturation of the canal without apical extrusion of gutta-percha.

Prognosis

The prognosis depends on the ability of the operator to renegotiate the original canal and the remaining uninstrumented and unfilled portion of the main canal. Unless a perforation

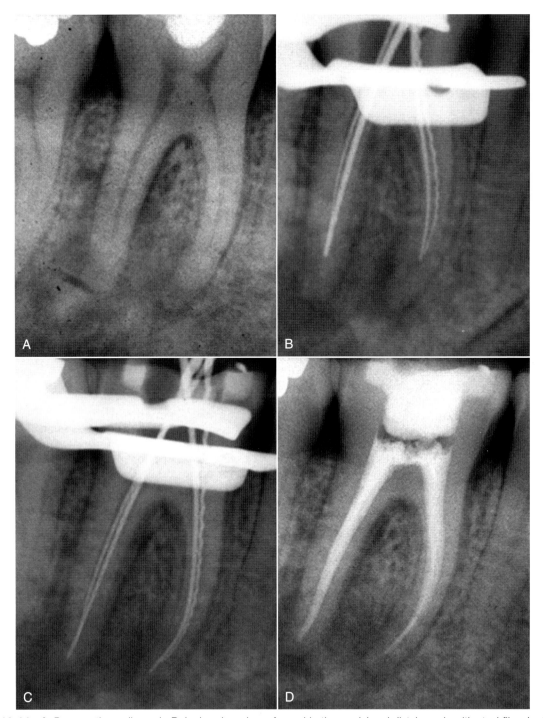

Fig. 19.11 **A,** Preoperative radiograph. **B,** Ledges have been formed in the mesial and distal canals with steel files. Ledges can be bypassed only with small, curved steel files. **C,** Ledges are bypassed and proper length is established. **D,** Final radiograph shows complete obturation of root canals.

exists, teeth in which the original canal can be renegotiated and obturated have a prognosis similar to that for teeth without procedural complications. In contrast, when a large portion of the main canal is uninstrumented and unobturated, the result is a poorer prognosis, and the tooth must be examined periodically. Failure usually means surgery will be required to resect the uninstrumented and unobturated root canal.

Root Perforations
Roots may be perforated at different levels during cleaning and shaping. The location of the perforation (apical, middle, or cervical) and the stage of treatment affect the prognosis.[17,28] The periodontal response to the injury is affected by the level and size of the perforation. Perforation in the early stages of cleaning and shaping affects the prognosis significantly.

Apical Perforations

Apical perforations occur through the apical foramen (over-instrumentation) or through the body of the root (perforated new canal).

Etiology and Indicators

Instrumentation of the canal beyond the apical constriction results in perforation. An incorrect working length or inability to maintain a proper working length causes "zipping"[4] or "blowing out" of the apical foramen. The appearance of fresh hemorrhage in the canal or on instruments, pain during canal preparation in a previously asymptomatic tooth, and sudden loss of the apical stop are indicators of foramen perforation. Extension of the largest (final) file beyond the radiographic apex is also a sign. An electronic apex locator may also confirm this procedural accident.

Prevention

To prevent apical perforation, proper working lengths must be established and maintained throughout the procedure. In curved canals, the flexibility of files with respect to size must be considered. Cleaning and shaping procedures straighten the canal somewhat and effectively decrease the working length by as much as 1 to 2 mm, thereby requiring compensation. To prevent apical perforation, the working length should be verified with an apex locator after completion of cleaning and shaping steps.

Treatment

Treatment includes establishing a new working length, creating an apical seat (taper), and obturating the canal to its new length. Depending on the size and location of the apical foramen, a new working length 1 to 2 mm short of the point of perforation should be established. The canal is then cleaned, shaped, and obturated to the new working length. The master cone must have a positive apical stop at the working length before obturation. Placement of MTA as an apical barrier can prevent extrusion of obturation materials

Prognosis

The success of treatment depends primarily on the size and shape of the defect. An open apex or reverse funnel is difficult to seal and also allows extrusion of the filling materials. In addition, the feasibility of repairing the perforation surgically may influence the final outcome.

Lateral (Midroot) Perforations
Etiology and Indicators

As discussed earlier, inability to maintain canal curvature is the major cause of ledge formation. Negotiation of ledged canals is not always possible, and misdirected pressure and force applied to a file may result in the formation of an artificial canal and eventually in an apical or midroot perforation. To avoid these perforations, the same factors mentioned earlier for prevention of ledge formation should be considered: (1) degree of canal curvature and size and (2) inflexibility of the larger files, especially stainless steel files.

Indicators of lateral perforation are similar to those of apical perforation (i.e., fresh hemorrhage in the root canal or sudden pain and deviation of instruments from their original course). Penetration of the instrument out of the root

radiographically (or as indicated by an apex locator) is the ultimate indicator.

Treatment

The optimal goal is to clean, shape, and obturate the entire root canal system of the affected tooth. After the perforation has been confirmed, the steps discussed previously for bypassing ledged canals are followed. If attempts to negotiate the apical portion of the canal are unsuccessful, the operator should concentrate on cleaning, shaping, and obturating the coronal segment of the canal. A new working length confined to the root is established, and the canal is then cleaned, shaped, and obturated to the new working length. A low concentration (0.5%) of sodium hypochlorite or saline should be used for irrigation in a perforated canal. Extrusion of concentrated irrigant into the surrounding periodontal tissues produces severe inflammation.

Prognosis

Success depends partially on the remaining amount of unebrided and unobturated canal. Obturation is difficult because of lack of a stop (matrix), and gutta-percha tends to be extruded during condensation. Teeth with perforations close to the apex after complete or partial debridement of the canal have a better prognosis than those with perforations that occur earlier. In addition to the length of uncleaned and unfilled portions of the canal, the size and surgical accessibility of perforations are important. In general, small perforations are easier to seal than large ones. Based on surgical accessibility, perforations toward the facial aspect are more easily repaired; therefore, these teeth have a better prognosis than those with perforations in other areas.

On recall, both radiographic and periodontal examinations for signs and symptoms are performed. Failure generally requires surgery or other approaches. These approaches depend on the severity of perforation, the strategic importance of the tooth, and the location and accessibility of the perforation. Corrective techniques include repair of the perforation site, root resection to the level of the perforation, root amputation, hemisection, replantation, and extraction.

Coronal Root Perforations
Etiology and Indicators

Coronal root perforations occur during access preparation as the operator attempts to locate canal orifices or during flaring procedures with files, Gates-Glidden drills, orifice openers, or Peeso reamers. Use of the methods described earlier in this chapter can minimize perforations during access preparation. Removal of restorations when possible, use of fiberoptic lights for illumination, magnification, and cautious exploration for calcified canals can prevent most problems during access preparation. Careful flaring (step-back) and conservative use of flaring instruments are required during cleaning and shaping procedures.

Treatment and Prognosis

Repair of a stripping perforation in the coronal third of the root has the poorest long-term prognosis of any type of perforation.[9] The defect is usually inaccessible for adequate repair. An attempt should be made to seal the defect internally, even though the prognosis is guarded. Patency of the canal system must be maintained during the repair process. Referral of the patient to a specialist is recommended.

Instrument Separation
Etiology
Limited flexibility and strength of intracanal instruments, along with improper use, may result in an intracanal instrument separation. Any instrument may break; stainless steel, nickel-titanium, hand, or rotary. Overuse or excessive force applied to files is the main cause of separation. Manufacturing defects in files are rare.

Recognition
Removal of a shortened file with a blunt tip from a canal and subsequent loss of patency to the original length are the main clues to the presence of a separated instrument. A radiograph is *essential* for confirmation. It is *imperative* that the patient be informed of the accident and its effect on the prognosis.[1] As with other procedural accidents, detailed documentation is also necessary for medical-legal considerations.

Prevention
Recognition of the physical properties and stress limitations of files is critical. Continual lubrication with either irrigating solution or lubricants is required. Each instrument is examined before use. If an unwound or twisted file is rotated and viewed, reflections from the chairside light magnify fluting distortions (Fig. 19.12). Small files must be replaced often. To minimize binding, each file size is worked in the canal until it is very loose before the next file size is used.[29] Nickel-titanium files usually do not show visual signs of fatigue

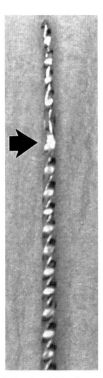

Fig. 19.12 Each steel file should be inspected for fluting distortion before use in the canal. Only untwisted files show a shiny spot *(arrow)*. This file must be discarded. Nickel-titanium files do not show this distortion and must be discarded after one or two uses, depending on wear.

similar to the "untwisting" of steel files. Many factors may affect the fatiguing of nickel-titanium files,[30] which should be discarded before visual signs of untwisting are seen. Preflaring of preparations through a passive step-back technique before the use of rotary instruments reduces the rates of separation of .04 taper nickel-titanium rotary instruments.[31] It is important to establish a glide path with hand files before rotary files are introduced into the canal.

Treatment
There are basically three approaches to managing intracanal instrument separation: (1) attempt to remove the instrument,[32] (2) attempt to bypass it, or (3) prepare and obturate the segment. Initial treatment is similar to that discussed earlier for a ledge. Using a small file and following the guidelines described for negotiating a ledge, the operator should attempt to bypass the separated instrument. After bypassing the separated instrument, ultrasonic files,[33] or Hedstrom files are used to remove the segment (Fig. 19.13). If removal of the separated piece is unsuccessful, the canal is cleaned, shaped, and obturated to its new working length.

When separated in a canal, files made of nickel-titanium present different circumstances from those seen with stainless steel files. Nickel-titanium files, because of their shape memory, tend to return to their straight shape in that portion of the file that is not bound in the canal, whereas stainless steel files tend to maintain any curvatures created in the instrument, either before placement in the canal or after use in the canal. Because of their properties, nickel-titanium file segments often lie against the outer canal wall, making them difficult to grasp with devices designed to remove separated files. On the other hand, stainless steel files may be more centered in the canal and may be more accessible to devices designed to grasp separated files.[34,35]

If a separated instrument is in the straight portion of a canal, it may be removed, if there is enough root structure present, by creating a staging platform and then using ultrasonic tips to either loosen the file or create space to bypass the separated instrument. The use of an operating microscope greatly improves visibility. The staging platform is created by flattening the end of a Gates-Glidden drill and then using it to the level of the coronal portion of the separated file. Ultrasonics can then be used in a counterclockwise direction to try to remove the separated instrument by "unscrewing" the separated file or by creating an area around the file, thereby allowing it to be grasped and removed (or bypassed).[34-36]

If the instrument has separated in an apical curved portion of the canal beyond the straight section, use of a staging platform should not be attempted because ledging, perforation, or excessive loss of dentin may result.[36]

If the instrument cannot be bypassed, preparation and obturation should be performed to the coronal level of the fragment.

For most cases involving separated instruments, the patient should be referred to an endodontist.

Prognosis
The prognosis depends on how much undebrided and unobturated canal apical to and including the instrument remains. The prognosis is best when separation of a large instrument occurs in the later stages of preparation close to the working length. The prognosis is poorer for teeth with undebrided

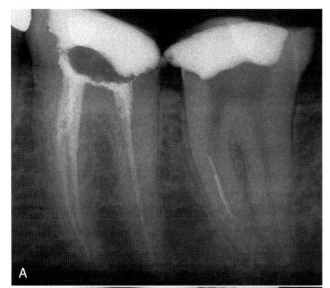

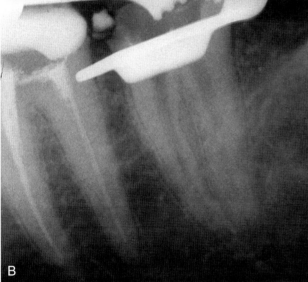

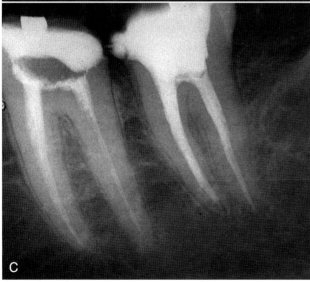

Fig. 19.13 **A,** A file is separated in the mesiobuccal canal of the second mandibular molar. **B,** The separated instrument is bypassed and removed. **C,** Both canals are cleaned, shaped, and obturated. The prognosis is good.

canals in which a small instrument is separated short of the apex or beyond the apical foramen early in preparation. For medical-legal reasons, the patient must be informed (with documentation in the record) of an instrument separation. Despite the concern of both patient and dentist,[37] clinical reports indicate that the prognosis is favorable in most procedures involving broken instruments that are managed properly.[38] The favorable prognosis also holds true for rotary files that are separated in canals.[39]

If the patient remains symptomatic or there is a subsequent failure, the tooth can be treated surgically. Accessible roots are resected, with placement of a root-end filling material (Fig. 19.14). Accessibility of the root apex for surgical intervention is critical to the final outcome.

Other Accidents
Aspiration or Ingestion

Aspiration or ingestion of instruments is a serious event but is easily avoided with proper precautions. *Use of the rubber dam is the standard of care to prevent such ingestion or aspiration and subsequent lawsuits.*[1]

The disappearance of an instrument that has slipped from the dentist's fingers, followed by violent coughing or gagging by the patient, and radiographic confirmation of a file in the alimentary tract or airway are the chief signs. These patients require immediate referral to a medical service for appropriate diagnosis and treatment. According to a survey by Grossman, 87% of these instruments are swallowed and the rest are aspirated.[40] Surgical removal is required for some swallowed (Fig. 19.15) and nearly all aspirated instruments.

Extrusion of Irrigant

Wedging of a needle in the canal[41,42] (or particularly out of a perforation) with forceful expression of irrigant (usually sodium hypochlorite [NaOCl]) causes penetration of irrigants into the periradicular tissues and inflammation and discomfort for patients. Extrusion of NaOCl into the periapical tissues can cause a life-threatening emergency.[43] Loose placement of irrigation needles, careful irrigation with light pressure, and use of a perforated needle[44] prevents irrigating solution from being forced into the periradicular tissues. Sudden, prolonged, and sharp pain during irrigation, followed by rapid, diffuse swelling ("sodium hypochlorite accident"), usually indicates penetration of solution into the periradicular tissues. The acute episode subsides spontaneously with time (Fig. 19.16). In teeth with open apices, the use of less concentrated irrigants, or saline, prevents the possibility of irrigant accidents.

Initially there is no reason to prescribe antibiotics or attempt surgical drainage. Treatment is palliative. Analgesics are prescribed, and the patient is reassured. Because the outcome is so dramatic, evaluation is performed frequently to follow progress.

ACCIDENTS DURING OBTURATION

Appropriate cleaning and shaping are the keys to preventing obturation problems because these accidents usually result from improper canal preparation. In general, adequately prepared canals are obturated without mishap. However, problems do occur. *The quality of obturation reflects the quality of canal preparation.*

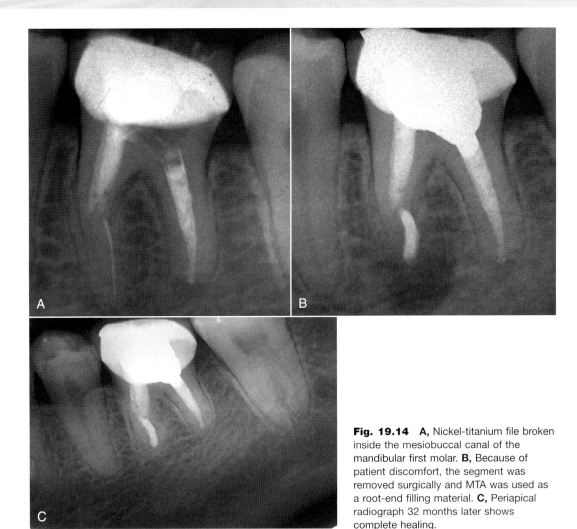

Fig. 19.14 **A,** Nickel-titanium file broken inside the mesiobuccal canal of the mandibular first molar. **B,** Because of patient discomfort, the segment was removed surgically and MTA was used as a root-end filling material. **C,** Periapical radiograph 32 months later shows complete healing.

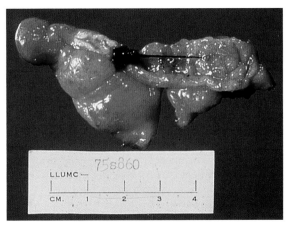

Fig. 19.15 A swallowed broach caused removal of a patient's appendix and a subsequent lawsuit against a dentist who did not use a rubber dam during root canal therapy. (Courtesy Dr. L. Thompsen.)

Underfilling

Etiology

Some causes of underfilling include a natural barrier in the canal, a ledge created during preparation, insufficient flaring, a poorly adapted master cone, and inadequate condensation pressure. Bypassing (if possible) any natural or artificial barrier to create a smooth funnel is one key to avoiding an underfill. The advent of nickel-titanium rotary files of increased taper has greatly improved the predictability of proper funnel and taper.

Treatment and Prognosis

Removal of underfilled gutta-percha and retreatment are preferred. Forcing gutta-percha apically by increased spreader or plugger pressure can fracture the root. If lateral condensation is the method of obturation, the master cone should be marked to indicate the working length. If displacement of the master cone during condensation is suspected, a radiograph is made *before* excess gutta-percha is removed. Removal can then be accomplished by pulling the cones in the reverse order of placement. Removal of gutta-percha in canals obturated with lateral condensation is easier than removal with other obturation techniques. However, warm gutta-percha techniques allow better obturation of irregularities within the canal.

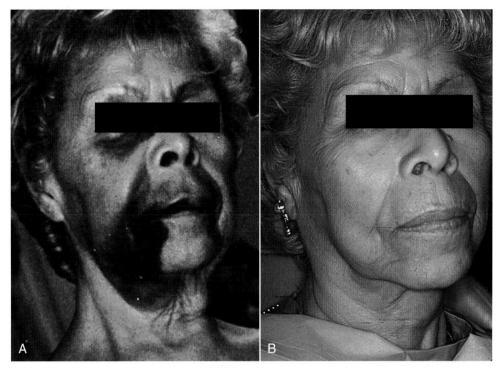

Fig. 19.16 A, NaOCl was inadvertently expressed through an apical perforation in a maxillary cuspid during irrigation. Hemorrhagic reaction was rapid and diffuse. **B,** No treatment was necessary; the swelling and hematoma disappeared within a few weeks. (Courtesy Dr. James Stick.)

Overfilling

Extruded obturation material causes tissue damage and inflammation. Postoperative discomfort (mastication sensitivity) usually lasts a few days.

Etiology

Overfilling is usually the consequence of overinstrumentation through the apical constriction or lack of proper taper in prepared canals. When the apex is open naturally by apical resorption or its constriction is removed during cleaning and shaping, there is no matrix against which to condense; uncontrolled condensation forces extrusion of materials (Fig. 19.17). Other causes include inflammatory resorption and incomplete development of the root.

Prevention

To avoid overfilling, guidelines for preventing apical foramen perforation should be followed. Tapered preparation with an apical "matrix" usually prevents overfill. The largest file and master cone at working length should have a positive stop. A customized master cone may be fabricated by briefly applying solvent on the tip. If overfilling is suspected, a radiograph should be made before excess gutta-percha is removed. As with underfilling, the gutta-percha mass may be removed if the sealer has not set.

Treatment and Prognosis

When signs or symptoms of endodontic failure appear, apical surgery may be required to remove the material from apical tissues and place root-end filling material. The long-term prognosis is dictated by the quality of the apical seal, the amount and biocompatibility of extruded material, host response, and toxicity and sealing ability of the root-end filling material.

Vertical Root Fracture

Complete vertical root fracture causes untreatable failure. Aspects of vertical root fracture are described in more detail in Chapter 8.

Etiology

Causative factors in vertical root fracture include root canal treatment procedures and associated factors, such as post placement. The main cause of vertical root fracture is post cementation. The secondary cause is overzealous application of condensation forces to obturate an underprepared or overprepared canal.[45]

Prevention

In root canal treatment procedures, the best means of preventing vertical root fractures are appropriate canal preparation and use of balanced pressure during obturation. A major reason for flaring canals is to provide space for condensation instruments. Finger spreaders produce less stress and distortion of the root than do their hand counterparts.[46-48] Furthermore, nickel-titanium finger spreaders produce less stress during compaction than do stainless steel finger spreaders.[49,50]

Indicators

Long-standing vertical root fractures are often associated with a narrow periodontal pocket or sinus tract stoma, as well as a **351**

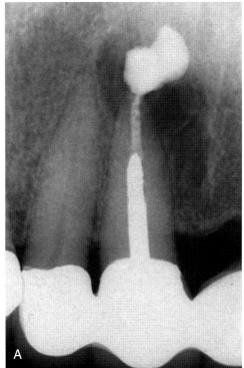

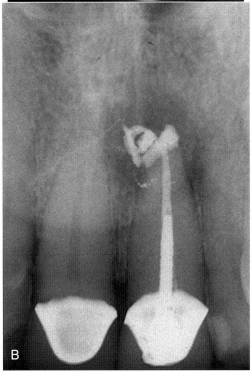

Fig. 19.17 Lack of proper length measurements can result in overfilling with root canal sealer **(A)** or with sealer and gutta-percha **(B)**.

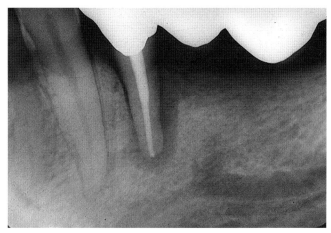

Fig. 19.18 A, A teardrop lateral radiolucency and a narrow probing defect extend to the apex of a tooth with vertical fracture.

or rule out vertical root fractures. However, scatter from posts or root canal filling materials may make interpretation of vertical root fractures difficult in CBCT images.[52,53]

Prognosis and Treatment

Complete vertical root fracture predicts the poorest prognosis of any procedural accident. Treatment is removal of the involved root in multirooted teeth and extraction of single-rooted teeth.

ACCIDENTS DURING POST SPACE PREPARATION

To prevent root perforation, gutta-percha may be removed to the desired level with heated pluggers or electronic heating devices, such as the Touch N Heat or System B (SybronEndo, Orange, California). This "pilot" post space provides a path of least resistance for sizing drills. Attempting to remove gutta-percha with a drill only can result in perforation. When a canal is prepared to receive a post, drills should be used sequentially, starting with a size that fits passively to the desired level. Miscalculation and incorrect preparation may result in perforation at any level. Knowledge of root anatomy is necessary for determining the size and depth of posts.

Indicators

The indicators of perforations and vertical root fractures are somewhat similar. The appearance of fresh blood during post space preparation is an indication of a root perforation. The presence of a sinus tract stoma or probing defects extending to the base of a post are frequently a sign of root fracture or perforation. Radiographs often show a lateral radiolucency along the root or perforation site.

Treatment and Prognosis

The prognosis for teeth with vertical root fractures resulting from post space preparation and post insertion is similar to that for teeth with fractures that develop during obturation; the involved root (or tooth) is hopeless and must be removed. As outlined earlier, the prognosis for teeth with a root perforation that occurs during post space preparation depends on the

lateral radiolucency (Fig. 19.18) extending to the apical portion of the vertical fracture.[51] To confirm the diagnosis, a vertical fracture must be visualized. Exploratory surgery or removal of the restoration is usually necessary to visualize this mishap. More recently, CBCT has been used to confirm

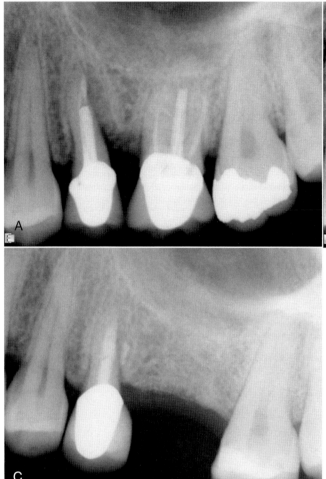
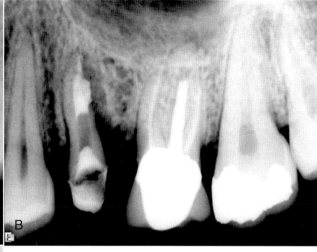

Fig. 19.19 **A,** Lateral root perforation is evident in a patient who had previous root canal therapy. **B,** After removal of the post and cleaning of the root canal, the apical portion of the root was filled with MTA. **C,** Postoperative radiograph taken 9 years later shows absence of any periradicular pathosis.

root size, the location of the perforation relative to the epithelial attachment, and the accessibility for repair. Management of the post perforation generally is surgical if the post cannot be removed. If the post can be removed, nonsurgical repair is preferred (Fig. 19.19). Teeth with small root perforations in the apical region that are accessible for surgical repair have a better prognosis than do teeth that have large perforations or perforations that are close to the gingival sulcus or inaccessible. Because of the complexity of diagnosis, surgical techniques, and follow-up evaluation, patients with post perforations should be referred to an endodontist for evaluation and treatment.

REFERENCES

1. Cohen S, Schwartz S: Endodontic complications and the law, *J Endod* 13:191, 1987.
2. Fishelberg G, Hook D: Patient safety during endodontic therapy using current technology: a case report, *J Endod* 29:683, 2003.
3. Lambrianidis T, Beltes P: Accidental swallowing of endodontic instruments, *Endod Dent Traumatol* 12:301, 1996.
4. Weine FS: Access cavity preparation and initiating treatment. In Weine F, editor: *Endodontic therapy*, ed 4, St Louis, 1989, Mosby.
5. Gorduysus MO, Gorduysus M, Friedman S: Operating microscope improves negotiation of second mesiobuccal canals in maxillary molars, *J Endod* 27:683, 2001.
6. de Carvalho MC, Zuolo ML: Orifice locating with a microscope, *J Endod* 26:532, 2000.
7. Baldassari-Cruz LA, Lilly JP, Rivera EM: The influence of dental operating microscope in locating the mesiolingual canal orifice, *Oral Surg Oral Med Oral Pathol Oral Radiol Endod* 93:190, 2002.
8. Lemon RR: Furcation perforation management: classic and new concepts. In Hardin JF, editor:

Clark's clinical dentistry, vol 1, Philadelphia, 1990, JB Lippincott.
9. Lemon RR: Nonsurgical repair of perforation defects: internal matrix concept, *Dent Clin North Am* 36:439, 1992.
10. Simon JH, Kelly WH, Gordon DG, et al: Extrusion of endodontically treated teeth, *J Am Dent Assoc* 97:17, 1978.
11. Lemon RR: Simplified esthetic root extrusion techniques, *Oral Surg Oral Med Oral Pathol* 54:93, 1982.
12. Suprabha BS, Kundabala M, Subraya M, et al: Reattachment and orthodontic extrusion in the management of an incisor crown-root fracture: a case report, *J Clin Pediatr Dent* 30:211, 2006.
13. Lee SJ, Monsef M, Torabinejad M: Sealing ability of a mineral trioxide aggregate for repair of lateral root perforations, *J Endod* 19:541, 1993.
14. Nicholls E: Treatment of traumatic perforations of the pulp cavity, *Oral Surg Oral Med Oral Pathol* 15:603, 1962.
15. Stromberg T, Hasselgren G, Bergstedt H: Endodontic treatment of traumatic root perforations

in man: a clinical and roentgenological follow-up study, *Sven Tandlak Tidskr* 65:457, 1972.
16. Harris WE: A simplified method of treatment for endodontic perforations, *J Endod* 2:126, 1976.
17. Benenati FW, Roane JB, Biggs JT, et al: Recall evaluation of iatrogenic root perforations repaired with amalgam and gutta-percha, *J Endod* 12:161, 1986.
18. Sinai IH: Endodontic perforations: their prognosis and treatment, *J Am Dent Assoc* 95:90, 1977.
19. Hartwell GR, England MC: Healing of furcation perforations in primate teeth after repair with decalcified freeze-dried bone: a longitudinal study, *J Endod* 19:357, 1993.
20. Aguirre R, el Deeb ME: Evaluation of the repair of mechanical furcation perforations using amalgam, gutta-percha, or indium foil, *J Endod* 12:249, 1986.
21. Oswald RJ: Procedural accidents and their repair, *Dent Clin North Am* 23:593, 1979.
22. Pitt Ford TR, Torabinejad M, McKendry DJ, et al: Use of mineral trioxide aggregate for repair of furcal

perforations, *Oral Surg Oral Med Oral Pathol Oral Radiol Endod* 79:756, 1995.

23. Hong CU, McKendry DJ, Pitt Ford TR, et al: Healing of furcal lesions repaired by amalgam or mineral trioxide aggregate (abstract), *J Endod* 20:197, 1994.

24. Noetzel J, Ozer K, Reisshauer BH, et al: Tissue responses to an experimental calcium phosphate cement and mineral trioxide aggregate as materials for furcation perforation repair: a histological study in dogs, *Clin Oral Invest* 10:77, 2006.

25. Tsatsas DV, Meliou HA, Kerezoudis NP: Sealing effectiveness of materials in furcation perforation in vitro, *Int Dent J* 55:133, 2005.

26. Yildirim T, Gencoglu N, Firat I, et al: Histologic study of furcation perforations treated with MTA or Super EBA in dogs' teeth, *Oral Surg Oral Med Oral Pathol Oral Radiol Endod* 100:120, 2005.

27. Main C, Mirzayan N, Shabahang S, et al: Repair of root perforations using mineral trioxide aggregate: a long-term study, *J Endod* 30:80, 2004.

28. Fuss Z, Trope M: Root perforations: classification and treatment choices based on prognostic factors, *Endod Dent Traumatol* 12:255, 1996.

29. Grossman LI: Guidelines for the prevention of fracture of root canal instruments, *Oral Surg Oral Med Oral Pathol* 28:746, 1969.

30. Di Fiore PM, Genov KI, Komaroff E, et al: Fracture of ProFile nickel-titanium rotary instruments: a laboratory simulation assessment, *Int Endod J* 39:502, 2006.

31. Roland DD, Andelin WE, Browning DF, et al: The effect of preflaring on the rates of separation for 0.04 taper nickel titanium rotary instruments, *J Endod* 28:543, 2002.

32. Shen Y, Peng B, Cheung GS: Factors associated with the removal of fractured NiTi instruments from root canal systems, *Oral Surg Oral Med Oral Pathol Oral Radiol Endod* 98:605, 2004.

33. Suter B, Lussi A, Sequeira P: Probability of removing fractured instruments from root canals, *Int Endod J* 38:112, 2005.

34. Ruddle CJ: Micro-endodontic nonsurgical retreatment, *Dent Clin North Am* 41:429, 1997.

35. Ruddle CJ: Nonsurgical retreatment, *J Endod* 30:827, 2004.

36. Ward JR, Parashos P, Messer HHL: Evaluation of an ultrasonic technique to remove fractured rotary nickel-titanium endodontic instruments from root canals: an experimental study, *J Endod* 29:756, 2003.

37. Frank AL: The dilemma of the fractured instrument, *J Endod* 9:515, 1983.

38. Crump MC, Natkin E: Relationship of broken root canal instruments to endodontic case prognosis: a clinical investigation, *J Am Dent Assoc* 80:1341, 1970.

39. Spili P, Parashos P, Messer HH: The impact of instrument fracture on outcome of endodontic treatment, *J Endod* 31:845, 2005.

40. Grossman LI: Prevention in endodontic practice, *J Am Dent Assoc* 82:395, 1971.

41. Bradford CE, Eleazer PD, Downs KE, et al: Apical pressures developed by needles for canal irrigation, *J Endod* 28:333, 2002.

42. Kahn FH, Rosenberg PA, Gliksberg J: An in vitro evaluation of the irrigating characteristics of ultrasonic and subsonic handpieces and irrigating needles and probes, *J Endod* 21:277, 1995.

43. Bowden JR, Ethunandan M, Brennan PA: Life-threatening airway obstruction secondary to hypochlorite extrusion during root canal treatment, *Oral Surg Oral Med Oral Pathol Oral Radiol Endod* 101:402, 2006.

44. Goldman M, Kronman JH, Goldman LB, et al: New method of irrigation during endodontic treatment, *J Endod* 2:257, 1976.

45. Obermayr G, Walton RE, Leary JM, et al: Vertical root fracture and relative deformation during obturation and post cementation, *J Prosthet Dent* 66:181, 1991.

46. Murgel CA, Walton RE: Vertical root fracture and dentin deformation in curved roots: the influence of spreader design, *Endod Dent Traumatol* 6:273, 1990.

47. Dang DA, Walton RE: Vertical root fracture and root distortion: effect of spreader design, *J Endod* 15:294, 1989.

48. Lertchirakarn V, Palamara JE, Messer HH: Load and strain during lateral condensation and vertical root fracture, *J Endod* 25:99, 1999.

49. Schmidt KJ, Walker TL, Johnson JD, et al: Comparison of nickel-titanium and stainless steel spreader penetration and accessory cone fit in curved canals, *J Endod* 25:506, 1999.

50. Gharai SR, Thorpe JR, Strother JM, et al: Comparison of generated forces and apical microleakage using nickel-titanium and stainless steel finger spreaders in curved canals, *J Endod* 31:198, 2005.

51. Walton RE, Michelich RJ, Smith GN: The histopathogenesis of vertical root fractures, *J Endod* 10:48, 1984.

52. Hassan B, Metska ME, Ozok AR, et al: Detection of vertical root fractures in endodontically treated teeth by a cone beam computed tomography scan, *J Endod* 35:719, 2009.

53. Ozer SY: Detection of vertical root fractures of different thicknesses in endodontically enlarged teeth by cone beam computed tomography versus digital radiography, *J Endod* 36:1245, 2010.

Retreatment

George Bogen, Robert Handysides

LEARNING OBJECTIVES

After reading this chapter, the student should be able to:

1. Recognize situations that might require nonsurgical root canal retreatment.
2. Identify the treatment options available for teeth with endodontic problems.
3. State the indications and contraindications for root canal retreatment.
4. Describe the risks and benefits of retreatment.
5. Describe techniques and materials used in endodontic retreatment.
6. Discuss restorative options and follow-up care.
7. Discuss the prognosis and outcomes for nonsurgical endodontic retreatment.

Root canal treatment using contemporary methods and materials has an excellent success rate, which maintains tooth function and retention.[1,2] However, initial root canal therapy may not always result in healing, and the recurrence of endodontic disease may also prevent a successful outcome. For instance, failure to adequately disinfect the root canal system can result in nonhealing. Bacteria may persist after initial treatment due to areas that were inaccessible to instrumentation and irrigation.[6,8-10] Additionally the reestablishment of root canal infection after initial treatment may lead to progression of disease.[3-5] The reintroduction of microorganisms is primarily caused by coronal microleakage and recurrent decay.[6-8] Other causes of treatment failure may include lack of tooth isolation; inadequate cleaning, shaping, and irrigation; and incomplete obturation. Root canal obstructions, including calcifications, can also be a problem (Fig. 20.1).[6,8,9]

Nonhealing after initial nonsurgical root canal therapy may also be related to procedural errors, complex anatomic variations in root canal anatomy, or the presence of extraradicular biofilms.[11] Procedural errors include perforations, canal transportation, separated instruments, and ledge formations, all of which can negatively impact the treatment outcome.[6,10] Furthermore, initial treatment may be compromised by long-term use of temporary materials before placement of definitive restorations.[12-14]

It is also important to recognize that vertical root fractures may sometimes appear as nonhealing lesions. These are longitudinal fractures that occur after root canal treatment and may be related to the weakening of roots from excessive dentin removal or simply from the stresses on teeth from normal function.[15-17]

TREATMENT OPTIONS

After initial root canal therapy, unsatisfactory short-term and long-term outcomes are primarily due to three causes: (1) nonhealing, (2) recurrence of endodontic disease, and (3) development of new disease and complications.

With nonhealing, a tooth with endodontic disease continues to have a problem after initial endodontic therapy. This may result from many factors, which are described in more detail throughout this chapter.

Recurrence of endodontic disease is found when healing occurs from the initial treatment, but bacteria subsequently regain entrance to the root canal system and reinfect the tooth. The tooth initially is comfortable, with no signs of disease, but later the patient may complain of symptoms. Both radiographic and clinical evidence of new endodontic concerns also may be seen.

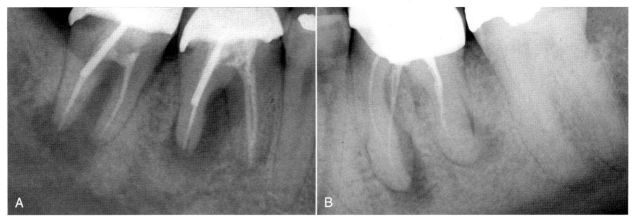

Fig. 20.1 **A,** Recall radiograph of mandibular right first and second molars 3 years after initial root canal treatment and coronal restorations. Both molars exhibit recurrent caries, coronal microleakage, and apical and lateral pathosis. The patient was symptomatic with the presence of a buccal sinus tract. **B,** Radiographic review of a mandibular left first molar showing apical pathosis associated with poor gutta-percha filling techniques and an untreated canal to the distal root. (© Dr. Robert Handysides. All rights reserved.)

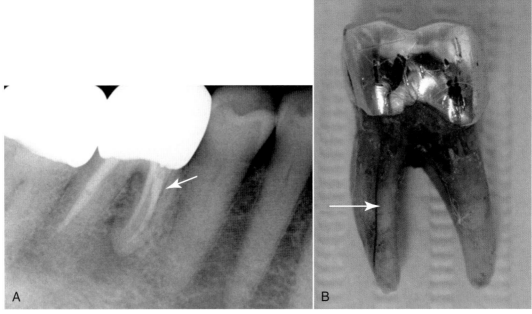

Fig. 20.2 **A,** Vertical root fractures occur mostly in endodontically treated teeth and typically originate from the apical end and progress toward the crown. They run mostly in a faciolingual direction, in contrast to infractions, which run mesiodistally. The radiograph shows a vertical root fracture *(arrow).* **B,** The extracted tooth also shows the presence of the fracture. (© Dr. Robert Handysides. All rights reserved.)

With the third main cause, namely development of a new problem after initial successful treatment of a tooth, complications arise that are not directly related to the root canal treatment. An example of such a situation is an endodontically treated tooth that develops a vertical root fracture (VRF). These fractures typically occur sometime after initial root canal treatment and may be recognized as lateral lesions instead of the usual apical lesions associated with root canal infections (Fig. 20.2). A VRF can occasionally be traced using a periodontal probe if the fracture extends coronally to the crestal bone. Although single-rooted teeth that develop VRFs usually need to be extracted, the failure in this case is not directly related to the root canal treatment. A similar situation is the endodontically treated tooth that may need to be

extracted for periodontal reasons; the reason for extraction is unrelated to the endodontic procedure. Other endodontic surgical procedures may be used to salvage portions of multirooted teeth that are not affected by the VRF.

When initial root canal treatment fails to promote healing, the treatment options to save the tooth include nonsurgical retreatment with or without apical surgery, apical surgery, intentional replantation, and extraction. If the tooth is restorable, nonsurgical retreatment is usually the preferred treatment strategy. This option may allow an opportunity to better disinfect the root canal system or to address areas of reinfection due to bacterial leakage associated with poor coronal restorations. Because orthograde endodontic retreatment may not allow access to all areas of canal infection, or if extraradicular infection is present, apical surgery may be a required part of the retreatment.

Surgical treatment may be considered a first choice in the presence of canal obstructions or extensive fixed prosthetic appliances or when removal of extruded filling materials is indicated. However, surgical endodontic treatment may not eliminate surviving microorganisms in inaccessible areas of the root canal system. Even when surgical treatment is required, nonsurgical retreatment prior to surgical treatment has been shown to improve healing and to help achieve a successful outcome.[9,18]

Intentional replantation of teeth is a treatment option that has a long history in dentistry. When properly planned and executed, intentional replantation has been shown to be quite successful in providing patients with additional years of service from their teeth.[19,20] This procedure can be considered for teeth that are not badly broken down but in which the initial root canal treatment has not allowed access to all of the root canal system, and apical surgery is complicated by anatomic difficulties. It also allows an opportunity to examine the roots of teeth for possible vertical fracture lines.[6,8,9]

Retreatment procedures are usually more difficult to perform than those used in the initial treatment. They frequently require advanced instrumentation, magnification systems, and special training.[9] Endodontists have extensive training and practice in evaluating and managing teeth with apparent lack of healing after initial root canal therapy and teeth developing new lesions. Much of this chapter discusses procedures performed by specialists. This discussion is intended to provide information on the techniques used by someone trained in such procedures. The emphasis in this chapter is on recognizing nonhealing and the recurrence of endodontic disease and on developing an understanding of what can be achieved.

INDICATIONS FOR NONSURGICAL ENDODONTIC RETREATMENT

The following describes a typical situation of a nonhealing initial root canal treatment based on a diagnosis of pulp necrosis and symptomatic apical periodontitis. The patient complains that the symptoms have not improved since the time of initial treatment and that the discomfort has in fact increased. Chewing and biting are painful, but the pain may also occur spontaneously. Radiographic examination reveals an emerging apical radiolucency not present at the time of initial treatment.

Clinical examination of teeth with nonhealing endodontic disease may reveal palpation and percussion sensitivity, localized swelling, recurrent caries, leaky provisional restorations, and substandard or missing coronal restorations. Radiographic evaluation may show the presence of untreated canals, poor canal obturation with voids, separated instruments, recurrent caries not located during the clinical examination, or defective restorations with open margins. All such findings can contribute to nonhealing associated with the previous treatment. Any combination of clinical symptoms and radiographic and clinical findings may indicate nonhealing. Nonhealing can also be present without any contribution from the aforementioned conditions.

Retreatment is considered the primary treatment option when the tooth is found to be periodontally stable; there is adequate remaining tooth structure with no detectable vertical fractures; and access to the root canal system is feasible. After disassembly of any defective restorations and post and core materials and the removal of all caries, tooth restorability must be determined. This initial assessment includes periodontal probing, mobility tests, and periapical and bitewing radiographs to determine the crown to root ratio, presence of supporting bone, health of the soft tissue, and need for crown lengthening procedures.

It is important for the chairside staff to be familiar with retreatment procedures so that endodontic care can be delivered in a professional and effective manner. The office must be equipped with the necessary illumination and magnification systems, ultrasonic units and appropriate tips, rotary handpieces, endodontic files, solvents, dental dams, various post extraction kits, and irrigation systems. The clinician must have high levels of skill, experience, and training to execute retreatment in an effective manner. Because these cases are commonly complex and challenging, the best interest of the patient should be considered when the decision is made to offer treatment or to recommend referral to a specialist.

CONTRAINDICATIONS TO NONSURGICAL ENDODONTIC RETREATMENT

A major factor when nonsurgical retreatment is considered is the restorability of the tooth after the necessary removal of preexisting restorative materials. Additional tooth structure may be lost during caries removal and removal of post and core materials. Lack of adequate tooth structure to support a postendodontic restoration is a contraindication to nonsurgical retreatment. The restorability decision often requires extensive disassembly of existing restorations and evaluation of the remaining root canal system. Other contraindications include the presence of extensive periodontal involvement of the tooth that weakens the tooth support and/or the presence of problematic coronal or radicular fractures.

INDICATIONS FOR SURGICAL RETREATMENT

Further contraindications to nonsurgical root canal retreatment include intracanal complications. For instance, access to the canals may not be possible due to the presence of obstructions. These obstructions include large, tight-fitting, prefabricated or cast posts and cores, root canal calcifications, and other obstructions that may prevent access. In such situations, surgical retreatment may offer the best available option.[6,10] Examples of possible root canal obstructions are the presence of separated instruments that cannot be bypassed or retrieved, filling materials that cannot be adequately removed, and teeth that after orthograde retreatment exhibit nonresponding periapical lesions.[21,22] Teeth with iatrogenic mishaps that cannot be adequately addressed, such as nonnegotiable ledges, transportation of the canal or apex, or perforations that cannot be repaired internally, also may be candidates for a surgical approach.[6,10]

Teeth with external root resorption associated with a history of trauma and infected pulp tissue that were inadequately **357** treated previously may be retreated in an orthograde approach. Surgical repair of resorptive areas on the external aspects of the roots is usually not indicated.

Extraction usually is indicated for teeth diagnosed with a VRF. An exception may be a multirooted maxillary molar that develops a VRF in one of the roots. Because replacement with a dental implant may be difficult due to the type or absence of alveolar bone, surgical amputation of the root with a VRF can provide a tooth that may serve satisfactorily for many years.[23-25] Each clinical situation is unique to the patient with the endodontic problem, and treatment options must be evaluated by carefully taking into account all aspects of the patient's situation.

RISKS AND BENEFITS OF RETREATMENT

The patient must be informed of the risks, benefits, alternatives, and consequences of the various treatment modalities prior to initiation of treatment. The discussion with the patient must include the importance of good oral hygiene and regular evaluation of the teeth. Because retreatment is often time-consuming, the cost of treatment must be explained.[26]

Nonsurgical root canal retreatment procedures have many potential risks. These include fracture of a porcelain crown during the access procedure, fracture of the root during post removal procedures, iatrogenic perforations during core and obturation material removal, and dislodgement of the crown that may necessitate replacement.[9,10,27] In addition, retreatment procedures may cause extensive removal of tooth structure that may further weaken the tooth, create ledges, or cause canal transportation. The separation of an instrument may impede the ability to completely remove obturation materials also. All of these complications may affect the retreatment outcome and potentially lead to necessary extraction. The benefits of retreatment include the preservation and retention of the patient's natural tooth structure and the avoidance of more extensive clinical treatment.

ENDODONTIC RETREATMENT PROCEDURES

Removal of Existing Restorations

Nonsurgical endodontic retreatment procedures are often more feasible if the coronal restorations are completely removed. This allows better visualization and access for post and core removal, caries excavation, assessment and management of coronal microleakage, and removal of obturation materials from the canals (Fig. 20.3).[9,28]

After disassembly of the coronal restoration, a clearer assessment of potential coronal microleakage can be made. If microleakage is evident, the entire remaining tooth structure can be inspected, including the canals and the pulpal floor. Disassembly also allows inspection for possible recurrent caries and fractures and evaluation of the tooth's restorability.[10,18,28] When posterior teeth have been restored with either composite resin or amalgam, the entire restoration should be removed. The remaining coronal structure can then be assessed for a new restoration that can provide adequate cuspal coverage and protection.

When a tooth presents with a full coverage restoration and exhibits recurrent caries, open margins, or loss of marginal integrity, complete removal of the restoration is also indicated. In many cases this is necessary for post and core disassembly.[9,10,28] Anterior teeth with cosmetic crowns that exhibit acceptable marginal integrity without the presence of recurrent caries may be retreated through a lingual access opening, but the risk of crown fracture is still present.[9,10,28] If there is a large metallic or nonmetallic post, crown removal most likely will be required to complete the treatment. Patients must be informed of the possibility of porcelain fracture, crown dislodgement, or root fracture, which may occur through any phase of retreatment. If the structural integrity of the prosthetic crown is compromised, the patient will most likely require a new restoration. If retreatment can be completed with the original full coverage restoration remaining intact, the access cavity can be filled with a permanent restorative material.

Removal of Canal Obstructions

Canal obstructions occasionally prevent successful negotiation of the root canal system during nonsurgical root canal treatment. Nonhealing is likely if these obstructions are not bypassed or removed. Surgical treatment may need to be included to manage these treatment challenges.

The four categories of canal obstructions are (1) posts and cores, (2) calcifications of the root canal system, (3) iatrogenic ledges and dentinal debris in the root canal system, and (4) separated instruments, silver points or metallic debris, and some paste materials.[6,9,10] These are typically complex treatment situations that frequently require extensive training and experience to manage. For the benefit of the patient, referral to a specialist should be considered and offered.[29] The following are general descriptions of the procedures used.

Post and Core Removal

Successful removal of posts and cores during retreatment depends on several factors that influence the outcome. These include the operator's level of skill, experience, and training and the availability of magnification, illumination, and ultrasonic systems. Other outcome considerations include the type of core material (cast versus resin or amalgam); the length and diameter of the preformed or cast post, post location, and post material (metallic or nonmetallic); and type of cement or bonding system used to secure the post and core system.[10,27,28] Any number of methods used to remove posts can compromise the existing tooth structure.[27] Some posts may be difficult or impossible to remove if they are long, well fitted, or cemented with bonding systems or resin cements (Fig. 20.4). Nonmetallic posts are very difficult to remove, particularly when they are tooth colored or made of zirconium (Fig. 20.5). Removal of long or large-diameter posts may be contraindicated if the existing root structure is thin or if perforation or a root fracture is likely to occur during the procedure.[9,28]

In preparation for post removal, the coronal core material must be carefully sectioned and removed incrementally to preserve the portion of the post that extrudes coronally from the root canal. Removal of the core material may require diamond, transmetal, and carbide burs or specifically designed ultrasonic tips.[10,27,28]

This procedure is best performed using illumination and magnification to help preserve adjacent tooth structure during the procedure. After core removal, any visible cement

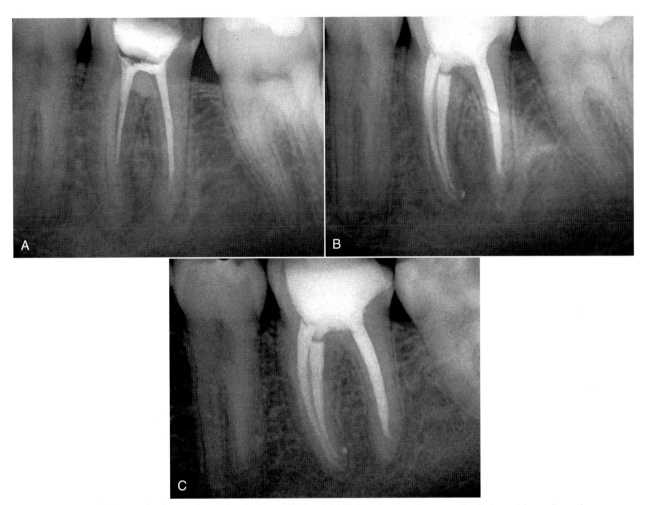

Fig. 20.3 **A,** Radiograph of a previously treated mandibular right first molar showing an untreated mesiobuccal canal, apical lesions, and substandard core buildup (note arrow showing void) in a 21-year-old, symptomatic female patient. **B,** Postoperative radiograph after nonsurgical retreatment and bonded core placement. **C,** Recall radiograph at 1.5 years showing complete healing of the original apical lesion. (© Dr. George Bogen. All rights reserved.)

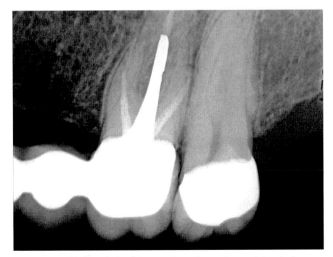

Fig. 20.4 Radiograph of a symptomatic root canal–treated maxillary left first molar with a large cast post and core. The molar is a distal abutment for a four-unit fixed bridge; therefore, surgical treatment may be a preferable treatment option, rather than attempting disassembly and post removal. (© Dr. George Bogen. All rights reserved.)

surrounding the post can be circumferentially removed using fine ultrasonic tips or a flame-tipped diamond bur.[10,30]

After the surrounding cement has been removed, the post can be loosened using specially designed ultrasonic tips at medium to high energy settings. This procedure must be executed with caution because it rapidly generates extremely high temperatures if performed without water coolant. Therefore, ultrasonic energy should be delivered in different locations around the exposed portion of the post at intervals lasting no longer than 15 seconds.[10,30-33] Ultrasonic tips used without water coolant and placed in contact with posts generate temperature increases of 10°C within 1 minute on the external root surface.[33] If this threshold temperature is reached, it can cause heat-induced bone necrosis, with possible loss of the tooth and supporting bone.

The time required to loosen posts depends on several factors, including the type of post (cast or preformed), the length and width of the post, and the luting agent used.[34] Posts cemented with zinc phosphate cement are generally easier to remove than those cemented with resin cements.[10,27,31-33,35,36] Posts cemented with resin cements are difficult or even impossible to remove.[28]

359

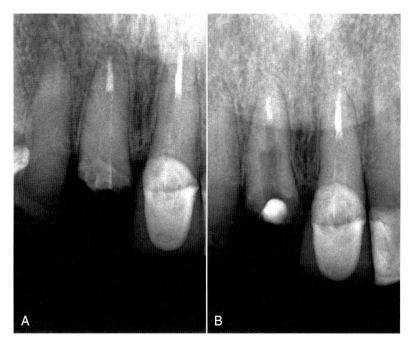

Fig. 20.5 **A,** Radiograph of a maxillary right central incisor with a fractured nonmetallic post in a 38-year-old female 10 years after placement. **B,** Working radiograph after post removal under the dental operating microscope (DOM). Note the gouging of the canal space and loss of tooth structure after post removal *(arrows).*

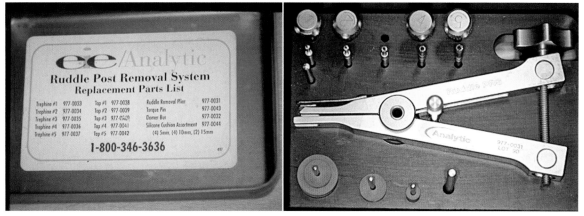

Fig. 20.6 Post removal system.

Once the post has been loosened, various-sized hemostats or small-tipped forceps or pliers can be used to grasp and remove it. In many cases the post can be dislodged using only ultrasonic energy. Screw posts can usually be removed with hemostats by turning them counterclockwise. When these methods are unsuccessful, post removal can be accomplished by using specially designed devices.[10,27,30,37] There is a greater risk of fracturing the tooth or removing excessive tooth structure using these instruments if the post is not first loosened with ultrasonics.[10,27,38] There does not seem to be any difference in the risk of root fracture between ultrasonic and post removal devices.[37,39] After post removal, any excess cement can be removed using a combination of solvents, rotary or hand instruments, or ultrasonic tips.[10,27,28]

The following is an example of post removal using a specially designed device (Fig. 20.6).[10,27,38] The coronal portion of the post is first reduced in size using a high-speed transmetal or diamond bur. After the reduction, a matching-size trepan bur is used to trough the post circumferentially, avoiding excess removal of tooth structure. The coronal portion of

the post is tapped with the matching-size extractor to firmly grasp the post, and the extractor is engaged with the specially designed pliers (Fig. 20.7). The remaining tooth structure is cushioned with rubber washers that allow the tooth to act as a fulcrum when the pliers are engaged. The technique is effective and has been shown to be relatively safe.[37] After the post and cement have been successfully removed, cleaning, shaping, and obturation of the canal system can proceed with the appropriate instruments and filling materials (Figs. 20.8 and 20.9).

Removal of Calcifications

Root canal calcifications may be noted radiographically, but internal visualization benefits from magnification and illumination using the dental operating microscope (DOM). Other obstructions must be removed before attempts are made to explore the calcified area. Once the area has been visualized, a combination of chelating agents, stiff hand files (e.g., C and C+ files), and ultrasonic tips or Mueller-type burs may be used to remove the calcified tissue to locate the root canal apical

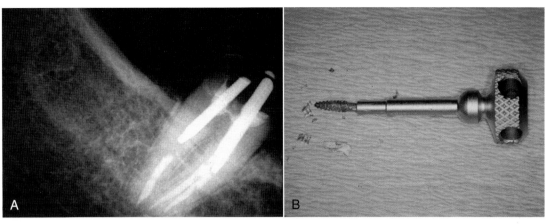

Fig. 20.7 **A,** Posts must be removed before retreatment. **B,** Post removed from the distal canal with the post removal system extractor.

to the calcification. Removal of the calcified barrier is restricted to the straight portion of the root canal when ultrasonic instrumentation or Mueller burs are used. If the canal is located with the aid of microexplorers and the DOM, a small bend can be placed on stiff, small-diameter hand files, and the curved portion of the canal can be carefully negotiated using various chelating agents and lubricants. The canal is then enlarged, using the crown-down technique, with a combination of hand files, Gates-Glidden drills, or a high-taper nickel-titanium rotary file system. If the canal cannot be negotiated due to extensive calcification or any other obstruction and an apical lesion is associated with the root, surgical intervention must be considered.

Management of Ledges

Ledges are generated during canal preparation if canal curvature is not maintained.[40] These canal problems typically occur when stainless steel files are not properly precurved to match the canal curvature. Stainless steel files have elastic memory and tend to straighten canals, thus creating ledges in the canal walls. This can lead to perforations if the situation is not recognized in a timely manner. Nickel-titanium rotary instruments reduce ledge formation because the files tend to stay centered during preparation of the canal curvature.[41]

If a ledge is encountered during the retreatment procedure, all obstructions and obturation materials must be removed and the ledge visualized after the canal has been opened up using the crown-down technique. A hand file with a sharp bend at the tip is applied with a watch-winding motion in an attempt to bypass the ledge apically. If the negotiation around the ledge is successful, the canal can be circumferentially filed until the irregularity is removed or smoothed enough to allow predictable instrumentation and obturation. Hedstrom files are an excellent option for ledges that may be more difficult to remove, but they should be used with extreme caution. After successful bypass and removal of the ledge, the apical portion of the canal can be cleaned and prepared using any of the instrumentation systems. It is worth noting that unsuccessful attempts at bypassing ledges do not always result in nonhealing (Fig. 20.10).

Instrument Fragment Removal

Successful removal of separated instrument fragments in the root canal system is influenced by various factors.[10,42-48] These

include the operator's experience and level of skill; the size, length, and location of the separated fragment; and the retrieval technique selected. Smaller instruments that are easily accessible in the coronal portion of the root canal system can be ground away or bypassed using burs or ultrasonic instruments.[28,49] Fragments deeper in the canal system may require the use of devices or kits designed specifically for this purpose (Fig. 20.11).[10,27,43]

Another approach for instrument removal is the braided file technique. Two or three small files can be used to engage the separated fragment at different locations by twisting the files together in a braiding manner and slowly pulling the files in a coronal direction. This technique works better with softer obstruction materials (e.g., silver points or plastic carriers) than with harder materials (e.g., separated instruments or metal carriers) (Fig. 20.12). As a general rule, however, the longer the fragment, the greater the probability of successful instrument removal with the braided technique. Using available instrument fragment removal kits can also be successful.[10,42,43,48,49]

The probability of successful instrument retrieval increases if the fragment is positioned coronal to the curvature and can be visualized using the DOM.[44] Separated fragments apical to the curvature are less likely to be removed, and bypassing the fragment may be attempted.[45-47] Attempts to remove canal fragments located apical to the curvature often result in canal transportation, perforations, and sometimes separation of additional instruments. Before removal procedures are initiated, the thickness of the dentin walls and the degree of curvature must be evaluated. The surgical approach may be a preferred option when the prognosis for successful removal is unfavorable.[27]

The primary goal in successful fragment removal is visualization of the coronal portion of the separated instrument, typically using the DOM. Illumination and magnification of the fragment are essential for viewing the segment. Access to the fragment can be accomplished using ultrasonic instruments, modified Gates-Glidden drills, hand files, or Mueller burs.[10,27,45-50] Small-diameter hand files are used to bypass and engage small fragments. Small-diameter ultrasonic tips can be helpful at dislodging the fragment or breaking it into smaller pieces that can be rinsed out and removed using a neutral irrigant. If the small fragment cannot be bypassed or removed, completing the treatment to the level of the **361**

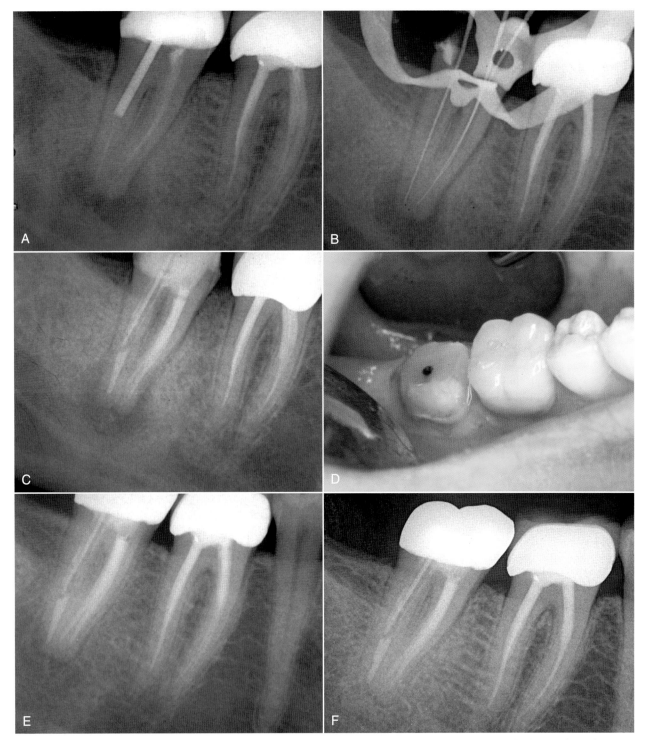

Fig. 20.8 **A,** Preoperative radiograph of a symptomatic mandibular right second molar exhibiting poorly obturated canals and an apical lesion. **B,** Initial working length radiograph after gutta-percha removal with Gates-Glidden drills and irrigation. **C,** Post-treatment radiograph of gutta-percha and sealer–retreated molar with nonmetallic (carbon fiber) post and bonded core buildup. **D,** Photograph after full crown preparation. **E,** Recall radiograph at 1 year showing remineralization of the previous apical lesion. **F,** Radiographic review at 11.5 years; the patient was asymptomatic, and the molar exhibited normal mobility and probing. (© Dr. George Bogen. All rights reserved.)

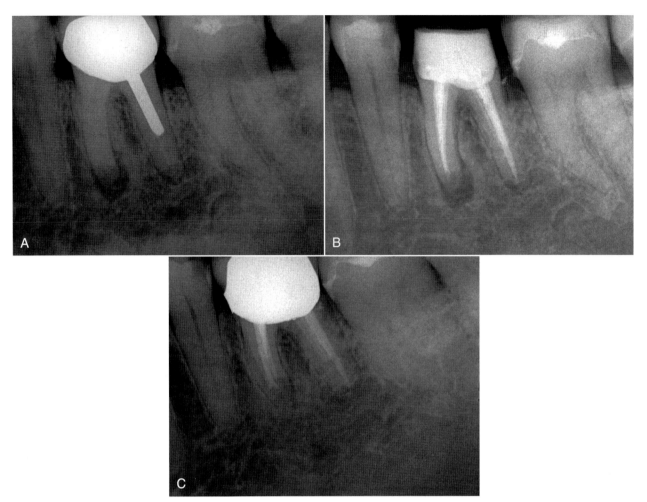

Fig. 20.9 **A,** Preoperative radiograph of a symptomatic mandibular left first molar with cast metal post and core showing a mesial root lesion and untreated mesial canals in a 41-year-old female patient. **B,** Final radiograph of nonsurgically retreated molar with laterally compacted gutta-percha and sealer restored with titanium Parapost and bonded core buildup. **C,** Recall radiograph at 4.5 years showing final full coverage restoration and apical healing of the previous mesial apical lesion. (© Dr. George Bogen. All rights reserved.)

obstruction may allow for monitoring of the outcome, in the absence of any other endodontic problems. Many teeth with inclusion of fractured instruments can succeed provided no other problems occur (Fig. 20.13).[51]

When a large, long fragment is firmly wedged in the straight portion of the canal, bypassing the object may be impossible. In these situations a staging platform is created adjacent to the coronal portion of the segment, using modified burs, rotary instruments, or Gates-Glidden drills, after the coronal portion of the fragment has been visualized.[42,45-47,50,52] The platform allows the operator to use small ultrasonic tips to carefully create space or trough around the top of the fragment. The separated segment can then be engaged and removed with a fragment removal kit or the braided file technique. The fragment may be dislodged and removed with the ultrasonic tip on higher energy settings if the tip is directed to the top of the fragment. In canals with small-diameter roots, caution must be exercised to prevent perforations. In these cases, kits that use soft metal microtubes paired with cyanoacrylate glue can be effective in fragment extraction.[10,27] Other extraction kits use microtubes with screw wedges or fine wires that can be

tightened to lock onto the head of the fragment and engage it for removal.[10,27,43,49]

If the fragment can be successfully removed, the apical portion of the canal can be cleaned and prepared with hand or rotary instrumentation. In the event that the segment is bypassed, the apical portion of the canal should be prepared using hand files. Rotary instrumentation is not recommended under these circumstances because the instrument design tends to bind against the retained fragment, causing fracture of the rotary file. The burden of additional separated instruments in the root canal system further complicates the long-term prognosis and successful outcome of nonsurgical root canal retreatment.[53]

Removal of Gutta-Percha

Gutta-percha is a universally used obturation material and therefore requires removal more frequently than all other materials during nonsurgical retreatment. The reason for removal may be to better prepare a root canal or to address a canal that has not been adequately filled. Removal of this filling material can be accomplished using hand and rotary

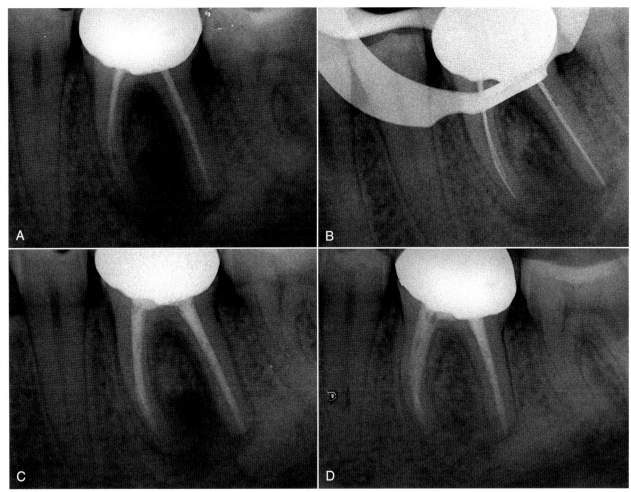

Fig. 20.10 **A,** Preoperative radiograph of a mandibular left first molar showing an inadequate obturation of the mesial roots and ongoing apical periodontitis in a symptomatic, 37-year-old male patient. **B,** Working file radiograph showing inability of operator to negotiate blocked apical 4-mm curvature. **C,** Post-treatment radiograph after placement of bonded core in the access cavity. **D,** Review radiograph at 1 year showing complete healing of the initial apical lesion. (© Dr. George Bogen. All rights reserved.)

instruments, ultrasonic instruments, heat systems, or solvents. Typically, removal of the material involves a combination of these methods.

Regular hand reamers, Hedstrom files, and Gates-Glidden drills are the instruments of choice to remove gutta-percha (Fig. 20.14).[49,54] If space exists or can easily be created between the canal wall and the obturation material, a hand reamer or Hedstrom file can be placed in the canal and the instrument twisted in a clockwise direction until the gutta-percha is engaged. The gutta-percha can occasionally be removed in one piece in a lifting motion. Remaining gutta-percha and sealer are removed during a crown-down instrumentation approach while using appropriate irrigants. Crown-down instrumentation avoids pushing debris apically and forcing material out the foramen into the periapical tissues. After canal instrumentation has been completed, inspection with the DOM and a radiograph are recommended to ensure that no residual gutta-percha or debris remains on the canal walls.[55]

Removal of gutta-percha can be more difficult when the material is densely packed and well adapted.[49,56] Flame-heated gutta-percha pluggers can be used to soften the material for removal with hand instruments. The pluggers cool quickly because the gutta-percha rapidly dissipates the heat; therefore, removal can be done only in short increments. This technique preserves internal canal tooth structure. However, the heated hand plugger technique is time-consuming, and when the apical portion of the canal is approached, it can increase the risk of pushing the gutta-percha beyond the apical foramen.

A more predictable alternative method involves using thermostatically heated pluggers that can be placed into the gutta-percha without cooling down.[54] These devices allow insertion into the gutta-percha toward the apical portion of the canal, increasing the probability that the mass of the material can be removed as the plugger is cooled down. This method also decreases the probability that gutta-percha will be extruded out of the apical foramen. After a large portion of the gutta-percha has been removed, the retreatment can be continued using irrigation and instrumentation in a crown-down manner.

Sonic and ultrasonic tips can also be used to remove gutta-percha.[49,56-58] The ultrasonic energy generated in the tips of the instruments is effective in softening the gutta-percha, but the actual removal of the filling material by this method is

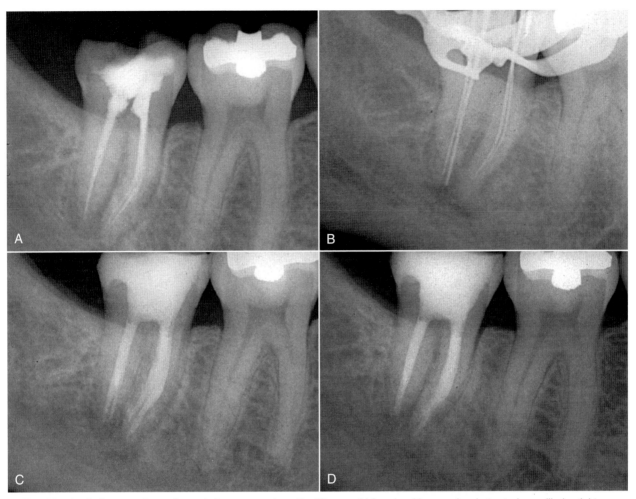

Fig. 20.11 **A,** Preoperative radiograph from a symptomatic, 52-year-old female with a previously treated mandibular right second molar. Note the separated K-file in the apical portion of the mesiobuccal root *(arrow)* associated with apical pathosis. **B,** Working length radiograph after file removal using the DOM and ultrasonic tips. Note the location and negotiation of the missed second distal canal. **C,** Final retreatment radiograph showing the obturated second distal canal *(arrow)* and bonded core buildup. **D,** Review radiograph at 6 months showing advanced healing of the previous apical periodontitis. (© Dr. George Bogen. All rights reserved.)

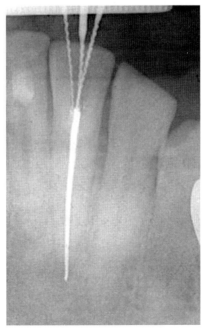

Fig. 20.12 Small Hedstrom files braided around a silver point obturation. (© Dr. Robert Handysides. All rights reserved.)

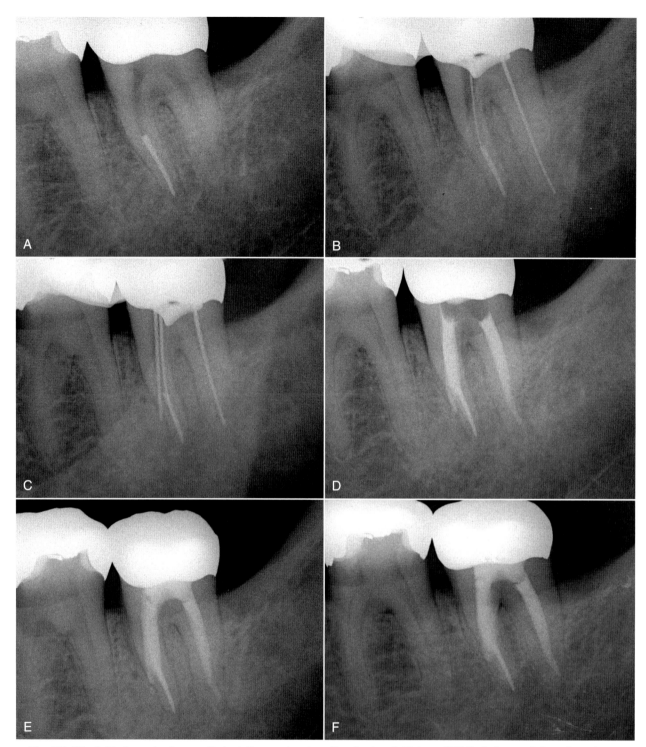

Fig. 20.13 **A,** Radiograph of a mandibular left second molar with a fractured .06 taper NiTi file in the mesiolingual root in an asymptomatic, 64-year-old male patient. **B,** Radiograph of working length files before "platforming." **C,** Working radiograph of files showing perforation to the mesial aspect of the mesiolingual canal after attempts were made to remove the file using ultrasonic tips. **D,** Postoperative radiograph after final obturation and mineral trioxide aggregate (MTA) repair. **E,** Recall radiograph at 1 year showing bonded core buildup. Note the absence of apical disease. **F,** Seven-year radiographic review. The tooth was firm and showed normal probing and mobility. (© Dr. George Bogen. All rights reserved.)

somewhat ineffective.[49] When used, this method must be coupled with hand and rotary instrumentation to successfully remove the existing gutta-percha. Ultrasonic tips are more effective at facilitating the removal of residual sealer and **366** debris after the bulk of the gutta-percha material has been removed.[59]

The quickest method of removing gutta-percha is with rotary files or Gates-Glidden drills.[54,60,61] Gates-Glidden drills are effective for this purpose but should probably be limited to the coronal portion of the canal, and excessive force must not be used due to the possible presence of apical root resorption and resultant material extrusion.[62,63] Rotary files modified

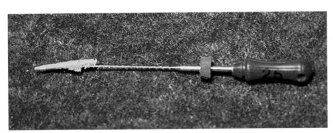

Fig. 20.14 Gutta-percha engaged with a Hedstrom file and removed in one piece.

by manufacturers specifically for gutta-percha removal can also be effective.[49,54,60,64-68]

The selected file system is directed to the most coronal aspect of the gutta-percha after a purchase point has been selected. At the appropriate speed setting, the files are directed apically; they remove the gutta-percha in a coronal direction as the files are advanced through the material. However, the technique is limited to roots with straight canals or the straight portions of curved canals. After the bulk of the material has been removed, the canal can be shaped and irrigated using the crown-down technique. It has been shown that this method is also effective in removing newly developed obturation materials, including synthetic polymers, silicone-based, glass ionomer, methacrylate, and epoxy-based materials.[65-67,69,70]

Removal of gutta-percha from the root canal system can be expedited by using solvents.[49,60,65,71] However, greater amounts of gutta-percha and sealer remnants can be found on the root canal walls when solvents are used.[68,71,72] If a solvent is indicated, a small amount of the solvent is carefully placed in contact with the exposed gutta-percha and allowed to soften the material. After the gutta-percha has softened, either rotary or hand files can be used to remove the material in a crown-down fashion. The most effective solvent has been shown to be chloroform.[49,60,65,73] The solvent works quickly, but care must be taken not to extrude the material out of the apical foramen.[74,75] A safer alternative to chloroform is halothane, which is slower to dissolve gutta-percha but shows acceptable results.[58,76,77] Methylchloroform is another alternative to chloroform. It is more effective than eucalyptol and xylene, shows less toxicity, and is not carcinogenic.[49] Xylene, eucalyptus oil, carbon disulfide, benzene, and orange oil have been used for this purpose but have been shown to be less effective at softening gutta-percha.[49,74,75]

Chloroform has been reported to have cytotoxic and carcinogenic properties, although it is considered relatively safe when used in small amounts.[78] Due to these properties, alternative solvents have been recommended, but their efficacy has met with mixed results. One investigation measured the amount of residual chloroform, halothane, and xylene expressed through the apical foramen during retreatment procedures.[74] It was determined that the amount of each solvent expressed was below the levels that may pose a health risk to patients. Solvents are helpful adjuncts to the removal of gutta-percha, especially when the material has hardened over time. After their use, treatment can proceed using the crown-down technique.

Removal of Carrier-Based Gutta-Percha Obturators

A popular method of root canal filling in recent years has been the use of carrier-based gutta-percha obturators. These devices

have a central core of plastic, metal, or other dense material that is coated with gutta-percha; they can be used typically as a single root canal filling cone. During nonsurgical retreatment, these obturators can be removed using a combination of techniques similar to those for removing posts, silver points, and gutta-percha. The initial treatment begins by creating a pathway that allows an instrument to engage the carrier by first softening the gutta-percha on the surface of the carrier with a heat source or solvent.[79,80-84] The solvents described earlier in this chapter are used for this purpose. If a heat source is used to soften the gutta-percha, a thermostatically controlled device, plugger, or endodontic heat carrier heated over an open flame is effective.[83] Care should be taken to avoid placing the heated tip in contact with the dentin wall for long periods because the rapid increase in temperature can damage the periodontium and surrounding bone.[84] Gutta-percha can also be softened using rotary instrumentation at higher speeds (1,500 to 2,500 rpm), but use of these instruments should be limited to straight canals because the possibility of file separation in a curved canal is high.[53,85]

Single or multiple files can be used to engage and remove the carrier once a pathway has been created.[79,80,82,83] Large-taper rotary files have also been recommended to engage and remove plastic-based carriers. These strategies can work well for plastic carriers but are less effective for metal-based carriers because of the difficulty of engaging the metal surface with files. Metal carriers are more easily removed using the braided file technique described previously or using modified hemostats, pliers, and ultrasonic instruments. After successful removal of the carriers and gutta-percha, canal preparation and obturation can be completed.

Removal of Silver Cones (Points)

The most important aspect of successfully removing silver cones is to ensure that as much of the coronal portion of the cone is accessible as possible.[86] Silver points are commonly embedded in a core material that must be carefully removed while preserving and not removing the coronal extent of the cone.[86-88] Illumination and magnification with the DOM are essential adjuncts during core or base material removal using burs or ultrasonic tips. After removal of the core material, solvents, ultrasonic instruments or hand files are used to create a space around the exposed silver point.[88-90] Silver points are soft, and attention must be paid to avoiding contact with ultrasonic tips that can easily cut through them. The removal strategy involves breaking the seal of the root canal cement and the silver cone. One or two files should be engaged and braided around the cone; then, ultrasonic energy is transferred to the files. When this technique is performed correctly, the ultrasonic energy facilitates cone removal by rapidly breaking down the cement seal.

The coronal portion of a loosened cone extending from the pulp chamber can then be grasped and pulled from the canal with a variety of devices. These include various types of specialized hemostats, modified or regular Steiglitz forceps, needle holders, gold foil pliers, Caufield silver point retrievers, or splinter forceps (Fig. 20.15).[27,49,89] If the coronal portion of the cone is not present or is accidentally removed during removal of the core material, one or more hand files can be used to engage and extract the cone, as described previously.[27,89] An alternative method to remove cones in this situation includes flexible metal tubes or needle-sleeve devices that grasp the cone with a file or wire or attach the cone head

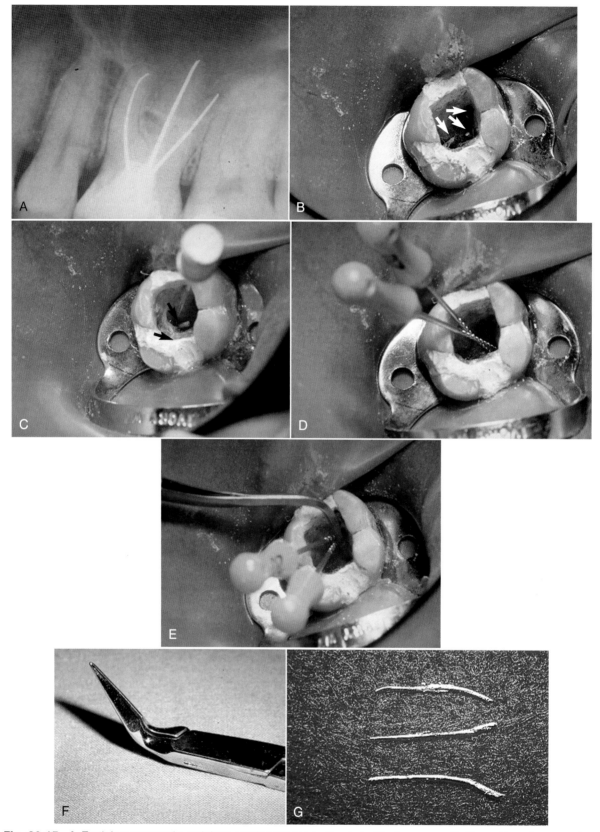

Fig. 20.15 **A,** Tooth is symptomatic, and three canals have been obturated with silver cones. **B,** Cement base is removed, and the coronal ends of the silver cones extending into the pulp chamber are exposed *(arrows).* **C,** A hand file is used to create space between the silver cone *(arrow)* and root canal wall. **D,** Hand files braided around one of the silver cones. **E,** An ultrasonic tip is activated while in contact with the files to deliver energy to the silver cone. This technique aids in breaking the seal between the silver cone and the root canal cement. **F,** Steiglitz forceps grasp the coronal ends of the loosened silver cones. **G,** All three silver cones were successfully removed intact.

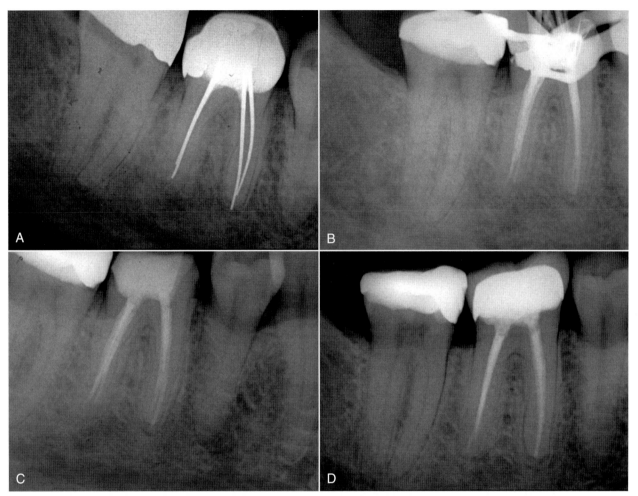

Fig. 20.16 **A,** Preoperative radiograph of a previously treated mandibular right first molar with silver cones in a 34-year-old, asymptomatic female patient. **B,** Radiograph of initial obturation using laterally compacted gutta-percha and sealer after silver point removal. **C,** Final radiograph of nonsurgically retreated molar with bonded core buildup. **D,** Two-year radiographic review showing full coverage restoration and absence of apical pathosis. (© Dr. George Bogen. All rights reserved.)

using cyanoacrylate glue.* These techniques require the use of a trepan bur to trough an access area for the devices.[27,49,86,91] After successful removal of the silver point, cleaning and shaping procedures can proceed (Fig. 20.16). Silver points that cannot be removed may necessitate surgical intervention to facilitate loosening of the point through a retrograde approach (Fig. 20.17).

Removal of Soft and Hard Pastes

Hand or rotary instruments can be used to easily penetrate and remove soft pastes used to obturate the root canal system.[49] It is important to use copious irrigation and a crown-down preparation technique when removing soft materials from the canal system.[49] This method can prevent potentially painful postoperative flare-ups caused when toxic or contaminated materials are inadvertently extruded into the apical tissues (Fig. 20.18).

The hard-setting pastes are more difficult (and in some cases may be impossible) to remove. One strategy is to remove

4 mm from the tip of a K-file, creating a sharp edge at the tip so as to better cut into and remove the hardened material.[92] Dental companies now manufacture files with hardened sharp points that can be used to penetrate these materials initially. If these devices are not successful, ultrasonic tips or burs with small-diameter heads can be used to try to remove the hardened paste.[28,49,93] Perforation and the creation of ledges are potential problems when attempting to remove hardened cements in the root canals, especially if the canals are curved.[49]

Various endodontic solvents have been investigated for their efficacy in softening hard obturation pastes to facilitate their removal. Although one investigation reported sodium hypochlorite to be effective in softening a resorcinol-formalin paste (Russian Red), a follow-up study comparing six different solvents, including sodium hypochlorite, found none to be more effective than water, which was used as the control (Fig. 20.19).[94,95] Ultrasonic instrumentation remains the most predictable means of hard paste removal. If removal of the hard paste is not successful or there is a high probability that procedural errors may occur during removal, the option of apical surgery or intentional replantation should be considered for tooth retention.

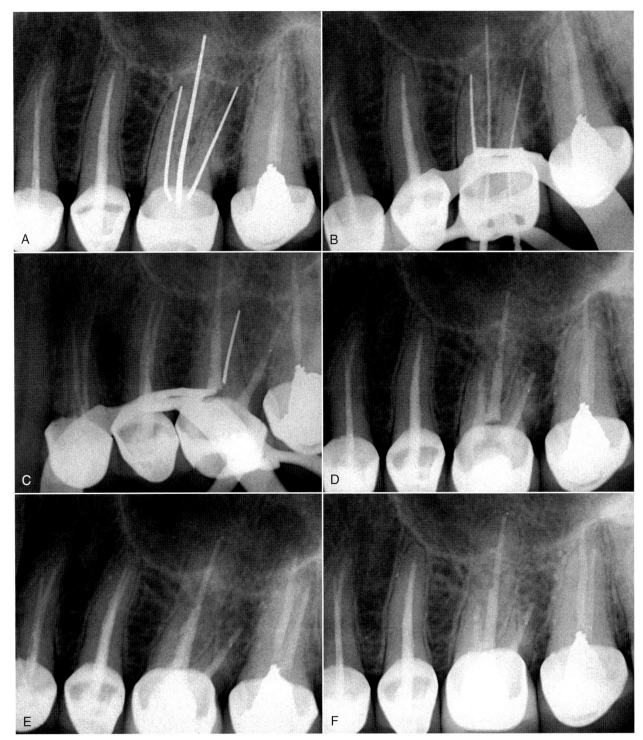

Fig. 20.17 **A,** Radiograph of a previously treated maxillary right first molar in a 62-year-old, symptomatic female patient. Note that the silver cones have been severed at the canal orifices. **B,** Working length radiograph **(B)** and obturation radiograph **(C)** showing irretrievable silver cone lodged in the mesiobuccal canal. **D,** Postoperative radiograph after removal of the silver point, resection of both buccal roots, and placement of MTA retrofills. Follow-up radiographs at 6 months **(E)** and 1 year **(F)** showing healing and repair of the osteotomy sites. The molar was firm and exhibited normal mobility and probing. (© Dr. George Bogen. All rights reserved.)

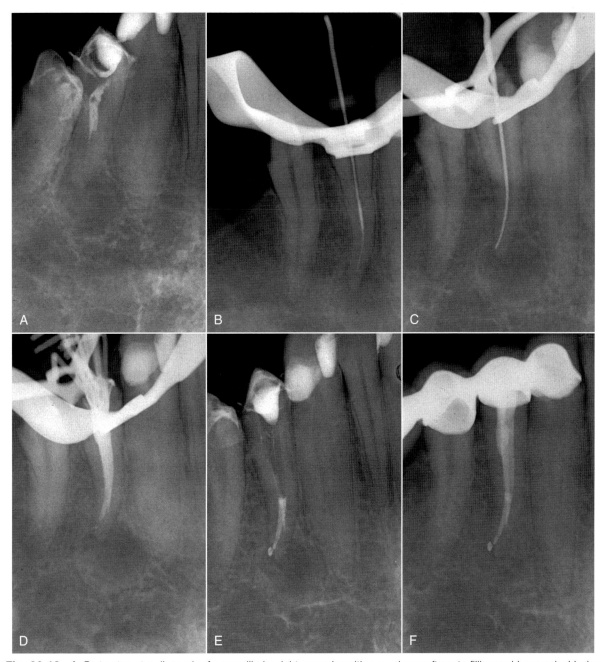

Fig. 20.18 **A,** Pretreatment radiograph of a mandibular right premolar with a previous soft paste filling and large apical lesion in a 29-year-old male. Radiograph of initial working length file **(B)** and with master apical file to length **(C)**. **D,** Radiograph of initial obturation using laterally compacted gutta-percha and AH26 sealer. **E,** Final radiograph with post space. **F,** One-year radiographic review showing nonmetallic post and placement of a five-unit fixed bridge. Note the presence of remineralization and healing of previous apical lesion. (© Dr. George Bogen. All rights reserved.)

POST-TREATMENT COMPLICATIONS

Post-treatment flare-ups occur more frequently in some but not all studies of retreatment cases, compared to teeth receiving initial root canal therapy.[96-98] Part of the explanation for an increase in flare-ups may be that procedures used in retreatment may result in extrusion of bacteria and other irritants into the apical tissues.[5] The crown-down technique, paired with frequent use of irrigants injected with side-venting needles, promotes debris removal in a coronal direction and helps prevent this complication. Other important preventive considerations include maintaining asepsis by using the dental dam, complete cleaning of the canal system initially, using intracanal medicaments (e.g., calcium hydroxide) between appointments, using advanced irrigants and evacuation systems, not leaving the tooth open for drainage between visits, and inspecting the canals with the DOM before obturation to ensure that all visible materials have been properly removed.[5,55,99,100] The clinician should consider scheduling more than one appointment for the retreatment process to gain the benefit of using intracanal medication and further irrigation to aid in canal disinfection.

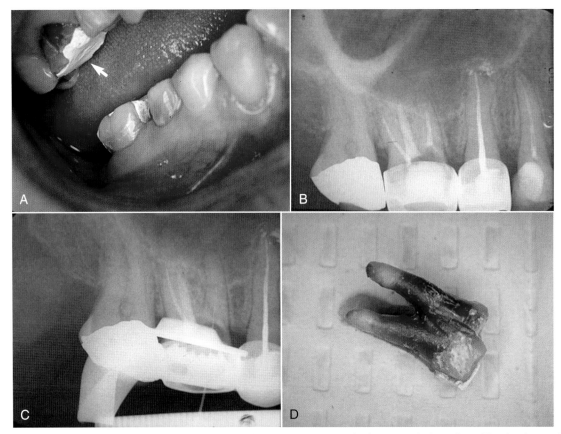

Fig. 20.19 **A,** Tooth *(arrow)* exhibits red discoloration of the crown as a result of root canal obturation with a hard resorcinol paste material. **B,** The resorcinol obturations are short of ideal length in all three canals of tooth #3. Resorcinol paste was also present in the premolars. **C,** The resorcinol material was successfully removed from the coronal portion of the mesiobuccal canal, but the canal was calcified apical to the level of the previous obturation. A root perforation occurred during attempts to remove the material from the palatal canal. The treatment plan was altered, and the tooth was extracted and replaced as part of a bridge. **D,** Note that the red discoloration of the roots extends to the level of the previous resorcinol obturations.

Repair of Perforations

Iatrogenic mishaps are addressed in Chapter 18; however, some of these mishaps are encountered during retreatment procedures. Retreatment outcomes have been shown to be less favorable when teeth have been perforated initially.[101,102] Such perforations need to be repaired during the retreatment. The prognosis for teeth with perforations depends on three critical factors: the size of the perforation, the location of the perforation, and the elapsed time since the injury.[102,103] In recent years mineral trioxide aggregate (MTA) and similar bioactive products have been shown to be favorable materials for repairing perforations (Fig. 20.20).[104,105] Preoperative radiographic assessment can aid in identifying previous areas of iatrogenic perforations prior to initiation of nonsurgical retreatment. The procedures for repairing perforations require careful evaluation of all factors involved; for the benefit of the patient, referral to a specialist should be considered.

RESTORATIVE OPTIONS

Successfully retreated teeth require the same attention to their restorative care as that provided for teeth receiving initial endodontic therapy. The key objective is to place a definitive restoration as soon as possible to prevent coronal microleakage, avoid propagation of existing coronal infractions if present, conserve remaining tooth structure, and prevent the need for additional retreatment or surgical procedures. Long-term provisional restorations can lead to recontamination of the filling material, which may necessitate tooth extraction.[106] Full coverage restorations are usually recommended for all posterior teeth and may be required for anterior teeth. If sufficient coronal tooth structure is present in anterior teeth, a bonded composite restoration usually is adequate.

FOLLOW-UP CARE

Follow-up visits are important for monitoring symptoms and ensuring that periapical healing occurs. A common schedule is a follow-up visit usually after the first 6 months and then yearly. Sometimes it is wise to schedule the first follow-up visit sooner than 6 months if there are questions about the condition of the tooth after treatment. Follow-up visits should include an assessment of mobility, periodontal probing, and palpation and percussion testing, in addition to radiographic examination of any periradicular pathosis present at the time of treatment. Patients should be advised to return if any symptoms recur.

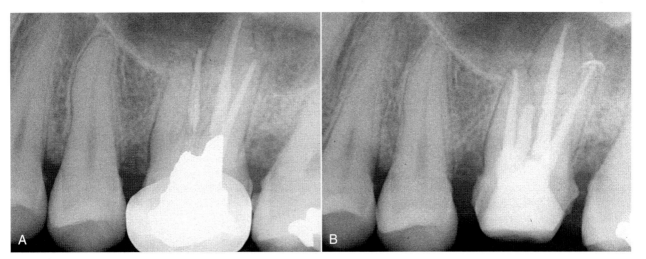

Fig. 20.20 **A,** Radiograph of a symptomatic maxillary left first molar exhibiting an untreated mesiobuccal canal, poorly adapted amalgam core, and substandard full coverage restoration in a 57-year-old male patient. **B,** Post-treatment radiograph showing nonsurgical retreatment of the molar with MTA repair *(arrow)* of the previous perforation, complete obturation of the mesiobuccal root, and a bonded composite core buildup. (© Dr. George Bogen. All rights reserved.)

PROGNOSIS

Advances in nonsurgical retreatment have improved the outcomes for cases completed using current technology, compared to past retreatment methods.[6,107-110] A meta-analysis of retreatment success rates that encompassed studies from 1956 until 1996 revealed success rates of 95% for teeth showing no apical pathology to 66% when apical pathosis was present. However, these same studies show that the tooth remains functional 86% to 92% of the time after endodontic therapy.[111-113]

It has been shown that long-term success rates for nonsurgical retreatment, compared to surgical treatment, is significantly higher at 4 to 6 years (83% versus 71.8%).[114] However, direct comparison of the two procedures using a randomized trial shows no significant differences.[115] Moreover, success rates for surgical endodontic procedures increase when these procedures are combined with nonsurgical retreatment.[9,18,21,90] One prospective study, which compared the periapical health of roots associated with initial treatment and retreatment over a 2- to 4-year period, found the rates for successful outcomes to be similar (83% and 80%, respectively).[101]

Some prognostic factors have been identified that improve periapical healing; these include the absence of a preoperative periapical lesion and sinus tract, achievement of apical patency and extension of canal cleaning to the apical terminus, proper irrigation protocols, absence of perforations or interappointment flare-ups, maintenance of the original shape of the canals radiographically, and satisfactory coronal restorations. A 4-year cumulative follow-up study comparing the survival of teeth after initial and retreatment procedures also showed similar success rates (95%) when the procedures were performed using contemporary protocols.[116]

Based on the findings of numerous studies, it is clear that retreatment of teeth that are associated with either initial nonhealing or recurrence of endodontic disease is quite predictable if the retreatment is carried out according to contemporary endodontic principles. It must be emphasized that favorable outcomes are enhanced by the use of good illumination and magnification, dental dam isolation, improved irrigation systems, and advanced instrumentation devices.[99,100]

REFERENCES

1. Alley BS, Kitchens GG, Alley LW, et al: A comparison of survival of teeth following endodontic treatment performed by general dentists or by specialists, *Oral Surg Oral Med Oral Pathol Oral Radiol Endod* 98:115, 2004.
2. Salehrabi R, Rotstein I: Epidemiologic evaluation of the outcomes of orthograde endodontic retreatment, *J Endod* 36:790, 2010.
3. Molander A, Reit C, Dahlen G, et al: Microbiological status of root-filled teeth with apical periodontitis, *Int Endod J* 31:1, 1998.
4. Sundqvist G, Figdor D, Persson S, et al: Microbiologic analysis of teeth with failed endodontic treatment and the outcome of conservative re-treatment, *Oral Surg Oral Med Oral Pathol Oral Radiol Endod* 85:86, 1998.
5. Siqueira JF Jr: Microbial causes of endodontic flare-ups, *Int Endod J* 36:453, 2003.

6. Allen RK, Newton CW, Brown CE Jr: A statistical analysis of surgical and nonsurgical endodontic retreatment cases, *J Endod* 15:261, 1989.
7. Sjögren U, Figdor D, Persson S, et al: Influence of infection at the time of root filling on the outcome of endodontic treatment of teeth with apical periodontitis, *Int Endod J* 30:297, 1997.
8. Hoen MM, Pink FE: Contemporary endodontic retreatments: an analysis based on clinical treatment findings, *J Endod* 28:834, 2002.
9. Friedman S, Stabholz A: Endodontic retreatment-case selection and technique. Part 1. Criteria for case selection, *J Endod* 12:28, 1986.
10. Ruddle CJ: Nonsurgical retreatment, *J Endod* 30:827, 2004.
11. Ricucci D, Siqueira JF Jr: Biofilms and apical periodontitis: study of prevalence and association with clinical and histopathologic findings, *J Endod* 36:1277, 2010.
12. Chong BS: Coronal leakage and treatment failure, *J Endod* 21:159, 1995.
13. Begotka BA, Hartwell GR: The importance of the coronal seal following root canal treatment, *Va Dent J* 73:8, 1996.
14. Hartwell GR, Loucks CA, Reavley BA: Bacterial leakage of provisional restorative materials used in endodontics, *Quintessence Int* 41:335, 2010.
15. Tamse A: Iatrogenic vertical root fractures in endodontically treated teeth, *Endod Dent Traumatol* 4:190, 1988.
16. Sedgley CM, Messer HH: Are endodontically treated teeth more brittle? *J Endod* 18:332, 1992.
17. Fuss Z, Lustig J, Katz A, et al: An evaluation of endodontically treated vertically fractured roots:

impact of operative procedures, *J Endod* 1:46, 2001.

18. Taschieri S, Machtou P, Rosano G, et al: The influence of previous non-surgical re-treatment on the outcome of endodontic surgery, *Minerva Stomatol* 59:625, 2010.

19. Kingsbury B, Weisenbaugh J: Intentional replantation of mandibular premolars and molars, *J Am Dent Assoc* 83:1053, 1971.

20. Koenig K, Nguyen N, Barkhordar RA: Intentional replantation: a report of 192 cases, *Gen Dent* 36:327, 1988.

21. Tsesis I, Faivishevsky V, Kfir A, et al: Outcome of surgical endodontic treatment performed by a modern technique: a meta-analysis of literature, *J Endod* 35:1505, 2009.

22. von Arx T, Hänni S, Jensen SS: Correlation of bone defect dimensions with healing outcome one year after apical surgery, *J Endod* 33:1044, 2007.

23. Klavan B: Clinical observations following root amputation in maxillary molar teeth, *J Periodontol* 46:1, 1975.

24. Kost WJ, Stakiw JE: Root amputation and hemisection, *J Can Dent Assoc* 57:42, 1991.

25. de Sanctis M, Prato GP: Root resection and root amputation, *Curr Opin Periodontol* PMID: 8401832, 1993.

26. Kim SG, Solomon C: Cost-effectiveness of endodontic molar retreatment compared with fixed partial dentures and single-tooth implant alternatives, *J Endod* 37:321, 2011.

27. Hülsmann M: Methods for removing metal obstructions from the root canal, *Endod Dent Traumatol* 9:223, 1993.

28. Stabholz A, Friedman S: Endodontic retreatment: case selection and technique. Part 2. Treatment planning for retreatment, *J Endod* 14:607, 1988.

29. Selbst AG: Understanding informed consent and its relationship to the incidence of adverse treatment events in conventional endodontic therapy, *J Endod* 16:387, 1990.

30. Machtou P, Sarfati P, Cohen AG: Post removal prior to retreatment, *J Endod* 15:552, 1989.

31. Smith BJ: Removal of fractured posts using ultrasonic vibration: an in vivo study, *J Endod* 27:632, 2001.

32. Dixon EB, Kaczkowski PJ, Nicholls JI, et al: Comparison of two ultrasonic instruments for post removal, *J Endod* 28:111, 2002.

33. Dominici JT, Clark S, Scheetz J, et al: Analysis of heat generation using ultrasonic vibration for post removal, *J Endod* 31:301, 2005.

34. Hauman CH: Factors influencing the removal of posts, *Int Endod J* 36:687, 2003.

35. Johnson WT, Leary JM, Boyer DB: Effect of ultrasonic vibration on post removal in extracted human premolar teeth, *J Endod* 22:487, 1996.

36. Yoshida T, Gomyo S, Itoh T, et al: An experimental study of the removal of cemented dowel-retained cast cores by ultrasonic vibration, *J Endod* 23:239, 1997.

37. Altshul JH, Marshall G, Morgan LA, et al: Comparison of dentinal crack incidence and of post removal time resulting from post removal by ultrasonic or mechanical force, *J Endod* 23:683, 1997.

38. Machtou P, Sarfati P, Cohen AG: Post removal prior to retreatment, *J Endod* 15:552, 1989.

39. Abbott PV: Incidence of root fractures and methods used for post removal, *Int Endod J* 35:63, 2002.

40. Jafarzadeh H: Ledge formation: review of a great challenge in endodontics, *J Endod* 33:1155, 2007.

41. Song YL, Bian Z, Fan B, et al: A comparison of instrument-centering ability within the root canal for three contemporary instrumentation techniques, *Int Endod J* 37:265, 2004.

42. Terauchi Y, O'Leary L, Suda H: Removal of separated files from root canals with a new file-removal system: case reports, *J Endod* 32:789, 2006.

43. Roig-Greene JL: The retrieval of foreign objects from root canals: a simple aid, *J Endod* 9:394, 1983.

44. Nevares G, Cunha RS, Zuolo ML, et al: Success rates for removing or bypassing fractured instruments: a prospective clinical study, *J Endod* 38:442, 2012.

45. Iqbal MK, Rafailov H, Kratchman SI, et al: A comparison of three methods for preparing centered platforms around separated instruments in curved canals, *J Endod* 32:48, 2006.

46. Thirumalai AK, Sekar M, Mylswamy S: Retrieval of a separated instrument using Masserann technique, *J Conserv Dent* 11:42, 2008.

47. Gencoglu N, Helvacioglu D: Comparison of the different techniques to remove fractured endodontic instruments from root canal systems, *Eur J Dent* 3:90, 2009.

48. Hülsmann M, Schinkel I: Influence of several factors on the success or failure of removal of fractured instruments from the root canal, *Endod Dent Traumatol* 15:252, 1999.

49. Friedman S, Stabholz A, Tamse A: Endodontic retreatment: case selection and technique. Part 3. Retreatment techniques, *J Endod* 16:543, 1990.

50. Souter NJ, Messer HH: Complications associated with fractured file removal using an ultrasonic technique, *J Endod* 31:450, 2005.

51. Panitvisai P, Parunnit P, Sathorn C, et al: Impact of a retained instrument on treatment outcome: a systematic review and meta-analysis, *J Endod* 36:775, 2010.

52. Nehme W: A new approach for the retrieval of broken instruments, *J Endod* 25:633, 1999.

53. Fishelberg G, Pawluk JW: Nickel-titanium rotary-file canal preparation and intracanal file separation, *Compend Contin Educ Dent* 25:17, 2004.

54. Hülsmann M, Stotz S: Efficacy, cleaning ability and safety of different devices for gutta-percha removal in root canal retreatment, *Int Endod J* 30:227, 1997.

55. Chauhan R, Tikku A, Chandra A: Detection of residual obturation material after root canal retreatment with three different techniques using a dental operating microscope and a stereomicroscope: an in vitro comparative evaluation, *J Conserv Dent* 15:218, 2012.

56. Wilcox LR, Krell KV, Madison S, et al: Endodontic retreatment: evaluation of gutta-percha and sealer removal and canal reinstrumentation, *J Endod* 13:453, 1987.

57. Wilcox LR: Endodontic retreatment: ultrasonics and chloroform as the final step in reinstrumentation, *J Endod* 15:125, 1989.

58. Ladley RW, Campbell AD, Hicks ML, et al: Effectiveness of halothane used with ultrasonic or hand instrumentation to remove gutta-percha from the root canal, *J Endod* 17:221, 1991.

59. Moshonov J, Trope M, Friedman S: Retreatment efficacy 3 months after obturation using glass ionomer cement, zinc oxide–eugenol, and epoxy resin sealers, *J Endod* 20:90, 1994.

60. Ferreira JJ, Rhodes JS, Ford TR: The efficacy of gutta-percha removal using ProFiles, *Int Endod J* 34:267, 2001.

61. Beasley RT, Williamson AE, Justman BC, et al: Time required to remove GuttaCore, Thermafil Plus and thermoplasticized gutta-percha from moderately curved root canals, *J Endod* 39:125, 2013.

62. Laux M, Abbott PV, Pajarola G, et al: Apical inflammatory root resorption: a correlative radiographic and histological assessment, *Int Endod J* 33:483, 2000.

63. Vier FV, Figueiredo JA: Prevalence of different periapical lesions associated with human teeth and their correlation with the presence and extension of apical external root resorption, *Int Endod J* 35:710, 2002.

64. Sae-Lim V, Rajamanickam I, Lim BK, et al: Effectiveness of ProFile .04 taper rotary instruments in endodontic retreatment, *J Endod* 26:100, 2000.

65. Ezzie E, Fleury A, Solomon E, et al: Efficacy of retreatment techniques for a resin-based root canal obturation material, *J Endod* 32:341, 2006.

66. de Oliveira DP, Barbizam JV, Trope M, et al: Comparison between gutta-percha and Resilon removal using two different techniques in endodontic retreatment, *J Endod* 32:362, 2006.

67. Schirrmeister JF, Meyer KM, Hermanns P, et al: Effectiveness of hand and rotary instrumentation for removing a new synthetic polymer-based root canal obturation material (Epiphany) during retreatment, *Int Endod J* 39:150, 2006.

68. Ma J, Al-Ashaw AJ, Shen Y, et al: Efficacy of ProTaper universal rotary retreatment system for gutta-percha removal from oval canals: a micro-computed tomography study, *J Endod* 38:1516, 2012.

69. Roberts S, Kim JR, Gu LS, et al: The efficacy of different sealer removal protocols on bonding of self-etching adhesives to AH plus-contaminated dentin, *J Endod* 35:563, 2009.

70. Kuga MC, Faria G, Rossi MA, et al: Persistence of epoxy-based sealer residues in dentin treated with different chemical removal protocols, *Scanning* 35:17, 2013.

71. Horvath SD, Altenburger MJ, Naumann M, et al: Cleanliness of dentinal tubules following gutta-percha removal with and without solvents: a scanning electron microscopic study, *Int Endod J* 42:1032, 2009.

72. Scelza MF, Coil JM, Maciel AC, et al: Comparative SEM evaluation of three solvents used in endodontic retreatment: an ex vivo study, *J Appl Oral Sci* 16:24, 2008.

73. Bueno CE, Delboni MG, de Araújo RA, et al: Effectiveness of rotary and hand files in gutta-percha and sealer removal using chloroform or chlorhexidine gel, *Braz Dent J* 17:139, 2006.

74. Chutich MJ, Kaminski EJ, Miller DA, et al: Risk assessment of the toxicity of solvents of gutta-percha used in endodontic retreatment, *J Endod* 24:213, 1998.

75. Hansen MG: Relative efficiency of solvents used in endodontics, *J Endod* 24:38, 1998.

76. Wourms DJ, Campbell AD, Hicks ML, et al: Alternative solvents to chloroform for gutta-percha removal, *J Endod* 16:224, 1990.

77. Wilcox LR: Endodontic retreatment with halothane versus chloroform solvent, *J Endod* 21:305, 1995.

78. McDonald MN, Vire DE: Chloroform in the endodontic operatory, *J Endod* 18:301, 1992.

79. Ibarrola JL, Knowles KI, Ludlow MO: Retrievability of Thermafil plastic cores using organic solvents, *J Endod* 19:417, 1993.

80. Imura N, Zuolo ML, Kherlakian D: Comparison of endodontic retreatment of laterally condensed gutta-percha and Thermafil with plastic carriers, *J Endod* 19:609, 1993.

81. Wilcox LR: Thermafil retreatment with and without chloroform solvent, *J Endod* 19:563, 1993.

82. Zuolo ML, Imura N, Ferreira MO: Endodontic retreatment of Thermafil or lateral condensation obturations in post space prepared teeth, *J Endod* 20:9, 1994.

83. Wolcott JF, Himel VT, Hicks ML: Thermafil retreatment using a new "System B" technique or a solvent, *J Endod* 25:761, 1999.

84. Lipski M, Wozniak K: In vitro infrared thermographic assessment of root surface temperature rises during Thermafil retreatment using system B, *J Endod* 29:413, 2003.

85. Rödig T, Hausdörfer T, Konietschke F, et al: Efficacy of D-RaCe and ProTaper universal retreatment NiTi instruments and hand files in removing gutta-percha from curved root canals: a micro-computed tomography study, *Int Endod J* 45:580, 2012.

86. Krell KV, Fuller MW, Scott GL: The conservative retrieval of silver cones in difficult cases, *J Endod* 10:269, 1984.

87. Stabholz A, Friedman S: Endodontic retreatment: case selection and technique. Part 2. Treatment planning for retreatment, *J Endod* 14:607,1988.

88. Suter B: A new method for retrieving silver points and separated instruments from root canals, *J Endod* 24:446, 1998.

89. Plack WF III, Vire DE: Retrieval of endodontic silver points, *Gen Dent* 32:124, 1984.

90. Friedman S: Considerations and concepts of case selection in the management of post-treatment endodontic disease, *Endo Topics* 1:54, 2002.

91. Spriggs K, Gettleman B, Messer HH: Evaluation of a new method for silver point removal, *J Endod* 16:335, 1990.

92. Fachin EV, Wenckus CS, Aun CE: Retreatment using a modified-tip instrument, *J Endod* 21:425, 1995.

93. Jeng HW, ElDeeb ME: Removal of hard paste fillings from the root canal by ultrasonic instrumentation, *J Endod* 13:295, 1987.

94. Vranas RN, Hartwell GR, Moon PC: The effect of endodontic solutions on resorcinol-formalin paste, *J Endod* 29:69, 2003.

95. Gambrel MG, Hartwell GR, Moon PC, et al: The effect of endodontic solutions on resorcinol-formalin paste in teeth, *J Endod* 31:25, 2005.

96. Torabinejad M, Kettering JD, McGraw JC, et al: Factors associated with endodontic interappointment emergencies of teeth with necrotic pulps, *J Endod* 14:261, 1988.

97. Trope M: Flare-up rate of single-visit endodontics, *Int Endod J* 24:24, 1991.

98. Walton R, Fouad A: Endodontic interappointment flare-ups: a prospective study of incidence and related factors, *J Endod* 18:172, 1992.

99. Miller TA, Baumgartner JC: Comparison of the antimicrobial efficacy of irrigation using the EndoVac to endodontic needle delivery, *J Endod* 36:509, 2010.

100. Innes N: Rubber dam use less stressful for children and dentists, *Evid Based Dent* 13:48, 2012.

101. Ng YL, Mann V, Gulabivala K: A prospective study of the factors affecting outcomes of nonsurgical root canal treatment. Part 1. Periapical health, *Int Endod J* 44:583, 2011.

102. Fuss Z, Trope M: Root perforations: classification and treatment choices based on prognostic factors, *Endod Dent Traumatol* 12:255, 1996.

103. Tsesis I, Fuss Z: Diagnosis and treatment of accidental root perforations, *Endod Topics* 13:95, 2006.

104. Pace R, Giuliani V, Pagavino G: Mineral trioxide aggregate as repair material for furcal perforation: case series, *J Endod* 34:1130, 2008.

105. Mente J, Hage N, Pfefferle T, et al: Treatment outcome of mineral trioxide aggregate: repair of root perforations, *J Endod* 36:208, 2010.

106. Begotka BA, Hartwell GR: The importance of the coronal seal following root canal treatment, *Va Dent J* 73:8, 1996.

107. Engstrom B, Hard AF, Segerstad L, et al: Correlation of positive cultures with the prognosis for canal treatment, *Odontol Rev* 15:257, 1964.

108. Bergenholtz G, Lekholm U, Milthon R, et al: Influence of apical overinstrumentation and overfilling on re-treated root canals, *J Endod* 5:310, 1979.

109. Bergenholtz G, Lekholm U, Milthon R, et al: Retreatment of endodontic fillings, *Scand J Dent Res* 87:217, 1979.

110. Paik S, Sechrist C, Torabinejad M: Levels of evidence for the outcome of endodontic retreatment, *J Endod* 30:745, 2004.

111. Friedman S, Mor C: The success of endodontic therapy-healing and functionality, *J Calif Dent Assoc* 32:493-503, 2004

112. de Chevigny C, Dao TT, Basrani BR, et al: Treatment outcome in endodontics—the Toronto study, phases 3 and 4: orthograde retreatment, *J Endod* 34:131, 2008.

113. de Chevigny C, Dao TT, Basrani BR, et al: Treatment outcome in endodontics—the Toronto study, phase 4: initial treatment, *J Endod* 34:258, 2008.

114. Torabinejad M, Corr R, Handysides R, et al: Outcomes of nonsurgical retreatment and endodontic surgery: a systematic review, *J Endod* 35:930, 2009.

115. Danin J, Strömberg T, Forsgren H, et al: Clinical management of nonhealing periradicular pathosis: surgery versus endodontic retreatment, *Oral Surg Oral Med Oral Pathol Oral Radiol Endod* 82:213, 1996.

116. Ng YL, Mann V, Gulabivala K: A prospective study of the factors affecting outcomes of non-surgical root canal treatment. Part 2. Tooth survival, *Int Endod J* 44:610, 2011.

Endodontic surgery

Mahmoud Torabinejad, Bradford R. Johnson

LEARNING OBJECTIVES

After reading this chapter, the student should be able to:
1. Discuss the role of endodontic surgery in treatment planning for a patient.
2. Recognize situations in which surgery is the treatment of choice.
3. Recognize medical or dental situations in which endodontic surgery is contraindicated.
4. Define the terms *incision for drainage, apical curettage, root-end resection, root-end preparation and filling, root amputation, hemisection,* and *bicuspidization.*
5. Briefly describe the step-by-step procedures involved in periapical surgery, including those for incision and reflection, access to the apex, apical curettage, root-end resection, root-end preparation and filling, flap replacement, and suturing.

6. Discuss the indications for each procedure listed in objective 4.
7. Discuss the prognosis for each procedure listed in objective 4.
8. State the principles of flap design.
9. Diagram the various flap designs and describe the indications, advantages, and disadvantages of each.
10. List the more common root-end filling materials.
11. Review the basic principles of suturing.
12. Describe general patterns of soft and hard tissue healing.
13. Write out instructions to be given to the patient concerning postoperative care after endodontic surgery.
14. List and describe conditions that indicate referral to a specialist for evaluation or treatment.

Nonsurgical root canal therapy is a highly successful procedure if diagnosis and technical aspects are carefully performed.[1-4] There is a common belief that if root canal therapy fails, surgery is indicated for correction. This is not necessarily true; most failures are best corrected by retreatment (revision). Studies have shown that between 77% and 89% of retreated cases are successful after retreatment of the original root canal therapy.[5-7] However, there are situations in which surgery is necessary to retain a tooth that would otherwise be extracted.

Endodontic surgery is not "oral surgery" in the traditional sense. Rather, it is actually "endodontic treatment through a surgical flap." Simply cutting off the apex of a root and placing a filling in the vicinity of the canal does not accomplish the goals of endodontic surgical treatment. The purposes of endodontic surgery include sealing of all portals of exit from the root canal system and the isthmuses, eliminating bacteria and preventing their byproducts from contaminating the periradicular tissues, and providing an environment that allows for regeneration of periradicular tissues.

During the past decade, the art and science of endodontic surgery have changed dramatically. Endodontic surgery was previously limited to the anterior teeth, where access was considered adequate. With the introduction of the operating microscope, ultrasonic tips, and new root-end filling materials, teeth that might otherwise be extracted now have a chance for retention.[8]

This chapter describes both the indications for and the procedures involved in incision for drainage, periapical surgery, and corrective surgical procedures, such as root amputation, hemisection, and bicuspidization.

INCISION FOR DRAINAGE

The objective of incision for drainage is to evacuate inflammatory exudates and purulence from a soft tissue swelling. Incision for drainage reduces discomfort resulting from the buildup of pressure and speeds healing.

Indications

The best treatment for swelling originating from a symptomatic apical abscess of pulpal origin (Fig. 21.1, *A*) is to establish drainage through the offending tooth (Fig. 21.1, *B*). When adequate drainage cannot be accomplished through the tooth itself, drainage is obtained through soft tissue incision. Occasionally, drainage is performed through the soft tissue even if it has also been obtained through the tooth (see Fig. 10.3 *B*; also Fig. 21.1, *B, C*). The reason for this is that there may be separate, noncommunicating abscesses—one at the apex and another in a submucosal location or in an anatomic space.

Drainage through the soft tissue is accomplished most effectively when the swelling is fluctuant. A fluctuant swelling is a fluid-containing mass in which a wavelike sensation (like pushing on a water balloon) is felt when pressure is applied (see Fig. 10, *B*; also Fig. 21.1, *A*). Incising a fluctuant swelling releases purulence immediately and provides rapid relief. If the swelling is nonfluctuant or firm, incision for drainage often results in drainage of only blood and serous fluids. Incision and drainage of a nonfluctuant abscess reduces pressure and facilitates healing by reducing irritants and increasing circulation in the area.

Contraindications

There are relatively few contraindications to the use of incision for drainage. Patients with prolonged bleeding or clotting times or those who are on bisphosphonates must be treated with caution, and hematologic screening is often indicated. An abscess in or near an anatomic space should be handled very carefully.

Procedures
Anesthesia

Profound anesthesia is difficult to obtain in the presence of inflammation, swelling, or exudates. Because direct subperiosteal infiltration is ineffective and may be quite painful, regional block anesthetic techniques are preferred. Mandibular blocks for posterior areas, bilateral mental blocks for the anterior mandible, posterior superior alveolar blocks for the posterior maxilla, and infraorbital blocks for the premaxilla area are the preferred choices. These injections may be supplemented by regional infiltration.

In addition to block anesthesia, one of the following methods may also be used. The first technique is infiltration that starts peripheral to the swelling. After the application of topical anesthetic, the solution is injected *slowly* with limited pressure and depth; this is followed by additional injections in previously anesthetized tissue, moving progressively closer to the center of the swelling. This procedure results in improved anesthesia without extreme discomfort.

The second technique is the use of topical ethyl chloride.[9] A stream of this solution is directed onto the swelling from a distance, and the liquid is allowed to volatilize on the tissue surface. Within seconds, the tissue at the site of volatilization turns white. The incision is quickly accomplished with continued ethyl chloride spray. This topical anesthesia is a supplement to block anesthesia when a quick incision is required.

If neither of these procedures work, nitrous oxide/oxygen sedation or intravenous (IV) sedation can be used for incision and drainage.

Incision

After anesthesia has been induced, the incision is made vertically with a No. 11 scalpel. Vertical incisions are made parallel to the major blood vessels and nerves and leave very little scarring. The incision should be made firmly through periosteum to bone. If the swelling is fluctuant, pus usually flows immediately, followed by blood. If the swelling is nonfluctuant, the predominant drainage is blood.

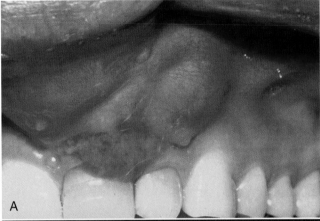

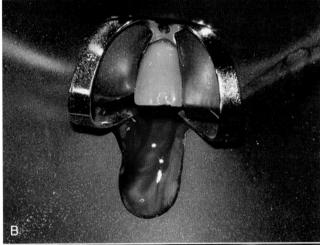

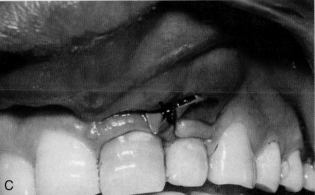

Fig. 21.1 **A,** Fluctuant swelling is present as a result of an infection in the left lateral incisor. **B,** Establishment of drainage through an offending tooth. **C,** Incision for drainage is made horizontally into the swelling, and a rubber drain is sutured in place to prevent immediate closure of the incision.

Drainage

After the initial incision, a small, closed hemostat may be placed in the incision and then opened to enlarge the draining tract.[10] This procedure is indicated with more extensive swelling. To maintain a path for drainage, an I-shaped or "Christmas tree" drain cut from a rubber dam or a piece of iodoform gauze can be placed (suturing is optional) in the incision (see Fig. 10.5). The drain should be removed after 2 to 3 days; if it is not sutured, the patient may remove the drain at home.

PERIAPICAL SURGERY

Periapical surgery (PAS) is commonly performed to remove a portion of the root with undebrided canal space or to seal the canal apically when a complete seal cannot be accomplished with nonsurgical root canal treatment through an orthograde approach.

Indications

The main indications for PAS are anatomic complexity of the root canal system, procedural accidents, irretrievable materials in the root canal, symptomatic cases, and horizontal apical fracture, in addition to biopsy and corrective surgery.

Anatomic Problems

A nonnegotiable, blocked canal or severe root curvature may prevent adequate cleaning and shaping or obturation. Nonsurgical (and surgical) endodontic treatments are indicated in these cases (Fig. 21.2). Nonsurgical root canal therapy or revision (if possible) before surgery improves the surgical success rate.[11,12] However, if neither is feasible, removal of the uninstrumented and unfilled portion of the root or PAS may be necessary (Fig. 21.3).

Anatomic perforation of the root apex through the bone (fenestration), although infrequent, may necessitate PAS after root canal treatment. Reducing the root apex to place it within

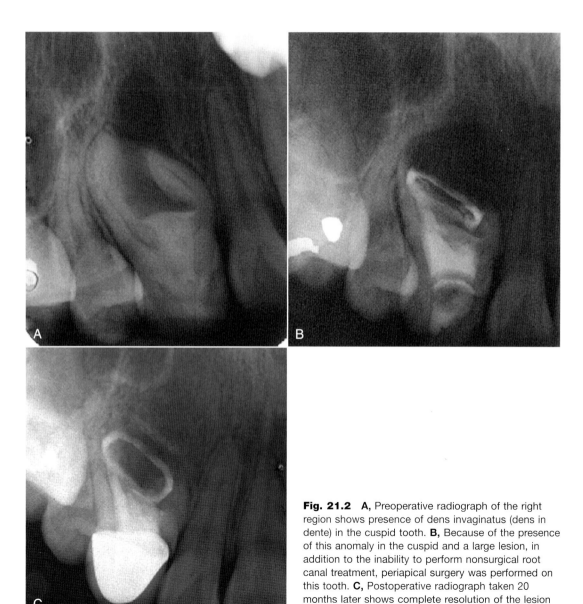

Fig. 21.2 **A,** Preoperative radiograph of the right region shows presence of dens invaginatus (dens in dente) in the cuspid tooth. **B,** Because of the presence of this anomaly in the cuspid and a large lesion, in addition to the inability to perform nonsurgical root canal treatment, periapical surgery was performed on this tooth. **C,** Postoperative radiograph taken 20 months later shows complete resolution of the lesion in the cuspid.

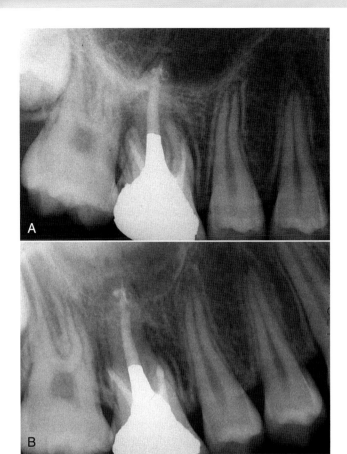

Fig. 21.3 **A,** A nonnegotiable ledge is present in the mesiobuccal root of the first maxillary molar. **B,** Endodontic surgery was performed to correct this accidental procedure on this root and deficiencies present in the distobuccal root.

the bone corrects this condition. Occasionally, adequate root canal therapy is compromised by extensive apical root resorption. It may then be necessary to expose the root, remove the resorbed area, and repair it.

Procedural Accidents

Separated instruments, ledging, perforations, and gross overfills may cause failure of root canal treatment, requiring surgical intervention. If symptoms or lesions develop or persist after the accidents, PAS is usually necessary (see Fig. 19.14; also Fig. 21.4).

Irretrievable Materials in the Root Canal

Retreatment (revision) is recommended for treatment of failures. However, irretrievable posts or dowels or root filling materials, such as silver cones, amalgam, or nonabsorbable pastes, often prevent revision, or their removal would result in further damage to the root structure. The best alternative is a surgical approach and placement of a root-end filling material (Fig. 21.5).

Symptomatic Cases

Most symptoms disappear after complete cleaning and obturation of root canals. However, when symptoms persist after meticulous performance of these procedures, PAS should be considered to identify the cause or causes of the persistence of the symptoms. The main cause of the persistence of pain

in these cases is usually inflammation that results from the inability of the operator to completely clean the root canal or canals. Exploratory surgery may identify undetected vertical root fractures (Fig. 21.6), additional apical and lateral foramina (possible missed canals), perforations, apical ramifications, overfills, or other causes of failure. Once the cause has been eliminated, the symptoms disappear.

Horizontal Apical Fracture

Although most traumatic horizontal apical fractures usually heal without intervention, occasionally the apical portion of a root becomes necrotic and cannot be treated nonsurgically. In these cases, the apical portion of the root should be removed and the apical seal should be evaluated.

Biopsy

Although most periapical lesions are of pulpal origin, nonpulpal lesions do exist (see Chapter 5 for diagnosis and treatment planning). The presence of a vital pulp in a tooth with a radicular radiolucency (Fig. 21.7), undefined periapical lesions in teeth with vital pulps in patients with a history of previous malignancy, and lip paresthesia or anesthesia are indications for biopsy.

Contraindications

The four major contraindications to PAS are (1) anatomic factors, (2) medical or systemic complications, (3) indiscriminate use of surgery, and (4) an unidentified cause of treatment failure.[10]

Anatomic Factors

Inaccessibility of the surgical site because of tooth location, spaces (e.g., maxillary sinus or nasal fossa), unusual bony configuration, or proximity of neurovascular bundles may be a contraindication or at least require caution or special approaches (Fig. 21.8). For example, a thick external oblique ridge associated with a mandibular molar or apices contiguous with the mandibular canal may compromise surgical access. Other situations that may contraindicate PAS or modify the approaches used include very short root length (precluding root-end resection), severe periodontal disease (prognosis hopeless, even with surgery), and unrestorable teeth.

Medical or Systemic Complications

Serious systemic health problems or extreme apprehension make the patient a poor candidate for PAS. Surgery may also be contraindicated in patients with blood disorders, terminal disease, uncontrolled diabetes, or severe heart disease and in those whose immune systems are compromised.

Indiscriminate Use of Surgery

As previously stated, surgery is not indicated when a nonsurgical approach is possible and would probably result in success Fig. 21.9. The practice of managing all accessible periapical lesions or large periradicular lesions surgically is unethical and contraindicated. A recent systematic review comparing treatment outcomes for endodontic surgery and nonsurgical retreatment found an initial higher success rate for surgery at 2 to 4 years, but a significant shift in favor of nonsurgical retreatment at 4 to 6 years.[6] This finding supports the position that nonsurgical retreatment should usually be the first choice when possible.

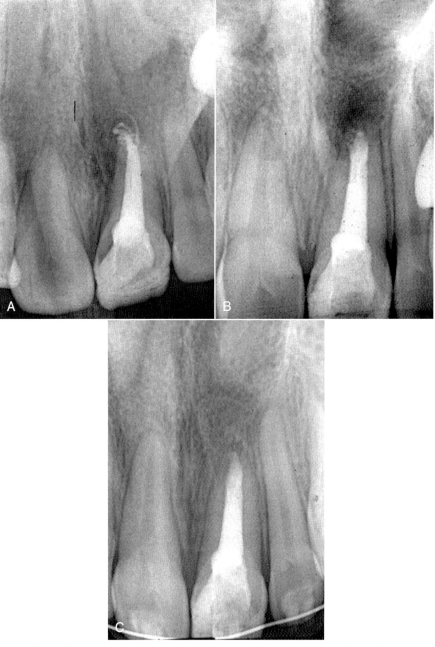

Fig. 21.4 **A,** Preoperative radiograph of a maxillary central incisor shows presence of gutta-percha segments in the bone. **B,** Because of the patient's discomfort and pain, periapical surgery was performed on this tooth. **C,** Postoperative radiograph taken 18 months later shows complete resolution of the lesion.

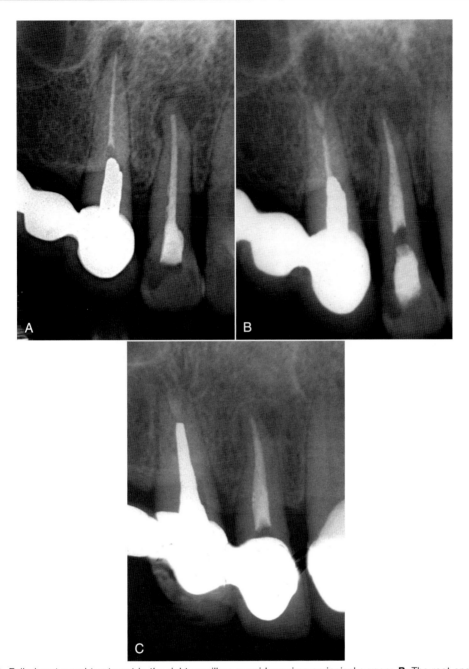

Fig. 21.5 **A,** Failed root canal treatment in the right maxillary cuspid requires periapical surgery. **B,** The root end is resected, and a cavity is prepared and filled with mineral trioxide aggregate (MTA). **C,** Postoperative film after 5 years showing complete healing. (Courtesy Dr. CCU Hong.)

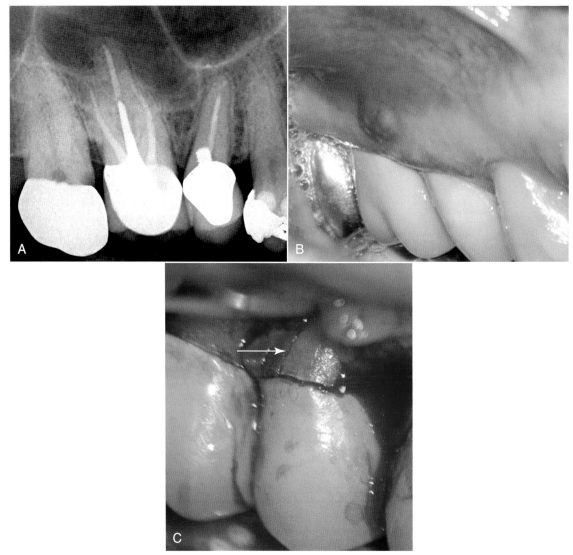

Fig. 21.6 Based on the radiographic findings **(A)** and clinical exam **(B),** a perforation or root fracture of the maxillary right second premolar was suspected. **C,** A vertical root fracture was confirmed during exploratory surgery. (Case courtesy Dr. Martin Rogers.)

Unidentified Cause of Treatment Failure

Using surgery to correct a treatment failure for which the cause cannot be identified is unlikely to be successful.

Recent Advances in Endodontic Surgery

Many advances in surgical technique and instrumentation have occurred over the past 10 to 15 years.[8,13] These include enhanced magnification and illumination, ultrasonic tips, microinstruments, and newer root-end filling materials. Enhanced illumination and magnification have greatly improved the procedures that practitioners can perform. Magnification in endodontic surgery has led to miniaturization of endodontic surgical instruments (Figs. 21.10 to 21.13). Developments in root-end filling materials have increased both the quality and biocompatibility of the apical seal. Cone beam volumetric tomography (CBVT) is an emerging technology with many applications in endodontic diagnosis and treatment, including presurgical treatment planning. Compared to traditional two-dimensional imaging, CBVT has the unique ability to provide high-resolution images in three dimensions while eliminating superimposition of surrounding anatomic structures.[14]

Together, these advances have significantly improved the state of the art and science of endodontic surgery, giving a second chance to a tooth that traditionally would have been considered for extraction.

Procedures Involved in Periapical Surgery

The typical sequence of procedures in PAS is as follows: flap design, incision and reflection, apical access, periradicular curettage, root-end resection, root-end cavity preparation, root-end filling, flap replacement and suturing, postoperative care and instructions, and suture removal and evaluation.

Flap Design

The first step in PAS is designing a flap that allows adequate exposure of the site of the surgery. The following general guidelines and principles should be used during flap design.[15,16]

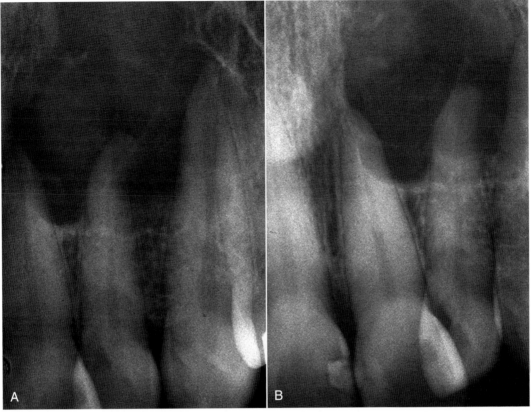

Fig. 21.7 **A,** Presence of vital pulps in the left anterior teeth and a multilocular large radiolucency indicated a possible lesion of nonpulpal origin. **B,** Another radiograph shows the extent of this lesion. A biopsy revealed the presence of a keratocyst.

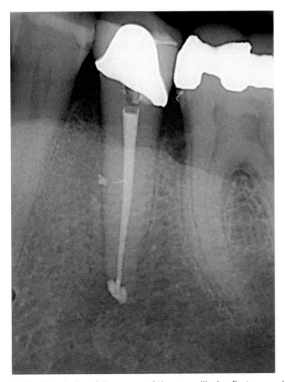

Fig. 21.8 Proximity of the apex of the mandibular first premolar to the neurovascular bundle dictates caution during endodontic surgery.

1. The flap should be designed for maximum access to the site of surgery.
2. An adequate blood supply to the reflected tissue is maintained with a wide flap base.
3. Incisions over bony defects or over the periradicular lesion should be avoided; these might cause postsurgical soft tissue fenestrations or nonunion of the incision.
4. The actual bony defect is larger than the size observed radiographically.
5. A minimal flap, which should include at least one tooth on either side of the intended tooth, should be used.
6. Acute angles in the flap must be avoided. Sharp corners are difficult to reposition and suture and may become ischemic and slough, resulting in delayed healing and possibly scar formation.
7. Incisions and reflections include periosteum as part of the flap. Any remaining pieces or tags of cellular non-reflected periosteum will hemorrhage, compromising visibility.
8. The interdental papilla must not be split (incised through) and should be either fully included or excluded from the flap.
9. Vertical incisions must be extended to allow the retractor to rest on bone and not crush portions of the flap.

Although there are numerous flap designs, two meet most periapical surgery needs: the submarginal flap (curved, triangular, or rectangular) and the full mucoperiosteal flap (triangular or rectangular).

383

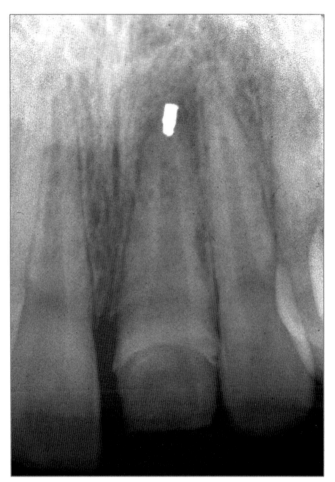

Fig. 21.9 Performing endodontic surgery without filling a canal is considered indiscriminate application of this procedure to treat pulp and periapical diseases

Submarginal Curved Flap

The submarginal curved flap is a slightly curved, half-moon–shaped, horizontal incision made in the attached gingiva with the convexity nearest the free gingival margin. It is simple and easily reflected and provides access to the apex without impinging on the tissue surrounding the crowns. Its disadvantages include restricted access with limited visibility, tearing of the incision corners if the operator tries to improve access by stretching the tissue, and leaving the incision directly over the lesion if the surgical defect is larger than anticipated. The incision margins of this flap frequently heal with scarring.[17] The submarginal curved flap is limited by the presence of the frenum, muscle attachments, or canine and other bony eminences. Because of its many disadvantages, this design is generally not indicated or used.

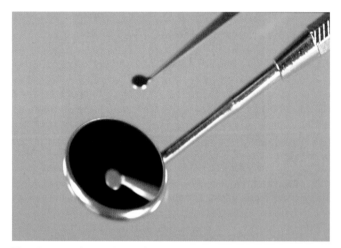

Fig. 21.11 Comparison of standard intraoral mirror and micromirror used for endodontic microsurgery

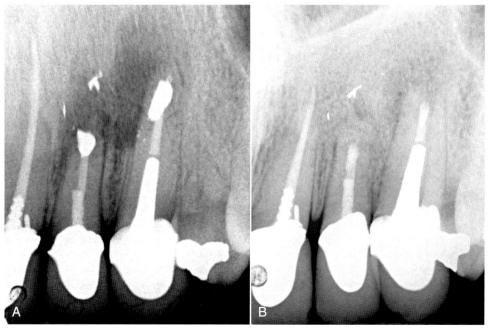

Fig. 21.10 **A,** Failure of previous surgery in teeth #10 and #11. Surgical revision was performed using current materials and techniques (dental operating microscope, perpendicular root-end resection, ultrasonic root-end preparation, and MTA filling). **B,** Good healing is observed at the 18-month follow-up. (Case courtesy Dr. Martin Rogers.)

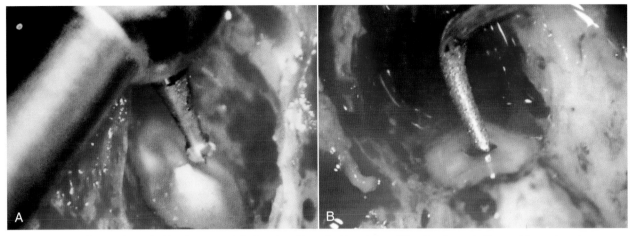

Fig. 21.12 Comparison of older, low-speed, "micro-head" surgical handpiece **(A)** with ultrasonic tip used for root-end preparation **(B)**.

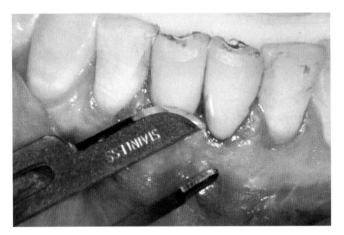

Fig. 21.13 Comparison of standard No. 15 scalpel *(top)* and microsurgical scalpel *(bottom)*.

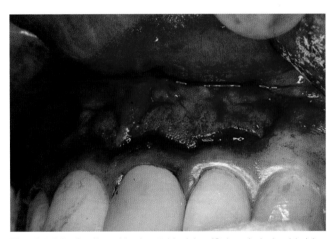

Fig. 21.14 Scalloped horizontal incision (Ochsenbein-Luebke) is made in the attached gingiva with two accompanying vertical incisions for surgery on the left central incisor.

Submarginal Triangular and Rectangular Flaps

Triangular and rectangular flaps are known as modified submarginal curved flaps. A scalloped horizontal incision (Ochsenbein-Luebke) is made in the attached gingiva with one or two accompanying vertical incisions (Fig. 21.14). This flap is used most successfully in maxillary anterior teeth with crowns. An alternative submarginal flap design is the papilla-based incision, in which the interdental papillae are left intact.[18] Prerequisites are 4 mm of attached gingiva, minimal probing depths, and good periodontal health.

This flap design provides better access and visibility compared to the submarginal curved flap and poses less risk of incising tissue over a bony defect. Disadvantages are possible scarring and hemorrhage from the cut margins to the surgical site.[19] This design also provides less visibility than the full mucoperiosteal flap.

Full Mucoperiosteal Flap

The full mucoperiosteal (intrasulcular) flap consists of an incision at the gingival crest with full elevation of the interdental papillae, free gingival margin, attached gingiva, and alveolar mucosa. It may have either one (triangular) or two (rectangular) vertical releasing incisions (Fig. 21.15). It allows maximal access and visibility, precludes incision over a bony defect, and has less of a tendency for hemorrhage. This design permits periodontal curettage, root planing, and bony reshaping, and it heals with minimal scar formation. Its disadvantages include the difficulty of replacing, suturing, and making alterations (height and shape) to the free gingival margin, in addition to possible gingival recession after surgery and exposure of the crown margins.[17,20]

Incision and Reflection

A firm incision is made with a CK-2, CK-3, or other suitable blade into the base of the sulcus or initiation of the horizontal incision. To prevent tearing during reflection, the incision must be made through periosteum to bone. Once the horizontal incision has been made, the same blade or a No. 15 scalpel can be used to place the vertical incision or incisions. The tissue is reflected with a sharp periosteal elevator. Because periosteum is reflected as part of the flap, the elevator must firmly contact bone as the tissue is relieved using firm, controlled force. The tissue is reflected beyond the mucogingival junction to a level that provides adequate access to the root apex and visibility of the surgical site and also allows a retractor to be placed on sound bone (Fig. 21.16).

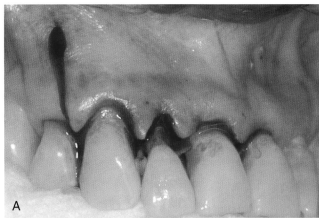

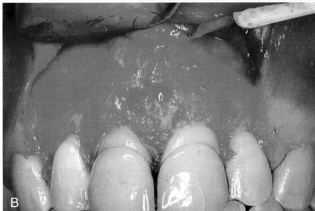

Fig. 21.15 **A,** Triangular full mucoperiosteal (sulcular) flap with one vertical incision made to access the right central incisor. **B,** Rectangular full mucoperiosteal flap with two vertical incisions made to access both central incisors.

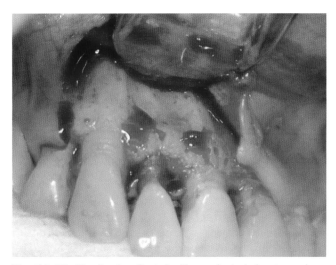

Fig. 21.16 The flap is reflected with a periosteal elevator and held with a retractor to allow visibility and access to the surgical site. The retractor must be placed on sound bone.

Osteotomy

In many cases, the presence of a periradicular lesion creates a defect in the cortical bone that is visible after flap reflection or is identified when firm probing with an explorer is applied on the bone. If the opening is small, a sharp round bur can be used to remove the bone until the apex is located (Fig. 21.17). If there is limited cortical bone destruction, after placement

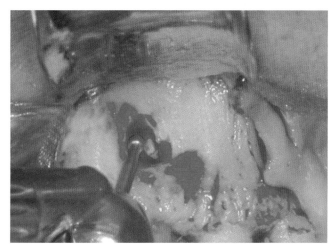

Fig. 21.17 A sharp round bur in a high-speed handpiece is used to remove the bone, with continuous spraying of sterile water to locate the tooth apex.

of a radiopaque object near the apex, a radiograph should be taken to locate the apex. Removal of bone with a bur is performed using a light brushing motion and copious sterile saline irrigation.[15,16,21]

Periradicular Curettage

Removal of pathologic soft tissue surrounding the apex has the following benefits:

- It provides access and visibility of the apex.
- It removes inflamed tissue.
- It provides a biopsy specimen for histologic examination.
- It reduces hemorrhage.

The tissue should be carefully peeled out, ideally in one piece, with a suitably sized sharp curette (Fig. 21.18). This process should leave a clean bony cavity. A sample of the tissue is usually submitted for biopsy. When the lesion is very large, portions of tissue can be left without compromising the blood supply to an adjacent tooth. This should not affect periradicular healing.

Root-End Resection

Root-end resection involves beveling the apical portion of the root. This step is often an integral part of PAS and serves two purposes:

- It removes the untreated apical portion of the root and enables the operator to determine the cause of failure.
- It provides a flat surface that allows the operator to create a root-end cavity preparation and pack it with a root-end filling material.

Apical sectioning is done with a tapered fissure bur in a high-speed handpiece and copious sterile saline irrigation (Fig. 21.19). The bevel should be made at as close to 0 degrees in a faciolingual direction as possible to still enable maximum visibility to the root apex.[15,16,19] In general, the amount of root removed depends on the reason for performing the root-end resection. However, sufficient resection must be performed to do the following:

- Provide access to the palatal-lingual root surface
- Place the canal in the center of the sectioned root
- Expose additional canals, apical deltas, or fractures

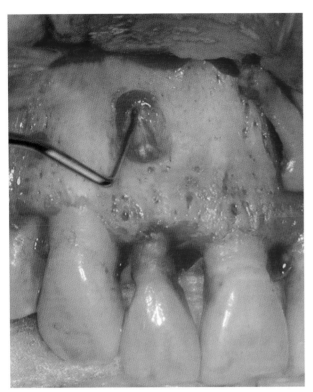

Fig. 21.18 Apical curettage and removal of diseased tissue at the apex enhance visualization of the apex and surrounding bone. This tissue should be submitted for histologic evaluation.

Root-End Cavity Preparation and Filling

Root-end cavity preparation and filling are indicated in most endodontic surgeries. Apical preparations are now made with ultrasonic tips. A variety of tips are available to accommodate virtually all access situations (Fig. 21.20). When used, the tips are placed so that the walls of the preparation will be parallel to the long axis of the root. A Class I–type preparation is made with ultrasonic tips to a minimum depth of 3 mm into the canal (Fig. 21.21).[19,22,23] More complicated apical root anatomy may require other types of preparation.[15] The ultrasonic instrument offers the advantages of control and ease of use and permits less apical root beveling and uniform depth of preparation.[22-24] In addition, the ultrasonic tips produce smaller apical preparations, allow easier preparation of an isthmus, follow the direction of the canals (Fig. 21.22), clean the canal surfaces better than burs, and create less fatigue for the operator.

After the apical preparation has been made and thoroughly examined, it should be filled with a root-end filling material (Fig. 21.23). Root-end filling materials should meet the following criteria:

1. Able to seal well
2. Biocompatible
3. Unresorbable
4. Easily inserted
5. Unaffected by moisture
6. Visible radiographically
7. Capable of regenerating periradicular tissues

Many materials have been used as root-end filling materials.[25-33] Root-end filling materials that are the consistency of cement, such as SuperEBA (Boswoth, Skokie, Illinois) and ProRoot MTA (Dentsply/Tulsa Dental, Johnson City, Tennessee), are currently the materials of choice.[8] In

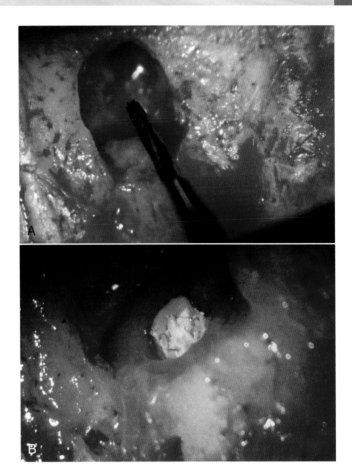

Fig. 21.19 **A,** Root-end resection (apicoectomy) is performed using a fissure bur in a high-speed handpiece. **B,** The entire resected portion of the tooth should be visible.

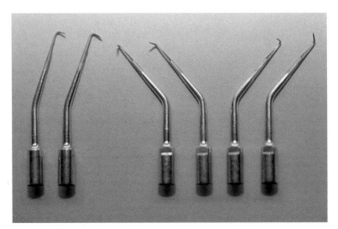

Fig. 21.20 A variety of ultrasonic tips are available to prepare root-end cavities for various roots.

several studies, histologic sections have shown the regeneration of new cementum over the mineral trioxide aggregate (MTA) root-end filling,[29,30,34] a phenomenon not seen with other commonly used root-end filling materials (Fig. 21.24).

Flap Replacement and Suturing

After the operator has placed a root-end filling material and taken a radiograph, the bone and soft tissues should be carefully inspected for remnants of filling material, hemostatic agents, or other foreign objects. The flap should then be **387** placed in its original position and held in place for 5 minutes with moistened gauze using moderate digital pressure. This allows expression of hemorrhage from under the flap, initial adaptation, easier suturing, and less postoperative swelling and bleeding.

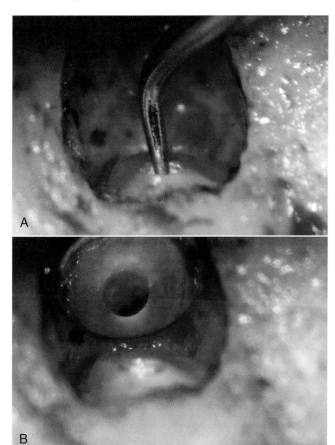

Fig. 21.21 **A,** An ultrasonic tip is used to prepare a class I preparation in the apical portion of the root canal. **B,** Mirror view of a root-end cavity preparation. (Courtesy Dr. R. Rubinstein.).

Suturing is commonly done with 5-0 Tevdek (Fig. 21.25), although other materials are acceptable.[35-37] There are many suturing techniques, including interrupted, continuous mattress, and sling sutures.[16] Interrupted sutures are commonly used (Fig. 21.26, *A*). For suturing, the needle passes first through reflected and then through attached tissue. The sutures are tied with a simple double surgeon's knot. The knot should not be placed over the incision line because it collects debris and bacteria, which promote inflammation, infection, and delayed healing. The sutures are usually removed 3 to 7 days after surgery (Fig. 21.26, *B*).

Postoperative Care and Instructions

Both oral and written postoperative instructions should be given to the patient. Instructions should be written in simple, straightforward language. They should minimize patient anxiety arising from normal postoperative symptoms by describing how to promote healing and comfort.

The following instructions are for patients.

1. Some swelling and discoloration are common. Use an ice pack with moderate pressure on the outside of your face (20 minutes on, 5 minutes off) until you go to bed tonight. Application of ice and pressure reduces bleeding and swelling and provides an analgesic effect.
2. Some oozing of blood is normal. If bleeding increases, place a moistened gauze pad or facial tissues over the area and apply finger pressure for 15 minutes. If bleeding continues, call the dentist's office.
3. Do not lift your lip or cheek to look at the area. The stitches are tied, and you may tear them out.
4. Starting tomorrow, dissolve 1 teaspoon of salt in a glass of warm water and gently rinse your mouth three or four times daily. Rinsing with a 0.12% chlorhexidine mouthwash may promote healing. Mouthwashes containing alcohol should be avoided for the first several days after surgery. Careful brushing is important, but vigorous brushing may damage the area. Tonight you should brush and floss all areas except the surgery site. Tomorrow night, carefully brush the surgery site.

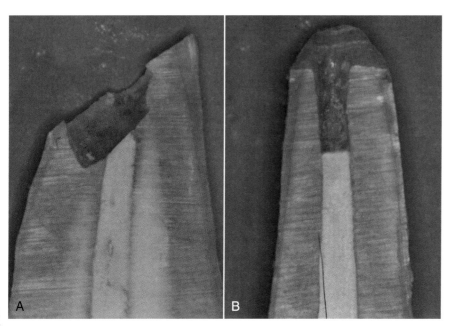

Fig. 21.22 **A,** Root-end cavity prepared by a small inverted bur. **B,** Root-end cavity prepared by an ultrasonic bur.

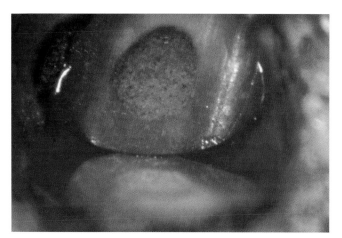

Fig. 21.23 MTA (3 mm) is placed in the root-end cavity preparation to provide a fluid-tight apical seal. (Courtesy Dr. R. Rubinstein.)

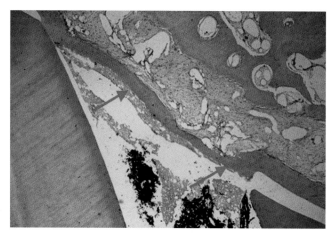

Fig. 21.24 Complete periapical healing and formation of cellular cementum *(arrows)* adjacent to the MTA were seen when MTA was used as a root-end filling material in monkeys.

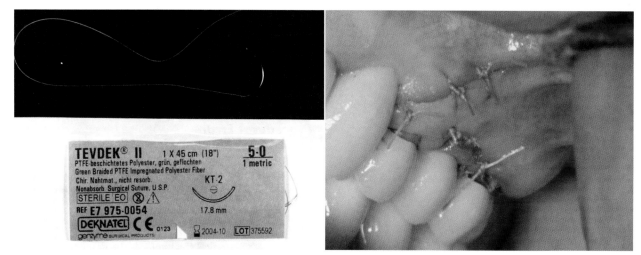

Fig. 21.25 Tevdek suture material.

5. Proper diet and fluid intake are essential after surgery. Eat a soft diet and chew on the opposite side of your mouth. Drink lots of fluids and eat soft foods such as cottage cheese, yogurt, eggs, and ice cream.

6. Pain is usually minimal after PAS, and strong analgesics are normally not required. Some discomfort is normal. If pain medication was prescribed, follow the instructions. If no medication was prescribed, take your preferred nonprescription pain remedy if needed. If this is not sufficient, call the dentist's office.

7. If you are a smoker, do not smoke for the first 3 days after the procedure.

8. If you experience excessive swelling or pain or if you run a fever, call the dentist's office immediately.

9. Keep your appointment to have the stitches removed. (sutures are removed 3 to 7 days after surgery.)

10. Call the dentist's office if you have any concerns or questions.

Healing

Surgery involves the manipulation of soft and hard tissues. Handling of both soft tissues (periosteum, gingiva, periodontal ligament, and alveolar mucosa) and hard tissues (dentin, cementum, and bone) is accomplished by incision, dissection, and excision.

Soft Tissue

Healing of soft tissue involves clotting, inflammation, epithelialization, and connective tissue healing, in addition to maturation and remodeling.[38] Clotting and inflammation consist of both chemical and cellular phases. The clotting mechanism is important because it is based on the conversion of fibrinogen to fibrin. Under pressure, the clot should be a thin layer. Failure of the clot to form results in leakage of blood into the wound site. The inflammatory components of healing are a complex network of both extrinsic and intrinsic elements.[38]

Initial epithelial healing consists of the formation of the epithelial barrier, which is made up of layers of epithelial cells that depend on the underlying connective tissue for nutrients. This epithelial layer migrates along the fibrin surface until it makes contact with epithelial cells from the opposite border of the wound, forming an epithelial bridge.

The connective tissue component comes from fibroblasts, which are differentiated from ectomesenchymal cells and are attracted to the wound site. Adjacent blood vessels provide nutrients for the fibroblasts and their precursors, **389**

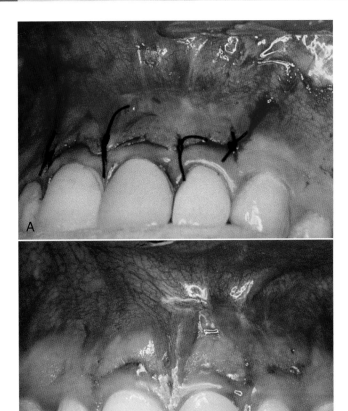

Fig. 21.26 **A,** Interrupted sutures are commonly used to hold the soft tissue flap in its original location. **B,** Sutures are removed 3 to 7 days after surgery.

which elaborate collagen, initially type III, followed by type I. Macrophages are an important part of these processes. As healing matures, there is a decrease in the amount of inflammation and numbers of fibroblasts, accompanied by deaggregation and reaggregation of collagen with formation of collagen fibers into a more organized pattern.[38-41]

Hard Tissue
As with healing in soft tissue, the hard tissue response is based on the presence of cells such as fibroblasts, osteoblasts, and cementoblasts, which produce ground substance, cementum, and bone matrix formation. New cementum deposition from cementoblasts begins about 12 days after surgery; eventually, a thin layer of cementum may cover resected dentin and even certain root-end filling materials (see Fig. 21.24). The exposed dentin acts as an inductive force, with new cementum forming from the periphery to the center.

Osseous healing begins by the proliferation of endosteal cells into the coagulum of the wound site. At 12 to 14 days, woven trabeculae and osteocytes appear, leading to early maturation of the collagen matrix at about 30 days. This process occurs from inside to outside, ending in the formation of mature lamellar bone,[42-44] which is visible radiographically (see Fig. 21.5, *C*).

Research is emerging to suggest that the addition of autologous platelet concentrate to the surgical site decreases postsurgical pain and the need for analgesics. The platelet concentrate supplies growth factors to the surgical area and may also accelerate the healing process.[45]

Guided Tissue Regeneration
In certain situations, the use of bone grafting and/or barrier membranes may facilitate healing after endodontic surgery. An apicomarginal bony defect (as may be seen with a true endodontic-periodontic lesion) or loss of cortical plate on both sides of the lesion (a through-and-through lesion) may be an indication for guided tissue regeneration.[13] The general concept of guided tissue regeneration is to create an environment that controls rapid epithelial proliferation and allows time for the slower-occurring regeneration of normal periodontal attachment and bone. Grafting materials include autogenous bone, allografts (e.g., demineralized freeze-dried human bone), xenografts (e.g., inorganic bovine bone), synthetic materials (e.g., calcium sulfate, bioactive glasses), and combination materials. Membranes used for guided tissue regeneration fall into two broad categories, nonresorbable and resorbable.

CORRECTIVE SURGERY

Corrective surgery procedures are specially designed to correct pathologic or iatrogenic conditions.

Indications
Procedural Errors
Root perforations typically occur during access, canal preparation, or restorative procedures (usually post placement). They require restorative and endodontic management. Most perforations can be managed using MTA via an orthograde approach (see Chapter 19). However, there are some cases that need to be managed surgically.

The location of the perforation is often the factor limiting the success of surgical treatment. If the defect is on the proximal root surfaces in close proximity to adjacent teeth, repair is a problem because access to the site is difficult without damaging adjacent teeth (Fig. 21.27). This is particularly true of the lingual surface of mandibular teeth. However, defects on the facial surface are easier to treat.

Resorptive Perforations
Resorptive root perforations typically occur as a result of trauma or internal bleaching procedures. The defects may be localized to the root surface or communicate with the canal.

Techniques
Repair of these defects presents unique problems. Often a defect on the root surface wraps onto the palatal or lingual surface, compromising access and homeostasis. Repair can be accomplished with various materials. If the field can be kept dry, a glass ionomer, a dentin-bonding agent with composite resin, or White ProRoot MTA can be used. Esthetically pleasing materials are preferred for facial repairs because dark materials, such as amalgam or gray MTA, may stain the teeth.

If a post perforates the root, it must be reduced so that it is well within the root structure. Then the defect is repaired with ProRoot MTA.

Repairs in the cervical portion of the root are often difficult to manage and maintain because communication with the gingival sulcus leads to periodontal breakdown. This often

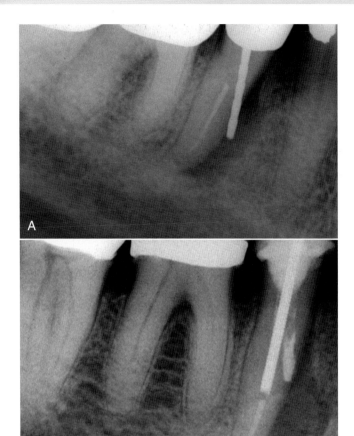

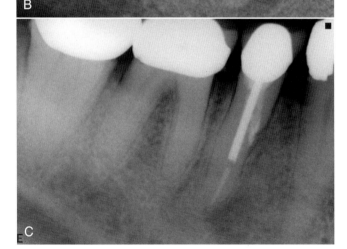

Fig. 21.27 Perforation repair. **A,** An off-center post has perforated the root and caused a bony lesion. **B,** Internal and external perforation repairs with MTA. **C,** Complete repair of the bony lesion in 3 years. (Courtesy Dr. N. Chivian.)

Box 21.1 Indications and Contraindications in Root Amputation, Hemisection, and Bicuspidization

Indications for root amputation or hemisection
- Severe bone loss in a periodontally involved root or furcation that cannot be surgically treated
- Untreatable roots with broken instruments, perforations, caries, resorption, and vertical root fracture or calcified canals
- Preservation of a strategically important root (or roots) and its crown

Contraindications to root amputation or hemisection
- Insufficient bony support for the remaining root or roots
- Root fusion or proximity so that root separation is not possible
- Availability of strong abutment teeth (the involved tooth should be extracted and a prosthesis fabricated)
- Inability to complete root canal treatment on the remaining root or roots

Indications for bicuspidization
- Furcation perforation
- Furcation pathosis from periodontal disease
- Buccolingual cervical caries or fracture into furcation

Contraindications to bicuspidization
- Deep furcation (thick floor of pulp chamber)
- Unrestorable half
- Periodontal disease (each half must be periodontally sound)
- Inability to complete root canal treatment on either half
- Root fusion
- Severe periodontal disease

soft tissue, and root. Root amputation, hemisection, and bicuspidization involve the resection of one or more roots and the crown.[48] Box 21.1 lists the indications and contraindications in root amputation, hemisection, and bicuspidization.

Root amputation is the removal of one or more roots of a multirooted tooth. The involved root (or roots) is separated at the junction of the root and the crown (Fig. 21.28). In general, this procedure is performed in maxillary molars but can be performed for mandibular molars.

Hemisection is the surgical division of a multirooted tooth. In mandibular molars the tooth is divided buccolingually through the bifurcation (Fig. 21.29). In maxillary molars the cut is made mesiodistally, also through the furcation. The defective or periodontally involved root (or roots) and its coronal crown are then removed.[49]

Bicuspidization is typically a surgical division of a mandibular molar. The crown and root of both halves are retained. If severe bone loss or destruction of tooth structure is confined primarily to the furcation area, hemisection and furcal curettage may allow retention of both halves (Fig. 21.30). Each half may be restored to approximate a bicuspid; thus the term *bicuspidization* is used for this procedure.

Techniques

Root amputation is performed by making a horizontal cut to separate the root from the crown. The crown remains intact, and the root segment is removed. Therefore the crown is cantilevered over the extracted root segment (see Fig. 21.28). A second approach is to use an angled vertical cut in which the crown above the root to be amputated is recontoured, decreasing the occlusal forces and making the procedure

means that guided bone regeneration (GBR) procedures,[46] along with endodontic surgical treatment, periodontal treatment (e.g., crown lengthening), orthodontic extrusion, or a combination thereof, may be necessary in conjunction with the repair.[47]

ROOT AMPUTATION, HEMISECTION, AND BICUSPIDIZATION

The three categories described previously (i.e., incision for drainage, PAS, and corrective surgery) involve cutting bone,

21-3

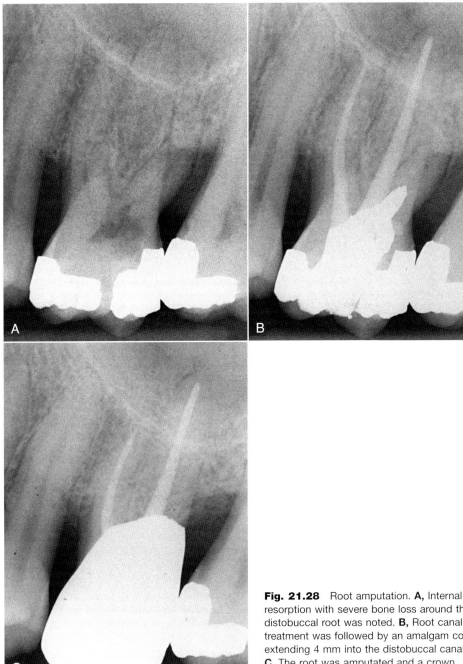

Fig. 21.28 Root amputation. **A,** Internal resorption with severe bone loss around the distobuccal root was noted. **B,** Root canal treatment was followed by an amalgam core extending 4 mm into the distobuccal canal. **C,** The root was amputated and a crown subsequently placed.

easier. As the crown is shaped, the bur is gradually angled into the root, resulting in good anatomic contour.

21-4

Hemisection is carried out by making a vertical cut through the crown into the furcation, which results in complete separation of the hemisected section (crown and root) from the tooth segment that is retained. These techniques may or may not require a flap. Often, if the root is periodontally involved, it is removed without a flap (see Fig. 21.29). If bony recontouring is indicated, a flap is necessary before root resection is carried out. A sulcular flap design is often adequate without a vertical releasing incision. However, when in doubt, a flap should be raised because doing so always helps.

21-5

Bicuspidization is performed after making a vertical cut through the crown into the furcation with a fissure bur. This

procedure results in complete separation of the roots and creation of two separate crowns. After healing of tissues the teeth can be restored as for two separate premolars (see Fig. 21.30).

Prognosis

Each case is unique and has a different prognosis according to the situation. The results of root removal have been reported as good by some but only fair by others.[50] Success is defined by tooth retention with absence of pathosis. Success depends on the following factors:

- Case selection
- Cutting and preparation of the tooth without additional damage

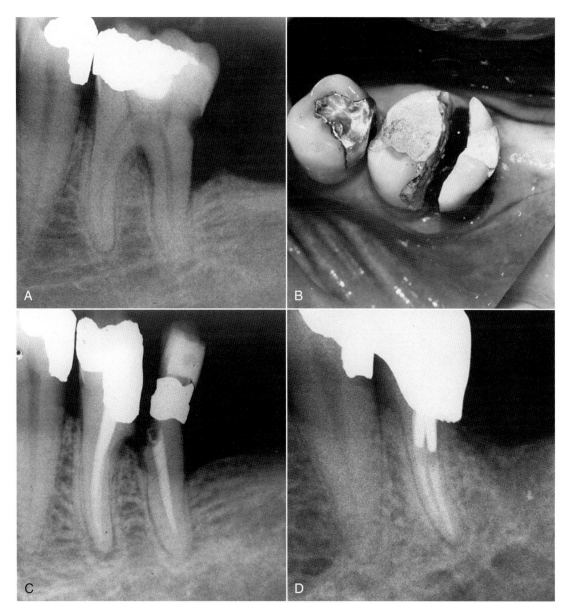

Fig. 21.29 Hemisection. **A,** Furcation caries and bone loss have compromised the distal root. **B,** After root canal treatment, the crown was divided through the furcation **(C). D,** Twenty-month recall, after posts and core and a crown were placed. The extraction socket has healed.

- Good restoration
- Good oral hygiene
- Absence of the following conditions:
  - Caries (the most frequent cause of failure)
  - Root fractures
  - Excessive occlusal forces
  - Untreatable endodontic problems
  - Periodontal disease

If reparative procedures are performed correctly and the tooth is restored properly, the major factor affecting success is the patient's oral hygiene. The patient must be willing and able to perform extra procedures to prevent plaque accumulation, particularly in the area adjacent to what was once the furcation. Failure to do so results in untreatable caries or periodontal disease. The dentist must work carefully with the patient to render this area plaque free. A procedure that appears to be a success at 5 years may fail later. Thus the judgment of success or failure should be guarded and should extend over many years.

Outcome of Endodontic Surgery

Mead and associates searched clinical articles pertaining to success and failure of PAS and assigned levels of evidence to these studies.[51] Their search located many clinical studies, most of which were case series. In a prospective study, Rubinstein and Kim showed that the 1-year healing rate for endodontic surgery performed under the surgical operating microscope (SOM) in conjunction with microsurgical technique was 96.8%.[52] Long-term follow-up of these cases showed that 91.5% of them remained healed after 5 to 7 years.[53] Maddalone and Gagliani, who monitored the outcome of periradicular surgery in teeth treated with microsurgical technology and ultrasonic root-end preparation, reported a similar high success rate.[54]

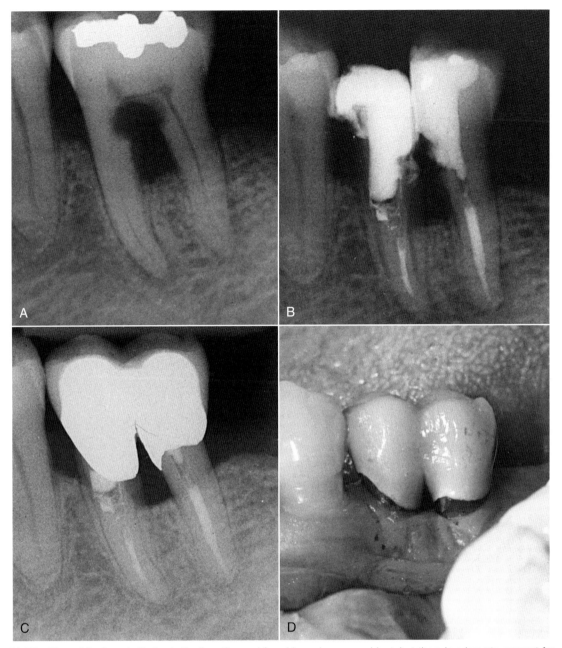

Fig. 21.30 Bicuspidization. **A,** Caries in the furcation and furcal bone loss are evident, but there is adequate support for both roots. **B,** Root canal treatment and bur separation through furcation and crown. **C,** Restoration with a porcelain fused to metal crown splinting the two roots. **D,** Good gingival response at 30-month recall with no probing defects. Note that the furcation is open to facilitate special oral hygiene procedures.

Although it is impossible to tell whether the unusually high success rate resulted from the technique or the material, the clinical impression is that it was both the technique and the material, with the emphasis on the technique. Sechrist[55] reviewed the clinical records of 294 patients in whom MTA was used during endodontic treatment from 1996 to 2001. Of these, 75 patients whose root-end cavities had been filled with MTA were identified for recall. Twenty-five patients responded for clinical and radiographic evaluations. Twenty-five (93%) of the recalled cases were functional and asymptomatic. Based on Sechrist's results, it appears that the use of MTA should promote healing in the majority of surgical endodontic cases.

recent systematic review by Setzer and colleagues[56] compared the outcomes of traditional endodontic surgery with those of current endodontic microsurgery techniques and materials (e.g., ultrasonic root-end preparation; root-end filling with intermediate restorative material [IRM], Super EBA, or MTA; and high-power illumination and magnification). These researchers found a 94% success rate with endodontic microsurgery compared to a 59% success rate for older techniques and materials. The value of using the dental operating microscope for endodontic microsurgery, especially for molar surgery, has also been confirmed in a recent systematic review.[57] Careful case selection is a key element in predicting a successful outcome. For example, the presence of a combined periodontal-endodontic lesion significantly lowers the probability of successful healing.[58]

CONDITIONS INDICATING REFERRAL

Except for incision for drainage, remaining endodontic surgical procedures should be referred to an endodontist. Although the procedures described in this chapter may appear straightforward, endodontic surgery requires advanced training and experience, in addition to considerable surgical skill. The concern about standard of care and litigation in today's society, coupled with the availability of experienced specialists, means that general dentists must carefully examine their own expertise and accurately assess the difficulty of the case before attempting a surgical procedure. These procedures are often the last hope for retaining the tooth and require the highest level of skill and expertise to achieve success. Lack of training may result not only in the loss of the tooth, but also in damage to adjacent structures, paresthesia from nerve injury, sinus perforations, soft tissue fenestrations, and postoperative complications, such as hemorrhage and infection.

In many situations, access to the surgical site is limited and potentially hazardous. Long-standing, large lesions may impinge on adjacent structures, requiring special

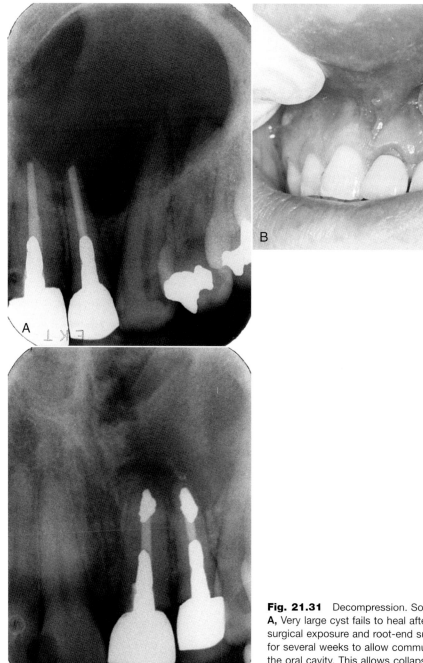

Fig. 21.31 Decompression. Some cases require special procedures. **A,** Very large cyst fails to heal after root canal treatment. **B,** After surgical exposure and root-end surgery, a polyethylene tube is placed for several weeks to allow communication between the cyst cavity and the oral cavity. This allows collapse of the cyst wall. **C,** The lesion has resolved 1 year later, and regeneration of bone is seen. (Courtesy Dr. S. Gish.)

techniques for resolution (Fig. 21.31). The neurovascular bundle near the apices of mandibular molars, premolars, and maxillary palatal roots predisposes the patient to postoperative surgical paresthesia or excessive hemorrhage. The treatment of endodontic problems in these areas requires careful preoperative assessment and considerable surgical skill. The presence of thick cortical bone and bony eminences throughout the mandible and in the palate, frenum, and muscle attachments; fenestrations of the cortical bone; and sinus cavities all require considerable surgical skill and experience in gaining access to most teeth.

Most important is the need for appropriate diagnosis, treatment planning, case assessment, prognostication, and follow-up evaluation. The general dentist should have knowledge in these areas but may prefer to refer the patient to or request input from an endodontist. The specialist is better able to accomplish these goals and assess the short-term and long-term outcomes.[59]

REFERENCES

1. Lazarski M, Walker W III, Flores C, et al: Epidemiological evaluation of the outcomes of nonsurgical root canal treatment in a large cohort of insured dental patients, *J Endod* 27:791, 2001.
2. Salehrabi R, Rotstein I: Endodontic treatment outcomes in a large patient population in the USA: an epidemiological study, *J Endod* 30:846, 2004.
3. Ng YL, Mann V, Gulabivala K: Tooth survival following non-surgical root canal treatment: a systematic review of the literature, *Int Endod J* 43:171, 2010.
4. Torabinejad M, Anderson P, Bader J, et al: Outcomes of root canal treatment and restoration, implant supported single crowns, fixed partial dentures, and extraction without replacement: a systematic review, *J Prosthet Dent* 98:285, 2007.
5. Salehrabi R, Rotstein I: Epidemiological evaluation of the outcomes of orthograde endodontic retreatment, *J Endod* 36:790, 2010.
6. Torabinejad M, Corr R, Handysides R, et al: Outcomes of nonsurgical retreatment and endodontic surgery: a systematic review, *J Endod* 35:930, 2009.
7. Ng YL, Mann V, Gulabivala K: Outcome of secondary root canal treatment: a systematic review of the literature, *Int Endod J* 41:1026, 2008.
8. Rubinstein R, Torabinejad M: Contemporary endodontic surgery, *J Calif Dent Assoc* 32:485, 2004.
9. Siskin M: Surgical techniques applicable to endodontics, *Dent Clin North Am* 74-69, 1967.
10. Bellizzi R, Loushine R: *Clinical atlas of endodontic surgery*, Chicago, 1991, Quintessence Publishing.
11. Molven O, Halse A, Grung B: Surgical management of endodontic failures: indications and treatment results, *Int Dent J* 41:33, 1991.
12. Friedman S: Retrograde approaches in endodontic therapy, *Endod Dent Traumatol* 7:97, 1991.
13. Kim S, Kratchman S: Modern endodontic surgery concepts and practice: a review, *J Endod* 32:601, 2006.
14. Cotton TP, Geisler TM, Holden DT, et al: Endodontic applications of cone-beam volumetric tomography, *J Endod* 33:1121, 2007.
15. Gutmann J, Harrison J: *Surgical endodontics*, Boston, 1991, Blackwell Scientific.
16. Arens D, Torabinejad M, Chivian N, et al: *Practical lessons in endodontic surgery*, Chicago, 1998, Quintessence Publishing.
17. Kramper B, Kaminski E, Osetek E, et al: A comparative study of the wound healing of three types of flap design used in periapical surgery, *J Endod* 10:17, 1984.
18. Velvart P: Papilla base incision: a new approach to recession-free healing of the interdental papilla after endodontic surgery, *Int Endod J* 35:453, 2002.
19. Gilheany P, Figdor D, Tyas M: Apical dentin permeability and microleakage associated with root end resection and retrograde filling, *J Endod* 20:22, 1994.
20. Grung B: Healing of gingival mucoperiosteal flaps after marginal incision in apicoectomy procedures, *Int J Oral Surg* 2:20, 1973.
21. Fister J, Gross B: A histologic evaluation of bone response to bur cutting with and without water coolant, *Oral Surg Oral Med Oral Pathol* 49:105, 1980.
22. Morgan L, Marshall J: A scanning electron microscopic study of in vivo ultrasonic root-end preparations, *J Endod* 25:567, 1999.

23. Pileggi R, McDonald N: A qualitative scanning electron microscopic evaluation of ultrasonically cut retropreparations, *J Dent Res* 73:383, 1994.
24. Wuchenich G, Meadows D, Torabinejad M: A comparison between two root end preparation techniques in human cadavers, *J Endod* 20:279, 1994.
25. Pantschev A, Carlsson A, Andersson L: Retrograde root filling with EBA cement or amalgam: a comparative clinical study, *Oral Surg Oral Med Oral Pathol* 78:101, 1994.
26. Marcotte L, Dowson J, Rowe N: Apical healing with retrofilling materials amalgam and gutta-percha, *J Endod* 1:63, 1975.
27. Flanders D, James G, Burch B, et al: Comparative histopathologic study of zinc free amalgam and Cavit in connective tissue of the rat, *J Endod* 1:56, 1975.
28. Witherspoon D, Gutmann J: Analysis of the healing response to gutta-percha and Diaket when used as root-end filling materials in periradicular surgery, *Int Endod J* 33:37, 2000.
29. Torabinejad M, Hong C, Lee S, et al: Investigation of mineral trioxide aggregate for root-end filling in dogs, *J Endod* 21:603, 1995.
30. Torabinejad M, Pitt Ford T, McKendry D, et al: Histologic assessment of mineral trioxide aggregate as a root-end filling in monkeys, *J Endod* 23:225, 1997.
31. De Bruyne MA, De Moor RJ: The use of glass ionomer cements in both conventional and surgical endodontics, *Int Endod J* 37:91, 2004.
32. Shahi S, Rahimi S, Lotfi M, et al: A comparative study of the biocompatibility of three root-end filling materials in rat connective tissue, *J Endod* 32:776, 2006.
33. Al-Rabeah E, Perinpanayagam H, MacFarland D: Human alveolar bone cells interact with ProRoot and tooth-colored MTA, *J Endod* 32:872, 2006.
34. Maguire H, Torabinejad M, McKendry D, et al: Effects of resorbable membrane placement and human osteogenic protein-1 on hard tissue healing after periradicular surgery in cats, *J Endod* 21:720, 1998.
35. Racey G, Wallace W, Cavalaris C, et al: Comparison of a polyglycolic–polylactic acid suture to black silk and plain catgut in human oral tissues, *J Oral Surg* 36:766, 1978.
36. Lilly G, Salem J, Armstrong J, et al: Reaction of oral tissues to suture materials. Part 3, *Oral Surg Oral Med Oral Pathol* 28:432, 1969.
37. von Recum AF, Imamura H, Freed PS, et al: Biocompatibility tests of components of an implantable cardiac assist device, *J Biomed Mater Res* 12:743, 1978.
38. Harrison J, Jurosky K: Wound healing in the tissues of the periodontium following periradicular surgery. I. The incisional wound, *J Endod* 17:425, 1991.
39. Robbins S, Kumar V: Inflammation and repair. In Robbins SL, Kumar V, editors: *Basic pathology*, ed 4, Philadelphia, 1987, WB Saunders.
40. Hunt T, Knighton D, Thakral K, et al: Studies on inflammation and wound healing: angiogenesis and collagen synthesis stimulated in vivo by resident and activated wound macrophages, *Surgery* 96:48, 1984.

41. Melcher A, Chan J: Phagocytosis and digestion of collagen by gingival fibroblasts in vivo: a study of serial sections, *J Ultrastruct Res* 77:1, 1981.
42. Harrison J, Jurosky K: Wound healing in the tissues of the periodontium following periradicular surgery. III. The osseous incisional wound, *J Endod* 18:76, 1992.
43. Iglhaut J, Aukhil I, Simpson D, et al: Progenitor cell kinetics during guided tissue regeneration in experimental periodontal wounds, *J Periodontal Res* 23:107, 1988.
44. Melcher A, Irving J: The healing mechanism in artificially created circumscribed defects in the femora of albino rats, *J Bone Joint Surg* 44:928, 1962.
45. Del Fabbro M, Ceresoli V, Lolato A, et al: Effect of platelet concentrate on quality of life after periradicular surgery: a randomized clinical study, *J Endod* 38:733, 2012.
46. Yoshikawa G, Murashima Y, Wadachi R, et al: Guided bone regeneration (GBR) using membranes and calcium sulphate after apicectomy: a comparative histomorphometrical study, *Int Endod J* 35:255, 2002.
47. Davis WL: *Oral histology: cell structure and function*, Philadelphia, 1986, WB Saunders.
48. American Association of Endodontists: *Glossary of endodontic terms*, ed 8, Chicago, 2012, The Association.
49. Bergenholtz A: Radectomy of multirooted teeth, *J Am Dent Assoc* 85:870, 1972.
50. Langer B, Stein S, Wagenberg B: An evaluation of root resections: a ten-year study, *J Periodontol* 52:719, 1981.
51. Mead C, Javidan-Nejad S, Mego M, et al: Levels of evidence for the outcome of endodontic surgery, *J Endod* 31:19, 2005.
52. Rubinstein R, Kim S: Short-term observation of the results of endodontic surgery with the use of a surgical operation microscope and Super-EBA as root-end filling material, *J Endod* 25:43, 1999.
53. Rubinstein R, Kim S: Long-term follow-up of cases considered healed one year after apical microsurgery, *J Endod* 28:378, 2002.
54. Maddalone M, Gagliani M: Periapical endodontic surgery: a 3-year follow-up study, *Int Endod J* 36:193, 2003.
55. Sechrist C: *The outcome of MTA as a root end filling material: a long term evaluation*, Loma Linda, Calif, 2005, Loma Linda University.
56. Setzer FC, Shah SB, Kohli MR, et al: Outcome of endodontic surgery: a meta-analysis of the literature. Part 1. Comparison of traditional root-end surgery and endodontic microsurgery, *J Endod* 36:1757, 2010.
57. Setzer FC, Kohli MR, Shah SB, et al: Outcome of endodontic surgery: a meta-analysis of the literature. Part 2. Comparison of endodontic microsurgical techniques with and without the use of higher magnification, *J Endod* 38:1, 2012.
58. Kim E, Song J-S, Jung I-L, et al: Prospective clinical study evaluating endodontic microsurgery outcomes for cases with lesions of endodontic origin compared with cases with lesions of combined periodontic-endodontic origin, *J Endod* 34:546, 2008.
59. Zuolo M, Ferreira M, Gutmann J: Prognosis in periradicular surgery: a clinical prospective study, *Int Endod J* 33:91, 2000.

Evaluation of endodontic outcomes

Mahmoud Torabinejad, Shane N. White

LEARNING OBJECTIVES

After reading this chapter, the student should be able to:

1. Describe signs of successful and unsuccessful root canal treatment.
2. Describe the most common modalities used to determine success or failure.
3. State the approximate range of expected outcomes of routine, uncomplicated root canal treatment based on pretreatment conditions.
4. State predictors of success and failure.
5. Identify endodontic and nonendodontic causes of treatment failure.
6. State the outcomes of retreatment, endodontic surgery, and intentional replantation.
7. State the outcomes of fixed partial denture and single tooth implant treatments.
8. Approach treatment planning of root canal failure, recognizing the advantages and disadvantages of different treatment modalities.

T he highest possible long-term levels of comfort, function, and esthetics are the primary objectives of root canal treatment in patients with inflammation or infection arising from disease of pulpal origin or trauma. These objectives are achieved by eliminating or significantly reducing bacteria and preventing recontamination.[1-3] Rubber dam isolation and aseptic technique provide a hygienic environment. Thorough chemomechanical cleaning and shaping eliminate or significantly reduce pathogenic bacteria. Complete obturation eliminates a habitat for bacteria. Leak-resistant restoration prevents bacterial recontamination and achieves functional and esthetic rehabilitation.

Optimal outcomes are dependent on attainment of these technical goals. Because of the complexity of root canal systems,[4,5] less than perfect instrumentation and obturation methods, and leakage of permanent restorations, elimination of bacteria from the root canal systems cannot be achieved in some cases. Adherence to proper protocol significantly improves the prognosis of root canal–treated teeth; however, because of the complex interactions between host and pathogen, unexpected results are occasionally seen, regardless of whether proper or improper protocols were followed.

The purposes of this chapter are to (1) define success and failure, (2) describe methods for evaluation of endodontic outcomes, (3) provide success rates, (4) explain the signs and symptoms of negative outcomes, (5) discuss factors influencing outcomes, and (6) compare the outcomes of initial nonsurgical root canal treatment with those of retreatment, endodontic surgery, and alternative treatments, such as single tooth implants.

DEFINITIONS OF SUCCESS AND FAILURE

Patients, third-party payers, and dentists, all stakeholders in the dental delivery system, have differing perspectives on and expectations for the outcomes of root canal treatment.[6] Patients are usually satisfied if their teeth are comfortable, functional, and esthetically pleasing. Insurance companies measure success by access to care, quality of care, cost, and the longevity of the treatment provided. Dentists are usually most concerned with the delivery of optimal care, predictable elimination of disease as measured clinically and radiographically, and fair compensation. The real art of dentistry is to coordinate and interface these perspectives and expectations among the stakeholders without sacrificing the quality of care.

Over the years, many terms have been used to describe endodontic outcomes. Sometimes the same words have been defined in different ways by different authors. Therefore, it is important to understand the definitions of the words being used. The simple terms "success" and "failure" may be clear to all. The absence of clinical symptoms and apical lesions is the principal indicator of successful root canal treatment. It is important to remember that apical periodontitis is frequently asymptomatic and can often only be demonstrated radiographically.[7]

For a treated tooth with a previously vital pulp and no preexisting apical lesion, success means that the tooth remains asymptomatic and an apical lesion does not form. New symptoms or the appearance of an apical lesion is a sign of a failed root canal in a tooth with a previously vital pulp and no preexisting apical lesion.

For a tooth with a previously necrotic pulp, the treatment is considered successful if the tooth remains asymptomatic, its preexisting apical lesion heals, and no new apical lesion develops. The presence of symptoms or a new or enlarging lesion in a tooth with necrotic pulp indicates failure.

As an alternative to the terms "success" and "failure," the American Association of Endodontists has proposed the following terms:

- *Healed*—Functional, asymptomatic teeth with no or minimal radiographic periradicular pathosis
- *Nonhealed*—Nonfunctional, symptomatic teeth with or without radiographic periradicular pathosis
- *Healing*—Teeth with periradicular pathosis that are asymptomatic and functional, or teeth with or without radiographic periradicular pathosis that are symptomatic but for which the intended function is not altered
- *Functional*—A treated tooth or root that is serving its intended purpose in the dentition

Because the path to bony periradicular healing may be long and irregular, determination of success or failure may be difficult. Many asymptomatic root canal–treated teeth have varying degrees of radiolucency. The dentist must judge whether these teeth are in progress to success or to failure and then advise the patient and manage the teeth appropriately.

WHEN TO EVALUATE

Recommended follow-up periods have ranged from 6 months to 5 years.[8-13] Six months is a widely accepted and reasonable interval for a recall evaluation for most patients. The key question is: At what point is it likely that a treatment outcome will not change? In other words: When can it be determined that treatment has either succeeded or failed, and the outcome is unlikely to change, so that no further recall is necessary? A radiographic lesion that is unchanged or has increased in size after 1 year is unlikely to ever resolve; therefore, the treatment may be considered to be unsuccessful. If at 6 months the lesion is still present but smaller, it is likely to be in progress to healing, and additional recall is needed. It takes longer for larger periradicular lesions to heal than smaller lesions. Unfortunately, apparent success may revert to failure at a later time (often as a result of reinfection through coronal leakage). Late healing may also occur. Therefore, an endodontic evaluation, including a patient history, clinical examination, and radiography of teeth treated with root canals, should be part of every comprehensive patient examination.

METHODS FOR EVALUATION OF ENDODONTIC OUTCOMES

The patient history, clinical findings, and radiographic examinations are the commonest metrics of root canal treatment outcomes. Evaluation of endodontic outcomes follows the same diagnostic pathway as for initial treatment (see Chapter 5). Biopsy of periradicular tissues during endodontic surgery provides a histologic diagnosis, another method for evaluation of success or failure of root canal treatment. This method is not routinely used and is an impractical approach to determine clinical outcomes of root canal treatments.

Patient History
Complaints of persistent or worsening symptoms months or years after root canal treatment has been completed are usually an indication of treatment failure and continuing disease. Symptoms related to discomfort or pain on chewing, aching, and so forth are generally an indication of periradicular inflammation or infection. It must be remembered that bony healing takes time and that a tooth that feels "different" on biting may be en route to healing; this should be confirmed clinically and radiographically. Pain on release may indicate a cracked tooth. A bad taste may indicate a draining abscess. Occasionally a patient reports sensitivity to cold or heat; this is most likely related to an adjacent untreated tooth but could be an indication of a missed vital canal in a treated tooth.

Clinical Examination
Presence of persistent signs or symptoms is usually an indication of disease and failure. However, absence of symptoms does not signify success. Periapical pathosis without significant symptoms is usually present in teeth before and after root canal treatment until healing has occurred.[7] There is little correlation between the presence of pathosis and corresponding symptoms; yet when adverse signs or symptoms are evident, there is a strong likelihood that a pathosis is present.[14] Persistent signs (e.g., swelling, probing defect, or sinus tract) or symptoms usually indicate failure.

Clinical criteria for success generally include the following[14]:

- Absence of swelling and other signs of infection and inflammation
- Disappearance of sinus tract or narrow, isolated probing defect
- No evidence of soft tissue destruction, including probing defects
- The tooth has been restored and is in function.

Radiographic Findings
Radiograph findings can classify the outcome of each treatment as success, failure, or unknown status. Radiographs made at different times must be made in a reproducible fashion and with minimal distortion so that valid longitudinal comparisons can be made over time. The best way to ensure reproducibility is to use a radiographic paralleling device (see Chapter 12). Teeth with multiple roots or canals should be

examined using both straight-on and off-angle periapical views.

Radiographic success is the absence of an apical radiolucent lesion. This means that a lesion present at the time of treatment has resolved or, if there was no lesion present at the time of treatment, none has developed. Thus radiographic success is evident by the elimination or lack of development of an area of radiolucency for a minimum of 1 year after treatment (Fig. 22.1).

Radiographic failure is the continued persistence or development of radiolucency. Specifically, a radiolucent lesion has remained the same, enlarged, or has developed since treatment (Fig. 22.2). Nonfunctional, symptomatic teeth with or without radiographic lesions are considered failures.

Radiographically unknown status indicates a state of uncertainty. This classification includes teeth with radiolucency that are asymptomatic and functional. The preexisting radiolucent lesion in these teeth has not yet decreased or become larger in size. Teeth with radiolucencies that were treated elsewhere and for which there are no prior radiographs for comparison are often assigned to this category (Fig. 22.3).

A shortcoming of radiographic evaluation is that radiographs may not be made or interpreted in standardized ways.

As early as 1966, Bender and coworkers[14] noted that radiographic interpretation is often subject to personal bias and that a change in angulation can give a completely different appearance to the lesion, making it appear either smaller or larger. Also, different observers may not agree on what they see in a radiograph, and the same observer may disagree with his or her earlier interpretation if asked to review the same radiograph at a different time.[15]

Long ago, in order to study predictors of endodontic treatment outcomes, Larz Strindberg created a three-step scale based on the history of symptoms, the clinical examination, and radiographic signs.[16] These criteria were extremely strict, designed for predicting future outcomes, not current outcomes; even the appearance of a poorly defined lamina dura was reason for assignment as failure. Later, Ørstavik and associates[17] suggested a five-step periapical index (PAI) for use in epidemiologic studies of root canal treatment. A current patient radiograph is compared to a set of five standard radiographic images ranging from a radiographically healthy periapex to a large periapical lesion.[18] Preoperative and recall radiographs are assigned scores according to their resemblance to one of the five reference images. The PAI can classify root canal treatments as "healing" if the lesion size is

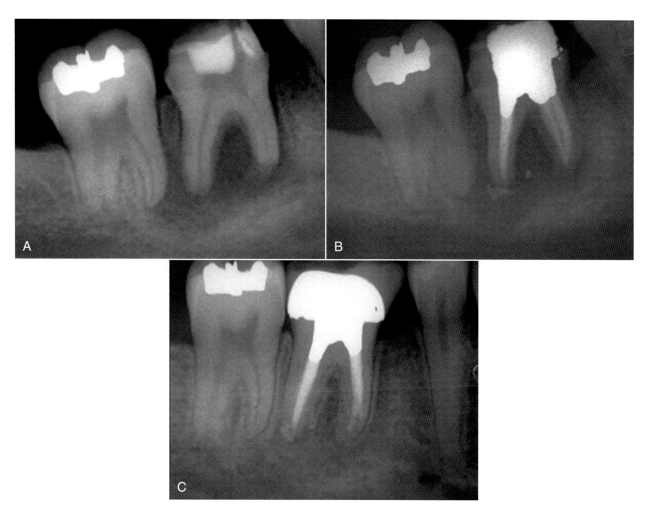

Two years later

Fig. 22.1 Success. **A,** The initial radiograph shows the presence of bone loss from the crest of the ridge around the apices of all roots in the tooth. Periodontal probing demonstrates that the gingival sulcus is intact. There is no response to pulpal vitality tests. **B,** Root canal treatment completed. **C,** A 2-year recall radiograph shows resolution of the radiolucency.

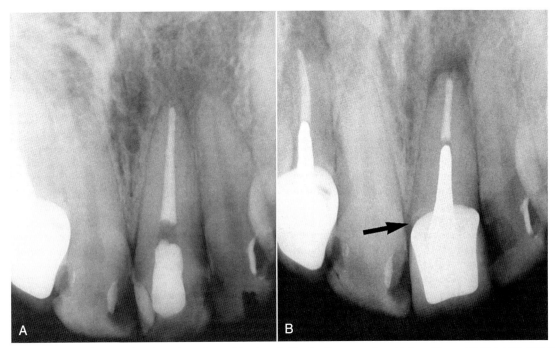

Fig. 22.2 Failure. **A,** Apparently adequate root canal treatment. The tooth was restored later with a post and core and crown. **B,** The patient reports persistent discomfort after 2 years. A periradicular radiolucency indicates failure, probably a result of coronal leakage at a defective margin *(arrow)*.

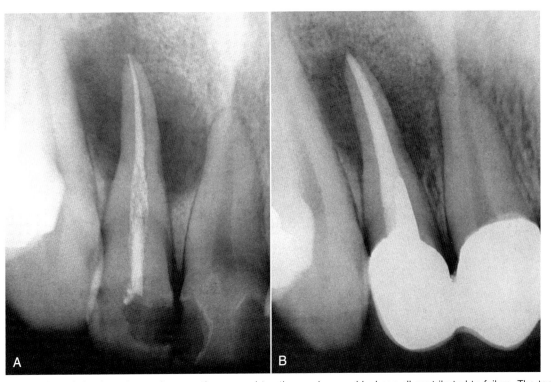

Fig. 22.3 Failure. **A,** Inadequate canal preparation, poor obturation, and coronal leakage all contributed to failure. The tooth is suitable for conventional retreatment and restoration. **B,** Twelve-month recall after retreatment. A sinus tract has disappeared, and the patient reports absence of symptoms. The radiolucent lesion is decreasing in size but has not resolved. Because the final outcome is still unknown, additional recall evaluation is necessary. (Courtesy Dr. A. Stabholz.)

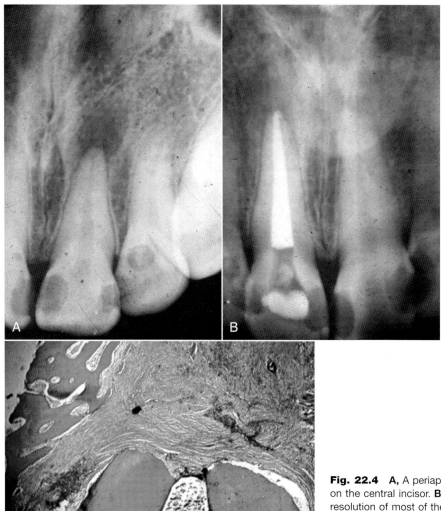

Fig. 22.4 **A,** A periapical radiograph revealed an apical radiolucency on the central incisor. **B,** A periapical film taken 6 months later shows resolution of most of the apical radiolucency. Despite radiographic change, the patient stayed symptomatic, and surgery had to be performed. **C,** Histologic examination of this tooth shows resolution of most of the inflammatory cells near the apex. (Courtesy Dr. A. Khayat.)

reduced, "healed" if the lesion has been completely eliminated, or "developing" if a new lesion has formed. The PAI correlates with the histology and radiodensity; it is accurate, reproducible, and discriminatory. However, root canal treatments measured using the PAI typically do not reach complete healing for several years. As late as 4 to 5 years after surgery, according to the PAI, slow healers tend to outnumber late failures.

Cone beam computed tomography (CBCT) can be used for endodontic diagnosis and for assessment of healing. CBCT may sometimes reveal pathology not seen using periapical radiography.[19] However, healing must be judged over time using a comparable baseline preoperative view; it cannot be assessed by a single snapshot nor by comparison of dissimilar images. Currently, CBCT has lower resolution, greater expense, and considerably higher radiation exposure than conventional periapical films and digital images.

Histologic Examination
Routine histologic evaluation of periapical tissues after root canal treatment is impractical and impossible without

surgery.[20] If a treated tooth were to be evaluated histologically, success would be signified by reconstitution of the periradicular tissue structure and absence of inflammation (Fig. 22.4).

The degree of correlation between histologic findings and radiographic appearance is unclear. Two cadaver-based histologic investigations of teeth treated with root canals reached different conclusions.[18,21] Brynolf concluded that most root canal–treated teeth showed some periradicular histological inflammation despite the appearance of radiographic success.[18] In contrast, Green and colleagues[21] observed that most root canal–treated teeth with radiographically normal periapices were indeed free of histologic inflammation. Thus, with current technology, the patient history, clinical evaluation, and radiography are the only practical means of assessing healing after root canal treatment.

SUCCESS RATES

As is the case for all dental and medical procedures, some root canal treatments may be unsuccessful. Prompt **401** recognition and management of treatments that do not resolve and heal are critical but can be difficult and complex. Historically, it has been thought that success rates for root canal treatment, using highly discriminatory instruments such as the Strindberg criteria or the PAI, range from 80% to 95%. However, general percentages should be taken with caution, and *each case should be individually assessed to determine its probability of success.*

Torabinejad and colleagues[22] performed a systematic review of the literature pertaining to success and failure of nonsurgical root canal therapy and assigned levels of evidence (LOE) to the studies. In the prior 40 years, 306 articles had been published related to the outcome of nonsurgical root canal treatment. Fifty-one studies included at least 100 teeth; meta-analysis of these studies suggested an overall radiographic success rate of 81.5% over a period of 5 years. Others who assessed the 4- to 6-year outcomes of initial endodontic treatment have reported similar overall healing rates.[23] In a recent systematic review, Torabinejad and colleagues[24] compared the outcomes of endodontically treated teeth with those of single implant crowns, fixed dental prostheses, and no treatment after extraction. Success data in that review consistently ranked implant therapy as superior to endodontic treatment, which in turn was ranked as superior to fixed prosthodontic treatment (Table 22.1). However, very different criteria for success are used in implant dentistry, endodontics, and prosthodontics; therefore, such comparisons lack validity. Comparison of survival rates is much more meaningful.

SURVIVAL RATES

Long-term survival rates for endodontically treated teeth are very high, over 90%.[24-28] A recent systematic review by Torabinejad and colleagues showed that both root canal and implant treatments resulted in a very high survival rate (97% at more than 6 years), compared to only 80% for a fixed dental prosthesis, a three- or four-unit bridge (see Table 22.1).[24] Iqbal and Kim reported similar findings in a systematic review when they compared the survival rates of restored endodontically treated teeth with those of implant-supported restorations.[25] Several very large studies have all reported extremely high long-term survival rates for teeth with root canal treatment: Lazarski and colleagues,[26] 94% functional survival for 44,613 cases at 3.5 years in the United States; Salehrabi and Rotstein,[27] 97% survival for 1.1 million patients at 8 years in the United States; and Chen and colleagues,[28] 93% survival for 1.5 million teeth at 5 years in Taiwan. Teeth with root canal treatments have remarkably high long-term survival rates.

PATIENT-BASED OUTCOMES

Patients choose root canal treatment (RCT) to retain teeth (and thus preserve the natural esthetics of their smile) and to relieve pain. Anticipation and experience of root canal–associated pain are major sources of fear for patients and a very important concern of dentists. Pain is anticipated, experienced, remembered, and shared by patients. A recent systematic review found that the severity of pretreatment root canal–associated pain was moderate, dropped substantially

Table 22.1 Percentages of pooled and weighted survival and success rates of dental implants, root canal treatment, and three- or four-unit bridges over 2 to 4, 4 to 6, and 6+ years

Procedure	Success (%)	Survival (%)
2 to 4 Years		
Dental implant (pooled)	98 (95-99)	95 (93-97)
Dental implant (weighted)	99 (96-100)	96 (94-97)
Root canal treatment (pooled)	90 (88-92)	94
Root canal treatment (weighted)	89 (88-91)	—
Three-unit bridge (pooled)	79 (69-87)	94
Three-unit bridge (weighted)	78 (76-81)	—
4 to 6 Years		
Dental implant (pooled)	97 (96-98)	97 (95-98)
Dental implant (weighted)	98 (97-99)	97 (95-98)
Root canal treatment (pooled)	93 (87-97)	94 (92-96)
Root canal treatment (weighted)	94 (92-96)	94 (91-96)
Three-unit bridge (pooled)	82 (71-91)	93
Three-unit bridge (weighted)	76 (74-79)	—
6+ Years		
Dental implant (pooled)	95 (93-96)	97 (95-99)
Dental implant (weighted)	95 (93-97)	97 (96-98)
Root canal treatment (pooled)	84 (82-87)	92 (84-97)
Root canal treatment (weighted)	84 (81-87)	97 (97-97)
Three-unit bridge (pooled)	81 (74-86)	82
Three-unit bridge (weighted)	80 (79-82)	—

within 1 day of treatment, and continued to drop to minimal levels in 7 days.[29] The prevalence of pretreatment root canal–associated pain was high but dropped moderately within 1 day and substantially to minimal levels in 7 days. Supplemental anesthesia is often required during treatment. Pain during RCT was usually less than anticipated.[30] High percentages of patients reported a willingness to choose root canal treatment again.[31] Overall satisfaction ratings for root canal treatment are extremely high, generally above the 90th percentile.[32] Satisfaction is higher when endodontic treatment is provided by specialists, probably a reflection of effective communication and efficient management. Initial costs for root canal treatment and restoration are substantially lower than for replacement with an implant single crown or fixed dental prostheses.[24,33] Although longitudinal studies show excellent long-term outcomes, it is to the detriment of individual patients that community care may often not follow accepted standards and protocols as described in standard texts, such as this one.[34,35]

POSTOPERATIVE COMPLICATIONS

As with all dental procedures, complications may occur after root canal treatment. However, the incidence of long-term postoperative complications appears to be lower than for the alternatives, single tooth implants and fixed dental prostheses.[36,37] The 10-year complication rate for retained root canal–treated teeth is approximately 4%, compared to approximately 18% for retained single tooth implant restorations.[37] Typical complications include symptoms, swelling, and the need for retreatment.[37] In endodontics, complications are recorded as failures according to the criteria described previously; in other disciplines, complications are generally not recorded as failures.

PROGNOSTIC INDICATORS

The classic landmark study published by Larz Strindberg in 1956 related treatment outcomes to biologic and therapeutic factors.[16] Factors now considered to be predictors of success and failure include (1) apical pathosis, (2) bacterial status of the canal, (3) extent and quality of the obturation, and (4) quality of the coronal restoration. The role of these factors should be discussed with the patient before and after treatment.

Several investigations have shown that the following factors result in a slightly less favorable prognosis: the presence of periradicular lesions and larger lesion size[22,38]; the presence of bacteria in the canal before obturation[39]; and obturations that are short, long, contain voids, or lack density.[40-44] Some evidence suggests that the use of a calcium hydroxide intracanal medicament may improve the prognosis.[45-47] The quality of the coronal restoration plays a key role in the outcomes of root canal treatment.[48-50]

Factors such as the tooth type, age and gender of the patient, and obturation technique have minimal if any influence on the prognosis.[51] Most medical conditions have no significant bearing on the prognosis.[52] However, patients with insulin-dependent diabetes mellitus have a significantly lower healing rate after root canal therapy in teeth with apical lesions.[53] Interestingly, diabetes mellitus, hypertension, and coronary artery disease are associated with an increased risk of extraction after root canal treatment.[54] Although this finding does not indicate causality, the systemic disease burden has broad effects on the patient's welfare, morbidity, and behavior. Obviously, a patient with a complex medical history, serious illness, or disability may present a high degree of difficulty in management and demands high levels of experience and expertise. However, root canal treatment may greatly benefit some patients by preventing the need for high-risk extractions or other surgical procedures; such patients include those with bleeding disorders, those who have undergone head and neck irradiation, and those treated with high-dose bisphosphonates.

CAUSES OF NONHEALED, FAILED ROOT CANAL TREATMENT

The persistent presence of bacteria is the primary cause of endodontic pathology.[55] Ideally, after preparation the root canal should be free of bacteria.[56] If the pulp was vital, isolation, disinfection and root canal treatment are more likely to prevent bacterial contamination and to achieve a superior prognosis. If the pulp was necrotic and an apical lesion was present, removal of bacteria and their toxins, metabolites, antigens, and byproducts is both essential and even more challenging. Unfortunately, complete mechanical debridement of the canal and all its complex ramifications is virtually impossible.[57,58] Therefore, bacterial counts are minimized by careful chemomechanical instrumentation using copious gentle and frequent sodium hypochlorite irrigation.[59] The interappointment medicament, calcium hydroxide, reduces the number of bacteria,[60] enhances the speed of healing, and reduces inflammation.[45,46] However, there is uncertainty whether use of this medicament ultimately results in a better prognosis.[47]

The most common errors leading to bacterial persistence and failure are (1) errors in diagnosis and treatment planning; (2) lack of knowledge of pulp anatomy, resulting in missed canals; (3) inadequate debridement and/or disinfection of the root canal system, resulting in persistent bacteria; (4) operative errors; (5) obturation deficiencies; (6) absence of cuspal coverage in posterior teeth, allowing vertical root fracture; (7) excessive removal of tooth structure, predisposing teeth to fracture; and (8) coronal leakage through inadequate provisional or definitive restorations. These factors can be linked to the preoperative, operative, and postoperative phases of root canal treatment.

Preoperative Causes

Failure of root canal treatment is often traced to misdiagnosis; errors in treatment planning; poor case selection (i.e., dentists attempting treatment beyond their experience and skill levels); and treatment of a tooth with a poor initial prognosis. Diagnosis should be based on all available information: the patient's history, signs, and symptoms; a current, comprehensive endodontic evaluation (e.g., palpation, percussion, probing, and heat/cold and electrical tests); and radiographic evaluation (see Chapter 5). The clinician must assess all factors and form a clear diagnosis; otherwise, there is a risk of inappropriate treatment or even of treating the wrong tooth.

Failure to use good radiographic projections, including multiple views with different mesiodistal angulations, to determine various root canal system aberrations, such as extra canals (e.g., MB2 canals in maxillary molars, DB canals in mandibular molars, and lingual canals in mandibular incisors), often results in failure, even with correct pulpal and periapical diagnoses (Fig. 22.5).

Root fractures are also often misdiagnosed or escape early detection. Periodontal defects with associated bone loss often appear after the fracture has been in the crown and root long enough for the crack to become infected (see Chapter 7).[16,39-41] If an isolated, deep probing defect is associated with the suspect tooth, vertical root fracture must be considered (Fig. 22.6).

Operative Causes

Many failures result from errors in operative procedure (see Chapter 19). Chemomechanical cleaning and shaping of the

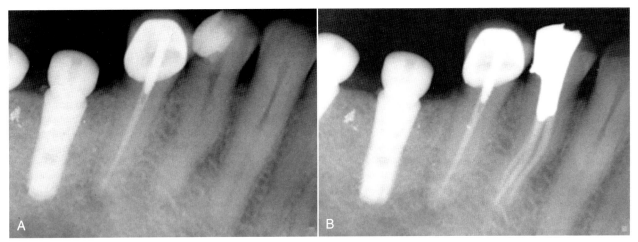

Fig. 22.5 **A,** Sudden disappearance of the canal "fast break" in the mandibular first premolar indicates the presence of a division in the canal or the root. **B,** A postoperative radiograph revealed three canals and two separate roots in this tooth. (Courtesy Dr. Shawn Anderson.)

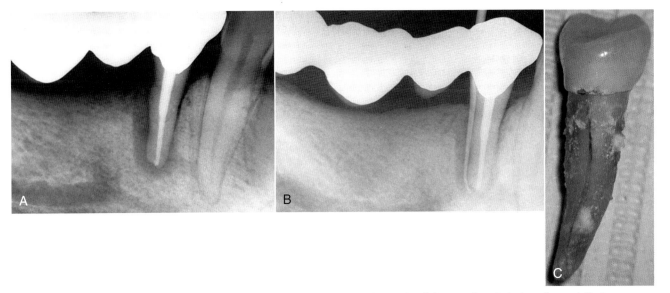

Fig. 22.6 Indicators of vertical root fracture. **A,** A teardrop or J-shaped lateral radiolucency is noted along the root. **B,** A narrow probing defect extends to the apex. **C,** Confirmation of a vertical fracture after tooth extraction.

root canal space, followed by complete obturation of the root canal system, are necessary for success.

Straight-line access preparation to facilitate debridement and obturation is often overlooked. Access is even more important when using rotary nickel-titanium file systems. If the access preparation is underextended, canals may be missed, and the treatment is likely to fail. If the pulp horns are not opened, pulpal tissue, bacteria, debris, and sealer may remain in the coronal pulp space. Such remnants often result in persistent infection or coronal discoloration.

Underextended access preparations limit instrument maneuverability, resulting in insufficient cleaning, aberrant shaping, and instrument breakage. Overextended access cavities, with excessive loss of dentin, weaken the tooth, increase the risk of fracture and perforation, and complicate restoration.[61,62]

Failure to maintain apical canal curvature (which can occur because files cut to the outside of the apical curve) results in transportation, ledging, and apical perforation. This alters canal morphology, leaves potentially infected debris in the canal system, and makes obturation more difficult. Stainless steel files must be precurved. Marked deviation or overzealous flaring or overpreparation in the furcal danger zone or in the apical third may result in perforation (see Figs. 16.15 and 19.8). Most of these perforations can be repaired nonsurgically using mineral trioxide aggregate (MTA), but some may require endodontic surgery (see Fig. 22.4).[63] Leakage or mechanical irritation may result, and a lesion may develop.[64]

The consequences of a separated instrument or broken endodontic file lodged in a root canal system depends on the stage of canal preparation and the pretreatment pulp status (vital or necrotic) (see Figs. 19.13 and 19.14).[65,66] The outcome may be unaffected if the biologic objectives of bacterial removal and exclusion can be attained through chemomechanical debridement and obturation, even if the instrument cannot be bypassed or removed.

Underinstrumentation short of the apical constriction leaves the most important part of the canal uncleaned and is associated with increased failure rates.[12,44] Confining operative procedures and materials to the canal space facilitates repair of periradicular tissues.[40,67] Overinstrumentation causes some tissue damage, periradicular hemorrhage, and transitory inflammation. Continuous overinstrumentation can provoke a persistent inflammatory response capable of resorbing dental and osseous tissues.[68] Overinstrumentation may also transfer microorganisms from the canal to the periapical tissues, possibly compromising the outcome.[69]

Overextended obturation also may lead to treatment failure. In many cases the material does not cause an apical lesion to develop because gutta-percha is relatively inert. Rather, inadequate apical cleaning or sealing causes failure. A gutta-percha cone may slip through the apex because the preparation taper or the apical stop was inadequate. Additionally, sealers can be irritating or toxic to tissues.[20,70,71]

Errors in obturation frequently result from poor canal shaping and poor obturation techniques. An obturation that is poorly condensed (i.e., short or contains voids) can result in apical and/or coronal leakage.[20,72,73] Both short and long obturations are associated with failure, particularly in the presence of previously necrotic pulps, bacteria, and apical lesions.[74]

Postoperative Causes

Regrettably, lack of a timely or durable coronal seal is a common problem. A high-quality, durable coronal restoration definitively protects and seals the tooth, preventing ingress and apical percolation of bacteria and salivary contaminants (Fig. 22.7).[45-50,56-60,74-78] The coronal access to a root canal–treated tooth must be sealed completely for the lifetime of this organ.

Restoration should occur at the time of obturation or immediately thereafter, using rubber dam isolation in a saliva-free environment. Temporary restorations and cotton pledgets must be completely removed before restoration. Gutta-percha and sealer should be removed from the floor of the access

cavity. No space should remain between the coronal filling or buildup and the obturation because such a space provides a habitat for bacterial colonization and growth.

Restorative errors also compromise success. For example, dentin removal for posts weakens teeth and increases susceptibility to fracture (Fig. 22.8).[61] All too often, post preparations cause perforations. Coronal coverage (i.e., a crown or an onlay) improves the prognosis for posterior teeth by reducing the incidence of root fracture. However, preparing anterior root canal–treated teeth for a crown removes much precious remaining tooth structure and results in a less favorable prognosis. Internal bleaching, layered composite restorations, and porcelain veneers are preferred to crowns on anterior teeth.

OUTCOMES OF TREATMENTS AFTER FAILURE OF INITIAL NONSURGICAL ENDODONTICS

For decades a primary goal of dentistry was to preserve the natural dentition. In previous years all efforts would have been made to save teeth with pulpal and periodontal diseases or to extract hopeless teeth and replace them with fixed or removable prostheses. The high success and survival rates of dental implants have created a paradigm shift in treatment planning. Clinicians are regularly confronted with difficult choices after failure of root canal treatment. Treatment options now include (1) nonsurgical retreatment, (2) endodontic surgery, (3) extraction and replacement using a single tooth implant, (4) extraction and replacement using a fixed dental prosthesis, (5) intentional replantation or autotransplantation, and (6) extraction without replacement. It must be remembered that the vast majority of teeth with root canal treatment heal without any further intervention and that the options discussed in the following sections represent additional "safety nets."

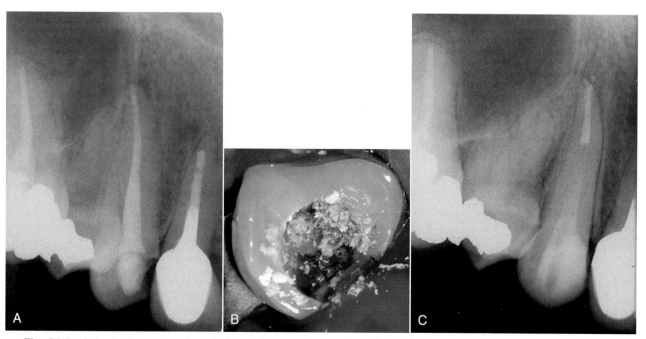

Fig. 22.7 **A,** Lack of coronal seal resulted in clinical symptoms and a periapical lesion in the maxillary right cuspid. **B,** A clinical photograph shows lack of permanent restoration and coronal decay. **C,** After retreatment of the previous root canal treatment and placement of a C-fiber post, the coronal access to the root canal–treated tooth was sealed permanently. (Courtesy Dr. D. Roland.)

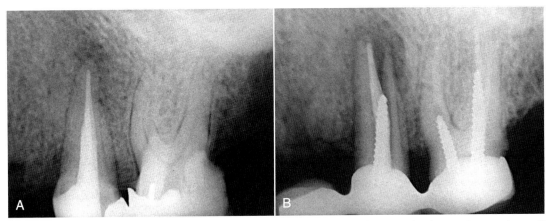

Fig. 22.8 **A,** Overenlargement of a canal has weakened the root. **B,** Placement of an oversized screw-type post, possibly combined with prior excessive condensation forces, resulted in a vertical fracture and apical-lateral pathosis. The tooth had to be extracted.

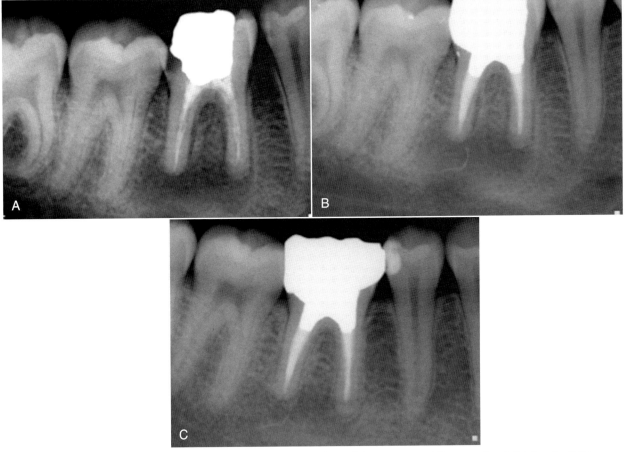

Fig. 22.9 **A,** A preoperative periapical radiograph shows extensive radiolucency around the mesial and distal roots of the first mandibular molar with previous inadequate root canal treatment. **B,** The root canal treatment was retreated nonsurgically; the canals were filled with mineral trioxide aggregate (MTA) and restored permanently. **C,** A radiograph 4 years later shows complete resolution of the periapical lesions. (Courtesy Dr. M. Pouresmail.)

Nonsurgical Retreatment

A thorough search of published literature related to clinical studies on the success and failure of nonsurgical retreatment identified 31 clinical studies since 1970.[79] The success rate of nonsurgical retreatment ranged between 40% and 100%.[79] In the prospective Toronto Study, the "healed" rate of endodontic retreatment cases was reported to be 81%.[80] Recently, Torabinejad and colleagues performed a systematic review to compare the clinical and radiographic outcomes of nonsurgical retreatment with those of endodontic surgery. They found that although endodontic surgery offers more favorable initial success rates, nonsurgical retreatment offers more favorable long-term outcomes.[81] Based on these results, it appears that if a failure is retreated by conventional means (Fig. 22.9), the success rate is very high, especially in teeth without periapical lesions and *when the cause of failure is identified and corrected* (see Chapter 20).[82]

Endodontic Surgery

In a Loma Linda University study, investigators searched the literature for clinical articles pertaining to the success and failure of periapical surgery.[83] Their electronic and manual searches showed that the majority of frequently quoted "success and failure" studies are case series, a low level of evidence. Recent long-term follow-up studies of endodontic surgery show high success rates (Fig. 22.10) (see Chapter 21).[84-86] However, the recent systematic review comparing the outcomes of nonsurgical retreatment with those of endodontic surgery demonstrated that retreatment has superior long-term results.[81] Therefore, endodontic surgery should be reserved for cases in which retreatment has failed to produce healing or retreatment may be precluded for technical reasons.

Single Tooth Implant

Implant dentistry provides functional, durable, and esthetic tooth replacement. This has had profound effects on endodontic, periodontic, and prosthodontic treatment planning and provision.[87] Implant-supported restorations have obviated the need for crown preparations on intact abutment teeth (Fig. 22.11) and have allowed fixed prosthodontic replacement when suitable abutments are absent.[88,89]

Criteria for implant success are generally not directly comparable to those used for other treatment modalities; for example, the integrity of the prosthesis is not usually included, nor are complications requiring surgical or prosthodontic intervention. Success and survival rates for single tooth implants are now generally very high. The mean success and survival rates (at more than 6 years) for single tooth implants, as determined by systematic review, are 95% and 97%, respectively (see Table 22.1). However, a wide range of success rates has been reported in the literature.[90-101] Nonetheless, it is clear that both endodontic and implant success and survival rates are substantially superior to those for fixed dental prostheses (see Table 22.1).

Several factors affect the decision on whether a tooth should receive root canal treatment or be extracted and replaced by an implant-supported restoration. These factors are related to the patient, tooth, periodontium, site, and type of treatment required. Considering these factors during treatment planning enables the clinician to provide the highest possible level of comfort, function, longevity, and esthetics for patients with oral diseases or traumatic injuries.[102-104] It must be remembered that the artificial alternative to the natural condition should only be chosen when the artificial alternative is superior or less costly than maintaining the natural state.[24]

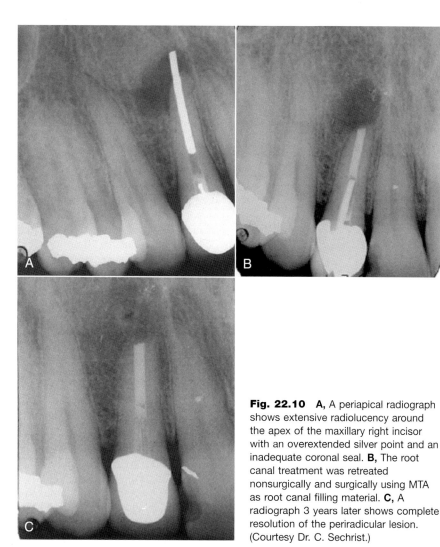

Fig. 22.10 A, A periapical radiograph shows extensive radiolucency around the apex of the maxillary right incisor with an overextended silver point and an inadequate coronal seal. **B,** The root canal treatment was retreated nonsurgically and surgically using MTA as root canal filling material. **C,** A radiograph 3 years later shows complete resolution of the periradicular lesion. (Courtesy Dr. C. Sechrist.)

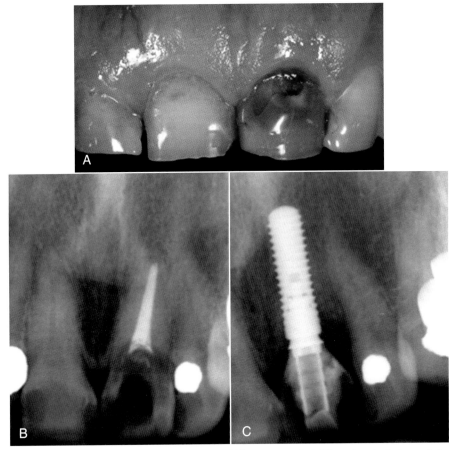

Fig. 22.11 A badly discolored and nonrestorable tooth (**A** and **B**) was extracted (**C**), and a single immediate implant was placed.

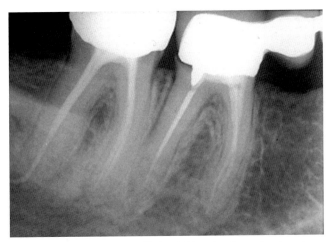

Fig. 22.12 Restored mandibular right molars have developed pulpal and periapical problems, in addition to caries under the margins of the crowns. Coronal leakage likely contributed to the development of the new periapical lesions.

Fixed Dental Prostheses

Traditionally, after extraction of hopeless teeth, adjacent teeth were prepared as abutments for fixed or removable prostheses. These teeth are prone to future disease, such as caries and pulpal and periodontal problems, in addition to complications such as porcelain or root fracture (Fig. 22.12).[105] Success and survival rates for fixed dental prostheses have been reported as 48% to 95%. A meta-analysis of the literature reported an 87% 10-year survival rate and a 69% 15-year survival rate for fixed dental prostheses.[106] Other investigators have reported similar results.[24,107,108] The definitive systematic review comparing endodontics with implant single crowns and fixed dental prostheses reported a success rate at more than 6 years of only 82% (see Table 22.1). Treatment planning in prosthodontics has changed significantly because of the recent advances in the success rate of single tooth implants.[109] Implant-supported prostheses are now broadly preferred to tooth-supported prostheses.

Intentional Replantation and Autotransplantation

Intentional replantation is the reinsertion of a tooth into its alveolus after extraction of the tooth to allow root-end surgery in the hand while the tooth is out of the socket.[110] Intentional replantation is indicated when there is no other treatment alternative to maintain a strategic tooth (see Fig. 19.10). Intentionally replanted teeth are often successful long term[111-113] but require careful case selection (see Chapter 21).

Autotransplantation is the transfer of a tooth from one alveolar socket to another in the same patient.[114-115] The clinical procedures involved include socket preparation, extraction, transplantation, and stabilization (Fig. 22.13). When autotransplantation is appropriately indicated and performed, these teeth may have a good prognosis.[116-119]

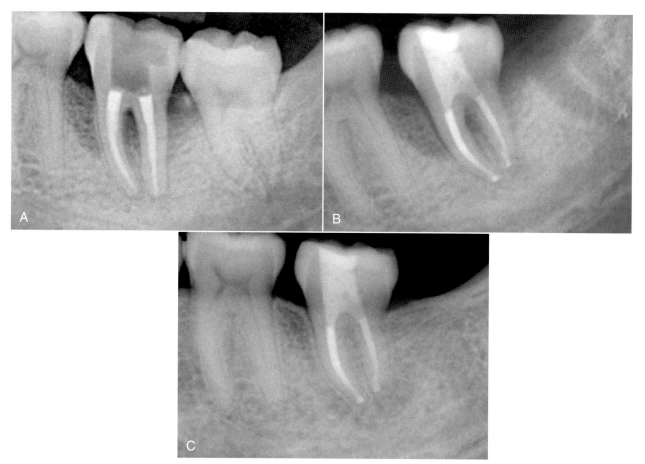

Fig. 22.13 A, A periapical radiograph shows a nonrestorable mandibular second left molar. **B,** After root canal treatment and endodontic surgery using MTA as root-end filling on the third molar on the same side, the second molar was extracted and the third molar was autotransplanted into its socket. **C,** A radiograph 46 months later shows complete healing of periradicular tissues.

Ankylosis and resorption are the most common failure modes of intentionally replanted and autotransplanted teeth.

Extraction Without Replacement

Surprisingly little information is available about the beneficial or harmful effects (and the psychosocial and economic outcomes) of extracting and not replacing individual teeth. What information there is suggests that a shortened or even an interrupted dental arch has little adverse effect. However, the loss of visible teeth without replacement has a tremendous adverse psychosocial impact.[24]

REASONS FOR EXTRACTION OF ENDODONTICALLY TREATED TEETH

Only a very small proportion of endodontically treated teeth are extracted; of these, very few are extracted for endodontic reasons.[28,37,54] Common reasons for extraction are decay, periodontal disease, nonrestorability, prosthodontic failure, and fracture.[28,37,54,120,121] Therefore, it is critical that risk factors for all of these problems be considered during comprehensive patient assessment and treatment planning.[102-104]

REFERENCES

1. Sundqvist G: *Bacteriological studies of necrotic dental pulps,* odontol dissertation no 7, Umeå, Sweden, 1976, University of Umeå.
2. Bergenholtz G: Micro-organisms from necrotic pulp of traumatized teeth, *Odontol Rev* 25:347, 1974.
3. Kantz WE, Henry CA: Isolation and classification of anaerobic bacteria from intact pulp chambers of non-vital teeth in man, *Arch Oral Biol* 19:91, 1974.
4. Hess W: The permanent dentition. I. In Hess W, Zürcher E, editors: *The anatomy of the root-canals of the teeth,* London, 1925, John Bale, Sons & Danielsson.

5. Davis SR, Brayton SM, Goldman M: The morphology of the prepared root canal: a study utilizing injectable silicone, *Oral Surg Oral Med Oral Pathol* 34:642, 1972.
6. Anderson MH: Use of evidence-based data by insurance companies, *J Evid Base Dent Pract* 4:120, 2004.
7. Lin LM, Pascon EA, Skribner J, et al: Clinical, radiographic, and histologic study of endodontic treatment failures, *Oral Surg Oral Med Oral Pathol* 71:603, 1991.
8. Reit C: Decision strategies in endodontics: on the design of a recall program, *Endod Dent Traumatol* 3:233, 1987.

9. Ørstavik D: Time-course and risk analyses of the development and healing of chronic apical periodontitis in man, *Int Endod J* 29:150, 1996.
10. Adenubi JO, Rule DC: Success rate for root fillings in young patients, *Br Dent J* 141:237, 1976.
11. Byström A, Happonen RP, Sjögren U, et al: Healing of periapical lesions of pulpless teeth after endodontic treatment with controlled asepsis, *Endod Dent Traumatol* 3:58, 1987.
12. Sjögren U, Hägglund B, Sundqvist G, et al: Factors affecting the long-term results of endodontic treatment, *J Endod* 16:498, 1990.

13. Molven O, Halse A: Success rates for gutta-percha and Kloroperka N-Ø root fillings made by undergraduate students: radiographic findings after 10-17 years, *Int Endod J* 21:243, 1988.

14. Bender IB, Seltzer S, Soltanoff W: Endodontic success: a reappraisal of criteria. Part 1, *Oral Surg Oral Med Oral Pathol* 22:780, 1966.

15. Goldman M, Pearson AH, Darzenta N: Endodontic success: who's reading the radiograph? *Oral Surg Oral Med Oral Pathol* 33:432, 1972.

16. Strindberg LL: The dependence of the results of pulp therapy on certain factors, *Acta Odontol Scand* 14:175, 1956.

17. Ørstavik D, Kerekes K, Eriksen HM: The periapical index: a scoring system for radiographic assessment of apical periodontitis, *Endod Dent Traumatol* 2:20, 1986.

18. Brynolf I: A histological and roentgenological study of the periapical region of human upper incisors, *Odontol Rev* 18(Suppl 11):1-33, 1967.

19. Liang Y, Li G, Shemesh H, et al: The association between complete absence of post-treatment periapical lesion and quality of root canal filling, *Clin Oral Investig* 16:1619, 2012.

20. Ricucci D: Apical limit of root canal instrumentation and obturation. Part 1. Literature review, *Int Endod J* 31:384, 1998.

21. Green TL, Walton RE, Taylor JK, et al: Radiographic and histologic periapical findings of root canal treated teeth in cadaver, *Oral Surg Oral Med Oral Pathol Oral Radiol Endod* 83:707, 1997.

22. Torabinejad M, Kutsenko D, Machnick TK, et al: Levels of evidence for the outcome of nonsurgical endodontic treatment, *J Endod* 31:637, 2005.

23. Friedman S, Abitbol S, Lawrence HP: Treatment outcome in endodontics: the Toronto Study—phase 1: initial treatment, *J Endod* 29:787, 2003.

24. Torabinejad M, Anderson P, Bader J, et al: The outcomes of endodontic treatment, single implant, fixed partial denture and no tooth replacement: a systematic review, *J Prosthet Dent* 98:285, 2007.

25. Iqbal MK, Kim S: For teeth requiring endodontic therapy, what are the differences in the outcomes of restored endodontically treated teeth compared to implant-supported restorations? *Int J Oral Maxillofac Implants* 221(Suppl):96, 2007.

26. Lazarski MP, Walker WA III, Flores CM, et al: Epidemiological evaluation of the outcomes of nonsurgical root canal treatment in a large cohort of insured dental patients, *J Endod* 27:791, 2001.

27. Salehrabi R, Rotstein I: Endodontic treatment outcomes in a large patient population in the USA: an epidemiological study, *J Endod* 30:846, 2004.

28. Chen S, Chueh L, Hsiao CK, et al: An epidemiologic study of tooth retention after nonsurgical endodontic treatment in a large population in Taiwan, *J Endod* 33:226, 2007.

29. Pak JG, White SN: Pain prevalence and severity before, during, and after root canal treatment: a systematic review, *J Endod* 37:429, 2011.

30. Watkins CA, Logan HL, Kirchner HL: Anticipated and experienced pain associated with endodontic therapy, *J Am Dent Assoc* 133:45, 2002.

31. Lobb WK, Zakariasen KL, McGrath PJ: Endodontic treatment outcomes: do patients perceive problems? *J Am Dent Assoc* 127:597, 1996.

32. Dugas NN, Lawrence HP, Teplitsky P, et al: Quality of life and satisfaction outcomes of endodontic treatment, *J Endod* 28:819, 2002.

33. Kim SG, Solomon C: Cost-effectiveness of endodontic molar retreatment compared with fixed partial dentures and single-tooth implant alternatives, *J Endod* 37:321, 2011.

34. Eriksen HM: Endodontology: epidemiologic considerations, *Endod Dent Traumatol* 7:189, 1991.

35. Pak JG, Fayazi S, White SN: Prevalence of periapical radiolucency and root canal treatment: a systematic review of cross-sectional studies, *J Endod* 38:1170, 2012.

36. Goodacre CJ, Bernal G, Rungcharassaeng K, et al: Clinical complications in fixed prosthodontics, *J Prosthet Dent* 90:31, 2003.

37. Doyle SL, Hodges JS, Pesun IJ, et al: Retrospective cross sectional comparison of initial nonsurgical endodontic treatment and single-tooth implants, *J Endod* 32:822, 2006.

38. Chugal NM, Clive JM, Spangberg LS: A prognostic model for assessment of the outcome of endodontic treatment: effect of biologic and diagnostic variables, *Oral Surg Oral Med Oral Pathol Oral Radiol Endod* 91:342, 2001.

39. Sjögren U, Figdor D, Persson S, et al: Influence of infection at the time of root filling on the outcome of endodontic treatment of teeth with apical periodontitis, *Int Endod J* 30:297, 1997.

40. Seltzer S, Bender IB, Turkenkopf S: Factors affecting successful repair after root canal therapy, *J Am Dent Assoc* 67:651, 1963.

41. Bergenholtz G, Lekholm U, Milthon R, et al: Influence of apical overinstrumentation and overfilling on re-treated root canals, *J Endod* 5:310, 1979.

42. Ørstavik D, Hörsted-Bindslev P: A comparison of endodontic treatment results at two dental schools, *Int Endod J* 26:348, 1993.

43. De Moor RJ, Hommez GM, De Boever JG, et al: Periapical health related to the quality of root canal treatment in a Belgian population, *Int Endod J* 33:113, 2000.

44. Chugal NM, Clive JM, Spangberg LS: Endodontic infection: some biologic and treatment factors associated with outcome, *Oral Surg Oral Med Oral Pathol Oral Radiol Endod* 96:81, 2003.

45. Katebzadeh N, Sigurdsson A, Trope M: Radiographic evaluation of periapical healing after obturation of infected root canals: an in vivo study, *Int Endod J* 33:60, 2000.

46. Katebzadeh N, Hupp J, Trope M: Histological periapical repair after obturation of infected root canals in dogs, *J Endod* 25:364, 1999.

47. Weiger R, Rosendahl R, Lost C: Influence of calcium hydroxide intracanal dressings on the prognosis of teeth with endodontically induced periapical lesions, *Int Endod J* 33:219, 2000.

48. Safavi KE, Dowden WE, Langeland K: Influence of delayed coronal permanent restoration on endodontic prognosis, *Endod Dental Traumatol* 1987:187, 1987.

49. Ray HA, Trope M: Periapical status of endodontically treated teeth in relation to the technical quality of the root filling and the coronal restoration, *Int Endod J* 28:12, 1995.

50. Chugal NM, Clive JM, Spangberg LS: Endodontic treatment outcome: effect of the permanent restoration, *Oral Surg Oral Med Oral Pathol Oral Radiol Endod* 104:576, 2007.

51. Stabholz A: Success rate in endodontics, *Alpha Omegan* 83:20, 1990.

52. Storms JL: Factors that influence the success of endodontic treatment, *J Can Dent Assoc (Tor)* 35:83, 1969.

53. Fouad AF, Burleson J: The effect of diabetes mellitus on endodontic treatment outcome: data from an electronic patient record, *J Am Dent Assoc* 134:43, 2003.

54. Wang C, Chueh L, Chen S, et al: Impact of diabetes mellitus, hypertension, and coronary artery disease on tooth extraction after nonsurgical endodontic treatment, *J Endod* 37:1, 2011.

55. Kakehashi S, Stanley HR, Fitzgerald R: The effects of surgical exposures of dental pulps in germ free and conventional laboratory rats, *Oral Surg Oral Med Oral Pathol* 20:340, 1965.

56. Grossman LI: Endodontic failures, *Dent Clin North Am* 16:59, 1972.

57. Mandel E, Machtou P, Friedman S: Scanning electron microscope observation of canal cleanliness, *J Endod* 16:279, 1990.

58. Dalton BC, Ørstavik D, Phillips C, et al: Bacterial reduction with nickel-titanium rotary instrumentation, *J Endod* 24:763, 1998.

59. Bystrom A, Sundqvist G: Bacteriologic evaluation of the effect of 0.5 percent sodium hypochlorite in endodontic therapy, *Oral Surg Oral Med Oral Pathol* 55:307, 1983.

60. Sjögren U, Figdor D, Spångberg L, et al: The antimicrobial effect of calcium hydroxide as a short-term intracanal dressing, *Int Endod J* 24:119, 1991.

61. Trope M, Maltz DO, Tronstad L: Resistance to fracture of restored endodontically treated teeth, *Endod Dent Traumatol* 1:108, 1985.

62. Salis SG, Hood JA, Stokes AN, et al: Patterns of indirect fracture in intact and restored human premolar teeth, *Endod Dent Traumatol* 3:10, 1987.

63. Hartwell GR, England MC: Healing of furcation perforations in primate teeth after repair with decalcified freeze-dried bone: a longitudinal study, *J Endod* 19:357, 1993.

64. Seltzer S, Sinai I, August D: Periodontal effects of root perforations before and during endodontic procedures, *J Dent Res* 49:332, 1970.

65. Fors UG, Berg JO: Endodontic treatment of root canals obstructed by foreign objects, *Int Endod J* 19:2, 1986.

66. Grossman LI: *Transactions: First International Conference on Endodontics*, Philadelphia, 1953, University of Pennsylvania Press.

67. Wu MK, Wesselink PR, Walton RE: Apical terminus location of root canal treatment procedures, *Oral Surg Oral Med Oral Pathol Oral Radiol Endod* 89:99, 2000.

68. Seltzer S, Soltanoff W, Sinai I, et al: Biologic aspects of endodontics. Part 3. Periapical tissue reactions to root canal instrumentation, *Oral Surg Oral Med Oral Pathol* 26:534, 1968.

69. Seltzer S: *Endodontology*, ed 2, Philadelphia, 1988, Lea & Febiger.

70. Morse DR, Wilcko JM, Pullon PA, et al: A comparative tissue toxicity evaluation of the liquid components of gutta-percha root canal sealers, *J Endod* 7:545, 1981.

71. Seltzer S: Long-term radiographic and histological observations of endodontically treated teeth, *J Endod* 25:818, 1999.

72. Pekruhn RB: The incidence of failure following single-visit endodontic therapy, *J Endod* 12:68, 1986.

73. Wu MK, De Gee AJ, Wesselink PR, et al: Fluid transport and bacterial penetration along root canal fillings, *Int Endod J* 26:203, 1993.

74. Smith CS, Setchell DJ, Harty FJ: Factors influencing the success of conventional root canal therapy: a five-year retrospective study, *Int Endod J* 26:321, 1993.

75. Swanson K, Madison S: An evaluation of coronal microleakage in endodontically treated teeth. I. Time periods, *J Endod* 13:56, 1987.

76. Magura ME, Kafrawy AH, Brown CE Jr, et al: Human saliva coronal microleakage in obturated root canals: an in vitro study, *J Endod* 17:324, 1991.

77. Khayat A, Lee SJ, Torabinejad M: Human saliva penetration of coronally unsealed obturated root canals, *J Endod* 19:458, 1993.

78. Alves J, Walton R, Drake D: Coronal leakage: endotoxin penetration from mixed bacterial communities through obturated, post-prepared root canals, *J Endod* 24:587, 1998.

79. Paik S, Sechrist C, Torabinejad M: Levels of evidence for the outcome of endodontic retreatment, *J Endod* 30:745, 2004.

80. Farzaneh M, Abitbol S, Friedman S: Treatment outcome in endodontics: the Toronto Study—phases I and II: orthograde retreatment, *J Endod* 30:627, 2004.

81. Torabinejad M, Corr R, Handysides R, et al: Outcomes of nonsurgical retreatment and endodontic surgery: a systematic review, *J Endod* 35:930, 2009.

82. Bergenholtz G, Lekholm U, Milthon R, et al: Retreatment of endodontic fillings, *Scand J Dent Res* 87:217, 1979.

83. Mead C, Javidan-Nejad S, Mego M, et al: Levels of evidence for the outcome of endodontic surgery, *J Endod* 31:19, 2005.

84. Rubinstein RA, Kim S: Long-term follow-up of cases considered healed one year after apical microsurgery, *J Endod* 28:378, 2002.

85. Maddalone M, Gagliani M: Periapical endodontic surgery: a 3-year follow-up study, *Int Endod J* 36:193, 2003.

86. Sechrist CM: The outcome of MTA as a root end filling material: a long term evaluation, Loma Linda, Calif, 2005, Loma Linda University.

87. American Academy of Periodontics: *Characteristics and trends in private periodontal practice*, Chicago, 2004, The Academy.

88. Brånemark PI, Zarb GA, Albrektsson T: *Tissue-integrated prostheses: osseointegration in clinical dentistry*, Chicago, 1985, Quintessence.

89. Schroeder A, Sutter F, Buser D, et al: *Oral implantology*, ed 2, New York, 1996, Thieme.

90. Schnitman PA, Shulman LB: Recommendations of the consensus development conference on dental implants, *J Am Dent Assoc* 98:373, 1979.

91. Cranin AN, Silverbrand H, Sher J, et al: The requirements and clinical performance of dental implants. In Smith DC, Williams DF, editors: *Biocompatibility of dental materials,* vol 4, Boca Raton, Fla, 1982, CRC Press.

92. McKinney R, Loth DL, Steflik DE: Conical standards for dental implants. In Clark JW, editor: *Clinical dentistry*, Harperstown, Md, 1984, Harper & Row.

93. Albrektsson T, Zarb GA, Worthington P, et al: The long-term efficacy of currently used dental implants: a review and proposed criteria of success, *Int J Oral Maxillofac Implants* 1:11, 1986.

94. Smith DE, Zarb GA: Criteria for success of osseointegrated endosseous implants, *J Prosthet Dent* 62:567, 1989.

95. van Steenberghe D: Outcomes and their measurement in clinical trials of endosseous oral implants, *Ann Periodontol* 2:291, 1997.

96. d'Hoedt B, Schulte W: A comparative study of results with various endosseous implant systems, *Int J Oral Maxillofac Implants* 4:95, 1989.

97. Buser D, Weber HP, Brägger U, et al: Tissue integration of one-stage ITI implants: 3-year results of a longitudinal study with hollow-cylinder and hollow-screw implants, *Int J Oral Maxillofac Implants* 6:405, 1991.

98. Spiekermann H, Jansen VK, Richter EJ: A 10-year follow-up study of IMZ and TPS implants in the edentulous mandible using bar-retained overdentures, *Int J Oral Maxillofac Implants* 10:231, 1995.

99. Roos J, Sennerby L, Lekholm U, et al: A qualitative and quantitative method for evaluating implant success: a 5-year retrospective analysis of the Bränemark implant, *Int J Oral Maxillofac Implants* 12:504, 1997.

100. Morris HF, Ochi S: Influence of two different approaches to reporting implant survival outcomes for five different prosthodontic applications, *Ann Periodontol* 5:90, 2000.

101. Andersson B, Taylor A, Lang BR, et al: Alumina ceramic implant abutments used for single-tooth replacement: a prospective 1- to 3-year multicenter study, *Int J Prosthodont* 14:432, 2001.

102. Torabinejad M, Goodacre CJ: Endodontic or dental implant therapy: the factors affecting treatment planning, *J Am Dent Assoc* 137:973, 2006.

103. White SN, Miklus VG, Potter KS, et al: Endodontics and implants: a catalog of therapeutic contrasts, *J Evid Based Dent Pract* 6:101, 2006.

104. Zitzmann NU, Krastl G, Hecker H, et al: Strategic considerations in treatment planning: deciding when to treat, extract, or replace a questionable tooth, *J Prosthet Dent* 104:80, 2010.

105. Brägger U, Aeschlimann S, Burgin W, et al: Biological and technical complications and failures with fixed partial dentures (FPD) on implants and teeth after four to five years of function, *Clin Oral Implants Res* 12:26, 2001.

106. Scurria MS, Bader JD, Shugars DA: Meta-analysis of fixed partial denture survival: prostheses and abutments, *J Prosthet Dent* 79:459, 1998.

107. Creugers NH, Kayser AF, van 't Hof MA: A meta-analysis of durability data on conventional fixed bridges, *Community Dent Oral Epidemiol* 22:448, 1994.

108. Walton TR: An up to 15-year longitudinal study of 515 metal-ceramic FPDs. Part 1. Outcome, *Int J Prosthodont* 15:439, 2002.

109. Curtis DA, Lacy A, Chu R, et al: Treatment planning in the 21st century: what's new? *J Calif Dent Assoc* 30:503, 2002.

110. American Association of Endodontists: *An annotated glossary of terms used in endodontics*, ed 6, Chicago, 1998, The Association.

111. Kingsbury BC Jr, Wiesenbaugh JM Jr: Intentional replantation of mandibular premolars and molars, *J Am Dent Assoc* 83:1053, 1971.

112. Bender IB, Rossman LE: Intentional replantation of endodontically treated teeth, *Oral Surg Oral Med Oral Pathol* 76:623, 1993.

113. Grossman LI: Intentional replantation of teeth, *J Am Dent Assoc* 72:1111, 1966.

114. Apfel H: Autoplasty of enucleated prefunctional third molars, *J Oral Surg Anesth Hosp Dent Serv* 8:289, 1950.

115. Miller HM: Transplantation; a case report, *J Am Dent Assoc* 40:237, 1950.

116. Tsukiboshi M: Autogenous tooth transplantation: a reevaluation, *Int J Periodontics Restorative Dent* 13:120, 1993.

117. Akiyama Y, Fukuda H, Hashimoto K: A clinical and radiographic study of 25 autotransplanted third molars, *J Oral Rehabil* 25:640, 1998.

118. Andreasen JO: Third molar autotransplantation relation between successful healing and stage of root development at time of grafting. Paper presented at the annual meeting of the Scandinavian Association of Oral and Maxillofacial Surgeons, August 15-19, 1990, Nyborg, Denmark.

119. Andreasen JO, Paulsen HU, Yu Z, et al: A long-term study of 370 autotransplanted premolars. II. Tooth survival and pulp healing subsequent to transplantation, *Eur J Orthod* 12:14, 1990.

120. Vire DE: Failure of endodontically treated teeth: classification and evaluation, *J Endod* 17:338, 1991.

121. Fuss Z, Lustig J, Tamse A: Prevalence of vertical root fractures in extracted endodontically treated teeth, *Int Endod J* 32:283, 1999.

23

Single implant

Mohammad A. Sabeti, Mahmoud Torabinejad

CHAPTER OUTLINE

History of Single Implants

Diagnosis and Treatment Planning for Single Implants

Tooth Extraction and Site Preparation

Single Implants in the Esthetic Zone

Single Implants in the Nonesthetic Zone

Dental Implant Maintenance Program

LEARNING OBJECTIVES

After reading this chapter, the student should be able to:

1. Relate the history of single tooth implants.
2. Enumerate the steps in the diagnosis and treatment planning for a single tooth implant.
3. Describe how to remove a tooth with minimal trauma and prepare the site for implant placement.
4. Describe the esthetic zone for single implants.
5. Explain the conditions that lend themselves to a single tooth implant without a flap.

6. Describe the steps in the surgical placement of a single tooth implant without a flap.
7. Identify the nonesthetic zones for single implants.
8. Describe hard and soft tissue considerations for placement of a single implant in nonesthetic zones.
9. Describe flap design and wound closure for a single implant in nonesthetic zones.
10. Describe the principles of maintaining single implants.

HISTORY OF SINGLE IMPLANTS

From the very beginning, humans have strived to retain their teeth (Fig. 23.1) and also to replace teeth when necessary. A pleasing smile has had enormous psychosocial importance since earliest times. Stone, metal, ivory, and sea shell implants are all cited in the archaeological records of China, Egypt, and the Americas. Success, however, was rare. In 1685, in the first modern textbook on dentistry (*The Operator for the Teeth*), Charles Allen[1] suggested that the teeth of dogs, baboons, and sheep be used for implantation. However, the possibility of disease transmission was recognized.

Transplantation was also described by Pare,[2] Fauchard,[3] and Hunter,[4] who used boiling for disinfection. Autotransplantation still has a place in clinical dentistry today. In 1807 Maggiolo developed a single-stage gold implant that was to be placed in fresh extraction sockets and allowed to heal passively without loading; however, pain and inflammation resulted.[5] At the beginning of the twentieth century, Greenfield[6] introduced latticelike, precious metal basket implants that were used to support complete dentures and single teeth. This hollow basket design continued to inspire implant designs used through the 1990s.

From the 1930s through the 1960s, new metallic alloys were used to form a variety of subperiosteal implants (Fig. 23.2) that are classified as *eposteal* (placed on or in bone) implants. Other types of implants include endosteal

blade implants (Fig. 23.3) and transmandibular, or staple, implants (Fig. 23.4). These approaches were generally directed toward supporting multiple prosthetic teeth. Most of these implants were one piece and were not fully submerged. Various one-stage endosteal root form pins, screws, and cylinder designs were also developed. In the 1930s, Strock[7] used immediate placement and a porcelain crown for single tooth replacement with a Vitallium implant. He reported a 15-year case study, noting the role of occlusion, and described the histology. Adams[8] considered a two-stage surgical procedure for placing a cylindrical screw implant with a healing cap.

In the late 1940s Formiggini[9] introduced a helicoidal screw tantalum implant. This design was modified by Chercheve in the 1960s to increase the distance between the screw threads and implant head (Fig. 23.5).[10] Some of these endosteal designs began to resemble contemporary solid, cylindrical, moderately tapered, and threaded osseointegrated implants (Fig. 23.6). Although the Dental Implants: Benefit and Risk Consensus Development and Technology Conference, held in 1978 at the Harvard School of Dental Medicine, set new standards for reporting implant data, an enthusiastic Brånemark began to publish a series of experimental studies on the use of intraosseous anchorage of dental prostheses in the late 1960s, leading to a landmark 10-year study in 1977.[11,12] His two-stage threaded titanium screw-type root form implant (Nobelpharma, now Nobel Biocare) was first presented in

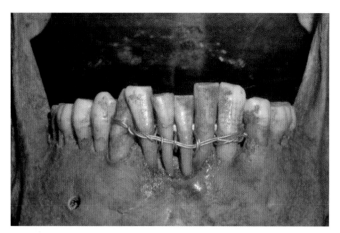

Fig. 23.1 Frontal view of a mandible from about 500 BC discovered in Lebanon at the ancient site of Sidon. The periodontally involved anterior teeth have been splinted together with gold wire. (Courtesy the Archaeological Museum, American University, Beirut, Lebanon.)

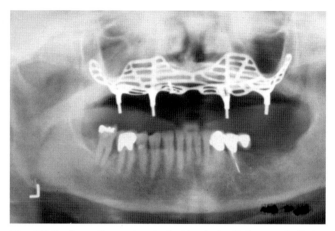

Fig. 23.2 A maxillary subperiosteal implant with four posts that will be used to support and retain a prosthesis. (Courtesy R. James.)

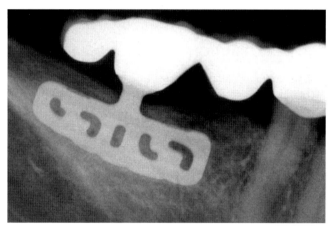

Fig. 23.3 Periapical radiograph of a blade implant that is supporting the distal aspect of a mandibular fixed partial denture.

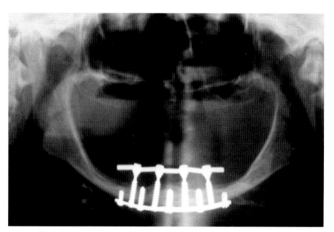

Fig. 23.4 Panoramic radiograph of a one-piece transosseous implant consisting of a metal plate located on the inferior border of the mandible, five posts that are placed into the mandible, and four posts that pass through the mandible. A bar attached to the four posts provides retention and stability for a mandibular implant overdenture.

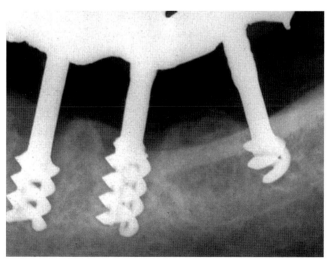

Fig. 23.5 Radiograph of implants placed by Dr. Rafael Chercheve. (Courtesy R. James.)

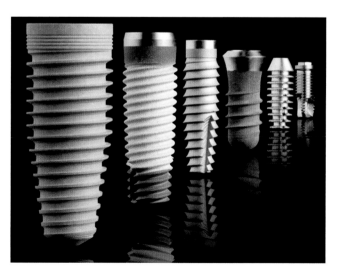

Fig. 23.6 A variety of endosseous root form implants have been aligned so that the different designs, thread patterns, and surfaces can be compared. The original Brånemark external hex implant can be seen at the end of the row.

North America in 1982 (Fig. 23.6) at the Toronto Implant Conference organized by Dr. George Zarb.[13]

Osseointegrated endosseous implants had been first used in the treatment of fully edentulous jaws more than four decades earlier. Brånemark's original protocol for dental implant placement in the anterior parts of edentulous jaws included a mucobuccal flap; a two-stage surgical approach, followed by 3 to 6 months of stress-free healing to allow for osseointegration; and restoration with complete implant-supported prostheses. By 1985 Zarb, Jansson, and Jemt were already investigating the longitudinal application of osseointegrated implants in the areas of overdenture application, treatment of partially edentulous patients, and single tooth implants.[14] Many innovations facilitated achievement of the current, predictable, widespread use of single tooth implants; however, future challenges may arise from the rapid launching of untested novelties or procedures.[15] The 1988 Consensus Development Conference on Dental Implants, held at the National Institutes of Health, added several more suggestions.

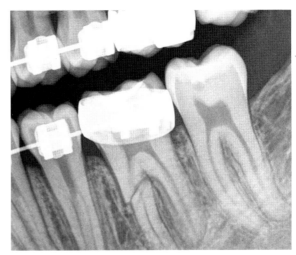

Fig. 23.7 Radiograph of a left mandibular first molar (#19) that was diagnosed with a root fracture and referred for extraction.

DIAGNOSIS AND TREATMENT PLANNING FOR SINGLE IMPLANTS

Even though there have been numerous advances in the field of dentistry, many teeth still develop decay and/or periodontal disease or are removed due to traumatic injuries. Traditional treatment options called for the restoration of diseased teeth with root canal or periodontal treatments and/or fixed or removable prostheses. When there is doubt that the teeth can be restored or treated, both practitioners and patients frequently ask whether the tooth should be saved by performing a root canal and periodontal treatment or whether extraction with replacement with an implant is the better choice.

Appropriate diagnosis of the patient's condition allows the dentist to create a suitable treatment plan that can be properly executed. All treatment planning must have a proven scientific basis to provide a successful result. Without anticipating potential failure, any immediate success is limited. A complete and accurate diagnosis must be performed systematically. This evaluation should include obtaining the patient's chief complaint, comprehensive pretreatment evaluation of the patient, a thorough radiographic examination, necessary tests, and a thorough review of the patient's dental and health history to identify any conditions that may interfere with implant therapy. The review should include cardiovascular health; any history of diabetes, osteopenia, or osteoporosis; anticoagulation therapy; and any history of smoking. A thorough examination of the patient's oral cavity also should be performed to identify areas of disease or tooth malposition that may affect the overall success of the final implant prosthesis. The evaluation should include decayed and missing teeth and the relationship of the opposing dentition and related interdental spacing. A thorough radiographic examination also is necessary for proper implant placement.

Diagnosis is important and has to be based on careful systematic examination and analysis of the data. Once the diagnosis has been made, proper treatment procedures usually can be carried out (Fig. 23.7). The patient's expectations and desires can often complicate the treatment planning. An ideal treatment plan tackles the patient's chief complaint, effectively meets the patient's expectations, addresses the biologic environment and scientific evidence, and restores or maintains the function and esthetic.

TOOTH EXTRACTION AND SITE PREPARATION

Dental implants are the preferred treatment for the replacement of missing teeth. Implant placement is a very predictable treatment for replacing lost or missing teeth, and long-term survival rates of 85% to 100% have been reported.[16] Today, osseointegration is not the only important goal of the treatment. Establishing a balance between the implant restoration and the surrounding soft tissues is also of great importance (Fig. 23.8). This is especially true in the esthetic zone. Tooth removal is often accompanied by varying degrees of loss of alveolar bone and soft tissue alterations that create a challenging situation for restoring soft tissue esthetics, ideal implant placement, and tissue management (Fig. 23.9). The loss of a tooth results in an immediate loss or fracture of alveolar bone, interproximal bone, and the papilla and may result in the recession of the marginal gingiva, formation of interproximal "black triangles" (Fig. 23.10), or a bulky restoration. Morphologic changes in the alveolar bone and soft tissue have been reported after extraction. An average loss of 2 mm of bone width may occur after loss of a tooth. Incomplete bone fill of a socket and reduction of alveolar bone height also have been reported.[17-19] If the situation is not corrected, this loss tends to impede ideal positioning of a dental implant replacement. Fortunately, this deficiency can be successfully overcome through the use of barrier membranes.

Minimally Traumatic Extraction

The tooth should be removed with a periotome instead of the conventional elevator that is associated with hard and soft tissue trauma. A periotome is typically used for extraction of a tooth in the esthetic area to prevent excess trauma to the interproximal papilla and marginal gingiva. A periotome has a thin, flat blade that conveniently facilitates tooth removal by severing the gingival attachment and luxating the tooth in the gingival sulcus. A periotome should be inserted into the periodontal ligament space along the root surfaces with the

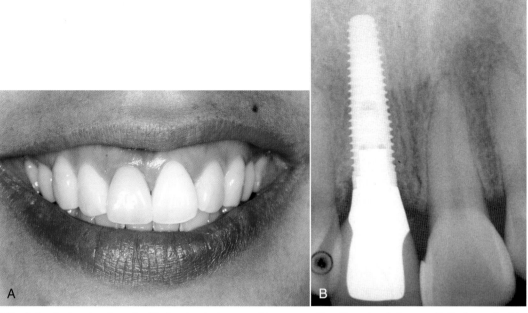

Fig. 23.8   **A,** Implant restoration site #8 showing balance and harmony with adjacent soft tissues. **B,** Radiograph of implant site #8 depicting excellent bone condition. (From Torabinejad M, Sabeti MA, Goodacre CJ: *Principles and practice of single implant and restoration,* St Louis, 2014, Saunders.)

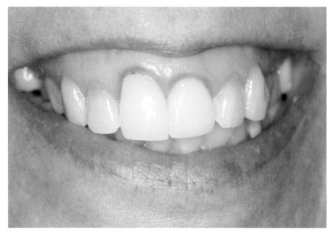

Fig. 23.9   Marginal recession around implant restoration site #8. (From Torabinejad M, Sabeti MA, Goodacre CJ: *Principles and practice of single implant and restoration,* St Louis, 2014, Saunders.)

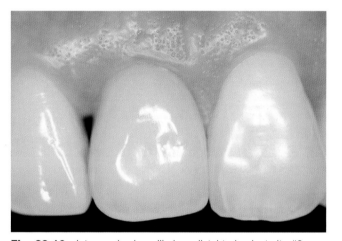

Fig. 23.10   Interproximal papilla loss distal to implant site #8. (From Torabinejad M, Sabeti MA, Goodacre CJ: *Principles and practice of single implant and restoration,* St Louis, 2014, Saunders.)

continued exertion of apical pressure. This pressure should be continued with or without using a surgical mallet until the periotome penetrates to a sufficient depth in the gingival sulcus to initiate tooth mobility (Fig. 23.11). A periotome is frequently used in the interproximal and palatal aspect of a tooth to prevent damage to the buccal plate in order to maintain integrity of the buccal wall and gingival margin.

Single Tooth Implant

During the clinical examination for implant placement, the dental practitioner may encounter horizontal, vertical, and intraalveolar bone defects (Fig. 23.12). These are common and therapeutically important. Proper diagnosis of the patient's condition allows the dental practitioner to devise a suitable treatment plan that can be predictably executed. The practitioner can choose either to perform guided bone regeneration (GBR) simultaneously with implant placement or to use a staged approach.

Single implants can replace any tooth in the dental arch. For purposes of single implant placement, the various areas of the oral cavity are broadly classified as comprising the esthetic zone (i.e., the central, lateral, canine, and first premolar areas in the maxilla) and the nonesthetic zone (i.e., the posterior maxilla, posterior mandible, and anterior mandible). This allows the characteristics of each area to be explained separately.

415

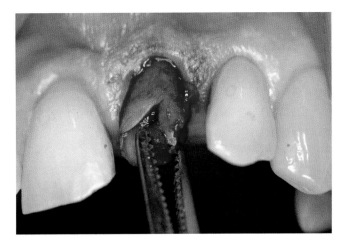

Fig. 23.11 Periotome penetration into the periodontal ligament (PDL) space initiates tooth mobility. (From Torabinejad M, Sabeti MA, Goodacre CJ: *Principles and practice of single implant and restoration,* St Louis, 2014, Saunders.)

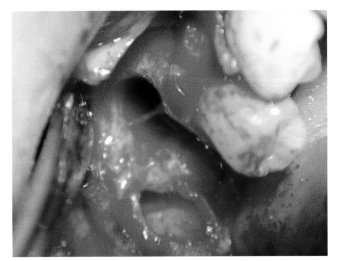

Fig. 23.12 Preoperative view of an alveolar ridge in which the hard and soft tissues available are inadequate for an implant procedure. (From Torabinejad M, Sabeti MA, Goodacre CJ: *Principles and practice of single implant and restoration,* St Louis, 2014, Saunders.)

SINGLE IMPLANTS IN THE ESTHETIC ZONE

As mentioned, the esthetic zone in the oral cavity consists of the central, lateral, canine, and first premolar areas in the maxilla. These areas are very important because of their role in the esthetic appearance of the patient. A large number of articles have been published on the subject from surgical and prosthetic viewpoints. The principles of implant surgery and osseous and soft tissue considerations in these areas are different from those in other areas of the oral cavity.

After necessary analysis of the region to undergo implant surgery, taking into account osseous and soft tissue considerations, the patient is ready for implant surgery. As described previously, the esthetic zone consists of the central, lateral, canine, and first premolar areas of the maxilla. The remaining mandibular and maxillary areas are not included in the esthetic zone. Before performing implant surgery, the dental surgeon must consider three important questions:

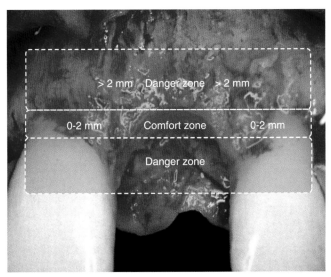

Fig. 23.13 Outline of comfort and danger zones in the vertical dimension. (From Torabinejad M, Sabeti MA, Goodacre CJ: *Principles and practice of single implant and restoration,* St Louis, 2014, Saunders.)

1. Will the implant surgery be immediate?
2. If the tooth has already been extracted, how long has it been since the extraction?
3. Are any bony defects present in the area? If so, is the defect vertical, horizontal, or both?

Immediate Implant Surgery without Any Flaps

If the tooth in question should be extracted because of endodontic problems or root fractures, immediate implant surgery can be carried out without any flaps if the following clinical characteristics are noted:

- Single-rooted tooth
- Healthy systemic condition
- Nonsmoking patient
- Low lip line
- Thick gingival biotype
- Intact and thick facial bones
- No acute infection
- Good vertical level at adjacent teeth

Surgical Technique

The tooth is removed with a periotome, and the buccal wall is inspected to make sure it is intact. Osteotomy then is carried out on the palatal wall of the socket to prepare the implant site. During the drilling procedure, care should be exercised to ensure that the implant is appropriately placed in its three-dimensional path. A proper implant site in the esthetic zone has the following characteristics:

- The implant platform is 3 to 4 mm apical to the cementoenamel junction (CEJ) of the two adjacent teeth (Fig. 23.13).
- The implant platform is 1 to 2 mm palatal to the profile of the two adjacent teeth (Fig. 23.14).
- The implant platform is placed in the bone so that it is 1.5 mm from the adjacent teeth (Fig. 23.15).

After the implant has been properly placed, the empty space between the implant and the buccal bone should be filled with

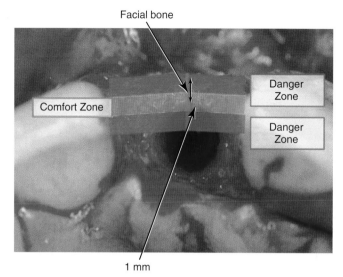

Facial bone

Comfort Zone

Danger Zone

Danger Zone

1 mm

Fig. 23.14 Outline of the comfort zone in the horizontal dimension. The comfort zone is the correct area for positioning of the implant platform in the horizontal dimension; the danger zone is the incorrect area for positioning of the implant platform.

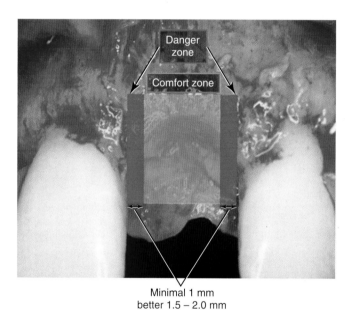

Danger zone

Comfort zone

Minimal 1 mm
better 1.5 – 2.0 mm

Fig. 23.15 Outline of the comfort zone in the mesiodistal dimension. The comfort zone is the correct area for positioning of the implant platform in the mesiodistal dimension; the danger zone is the incorrect area for positioning of the implant platform. (From Torabinejad M, Sabeti MA, Goodacre CJ: *Principles and practice of single implant and restoration,* St Louis, 2014, Saunders.)

autogenous bone[20] or other bone-filling materials to support the buccal osseous plate; this minimizes secondary resorption of the buccal bone. At this stage, if the insertion torque value is at least 35 N, the implant can be placed and a provisional prosthesis can be manufactured to support and preserve the soft tissue position in the area. Otherwise, the implant should be submerged, the second surgical procedure should be performed, and the prosthesis should be manufactured at the proper time (Fig. 23.16).

If the conditions that warrant surgery without flaps are not present, a flap surgical procedure should be performed. A mucoperiosteal flap is elevated so that the tooth can be removed less aggressively. The implant then is properly placed by observing the three-dimensional implant path. If the buccal bone requires reconstruction and reinforcement through the GBR technique, the necessary procedures are carried out with proper attention to all relevant surgical principles. The implant is submerged for 3 to 4 months to better preserve the graft, the second surgical procedure is carried out, and the prosthesis is manufactured (Fig. 23.17).

SINGLE IMPLANTS IN THE NONESTHETIC ZONE

The nonesthetic zone of the oral cavity consists of the remaining areas of the two arches, which are classified as the posterior maxilla, posterior mandible, and anterior mandible. Each of these regions has specific characteristics and anatomic features that should be taken into account during the surgical procedure. For example, the maxillary sinuses in the posterior maxilla and the inferior alveolar nerve in the posterior mandibular are two important anatomic structures in the nonesthetic zone. If they are ignored during surgery, irreparable injury to the patient may result. In addition, the spaces between the incisors in the mandible are very small, and the possibility of damaging the adjacent teeth is an important consideration during surgery for single implants. In the following sections, these problems are discussed further, and the surgical techniques for each area are explained.

Osseous Consideration

The fact that the process of bone resorption slows down after tooth extraction has been well established. The amount of bone resorbed during the first year after tooth extraction is much greater than that during the following years.[21] A complex osseous situation exists when bone volume is diminished and the quality of bone is not uniform in different regions of the jaw. These two important factors, the quality and quantity of bone, play an important role in determining implant location and position.

In 1985, Zarb and Lekholm created classification systems for the quality and quantity of jaw bones. They classified bone quality as type I to type IV and bone quantity as type A to type E (Fig. 23.18). From a qualitative viewpoint, type II and type III bones are the most appropriate for implant placement. Type I and type IV bones might pose problems in osseointegration and regenerative processes. From a quantitative viewpoint, type A and type B bones are ideal; however, more problems are encountered with an increase in bone resorption.

First, bone height is determined through radiographic evaluation of eligible jaw areas. Panoramic radiography is the method most commonly used to evaluate bone height. Bone height is measured from the crest of the edentulous ridge to anatomic landmarks. The maxillary sinus and mandibular canal restrict bone height. In general, the prognosis for the implant improves as the implant's length increases. However, implant lengths exceeding 13 to 14 mm currently are not recommended. Implants less than 8 mm in length belong to the short implant category; the prognosis for these implants **417**

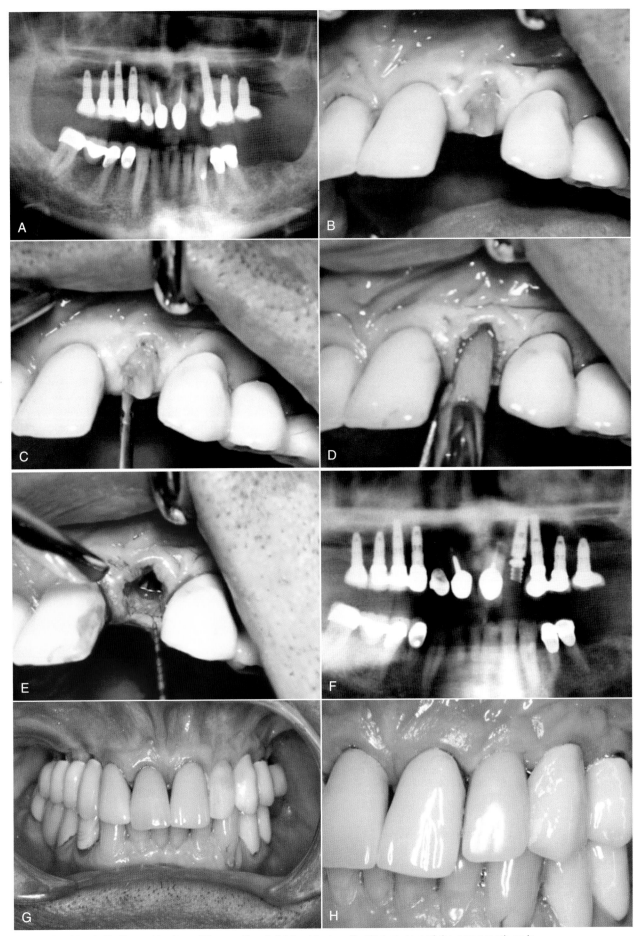

Fig. 23.16 **A,** Radiographic view of the maxillary left lateral incisor. **B,** Clinical view of the same tooth as in **A. C** to **E,** Traumatic extraction of the tooth using a periotome. **F,** Radiographic view of implant placement in correct three-dimensional position. **G** and **H,** Immediate provisional prosthesis. (From Torabinejad M, Sabeti MA, Goodacre CJ: *Principles and practice of single implant and restoration,* St Louis, 2014, Saunders.)

is less favorable than that for long implants. Therefore, if bone height is 8 to 14 mm and no impingement is made on anatomic structures, the condition is ideal for implant placement. It should be noted that a distance of at least 2 mm should exist between the apex of the implant and the roof of the mandibular canal. However, contact of the apex of the implant with the floor of the maxillary sinus or its perforation does not cause problems if the mucous membrane of the sinus is not ruptured.

Another important factor, which is crucial to the longevity of the implant, is bone width. Implants with a diameter of 4 mm require a minimum of 6 mm of bone width; with a bone width of 7 mm, the long-term prognosis is much better. If thick implants with a diameter of 5 mm are to be used, a bone diameter of 7 to 8 mm is required. If the remaining bone in the buccal aspect of the implant is less than 1 mm, the area should be reinforced with the GBR technique. This is more important in the anterior areas of the maxilla, because a thin buccal bone in this area leads to resorption of bone and subsequent gingival recession and exposure of the metallic margin of the implant, compromising the patient's esthetic appearance. To prevent such problems, all surgeries for single implants in the anterior area of the maxilla should be augmented with bone.

Soft Tissue Consideration

Similar to bone, which is an important determining factor for the long-term maintenance and success of an implant, keratinized soft tissue around the implant can play an important role in the longevity of the implant and in prevention of peri-implantitis. Considerable research has been dedicated to this issue. Some studies have shown that implants are durable even without keratinized gingiva, and no problems are encountered. Other studies have emphasized that attached keratinized gingiva is favorable and in fact necessary for implants.[22] Therefore, to prevent subsequent problems, the logical course is to provide an environment for implant placement in which sufficient keratinized gingiva is present. This environment can be provided during implant placement or subsequent to it. Advantages are associated with keratinized gingiva around implants (Box 23.1). During treatment planning for placement of implants, the presence of attached keratinized gingiva, which is very important, should be taken into account. This gingiva should be reconstructed during implant placement or after it if no keratinized gingiva is present. It has been empirically shown that at least 2 mm of attached keratinized gingiva around an implant is sufficient, and the prognosis improves with an increase of more than 2 mm. However, some authors think that the need for keratinized gingiva is patient specific.[23]

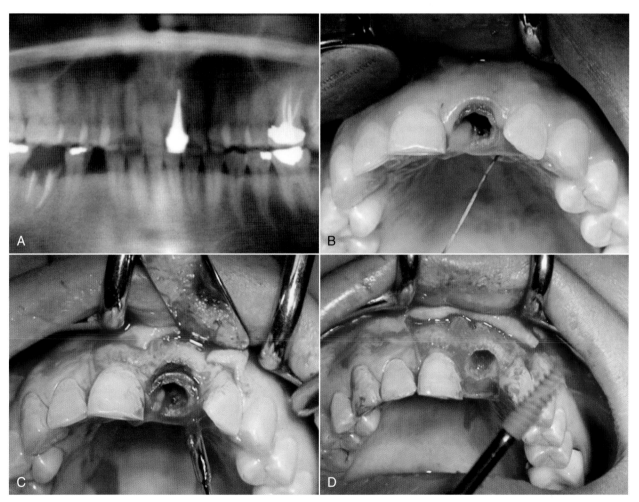

Fig. 23.17 **A,** Radiographic view of the maxillary left central incisor. **B,** Clinical view of the same tooth as in **A. C,** After creation of a mucoperiosteal flap. **D,** After extraction and site preparation.

Continued

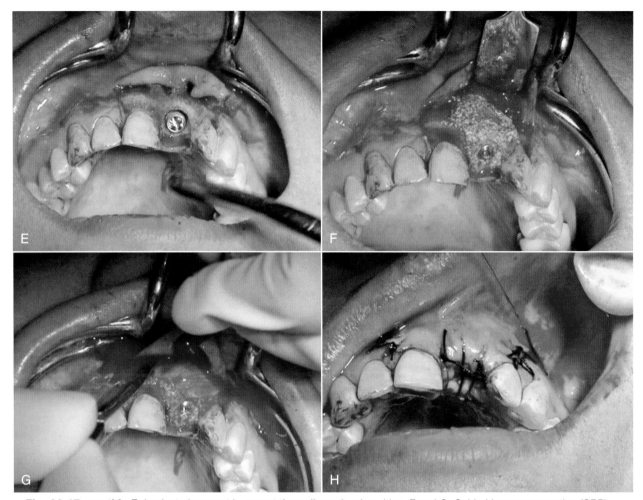

Fig. 23.17, cont'd **E,** Implant placement in correct three-dimensional position. **F** and **G,** Guided bone regeneration (GBR) technique with particulate bone graft and collagen membrane. **H,** Suturing and implant submerged. (From Torabinejad M, Sabeti MA, Goodacre CJ: *Principles and practice of single implant and restoration,* St Louis, 2014, Saunders.)

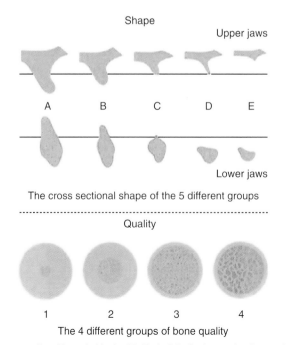

Shape

Upper jaws

A   B   C   D   E

Lower jaws

The cross sectional shape of the 5 different groups

Quality

1   2   3   4

The 4 different groups of bone quality

Fig. 23.18 The four types of bone quality. (From Lekholm U, Zarb GA: Patient selection and preparation. In Brånemark PI, Zarb GA, Albrektsson T, editors: *Tissue integrated prostheses: osseointegration in clinical dentistry,* Chicago, 1985, Quintessence.)

Therefore, during treatment planning, the amount of attached keratinized gingiva can be measured. If insufficient keratinized gingiva is present, measures can be taken to provide it. If sufficient keratinized gingiva is present, plans should be made so that this gingiva is located in its proper place around the implant. The techniques commonly used to provide attached keratinized gingiva around implants are the apically positioned flap, the free gingival graft, and the free connective tissue graft.

Guided Bone Regeneration for Implant Site Development

If adequate ridge width or height is not available at the onset of implant therapy, these often can be augmented at the time of implant placement. This procedure may involve grafting of excessive socket space after extraction with immediate implant insertion or more extensive augmentation of a horizontal or vertical ridge deficiency encountered at implant placement. Using the principles of GBR, a variety of methods can be used to repair these defects. For successful augmentation, a three-dimensional space must be maintained long enough for the regeneration process to take place and the final matrix to mineralize. This space can be created with a nonrigid or rigid

mesh or membrane material and a particulate bone graft. When a tooth is extracted and an implant is immediately placed in the resulting defect, a discrepancy often exists between the implant's surface and the surrounding bony housing. Augmentation may be used to establish an adequate thickness of facial bone to prevent future loss and compromise of implant esthetics.[24] This may be accomplished through placement of a graft in the socket housing or on the overlying facial bony plate immediately before implant insertion (Fig. 23.19). As an alternative, the graft material can be placed after fixture placement, although instrumentation and graft placement at the apex of the defect often are more difficult with this sequence.

Once the fixture and graft have been placed in the desired locations, particle containment and cellular exclusion can be performed with a resorbable or nonresorbable membranous material. If augmentation of the attached gingiva is desired, an autogenous or allogenic connective tissue graft is ideal for both functions. This not only provides adequate graft containment, but also serves as scaffolding for regeneration of the surrounding soft tissues. These materials also offer the benefit of not requiring primary closure of the wound site, thus requiring less tissue release for flap advancement (Fig. 23.20). If primary closure is not obtainable and soft tissue augmentation is not required or desired, a nonresorbable polytetrafluoroethylene (PTFE, or Teflon) membrane may be used (Fig. 23.21). This material may be left exposed during healing, but it provides insignificant enhancement of the soft tissues.[25]

If adequate attached gingiva is present at the time of placement and primary closure can be obtained at the site, a resorbable collagen membrane material may be used before closure. Often at the time of initial placement, inadequate bone is present adjacent to the implant. In such cases, lateral or vertical augmentation can be performed simultaneously, providing the implant has adequate initial stability in the proposed site. To offset the compressing pressures from the overlying flap and tissues, a rigid device must be used to provide three-dimensional space maintenance while the graft is maturing.

> ### Box 23.1 Advantages of Keratinized Gingiva Around Implants
>
> Some advantages of keratinized gingiva around implants are:
> 1. Keratinized gingiva stabilizes the crestal bone around the implant.
> 2. The patient can control plaque more easily.
> 3. The possibility of gingival recession and compromise of esthetic criteria decreases.
> 4. The dental practitioner can easily take impressions.
> 5. With an increase in gingival thickness, metallic surfaces are less likely to be visible.

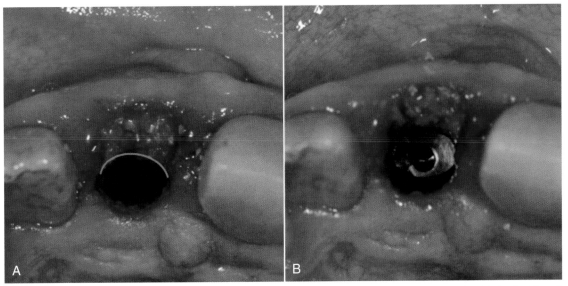

Fig. 23.19 **A,** Particulate graft placement in a fresh extraction site immediately before implant insertion. **B,** Implant insertion after graft placement. (From Torabinejad M, Sabeti MA, Goodacre CJ: *Principles and practice of single implant and restoration,* St Louis, 2014, Saunders.)

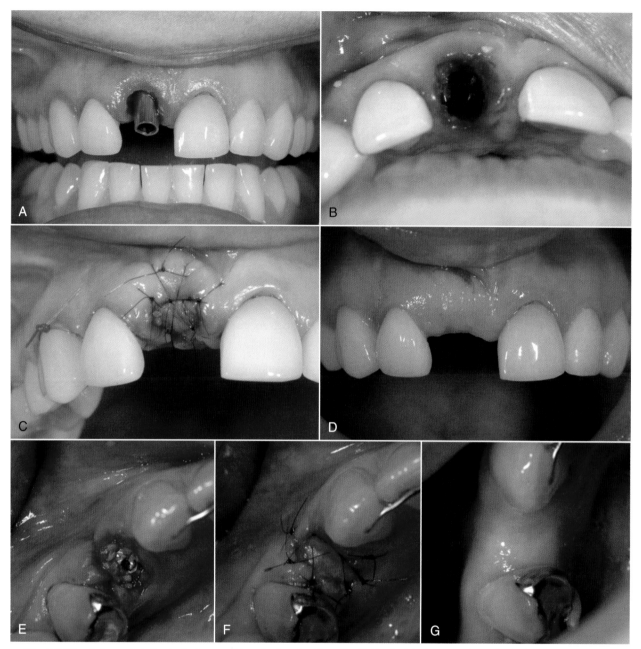

Fig. 23.20 **A,** Immediate implant placement in a fresh extraction site. **B,** Particulate bone graft on the facial surface of the implant. **C,** Autogenous connective tissue graft covers the surgical site and augments the soft tissue contours. **D,** Postoperative result, showing abundant soft tissue. **E,** Immediate implant placement in a fresh extraction site with particulate bone graft on the facial surface. **F,** Acellular dermal matrix graft covers the surgical site and augments the soft tissue contours. **G,** Postoperative result, showing abundant soft tissue. (From Torabinejad M, Sabeti MA, Goodacre CJ: *Principles and practice of single implant and restoration,* St Louis, 2014, Saunders.)

Traditionally, the primary rigid mesh material used for space maintenance in GBR has been made from titanium. The advantages of this material are proven biocompatibility, ease of contouring and stabilization at the surgical site, and maintenance of rigidity under reasonable load (Fig. 23.22). Although titanium mesh provides acceptable graft containment and stabilization, surgical reentry is always required to remove it. Oftentimes removal of the mesh can be a lengthy procedure because soft tissue can invade the latticework of the mesh, creating difficulty.

More recently, rigid, resorbable membranes have been used in GBR, eliminating the need for reentry removal surgery. Membranes made from thermoplastic D- and L-polymers of lactic acid have been successfully used to create three-dimensional shapes for placement of particulate bone graft material in the same method in which traditional titanium mesh has been used. Rather than with fixation screws or tacks that require removal, the membrane is fixed with a resorbable pin made from the same polymer, allowing for eventual resorption through hydrolysis (Fig. 23.23). This resorbable

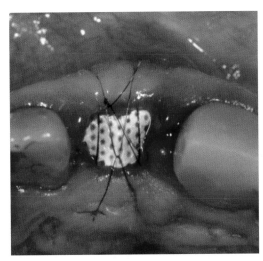

Fig. 23.21 A nonresorbable polytetrafluoroethylene (PTFE, or Teflon) membrane can be used to cover the surgical site when soft tissue augmentation is not required. (From Torabinejad M, Sabeti MA, Goodacre CJ: *Principles and practice of single implant and restoration,* St Louis, 2014, Saunders.)

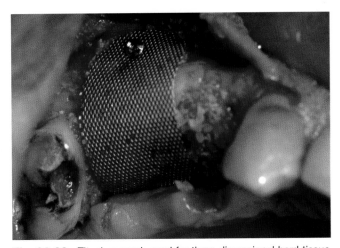

Fig. 23.22 Titanium mesh used for three-dimensional hard tissue augmentation. (From Torabinejad M, Sabeti MA, Goodacre CJ: *Principles and practice of single implant and restoration,* St Louis, 2014, Saunders.)

system uses an ultrasonic vibrating handpiece to create frictional heat that fixes the polymer pin into the host bone. Once the pin has been fixated, the polymer membrane is welded to the pinhead using the same sonic principle. Studies have shown that this frictional heat creates only a minimal elevation in temperature for short periods when the two hard surfaces are in contact.[26]

The introduction of rigid resorbable membranes has allowed for predictable hard tissue implant site development under a variety of circumstances, without the need for subsequent reentry into a surgical site to retrieve fixation screws, pins, or meshes. Although these materials offer the opportunity to avoid a second surgical entry for removal, as with any regenerative technique, adequate site access must be obtained for uncompromised initial graft placement. Surgical flap management is important not only to create uncompromised access

to the surgical site, but also to ensure proper closure at the completion of the procedure.

Flap Design

When surgical implant placement requires access through the oral soft tissues to the underlying alveolar bone, proper access design is important not only at the time of surgery, but also to minimize postoperative complications related to dehiscence or flap retraction. Typically, midcrestal or slightly palatal placement of the incision is appropriate for osteotomy preparation. Before this incision is made, however, the quality and quantity of the attached gingiva should be determined. When the incision is made in attached gingiva, the improved tissue density helps minimize marginal trauma during initial flap reflection. This improved density also facilitates suture placement and reduces the incidence of tearing upon completion of the procedure (see Fig. 23.24; also Fig. 23.25).

The initial incision should extend through the full thickness of the gingiva and periosteum to the underlying bony crest. This allows for a clean initial reflection of the mucoperiosteal flap in the surgical site. Failure to incise both layers carefully results in more difficulty with the initial reflection and leads to a higher incidence of tearing and trauma of the flap margin. This damage ultimately complicates the final wound closure because the blood supply to this critical area may be compromised, resulting in poor tissue stability postoperatively. If papillary reflection is required, the papilla should be split evenly to maintain as much thickness as possible in the reflection. By maintaining the integrity of the papilla in the reflection, compromise is reduced and postoperative vitality is enhanced (see Figs. 23.21 and 23.24).

Once the initial full-thickness reflection is complete, the practitioner may choose to incise the periosteum, thus creating a more mobile supraperiosteal reflection.[27] If access to the buccal surface for hard tissue regeneration is required, this periosteal release must be carried out more apically to allow access to the site. If hard tissue augmentation is not required or if a ridge-splitting procedure is to be carried out, the periosteal release should be performed more coronally in the reflection so as to maintain the periosteal blood supply to the cortical plate and limit postoperative remodeling. In keeping with traditional surgical principles, broad-based flaps should be created to minimize compromise of the blood supply to the reflected soft tissues. Microsurgical instruments can be used to gain minimized access through the creation of a reduced incision and minimal flap reflection. In this way, vertical incisions can be reduced or eliminated, as can the associated risk of postoperative dehiscence

Wound Closure

Once the surgical procedure is complete, passive wound closure is imperative for success. Because the periosteum provides for only a limited amount of mobility, periosteal release often is required for proper wound closure. After this release, tissue repositioning can be performed with greater ease. After positioning, the soft tissues should be carefully reapproximated at the desired locations with atraumatic suturing. For procedures that require short-term reapproximation, a resorbable or slowly resorbing material can be used (e.g., chromic gut). For procedures that require longer-term wound support, a nonresorbable material (e.g., polypropylene or PTFE) may be used and then removed at the practitioner's

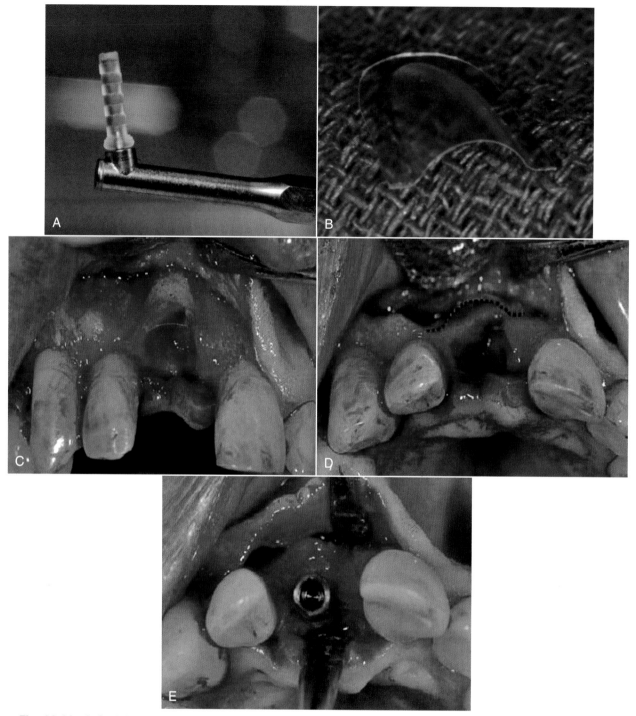

Fig. 23.23 **A,** SonicWeld Rx resorbable fixation pin. **B,** SonicWeld RX resorbable rigid membrane. **C,** The resorbable rigid membrane is used for buccal hard tissue ridge augmentation. **D,** Occlusal view showing space creation with the rigid membrane. **E,** Implant placed with buccal ridge augmentation. (From Torabinejad M, Sabeti MA, Goodacre CJ: *Principles and practice of single implant and restoration,* St Louis, 2014, Saunders.)

discretion. Adequate flap release should have been performed before closure; therefore, sutures should be able to be placed without creating tension on the flap margins.

DENTAL IMPLANT MAINTENANCE PROGRAM

Many principles and features of maintenance therapy apply to both the natural dentition and to dental implants. In patients who are partially edentulous with implant-supported restorations, maintenance visits combine traditional periodontal maintenance for the remaining natural teeth and dental implant maintenance. In fully edentulous patients with implant-supported restorations, the focus is on prevention or treatment of peri-implant mucositis or peri-implantitis because dental caries and endodontic pathologic conditions are not possible. Data collection includes measurement of probing depths, bleeding upon probing, suppuration, recession,

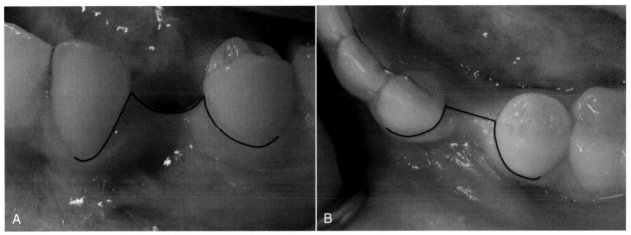

Fig. 23.24 **A,** Outline of an envelope flap design to minimize vertical releasing incisions and maximize available attached gingiva on the ridge crest. **B,** Outline of an alternate envelope flap design to minimize vertical releasing incisions and maximize available attached gingiva on the ridge crest. (From Torabinejad M, Sabeti MA, Goodacre CJ: *Principles and practice of single implant and restoration,* St Louis, 2014, Saunders.)

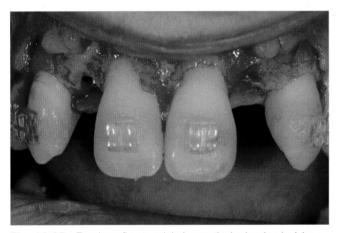

Fig. 23.25 Envelope flap to minimize vertical releasing incisions. (From Torabinejad M, Sabeti MA, Goodacre CJ: *Principles and practice of single implant and restoration,* St Louis, 2014, Saunders.)

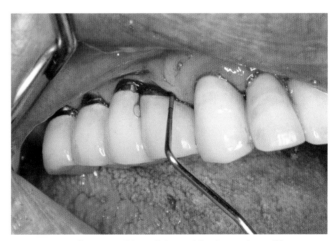

Fig. 23.26 Gentle probing of the peri-implant sulcus. (From Torabinejad M, Sabeti MA, Goodacre CJ: *Principles and practice of single implant and restoration,* St Louis, 2014, Saunders.)

mobility, response to percussion, and clinical appearance of peri-implant mucosa. Probing should be done with a very gentle force (not to exceed 0.15 N) because excessive force may disrupt the soft tissue attachment and has been shown to overestimate probing depths and the incidence of bleeding upon probing.[28,29] As with natural teeth, inflammation of peri-implant soft tissue results in greater apical penetration of the periodontal probe.[30] Hence, gentle probing has been shown to be an effective means to evaluate the stability of the peri-implant attachment and to detect peri-implantitis (Fig. 23.26).

Follow-up periapical radiographs are generally taken 1 year after loading; thereafter the frequency of radiographic evaluation is determined by the clinical findings.[31] Care should be taken to orient the film or digital sensor parallel to the long axis of the implant fixture; this can require special attention when an angled abutment has been used for the restoration. In general, any pain, edema, or suppuration indicates the need for radiographic evaluation; otherwise, routine radiographs

may be indicated only every few years. After examination and data collection, peri-implant conditions are documented. Instrumentation then is performed to reduce or eliminate bacterial plaque and calcified deposits.

Standard metal scalers and curettes are not recommended for implant debridement because of the risk of scratching the titanium surface. Although plastic scalers are available, their effectiveness in removing hard deposits is limited; gold, titanium, or vitreous carbon–tipped instruments are generally more effective. Ultrasonic and piezoelectric scalers with plastic or carbon tips have also proven effective and do not damage the implants' surfaces (see Fig. 23.26).[32-34] Air polishing devices and rotary rubber cups can be used to remove plaque and smooth implant collars.[35] Biofilm disruption in the peri-implant sulcus can be accomplished with air polishing devices using either sodium bicarbonate or amino acid glycine salt powders.[36] In addition to mechanical debridement with scalers and polishing devices, **425**

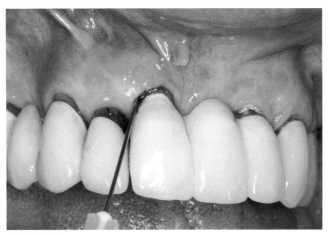

Fig. 23.27 Irrigation of the peri-implant sulcus with 10% povidone-iodine. (From Torabinejad M, Sabeti MA, Goodacre CJ: *Principles and practice of single implant and restoration*, St Louis, 2014, Saunders.)

adjunctive local antimicrobial therapy can be administered, although limited and often equivocal evidence of enhanced clinical outcomes has been published.[37-42] The peri-implant sulcus can be irrigated with antiseptic 10% povidone-iodine (Fig. 23.27).

Frequency of Maintenance Appointments

Periodic maintenance therapy is essential for long-term success of dental implants, but the optimum frequency of recall visits is largely intuitive.[43-45] Recall intervals should be individually determined for each patient, generally every 3 to 6 months. Factors to be considered in determining the frequency of maintenance visits include a history of periodontitis or peri-implantitis, the effectiveness of daily plaque control, tobacco use, the rate of calculus formation, the peri-implant probing depths, peri-implant bleeding upon probing, and suppuration.[46-53]

REFERENCES

1. Allen C: *The operator for the teeth*, York, 1685, White.
2. Pare A: *Oeuvres completes*, Ed. Malgaigne J-F, Paris,1840, Bailliere.
3. Fauchard P: *Le chirurgien dentiste, ou traité des dents*, Paris, 1728, Mariette.
4. Hunter J: *Natural history of human teeth*, London,1771, Johnson.
5. Jourdan AJL, Maggiolo L: *Le manuel de l'art du dentist*, Nancy, 1807, Le Seure.
6. Greenfield EJ: Implantation of artificial crown and bridge abutments, *Dental Cosmos* 55:364-369; 430-439; 1913.
7. Strock AE: Experimental work on a method for the replacement of missing teeth by direct implantation of a metal support into the alveolus: preliminary report, *Am J Orthod* 25:467-472, 1939.
8. Adams PB: Anchoring means for false teeth, US Patent #2,112,007, 1938.
9. Formiggini MS: Protesi dentale a mezzo di infibulazione diretta endoalveolare, *Riv It di Stomat* 4:193-195, 1947.
10. Driskell TD: History of implants, *Calif Dent Assoc J* 15:16-25, 1987.
11. Brånemark PI, Hansson BO, Adell R, et al: Osseointegrated implants in the treatment of the edentulous jaw: experience from a 10-year period, *Scan J Plast Reconstr Surg Suppl* 16:1-132, 1977.
12. Albrektsson T, Wennerberg A: The impact of oral implants: past and future, 1966-2042, *J Can Dent Assoc* 71:327-327d, 2005.
13. Zarb GA, editor: *Proceedings of the Toronto Conference on Osseointegration in Clinical Dentistry*, St Louis, 1983, Mosby.
14. Brånemark PI, Zarb GA, Albrektsson T: *Tissue integrated prostheses*, Chicago, 1985, Quintessence.
15. Wennerberg A, Albrektsson T: Current challenges in successful rehabilitation with oral implants, *J Oral Rehabil* 38:286-294, 2011.
16. Esposito M, Grusovin MG, Willings M, et al: The effectiveness of immediate, early, and conventional loading of dental implants: a Cochrane Systematic Review of randomized controlled clinical trials, *Int J Oral Maxillofac Implants* 22:893-904, 2007.
17. Araujo MG, Lindhe J: Dimensional ridge alterations following tooth extractions: an experimental study in the dog, *J Clin Periodontol* 32:212-218, 2005.
18. Amler MH: The time sequence of tissue regeneration in human extraction wounds *Oral Surg Oral Med Oral Pathol* 27:309-318, 1969.
19. Cardaropoli G, Araujo M, Lindhe J: Dynamics of bone tissue formation in tooth extraction sites: an experimental study in dogs, *J Clin Periodontol* 30:809-819, 2003.

20. Salama H, Salama MA: The role of orthodontic extrusive remodeling in the enhancement of soft and hard tissue profiles prior to implant placement: a systematic approach to the management of extraction sites defects, *In J Periodontics Restorative Dent* 13:312-334, 1993
21. Tan WL, Wong TL, Wong MC, et al: A systematic review of post-extractional alveolar hard and soft tissue dimensional changes in humans, *Clin Oral Implants Res* 23 (Suppl 5):1-21, 2012.
22. Grunder U: Crestal ridge width changes when placing implants at the time of tooth extraction with and without soft tissue augmentation after a healing period of 6 months: report of 24 consecutive cases, *Int J Periodontics Restorative Dent* 31:9-17, 2011.
23. Greenstein G, Cavallaro J: The clinical significance of keratinized gingiva around dental implants, *Compend Contin Educ Dent* 32:24-31; quiz, 32, 34; 2011.
24. Spray JR, et al: The influence of bone thickness on facial marginal cone response: stage 1 placement through stage 2 uncovering, *Ann Periodontol* 5:119-128, 2000.
25. Barboza EP, et al: Guided bone regeneration using nonexpanded polytetrafluoroethylene membranes in preparation for dental implant placements: a report of 420 cases, *Implant Dent* 19:2-7, 2010.
26. Pilling E, et al: An experimental in vivo analysis of the resorption to ultrasound activated pins and standard biodegradable screws in sheep, *Br J Oral Maxillofac Surg* 45:447-451, 2007. doi:10.1016/j.bjoms.2006.12.002.
27. Romanos GE: Periosteal releasing incision for successful coverage of augmented sites: a technical note, *J Oral Implantol* 36:25-30, 2010.
28. Eickholz P, Grotkamp FL, Steveling H, et al: Reproducibility of peri-implant probing using a force-controlled probe, *Clin Oral Implants Res* 12:153-158, 2001.
29. Gerber JA, Tan WC, Balmer TE, et al: Bleeding on probing and pocket probing depth in relation to probing pressure and mucosal health around oral implants, *Clin Oral Implants Res* 20:75-78, 2009.
30. Lang NP, Wetzel AC, Stich H, et al: Histologic probe penetration in healthy and inflamed peri-implant tissues, *Clin Oral Implants Res* 5:191-201, 1994.
31. Dula K, Mini R, van der Stelt PF, et al: The radiographic assessment of implant patients: decision-making criteria, *Int J Oral Maxillofac Implants* 16:80-89, 2001.
32. Sato S, Kishida M, Ito K: The comparative effect of ultrasonic scalers on titanium surfaces: an in vitro study, *J Periodontol* 75:1269-1273, 2004.

33. Kawashima H, Sato S, Kishida M, et al: Treatment of titanium dental implants with three piezoelectric ultrasonic scalers: an in vivo study, *J Periodontol* 78:1689-1694, 2007.
34. Ramaglia L, di Lauro AE, Morgese F, et al: Profilometric and standard error of the mean analysis of rough implant surfaces treated with different instrumentations, *Implant Dent* 15:77-82, 2006.
35. Mengel R, Buns CE, Mengel C, et al: An in vitro study of the treatment of implant surfaces with different instruments, *Int J Oral Maxillofac Implants* 13:91-96, 1998.
36. Petersilka GJ: Subgingival air-polishing in the treatment of periodontal biofilm infections, *Periodontol 2000* 55:124-142, 2011.
37. Renvert S, Lessem J, Dahlén G, et al: Topical minocycline microspheres versus topical chlorhexidine gel as an adjunct to mechanical débridement of incipient peri-implant infections: a randomized clinical trial, *J Clin Periodontol* 33:362-369, 2006.
38. Mombelli A: Microbiology and antimicrobial therapy of peri-implantitis, *Periodontol 2000* 28:177-189, 2002.
39. Porras R, Anderson GB, Caffesse R, et al: Clinical response to 2 different therapeutic regimens to treat peri-implant mucositis, *J Periodontol* 73:1118-1125, 2002.
40. Heitz-Mayfield LJ, Salvi GE, Botticelli D, et al: On behalf of the Implant Complication Research Group (ICRG): anti-infective treatment of periimplant mucositis—a randomised controlled clinical trial, *Clin Oral Implants Res* 22:237-241, 2011.
41. Mombelli A, Feloutzis A, Brägger U, et al: Treatment of peri-implantitis by local delivery of tetracycline: clinical, microbiological and radiological res results, *Clin Oral Implants Res* 12:287-294, 2001.
42. Zablotsky MH: Chemotherapeutics in implant dentistry, *Implant Dent* 2:19-25, 1993.
43. Heitz-Mayfield LJ: Peri-implant diseases: diagnosis and risk indicators, *J Clin Periodontol* 35(Suppl 8):292-304, 2008.
44. Eickholz P, Grotkamp FL, Steveling H, et al: Reproducibility of peri-implant probing using a force-controlled probe, *Clin Oral Implants Res* 12:153-158, 2001.
45. Gerber JA, Tan WC, Balmer TE, et al: Bleeding on probing and pocket probing depth in relation to probing pressure and mucosal health around oral implants, *Clin Oral Implants Res* 20:75-78, 2009.

46. Aglietta M, Siciliano VI, Rasperini G, et al: A 10-year retrospective analysis of marginal bone level changes around implants in periodontally healthy and periodontally compromised tobacco smokers, *Clin Oral Implants Res* 22:47-53, 2011.

47. Roccuzzo M, De Angelis N, Bonino L, et al: Ten-year results of a three-arm prospective cohort study on implants in periodontally compromised patients. Part 1. Implant loss and radiographic bone loss, *Clin Oral Implants Res* 21:490-496, 2010.

48. Anner R, Grossmann Y, Anner Y, et al: Smoking, diabetes mellitus, periodontitis, and supportive periodontal treatment as factors associated with dental implant survival: a long term retrospective evaluation of patients followed for up to 10 years, *Implant Dent* 19:57-64, 2010.

49. Rentsch-Kollar A, Huber S, Mericske-Stern R: Mandibular implant overdentures followed for over 10 years: patient compliance and prosthetic maintenance, *Int J Prosthodont* 23:91-98, 2010.

50. García-Bellosta S, Bravo M, Subirá C, et al: Retrospective study of the long-term survival of 980 implants placed in a periodontal practice, *Int J Oral Maxillofac Implants* 25:613-619, 2010.

51. Grusovin MG, Coulthard P, Worthington HV, et al: Maintaining and recovering soft tissue health around dental implants: a Cochrane Systematic Review of randomised controlled clinical trials, *Eur J Oral Implantol* 1:11-22, 2008.

52. Hultin M, Komiyama A, Klinge B: Supportive therapy and the longevity of dental implants: a systematic review of the literature, *Clin Oral Implants Res* 18(Suppl 3):50-62, 2007.

53. Humphrey S: Implant maintenance, *Dent Clin North Am* 50:463-478, 2006.

Bleaching discolored teeth

Ilan Rotstein, Richard E. Walton

CHAPTER OUTLINE

Causes of Discoloration
Endodontically Related Discolorations
Bleaching Materials
Internal (Nonvital) Bleaching Techniques

Complications and Safety
Intrinsic Discolorations
Extrinsic Discolorations
When and What to Refer

LEARNING OBJECTIVES

After reading this chapter, the student should be able to:
1. Identify the causes and nature of tooth discoloration.
2. Describe means of preventing coronal discolorations.
3. Differentiate between dentin and enamel discolorations.
4. Evaluate both the short-term and long-term prognoses of bleaching treatments.
5. Select the bleaching agent and technique according to the cause of discoloration.

6. Describe each step of the internal "walking bleach" technique.
7. Describe the indications for the microabrasion technique and the procedure.
8. Describe how bleaching agents may alter dentin.
9. Select the appropriate method to restore the access cavity after bleaching.
10. Recognize the potential adverse effects of bleaching and discuss means of prevention.

D iscoloration of anterior teeth is a cosmetic problem that is often significant enough to induce patients to seek corrective measures. Although restorative methods, such as crowns and veneers, are available, discoloration can often be corrected totally or partially by bleaching.

Bleaching procedures are more conservative than restorative methods, relatively simple to perform, and less expensive. Procedures may be internal (within the pulp chamber) or external (on the enamel surface) and involve various approaches.[1] The objectives of treatment are to reduce or eliminate discoloration, improve the degree of coronal translucency, and alleviate present and prevent future clinical signs and symptoms.[2]

To better understand bleaching techniques, it is important to know the causes of discoloration, location of the discoloring agent, and treatment modalities available. Also important is the ability to predict the outcome of treatment (i.e., how successfully various discolorations can be treated and how long the esthetic result will last). Therefore, before attempting to correct discoloration, there must be a diagnosis (to determine the cause and location of the discoloration), a treatment plan (internal or external bleaching and the technique), and a prognosis (anticipated short- and long-term success). Patients must be informed of these factors before undergoing the procedure; any discoloration treatment is tempered by the

explanation that bleaching is somewhat unpredictable and that substantial improvement may or may not occur. However, bleaching is worth a try because with proper and careful technique, no irreversible damage to the crown or root occurs.

This chapter reviews internal tooth discoloration and its prevention and correction. Discussed are the causes and management of discoloration as related to (1) the location of the discoloration, (2) the approach used for correction, and (3) the predicted short- and long-term success of bleaching. The following aspects of discoloration and bleaching procedures are discussed:

1. Causes and location of discoloration
2. Commonly used bleaching agents
3. Internal bleaching techniques (usually in conjunction with or after root canal treatment)
4. Microabrasion, (a technique for removing surface discolorations)
5. Predictability and permanence of each procedure
6. Possible complications and safety of the various procedures

CAUSES OF DISCOLORATION

Tooth discolorations may occur during or after enamel and dentin formation. Some discolorations appear after tooth eruption, and others are the result of dental procedures. Acquired (natural) discolorations may be on the surface or incorporated into tooth structure. Sometimes they result from flaws in enamel or a traumatic injury. Inflicted (iatrogenic) discolorations, which result from certain dental procedures, are usually incorporated into tooth structure and are largely preventable.

Acquired (Natural) Discolorations
Pulp Necrosis

Bacterial, mechanical, or chemical irritation of the pulp may result in necrosis. Tissue disintegration byproducts are then released, and these colored compounds may permeate tubules to stain surrounding dentin. The degree of discoloration is likely related to how long the pulp has been necrotic.[1] The longer the discoloration compounds are present in the pulp chamber, the greater the discoloration. This type of discoloration can be bleached internally, usually with both short- and long-term success (Fig. 24.1).

Intrapulpal Hemorrhage

Intrapulpal hemorrhage is usually associated with an impact injury to a tooth that results in disrupted coronal blood vessels, hemorrhage, and lysis of erythrocytes. It has been theorized that certain blood disintegration byproducts, presumably iron sulfides, permeate tubules to stain surrounding dentin. Discoloration tends to increase with time.

If the pulp becomes necrotic, the discoloration usually remains. If the pulp survives, the discoloration may resolve and the tooth regains its original shade. Sometimes, mainly in young individuals, the tooth remains discolored even if the pulp responds to vitality tests.

Internal bleaching of discoloration after intrapulpal hemorrhage is usually successful both short term and long term.[3,4]

Calcific Metamorphosis

Calcific metamorphosis is extensive formation of tertiary (irregular secondary) dentin in the pulp chamber or on canal walls. This phenomenon usually follows an impact injury that did not result in pulp necrosis. There is likely temporary disruption of the blood supply with partial destruction of odontoblasts. These are usually replaced by cells that rapidly form irregular dentin on the walls of the pulp chamber and root canal space. As a result, the crowns take on a "flat" appearance as they gradually decrease in translucency and acquire a yellowish or yellow-brown discoloration (Fig. 24.2). The pulp usually remains vital and does not require root canal treatment.

If the patient desires color correction, external bleaching should be attempted first. If this is unsuccessful, root canal treatment is performed (sometimes with difficulty), and internal bleaching is done. This may be carried out whether the pulp is vital or necrotic. The esthetic prognosis for such bleaching is fair (unpredictable).

Age

In older patients, color changes in the crown occur physiologically as a result of extensive dentin apposition and thinning of and optical changes in the enamel. Food and beverages also have a cumulative discoloring effect because of the inevitable cracking and other changes on the enamel surface and in the underlying dentin. In addition, previously applied restorations

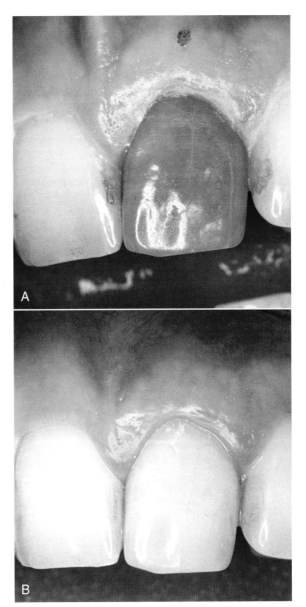

Fig. 24.1 **A,** Discoloration as a result of a traumatic injury followed by pulp necrosis. **B,** After root canal treatment, a paste of sodium perborate and water mixed to a consistency of wet sand was sealed in the pulp chamber. After 21 days of walking bleach, the tooth regained its original shade. (Courtesy Dr. A. Claisse.)

that degrade over time cause further discoloration. There is an increasing demand for bleaching among elderly patients. Bleaching is usually external because the discoloration is primarily on the enamel surface. Success may vary, depending on the causal factor of discoloration.

Developmental Defects

Discolorations may also result from development defects or from substances incorporated into enamel or dentin during tooth formation.

Endemic Fluorosis

Ingestion of excessive amounts of fluoride during tooth formation produces defects in mineralized structures, particularly enamel matrix, with resultant hypoplasia. The severity

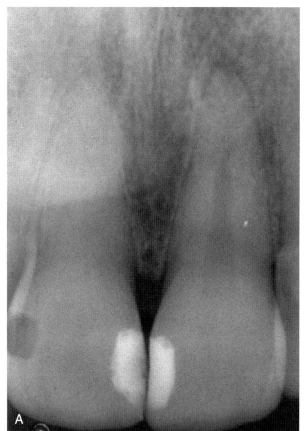

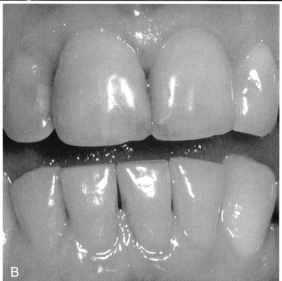

Fig. 24.2 Calcific metamorphosis. Impact trauma resulted in reversible pulp damage **(A)** with extensive tertiary dentin formation **(B)**. These teeth may present difficulties with root canal treatment and internal bleaching.

depends mainly on the degree and duration of the discoloration. Some regression and recurrence of discoloration tend to happen but can be corrected with future rebleaching.

Systemic Drugs

Administration or ingestion of certain drugs or chemicals (many of which have not yet been identified) during tooth formation may cause discoloration, which is occasionally severe.[6]

The most common and most dramatic discoloration of this type occurs after tetracycline ingestion, usually in children. Discoloration is bilateral, affecting multiple teeth in both arches. It may range from yellow through brownish to dark gray, depending on the amount, frequency, and type of tetracycline and the patient's age (stage of development) during administration.

Tetracycline discoloration has been classified into three groups according to severity.[7] First-degree discoloration is light yellow, light brown, or light gray and occurs uniformly throughout the crown without banding. Second-degree discoloration is more intense and is also without banding. Third-degree discoloration is very intense, and the clinical crown exhibits horizontal color banding. This type of discoloration usually predominates in the cervical region.

Tetracycline binds to calcium, which then is incorporated into the hydroxyapatite crystal in both enamel and dentin. Most of the tetracycline, however, is found in dentin. Chronic sun exposure of teeth with the incorporated drug may cause formation of a reddish purple tetracycline oxidation byproduct, resulting in further discoloration of permanent teeth.

A phenomenon of adult-onset tetracycline discoloration has also been reported.[8] This type of discoloration occurs occasionally in mature teeth in patients receiving long-term minocycline therapy, which was usually given for control of cystic acne. The discoloration is gradual because of incorporation of minocycline in continuously forming dentin.[5] Staining generally is not severe.

Two approaches have been used for bleaching tetracycline discoloration. The first, which involves bleaching the external enamel surface, is limited to lighter, yellowish discoloration and requires multiple appointments to achieve a satisfactory result.[9] The second, root canal treatment followed by internal bleaching, is a predictable procedure, is useful for all degrees of discoloration severity, and has proved successful in both the short term and long term.[10]

Defects in Tooth Formation

Defects in tooth formation are confined to the enamel and are either hypocalcific or hypoplastic. Enamel *hypocalcification* is common, appearing as a distinct brownish or whitish area, often on the facial aspect of a crown. The enamel is well formed and intact on the surface and feels hard to the explorer. Both the whitish and the brownish spots are amenable to correction with the pumice and acid technique (described later in this chapter) with good results.

Enamel *hypoplasia* differs from *hypocalcification* in that the enamel in the former is defective and porous. This condition may be hereditary (amelogenesis imperfecta) or may result from environmental factors. In the hereditary type, both deciduous and permanent dentitions are involved. Defects caused by environmental factors may involve only one or several teeth. Presumably during tooth formation the matrix is altered and

and degree of subsequent staining generally depend on the degree of hypoplasia, which depends in turn on the patient's age and the amount of fluoride ingested during odontogenesis.[5] The teeth are not discolored on eruption but may appear chalky. Their surface, however, is porous and gradually absorbs stains from chemicals in the oral cavity.

Because the discoloration is in the porous enamel, such teeth are bleached (or corrected) externally. Esthetic success does not mineralize properly. The porous enamel readily acquires stains from the oral cavity. Depending on the severity and extent of hypoplasia and the nature of the stain, these teeth may be bleached (or corrected by the acid pumice method) from the enamel surface with some degree of success.[11] The bleaching effect may not be permanent, and stains may recur with time. These stains, however, can be recorrected. As stated earlier, it is most important to inform the patient of the likely recurrence of discoloration of these teeth.

Blood Dyscrasias and Other Factors

Various systemic conditions may cause massive lysis of erythrocytes. If this occurs in the pulp at an early age, blood disintegration products are incorporated into and discolor the forming dentin. An example of this phenomenon is the severe discoloration of primary teeth that usually follows erythroblastosis fetalis. This disease in the fetus, or newborn, results from Rh incompatibility factors, which lead to massive systemic lysis of erythrocytes. Large amounts of hemosiderin pigment then stain the forming dentin of the primary teeth. This discoloration is not correctable by bleaching. However, this type of lysis is now uncommon because of new preventive measures.

High fever during tooth formation may result in linear defined hypoplasia. This condition, known as *chronologic hypoplasia,* is a temporary disruption in enamel formation that results in a banding type of surface defect that acquires stain. Porphyria, a metabolic disease, may cause deciduous and permanent teeth to show a red or brownish discoloration. Hyperbilirubinemia, thalassemia, and sickle cell anemia may cause intrinsic bluish, brown, or green discolorations. Amelogenesis imperfecta may result in yellowish or brownish discolorations. Dentinogenesis imperfecta can cause brownish violet, yellowish, or gray discoloration. These conditions are also not amenable to bleaching and should be corrected by minimally invasive restorative means.

Other staining factors related to systemic conditions or ingested drugs are rare and may not be identifiable.

Inflicted (Iatrogenic) Discolorations

Discolorations caused by various chemicals and materials used in dentistry are usually avoidable. Many of these discolorations respond well to bleaching, but some are more difficult to correct by bleaching alone.

ENDODONTICALLY RELATED DISCOLORATIONS

Obturating Materials

Obturating materials are the most common and severe cause of single tooth discoloration. Incomplete removal of materials from the pulp chamber upon completion of treatment often results in dark discoloration (Figs. 24.3 and 24.4). Removing all obturation materials to a level just cervical to the gingival margin can prevent such discoloration. Primary offenders are sealer remnants, whether of the zinc oxide–eugenol type or resins, which themselves also darken with time.[12-14] Sealer remnants gradually cause progressive coronal discoloration.[15] The prognosis of bleaching in such cases depends on the constituents of the sealer. Sealers with metallic components often do not bleach well, and the bleaching effect tends to regress with time.

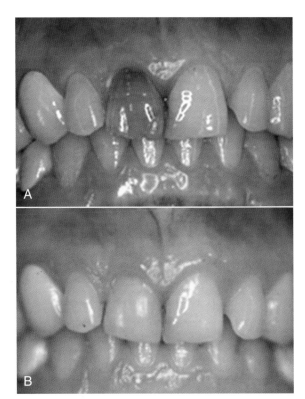

Fig. 24.3 **A,** Discoloration as a result of trauma and subsequent treatment. The patient was involved in an accident that caused a coronal fracture. Root canal treatment was performed, but gutta-percha and sealer were not completely removed from the pulp chamber. An additional discoloration factor was the defective leaking restoration. **B,** Two appointments of walking bleach and placement of a new, well-sealed composite restored esthetics. (Courtesy Dr. M. Israel.)

Remnants of Pulpal Tissue

Pulp fragments remaining in the crown, usually in pulp horns, may cause gradual discoloration. Pulp horns must be "opened up" and exposed during access preparation to ensure removal of pulpal remnants and to prevent retention of sealer at a later stage. Internal bleaching in such cases is usually successful (Fig. 24.5).

Intracanal Medicaments

Several medicaments have the potential to cause internal discoloration of the dentin.[16,17] Phenolic or iodoform-based intracanal medications, sealed in the root canal space, are in direct contact with dentin, sometimes for long periods, which allows penetration to dentin tubules and oxidization. These compounds have a tendency to discolor the dentin gradually. Fortunately, most such discolorations are not marked and are readily and permanently corrected by bleaching. Iodoform-induced discolorations tend to be more severe.

Coronal Restorations

Restorations are generally metallic or composite. The reasons for discoloration (and therefore the appropriate correction) are quite different.

Metallic Restorations

Amalgam is the worst offender because its dark metallic elements may turn dentin dark gray. If used to restore an access **431**

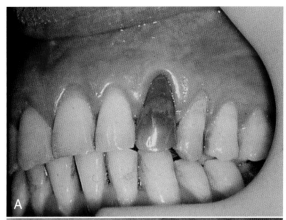

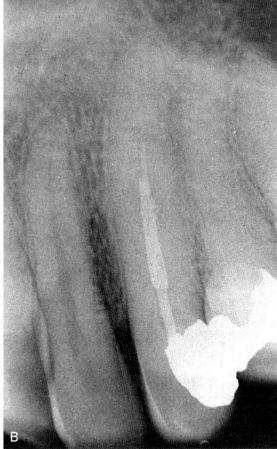

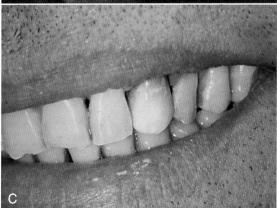

Fig. 24.4 **A,** Severely discolored canine. **B,** Poor root canal treatment, in which material extended into the pulp chamber, caused some of the discoloration. **C,** After retreatment and three appointments of walking bleach, esthetics has markedly improved. Although some cervical discoloration remains, this is largely hidden by the upper lip. (Courtesy Dr. H. Libfeld.)

preparation, amalgam often discolors the crown (Fig. 24.6). Such discolorations are difficult to bleach and tend to recur with time. However, bleaching them is worth a try. The result may be an improvement that satisfies the patient.

Discoloration from inappropriately placed metal pins and prefabricated posts in anterior teeth may sometimes occur. This is caused by metal that is visible through the composite or tooth structure. Occasionally, discoloration from amalgam is also caused by visibility of the restoration through translucent tooth structure. In such cases, replacement of old metallic restorations with an esthetically pleasing composite may suffice.

Composite Restorations

Microleakage of composites causes discoloration. Open margins may permit chemicals to permeate gaps between the restoration and tooth structure to stain the underlying dentin. In addition, composites may become discolored with time and alter the shade of the crown. These conditions can sometimes be corrected by replacing the old composite with a new, well-sealed esthetic restoration. In many cases, internal bleaching is carried out first with good results.

BLEACHING MATERIALS

Bleaching chemicals may act as either oxidizing or reducing agents. Most bleaching agents are oxidizers, and many preparations are available. Commonly used agents are solutions of hydrogen peroxide of different strengths, sodium perborate, and carbamide peroxide. Sodium perborate and carbamide peroxide are chemical compounds that are gradually degraded to release low levels of hydrogen peroxide. Hydrogen peroxide and carbamide peroxide are mainly indicated for external bleaching, whereas sodium perborate is mostly used for internal bleaching. All have proved effective.

Hydrogen Peroxide

Hydrogen peroxide is a powerful oxidizer that is available in various strengths, but 30% to 35% stabilized solutions (Superoxyl, Perhydrol) are the most common. These high-concentration solutions must be handled with care because they are unstable, lose oxygen quickly, and may explode unless they are refrigerated and stored in a dark container. Also, these are caustic chemicals and will burn tissue on contact.

Although 30% to 35% hydrogen peroxide bleaches quickly, other chemicals that release much lower levels of peroxide are available; usually they bleach effectively with longer application periods.[18]

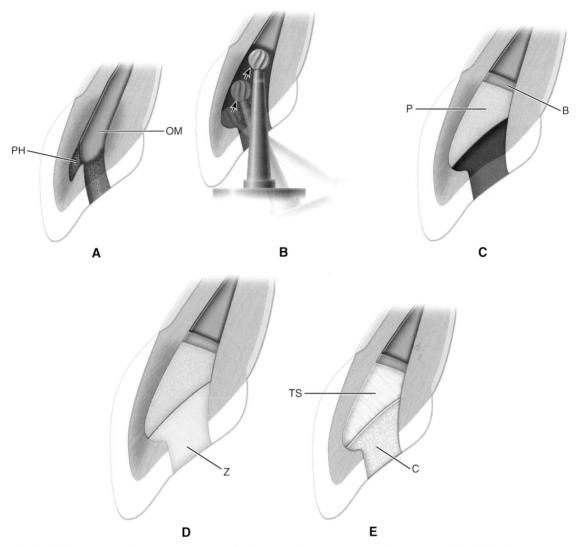

Fig. 24.5 Walking bleach. **A,** Internal staining of dentin caused by remnants of obturating materials *(OM)* in the pulp chamber and by materials and tissue debris in the pulp horns *(PH)*. **B,** Coronal restoration is removed completely, access preparation is improved, and gutta-percha is removed apically to just below the cervical margin. Next, the pulp horns are cleaned with a round bur. (Shaving a thin layer of dentin from the facial wall is optional and may be attempted at later appointments if discoloration persists.) **C,** An optional protective cement base *(B)* is placed over the gutta-percha, not extending above the cervical margin. After the removal of sealer remnants and materials from the chamber with solvents, a paste *(P)* composed of sodium perborate and water (mixed to the consistency of wet sand) is placed. The incisal area is undercut to retain the temporary restoration. **D,** A thick mixture of a zinc oxide–eugenol–type temporary filling *(Z)* seals the access. **E,** At a subsequent appointment, when the desired shade has been reached, a permanent restoration is placed. A suggested method is to fill the chamber with white temporary stopping *(TS)* or with light polycarboxylate or zinc phosphate base. Acid-etched composite *(C)* restores lingual access and extends into the pulp horns for retention and to support the incisal edge. (From Walton RE: Bleaching procedures for teeth with vital and nonvital pulps. In Levine N, editor: *Current treatment in dental practice,* Philadelphia, 1986, Saunders.)

Sodium Perborate

Sodium perborate is available in powder form or in various commercial proprietary combinations. When fresh, it contains about 95% perborate, corresponding to 9.9% available oxygen. Sodium perborate is stable when dry, but in the presence of acid, warm air, or water, it decomposes to form sodium metaborate, hydrogen peroxide, and nascent oxygen.[19] Various types of sodium perborate preparations are available: monohydrate, trihydrate, and tetrahydrate. They differ in oxygen content, which determines their bleaching efficacy.[20] Commonly used sodium perborate preparations are alkaline; their pH depends on the amount of hydrogen peroxide released and the residual sodium metaborate.[21]

Sodium perborate is more easily controlled and safer than concentrated hydrogen peroxide solutions.[3,4,19,22,23] Therefore, in most cases, it should be the material of choice for internal bleaching.

Carbamide Peroxide

Carbamide peroxide, also known as urea hydrogen peroxide, is usually available in concentrations varying between 3% and 15%. Popular commercial preparations contain about 10% **433**

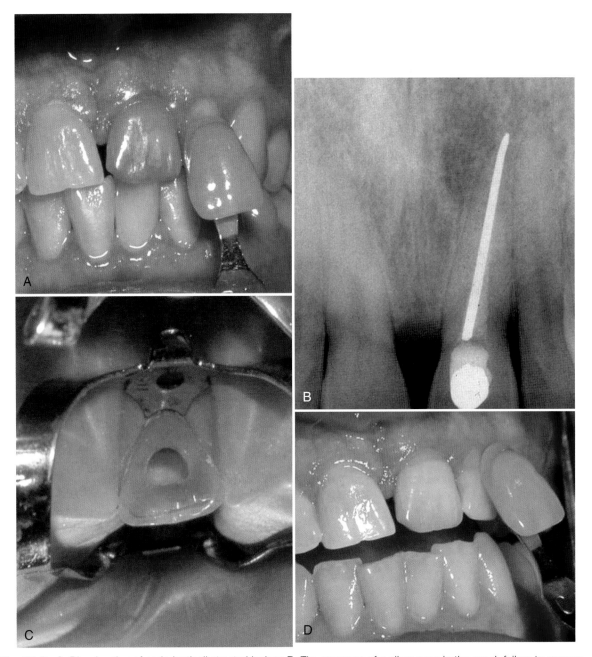

Fig. 24.6 **A,** Discoloration of endodontically treated incisor. **B,** The presence of a silver cone in the canal, failure to remove all remnants of pulpal tissue from the chamber and amalgam placed in the access cavity appear to be the causes of discoloration, **C,** Removal of amalgam and refinement of the access cavity. The silver cone was removed, and endodontic retreatment was performed. **D,** Internal bleaching, followed by placement of a new composite, restored esthetics.

carbamide peroxide and have an average pH of 5 to 6.5. They usually also include glycerin or propylene glycol, sodium stannate, phosphoric or citric acid, and flavor. In some preparations, Carbopol, a water-soluble resin, is added to prolong the release of active peroxide and to improve shelf-life. Ten percent carbamide peroxide breaks down into urea, ammonia, carbon dioxide, and approximately 3.5% hydrogen peroxide.

Carbamide peroxide and hydrogen peroxide–based systems are mostly used for external bleaching and have been associated with varying degrees (usually slight) of damage to teeth and surrounding mucosa.[24,25] They may adversely affect the bond strength of composite resins and their marginal seal.[24-27]

Therefore, these materials must be used with caution and usually under strict supervision of the dentist.

Other Agents

In the past, a preparation of sodium peroxyborate monohydrate (Amosan), which releases more oxygen than does sodium perborate, was recommended for internal bleaching.[28] Today, this product is not available in all countries and its clinical use is less common.

Sodium hypochlorite is a common root canal irrigant that is available commercially as a 3% to 6% household bleach. Although used as a household bleaching agent, it does not release enough oxidizer to be effective and is not recommended for routine bleaching.

Other nonperoxide bleaching agents have also been suggested for clinical use; however, these have been no more effective than traditional agents.[29,30]

INTERNAL (NONVITAL) BLEACHING TECHNIQUES

The methods most commonly used to bleach teeth in conjunction with root canal treatment are the *thermocatalytic* technique and the so-called walking bleach technique.[19,28] These techniques are somewhat different but produce similar results.[3,4,19] The walking bleach technique (described later in the chapter) is preferred because it requires the least chair time and is more comfortable and safer for the patient. Whatever technique is used, the active ingredient is the oxidizer, which is available in different chemical forms. The least potent form is preferred.

Indications for internal bleaching technique are (1) discolorations of pulp chamber origin, (2) dentin discolorations, and (3) discolorations that are not amenable to external bleaching. Contraindications are (1) superficial enamel discolorations, (2) defective enamel formation, (3) severe dentin loss, (4) presence of caries, and (5) discolored proximal composites (unless they are replaced after bleaching).

Thermocatalytic Technique

The thermocatalytic technique involves placing the oxidizing agent in the pulp chamber and then applying heat. Heat may be supplied by heat lamps, flamed instruments, or electrical heating devices, which are manufactured specifically to bleach teeth.[31]

Potential damage from the thermocatalytic approach includes the possibility of external cervical root resorption because of irritation to cementum and the periodontal ligament, possibly from the oxidizing agent in combination with heat.[32-34] Therefore the application of heat during internal bleaching is contraindicated. Also, the thermocatalytic technique has not proved more effective long term than other methods and is not recommended for routine internal bleaching.

A thermocatalytic variation is ultraviolet photo-oxidation. A 30% to 35% hydrogen peroxide solution is placed in the pulp chamber on a cotton pellet, followed by a 2-minute exposure to ultraviolet light applied to the coronal labial surface of the tooth. Supposedly this causes the release of oxygen similar to that seen in other thermocatalytic bleaching techniques.[35,36] There has been little clinical experience with ultraviolet photo-oxidation. It is probably no more effective than the walking bleach technique and requires more chair time. Because of toxicity considerations with concentrated hydrogen peroxide, this technique is not recommended.

Walking Bleach

The walking bleach technique should be used in all situations requiring internal bleaching. Not only is it as effective as the techniques previously described, but it also is the safest and has the shortest chair time requirement (Box 24.1).*

*References 2, 3, 10, 19, 21, 23, and 37.

It is commonly thought that "overbleaching" is desirable because of future recurrence of discoloration. However, bleaching a tooth to a lighter shade than its neighbors should be performed with caution because the overbleached tooth may not discolor again.[38] A tooth that is too light may be as unesthetic as one that is too dark.

Treatments at subsequent visits are similar. If early bleaching appointments do not provide satisfactory results, the following additional procedures may be attempted: (1) a thin layer of stained facial dentin is removed with a small round bur (see Box 24.1, step 7); and (2) the walking bleach paste is strengthened by mixing the sodium perborate with increasing concentrations of hydrogen peroxide (3% to 30%) instead of water. Heat is not used. The more potent oxidizer may enhance the bleaching effect but may increase the risk of subsequent root resorption.[32,39]

Carbamide peroxide has also been suggested for internal bleaching.[40] This agent, however, is probably not superior to sodium perborate.

Although usually the final results are excellent, occasionally only partial lightening is achieved. Surprisingly, the patient often is very pleased and satisfied with a modest improvement and does not expect perfection.[40] Therefore internal bleaching is worth the attempt.

Final Restoration

Proper tooth restoration is essential for long-term successful internal bleaching results.[41,42] The pulp chamber and access cavity are restored at the final visit (see Fig. 24.5, *E*). Although it has been proposed that substances such as acrylic monomer or silicones be placed in the chamber to fill the dentinal tubules, this is not beneficial. Furthermore, these substances may themselves lead to discoloration with time. However, it is important to restore the chamber carefully and to seal the lingual access to enhance the new shade and prevent leakage. The ideal method for filling the chamber after tooth bleaching has not been determined. However, the chamber must not be filled totally with composite; this may cause a loss of translucency of the tooth.[43]

It is easy and effective to fill the chamber with a light-colored gutta-percha temporary stopping, glass ionomer, or a light shade of zinc phosphate cement and then to restore the lingual access with a light-cured, acid-etched composite.[44] Composite resins have different levels of color and contrast ratio.[45] Awareness of such optical properties aids in material selection. An adequate depth of composite should be ensured to seal the cavity and provide some incisal support. Light curing from the labial, rather than the lingual, surface is recommended because this results in shrinkage of the composite resin toward the axial walls, reducing the rate of microleakage.[46] Coronal microleakage of lingual access restorations is a problem[47]; a leaky restoration may lead to recurrence of discoloration.

Residual peroxides of bleaching agents, mainly hydrogen peroxide and carbamide peroxide, may affect the bonding strength of composites to the tooth.[27,48-50] Sodium perborate mixed with water results in much less loss of bond strength than does concentrated hydrogen peroxide.[50] Therefore, it is not recommended that the tooth be restored with composite immediately after bleaching but only after an interval of a few days. The use of catalase and other agents has also been proposed for fast elimination of residual peroxides from the **435**

Box 24.1   Walking Bleach Technique

The steps of the walking bleach technique are as follows (see Fig. 24.5).

1. The patient is familiarized with the probable causes of discoloration, the procedure to be followed, the expected outcome, and the possibility of future recurrence of discoloration (regression). To avoid disappointment or misunderstanding, effective communication before, during, and after treatment is absolutely necessary.
2. Radiographs are made to assess the status of the periapical tissues and the quality of root canal treatment. Treatment failure or questionable obturation requires retreatment before bleaching.
3. The quality and shade of any restoration present are assessed. If defective, the restoration is replaced. Often tooth discoloration results from leaking or discolored restorations. Also, the patient is informed that the bleaching procedure may temporarily (or permanently) affect the seal and color match of the restoration, requiring its replacement.
4. Tooth color is evaluated with a shade guide, and clinical photographs are taken at the beginning of and throughout the procedure. These provide a point of reference for future comparison by both dentist and patient.
5. The tooth is isolated with a rubber dam. Interproximal wedges may also be used for better isolation. If Superoxol is used, a protective cream (e.g., petroleum jelly, Orabase, or cocoa butter) must be applied to the gingival tissues before dam placement. This protection is not required with sodium perborate use.
6. The restorative material is removed from the access cavity (see Fig. 24.5, B). Refinement of access and removal of all old obturating and restorative materials from the pulp chamber comprise the most important stage in the bleaching process. The clinician must check that pulp horns or other "hidden" areas have been opened and are free of pulp tissue remnants.

    A chamber totally filled with composite resin presents a clinical problem. First, this material is resistant to cutting with burs. Second, its shade is often indistinct from that of dentin. However, all composite must be removed to allow the bleaching agent to contact and penetrate the dentin. Care must be taken during restoration removal to avoid inadvertent cutting of sound dentin. The operating microscope or magnifying loupes are beneficial.
7. (Optional). This step may be necessary if the discoloration seems to be of metallic origin or if, on the second or third appointment, bleaching alone does not seem to be sufficient. A thin layer of stained dentin is carefully removed toward the facial aspect of the chamber with a round bur in a slow-speed handpiece (see Fig. 24.5, B). This removes much of the discoloration (which is concentrated in the pulpal surface area). It may also open the dentinal tubules for better penetration by the bleaching agents.
8. All materials should be removed to a level just apical to the gingival margin. Appropriate solvents (e.g., orange solvent, chloroform, or xylol on a cotton pellet) are used to dissolve remnants of the common sealers.
9. If 30% to 35% hydrogen peroxide is used, a sufficient layer of protective cement barrier (e.g., polycarboxylate, zinc phosphate, glass ionomer, intermediate restorative material [IRM], or Cavit at least 2 mm thick) is applied as a barrier on the obturating material. This is essential to minimize leakage of bleaching agents.[53] The barrier should protect the dentin tubules and conform to the external epithelial attachment.[54] It should not extend incisal to the gingival margin (see Fig. 24.5, C).

    Acid etching of dentin internally with phosphoric (or other) acid to remove the smear layer and open the tubules is not necessary.[55,56] The use of any caustic chemical in the chamber is unwarranted because periodontal ligament irritation or external root resorption may result.[56] The same reservation applies to solvents such as ether or acetone before application of the bleaching agent. The application of concentrated hydrogen peroxide with heat (thermocatalytic) has been suggested as the next step. This may not be more effective and also may be questionable from a safety standpoint.
10. The walking bleach paste is prepared by mixing sodium perborate and an inert liquid, such as water, saline, or anesthetic solution, to the consistency of wet sand (approximately 2 g/mL). Although sodium perborate mixed with 30% hydrogen peroxide bleaches faster, in most cases the long-term results are similar to those of sodium perborate mixed with water; therefore the former mixture should not be used routinely.[3,4,19,37] Another advantage of sodium perborate and inert liquid is that a protective cement barrier and gingival protection are unnecessary. With a plastic instrument, the pulp chamber is packed with the paste. Excess liquid is removed by tamping with a cotton pellet. This also compresses and pushes the paste into the recesses (see Fig. 24.5, C).
11. Excess oxidizing paste is removed from undercuts in the pulp horns and gingival area with an explorer. A cotton pellet is not used, but a thick mix of zinc oxide–eugenol (preferably IRM) or Cavit is packed carefully to a thickness of at least 3 mm to ensure a good seal (see Fig. 24.5, D).
12. The rubber dam is removed. The patient is informed that the bleaching agent works slowly and that significant lightening may not be evident for 2 or more weeks. It is common to see no change initially, but dramatic results occur in successive days or weeks or after a future reapplication.
13. The patient is scheduled to return approximately 2 to 6 weeks later, and the procedure is repeated. If at any future appointment (third or fourth) progressive lightening is not evident, further walking bleach treatments with sodium perborate and water solution may not prove beneficial.[37]

access cavity and for protection against potential hazardous effects[51,52]; this merits further investigation.

It has been suggested that packing calcium hydroxide paste in the chamber for a few weeks before the final restoration is placed would reverse the acidity caused by bleaching agents and prevent resorption; however, this procedure is ineffective and unnecessary.[21,39]

Other agents have been proposed to enhance the bleaching effect or to open tubules; none have been shown to be effective.[53-56]

Future Rediscoloration

Although initial bleaching is successful, many of these teeth rediscolor after several years.[38,57,58] Patients must be informed of this possible occurrence and that rebleaching usually will be successful.

When to Bleach

Internal bleaching may be performed at various intervals after root canal treatment (see Figs. 24.1 and 24.6). The appearance of the discolored tooth may be improved soon after treatment. However, the walking bleach technique may be initiated at the same appointment as the obturation. In fact, this may motivate the patient to accept bleaching because the appearance of the discolored tooth may be improved soon after treatment. Bleaching may also be attempted successfully many years after discoloration has occurred (see Figs. 24.3 and 24.4), even with porcelain veneer restorations (Fig. 24.7). Such teeth show no markedly greater tendency for recurrence of discoloration than teeth stained for shorter discoloration periods.[38] However, it is probable that a shorter discoloration period tends to improve the chances for successful bleaching and to reduce the likelihood of recurrence of discoloration.[58]

Other factors that may influence long-term success have also been evaluated clinically. The patient's age and the rate of discoloration have no major effect on the long-term stability of bleaching.[38]

COMPLICATIONS AND SAFETY

Patient safety is always the major concern in any procedure. Some possible adverse effects produced by chemicals and bleaching procedures are discussed in the following sections.

External Root Resorption

Clinical reports[33,34,59] and histologic studies[32,39] have shown that internal bleaching may induce external root resorption. The oxidizing agent, particularly 30% hydrogen peroxide, and heat may be the culprits. However, the exact mechanism by which periodontium or cementum is damaged has not been elucidated. Presumably, the irritating chemical diffuses through the dentinal tubules[60] and reaches the periodontium through defects in the cementoenamel junction.[61] Chemicals combined with heat are likely to cause necrosis of the cementum, inflammation of the periodontal ligament, and subsequent root resorption.[32,39] The process is liable to be enhanced in the presence of bacteria.[62] Previous traumatic injury and young age may also act as predisposing factors.[33] Therefore, injurious chemicals and procedures should be avoided if they are not essential for bleaching. Also, apical to the cervical margin, oxidizing agents should not be exposed to more of the pulp space and dentin than is absolutely necessary to obtain a satisfactory esthetic clinical result.

Coronal Fracture

Slightly increased brittleness of the coronal tooth structure, particularly when heat is applied, is also thought to result from bleaching. This supposedly is a result of either desiccation or alterations to the physicochemical characteristics of the dentin and enamel.[63-66] Clinical experience suggests that bleached teeth are no more susceptible to fracture, although this has not been proven conclusively.

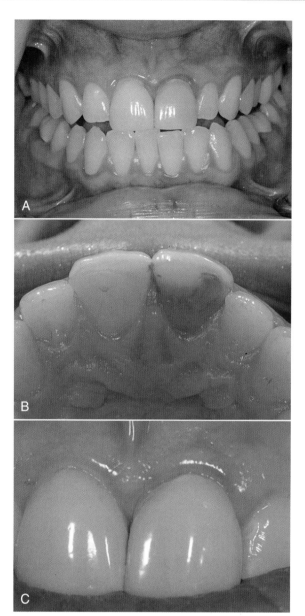

Fig. 24.7 **A,** Discoloration of endodontically treated incisor restored with a porcelain veneer. Discoloration is reflected through the veneer and is most evident at the cervical area. **B,** Lingual view reveals extensive discoloration of the dentin and composite that was used to restore the access cavity. **C,** Removal of discolored composite, internal bleaching, and placement of a new, well-sealed composite restored tooth esthetics. (Courtesy Dr. A. Sameni.)

Chemical Burns

As mentioned earlier, sodium perborate is safe, but 30% hydrogen peroxide is caustic and can cause chemical burns and sloughing of the gingiva. When this strong chemical is used, the soft tissues should be coated with an isolation cream such as petroleum jelly, Orabase, or cocoa butter. Animal studies suggest that catalase applied to oral tissues before hydrogen peroxide treatment fully prevents the associated tissue damage.[67]

INTRINSIC DISCOLORATIONS

Intrinsic discolorations are those incorporated into tooth structure during tooth formation.[68] Significantly, most of these discolorations are in dentin and are relatively difficult to treat externally.[69] A good example is staining from tetracycline, which is incorporated into the mineral structure of the developing tooth. The incorporated tetracycline imparts its color to the dentin.

Tetracycline

Both external and internal bleaching techniques have been advocated as a means of improving the appearance of tetracycline-discolored teeth. As noted earlier, the internal technique is more effective and has a very good long-term prognosis.[10,68,69] However, the best resolution for tetracycline discolorations is prevention.

The technique involves root canal treatment followed by an internal walking bleach technique, as outlined earlier in this chapter. If the procedure is explained to patients, they may accept this approach, with gratifying results (Fig. 24.8).

Other Intrinsic Discolorations

Other drugs or ingested chemicals are incorporated into teeth that are forming and cause discoloration. There are no reports of attempts to bleach these teeth. Presumably, attempts to lighten teeth with dentinal discolorations by the external application of bleaching agents would be only marginally effective.

EXTRINSIC DISCOLORATIONS

Extrinsic discolorations are more superficial and are obviously more amenable to external bleaching. The success of bleaching, however, depends more on the depth of the stain in the enamel rather than on the color of the stain itself.

Superficial Defects

Although a number of conditions may result in hypoplasia of enamel accompanied by porosity, the most common and often the most disfiguring is endemic fluorosis. This hypoplastic defect may result in various degrees and colors of superficial stains.

Mechanism of Discoloration

Ingestion of high levels of fluoride during tooth formation can lead to enamel hypoplasia and gradual tooth discoloration.[70] The appearance of such discolorations may be improved with bleaching or other measures, some dramatically. Although a variety of techniques involving different chemicals and procedures have been suggested, probably the most effective is

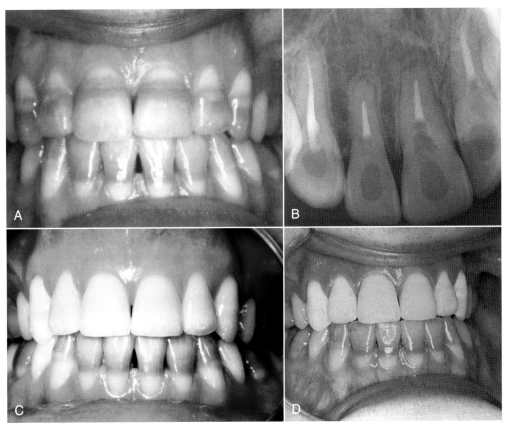

Fig. 24.8 **A,** Characteristic grayish discoloration and banding of tetracycline discolorations. Cervical regions on maxillary and mandibular teeth show no discoloration; tetracycline was not administered during those periods of tooth development. **B,** Root canal treatment has been completed on the maxillary anterior teeth, with subsequent walking bleach procedures. **C,** After the necessary number of bleaching appointments, the teeth are restored permanently. Note the marked contrast with the mandibular incisors, which remain untreated. **D,** At the 4-year follow-up, no regression and no recurrence of discoloration are seen. (Courtesy Dr. H. Wayne Mohorn.)

the microabrasion "controlled hydrochloric acid–pumice abrasion" technique (Fig. 24.9).[11] This is not a true bleaching (oxidizing) technique, but rather decalcification and removal of a thin layer of stained enamel. The technique has been modified somewhat since its development in the mid-1980s.[11,71] It is useful mainly for fluorosis and other extrinsic discolorations and has proved to be very effective.[72]

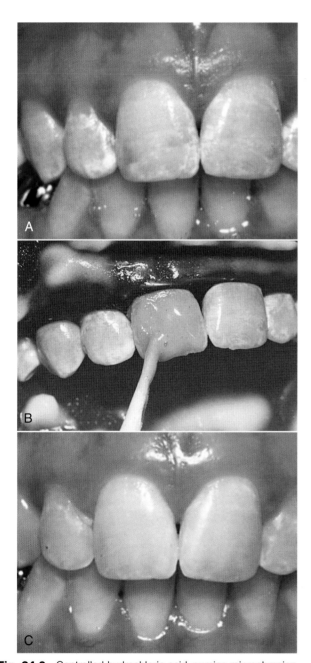

Fig. 24.9 Controlled hydrochloric acid–pumice microabrasion technique. **A,** Marked discoloration results from surface hypoplastic defects. **B,** Hydrochloric acid 18% is mixed with fine flour of pumice to form a thick paste, which is applied to the surface with a crushed orangewood stick. The paste is worked into the enamel with rubbing motions for 5 seconds and then followed with a water rinse. The paste is reapplied as necessary. Finally, acid is neutralized with sodium bicarbonate. **C,** The desired improvement was obtained in a single appointment. There was no regression. (Courtesy Dr. S. Goepferd.)

Microabrasion Technique

The steps in the controlled hydrochloric acid–pumice abrasion technique are as follows.

1. The teeth to be treated are photographed; this serves as a permanent record and a basis for future comparison.
2. The gingiva is protected, and the teeth are carefully isolated with an inverted rubber dam and ligatures. The rubber dam is extended over the patient's nostrils.
3. Exposed areas of the patient's face and eyes are covered with a suitable drape or towel for added safety from acid spatter.
4. A 36% hydrochloric acid solution is mixed with an equal volume of distilled water to make an 18% hydrochloric acid solution. A substantial amount of fine flour of pumice is added to form a thick paste. In another dappen dish, sodium bicarbonate and water are mixed to a thick paste, which is used later for acid neutralization. Ready-made commercial products are also available.
5. The hydrochloric acid and pumice paste is applied to the enamel surface with a piece of wooden tongue blade or crushed orangewood stick. Firm pressure is applied to work the paste into the enamel surface, using a scrubbing motion, for 5 seconds. The enamel surface is then rinsed for 10 seconds with water.
6. The paste is reapplied until the desired color is achieved.
7. The surface is neutralized with sodium bicarbonate and water. The rubber dam is removed, and the teeth are pumiced with a fine prophylactic paste to smooth the abraded surface. Usually the desired shade is obtained in a single appointment. If not, the stains may be too deep and may not be amenable to lightening.

Prognosis

The acid-pumice abrasion technique is relatively permanent if initial lightening is achieved. Many patients have been followed for long periods with no recurrence of discoloration.[11]

Safety

There are two areas in which safety is a concern: the effects on enamel (excessive decalcification) and chemical burns of soft tissue.

With care and judicious application of acid in either of the hydrochloric acid techniques, an insignificant amount of enamel is removed. Chemical burns of the gingiva by either concentrated acid or hydrogen peroxide may be easily prevented by coating the gingiva with isolating materials, inverting the rubber dam, and ligating the teeth. There are minimal to no pulpal effects.

WHEN AND WHAT TO REFER

Most bleaching procedures can be performed by general dentists, particularly if the cause of the discoloration is diagnosed. If the general practitioner cannot make this identification, referral to a specialist should be considered.

The practitioner may also wish to refer patients whose tooth discoloration does not respond to conventional methods of bleaching, either external or internal. Unidentified factors may be preventing the bleaching chemicals from effectively reaching the stain. The specialist may be able to identify and correct these factors.

REFERENCES

1. Rotstein I, Walton R: Bleaching discolored teeth: internal and external. In Torabinejad M, Walton RE, editors: *Endodontics: principles and practice,* ed 4, p. 391, St Louis, 2009, Saunders.

2. American Association of Endodontics: *Guide to clinical endodontics,* p 39, Chicago, 2010, The Association.

3. Rotstein I, Zalkind M, Mor C, et al: In vitro efficacy of sodium perborate preparations used for intracoronal bleaching of discolored non-vital teeth, *Endod Dent Traumatol* 7:177, 1991.

4. Rotstein I, Mor C, Friedman S: Prognosis of intracoronal bleaching with sodium perborate preparation in vitro: 1-year study, *J Endod* 19:10, 1993.

5. Driscoll WS, Horowitz HS, Meyers RJ, et al: Prevalence of dental caries and dental fluorosis in areas with optimal and above-optimal water fluoride concentrations, *J Am Dent Assoc* 107:42, 1983.

6. Tredwin CJ, Scully C, Bagan-Sebastian JV: Drug-induced disorders of teeth, *J Dent Res* 84:596, 2005.

7. Jordan RE, Boksman L: Conservative vital bleaching treatment of discolored dentition, *Compend Contin Educ Dent* 5:803, 1984.

8. Chiappinelli JA, Walton RE: Tooth discoloration resulting from long-term tetracycline therapy: a case report, *Quintessence Int* 23:539, 1992.

9. Leonard RH, Van Haywood B, Caplan DJ, et al: Nightguard vital bleaching of tetracycline-stained teeth: 90 months post treatment, *J Esthet Restor Dent* 15:142, 2003.

10. Walton RE, O'Dell NL, Lake FT, et al: Internal bleaching of tetracycline-stained teeth in dogs, *J Endod* 9:416, 1983.

11. Croll TP: Enamel microabrasion: observations after 10 years, *J Am Dent Assoc* 128(Suppl):45S, 1997.

12. Davis MC, Walton RE, Rivera EM: Sealer distribution in coronal dentin, *J Endod* 28:464, 2002.

13. Thomson AD, Athanassiadis B, Kahler B, et al: Tooth discoloration: staining effects of various sealers and medicaments, *Aust Endod J* 38:2, 2012.

14. Lenherr P, Allgayer N, Weiger R, et al: Tooth discoloration induced by endodontic materials: a laboratory study, *Int Endod J* 45:942, 2012.

15. Parsons JR, Walton RE, Ricks-Williamson L: In vitro longitudinal assessment of coronal discoloration from endodontic sealers, *J Endod* 27:699, 2001.

16. Kim JH, Kim Y, Shin SJ, et al: Tooth discoloration of immature permanent incisor associated with triple antibiotic therapy: a case report, *J Endod* 36:1086, 2010.

17. Kim ST, Abbott PV, McGinley P: The effects of Ledermix paste on discolouration of mature teeth, *Int Endod J* 33:227, 2000.

18. Lim MY, Lum SO, Poh RS, et al: An in vitro comparison of the bleaching efficacy of 35% carbamide peroxide with established intracoronal bleaching agents, *Int Endod J* 37:483, 2004.

19. Spasser H: A simple bleaching technique using sodium perborate, *NY State Dent J* 27:332, 1961.

20. Weiger R, Kuhn A, Lost C: In vitro comparison of various types of sodium perborate used for intracoronal bleaching of discolored teeth, *J Endod* 20:338, 1994.

21. Rotstein I, Friedman S: pH variation among materials used for intracoronal bleaching, *J Endod* 17:376, 1991.

22. Asfora KK, Santos C, Montes MA, et al: Evaluation of biocompatibility of sodium perborate and 30% hydrogen peroxide using the analysis of the adherence capacity and morphology of macrophages, *J Dent* 33:155, 2005.

23. Maleknejad F, Ameri H, Kianfar I: Effect of intracoronal bleaching agents on ultrastructure and mineral content of dentin, *J Conserv Dent* 15:174, 2012.

24. Swift EJ Jr, Perdigao J: Effects of bleaching on teeth and restorations, *Compend Contin Educ Dent* 19:815; quiz, 22; 1998.

25. Goldberg M, Grootveld M, Lynch E: Undesirable and adverse effects of tooth-whitening products: a review, *Clin Oral Investig* 14:1, 2010.

26. Crim GA: Post-operative bleaching: effect on microleakage, *Am J Dent* 5:109, 1992.

27. Titley KC, Torneck CD, Ruse ND: The effect of carbamide-peroxide gel on the shear bond strength of a microfill resin to bovine enamel, *J Dent Res* 71:20, 1992.

28. Nutting EB, Poe GS: Chemical bleaching of discolored endodontically treated teeth, *Dent Clin North Am* 11:655, 1967.

29. Marin PD, Heithersay GS, Bridges TE: A quantitative comparison of traditional and non-peroxide bleaching agents, *Endod Dent Traumatol* 14:64, 1998.

30. Kaneko J, Inoue S, Kawakami S, et al: Bleaching effect of sodium percarbonate on discolored pulpless teeth in vitro, *J Endod* 26:25, 2000.

31. Buchalla W, Attin T: External bleaching therapy with activation by heat, light or laser: a systematic review, *Dent Mater* 23:586, 2007.

32. Madison S, Walton R: Cervical root resorption following bleaching of endodontically treated teeth, *J Endod* 16:570, 1990.

33. Harrington GW, Natkin E: External resorption associated with bleaching of pulpless teeth, *J Endod* 5:344, 1979.

34. Friedman S, Rotstein I, Libfeld H, et al: Incidence of external root resorption and esthetic results in 58 bleached pulpless teeth, *Endod Dent Traumatol* 4:23, 1988.

35. Howell RA: Bleaching discoloured root-filled teeth, *Br Dent J* 148:159, 1980.

36. Lin LC, Pitts DL, Burgess LW Jr: An investigation into the feasibility of photobleaching tetracycline-stained teeth, *J Endod* 14:293, 1988.

37. Holmstrup G, Palm AM, Lambjerg-Hansen H: Bleaching of discoloured root-filled teeth, *Endod Dent Traumatol* 4:197, 1988.

38. Howell RA: The prognosis of bleached root-filled teeth, *Int Endod J* 14:22, 1981.

39. Rotstein I, Friedman S, Mor C, et al: Histological characterization of bleaching-induced external root resorption in dogs, *J Endod* 17:436, 1991.

40. Vachon C, Vanek P, Friedman S: Internal bleaching with 10% carbamide peroxide in vitro, *Pract Periodontics Aesthet Dent* 10:1145; 50; 52 passim; 1998.

41. Attin T, Paque F, Ajam F, et al: Review of the current status of tooth whitening with the walking bleach technique, *Int Endod J* 36:313, 2003.

42. Deliperi S: Clinical evaluation of nonvital tooth whitening and composite resin restorations: five-year results, *Eur J Esthet Dent* 3:148, 2008.

43. Freccia WF, Peters DD, Lorton L: An evaluation of various permanent restorative materials' effect on the shade of bleached teeth, *J Endod* 8:265, 1982.

44. Rivera EM, Vargas M, Ricks-Williamson L: Considerations for the aesthetic restoration of endodontically treated anterior teeth following intracoronal bleaching, *Pract Periodontics Aesthet Dent* 9:117, 1997.

45. de Costa J, Vargas M, Swift EJ, et al: Color and contrast ratio of resin composites for whitened teeth, *J Dent* 1:e27, 2009.

46. Lemon RR: Bleaching and restoring endodontically treated teeth, *Curr Opin Dent* 1:754, 1991.

47. Wilcox LR, Diaz-Arnold A: Coronal microleakage of permanent lingual access restorations in endodontically treated anterior teeth, *J Endod* 15:584, 1989.

48. Titley KC, Torneck CD, Ruse ND, et al: Adhesion of a resin composite to bleached and unbleached human enamel, *J Endod* 19:112, 1993.

49. Sundfeld RH, Briso AL, De Sa PM, et al: Effect of time interval between bleaching and bonding on tag formation, *Bull Tokyo Dent Coll* 46:1, 2005.

50. Timpawat S, Nipattamanon C, Kijsamanmith K, et al: Effect of bleaching agents on bonding to pulp chamber dentine, *Int Endod J* 38:211, 2005.

51. Rotstein I: Role of catalase in the elimination of residual hydrogen peroxide following tooth bleaching, *J Endod* 19:567, 1993.

52. Lima AF, Lessa FC, Mancini MN, et al: Transdentinal protective role of sodium ascorbate against the cytopathic effects of H_2O_2 released from bleaching agents, *Oral Surg Oral Med Oral Pathol Oral Radiol Endod* 109:e70, 2010.

53. Rotstein I, Zyskind D, Lewinstein I, et al: Effect of different protective base materials on hydrogen peroxide leakage during intracoronal bleaching in vitro, *J Endod* 18:114, 1992.

54. Steiner DR, West JD: A method to determine the location and shape of an intracoronal bleach barrier, *J Endod* 20:304, 1994.

55. Casey LJ, Schindler WG, Murata SM, et al: The use of dentinal etching with endodontic bleaching procedures, *J Endod* 15:535, 1989.

56. Camps J, Pommel L, Aubut V, et al: Influence of acid etching on hydrogen peroxide diffusion through human dentin, *Am J Dent* 23:168, 2010.

57. Dahl JE, Pallesen U: Tooth bleaching: a critical review of the biological aspects, *Crit Rev Oral Biol Med* 14:292, 2003.

58. Brown G: Factors influencing successful bleaching of the discolored root-filled tooth, *Oral Surg Oral Med Oral Pathol* 20:238, 1965.

59. Heithersay GS, Dahlstrom SW, Marin PD: Incidence of invasive cervical resorption in bleached root-filled teeth, *Aust Dent J* 39:82, 1994.

60. Rotstein I, Torek Y, Misgav R: Effect of cementum defects on radicular penetration of 30% H_2O_2 during intracoronal bleaching, *J Endod* 17:230, 1991.

61. Neuvald L, Consolaro A: Cementoenamel junction: microscopic analysis and external cervical resorption, *J Endod* 26:503, 2000.

62. Heling I, Parson A, Rotstein I: Effect of bleaching agents on dentin permeability to *Streptococcus faecalis,* *J Endod* 21:540, 1995.

63. Rotstein I, Lehr Z, Gedalia I: Effect of bleaching agents on inorganic components of human dentin and cementum, *J Endod* 18:290, 1992.

64. Lewinstein I, Hirschfeld Z, Stabholz A, et al: Effect of hydrogen peroxide and sodium perborate on the microhardness of human enamel and dentin, *J Endod* 20:61, 1994.

65. Chng HK, Ramli HN, Yap AU, et al: Effect of hydrogen peroxide on intertubular dentine, *J Dent* 33:363, 2005.

66. Eimar H, Siciliano R, Abdallah MN, et al: Hydrogen peroxide whitens teeth by oxidizing the organic structure, *J Dent* 40 suppl 2:e25, 2012.

67. Rotstein I, Wesselink PR, Bab I: Catalase protection against hydrogen peroxide–induced injury in rat oral mucosa, *Oral Surg Oral Med Oral Pathol* 75:744, 1993.

68. Walton RE, O'Dell NL, Myers DL, et al: External bleaching of tetracycline stained teeth in dogs, *J Endod* 8:536, 1982.

69. Lake FT, O'Dell NL, Walton RE: The effect of internal bleaching on tetracycline in dentin, *J Endod* 11:415, 1985.

70. Walton RE, Eisenmann DR: Ultrastructural examination of dentine formation in rat incisors following multiple fluoride injections, *Arch Oral Biol* 20:485, 1975.

71. de Araujo EB, Zis V, Dutra CA: Enamel color change by microabrasion and resin-based composite, *Am J Dent* 13:6, 2000.

72. Price RB, Loney RW, Doyle MG, et al: An evaluation of a technique to remove stains from teeth using microabrasion, *J Am Dent Assoc* 134:1066, 2003.

Geriatric endodontics

Richard E. Walton

CHAPTER OUTLINE

Biologic Considerations
Pulp Response
Periapical Response
Healing
Medically Compromised Patients
Diagnosis
Differential Diagnosis
Treatment Planning and Case Selection

Root Canal Treatment
Impact of Restoration
Retreatment
Endodontic Surgery
Bleaching
Restorative Considerations
Trauma

LEARNING OBJECTIVES

After reading this chapter, the student should be able to:

1. Identify biologic aspects in the elderly patient that are similar to and different from those in the younger patient.
2. Discuss age changes in the older dental pulp, both physiologic and anatomic.
3. Discuss differences in healing patterns in the older patient.
4. Describe complications presented by the medically compromised older patient.
5. Describe each step of the process of diagnosis and treatment planning in the elderly patient.

6. Identify factors that complicate case selection.
7. Discuss why there are differences and what those differences are when root canal treatment is performed in the older patient.
8. Recognize the complications of endodontic surgery.
9. Select the appropriate restoration after root canal treatment.
10. Identify those elderly patients who should be considered for referral.

Endodontic considerations in the elderly patient are similar in many ways to those in the younger patient, but there are some notable differences. This chapter discusses the similarities and concentrates on the differences. The topics include the biologic aspects of pulpal and periapical tissues, healing patterns, diagnosis, and treatment aspects in the geriatric patient.

The number of persons aged 65 or older in the United States exceeds 39 million, and they are expected to comprise 20% of the population by 2020. Their dental needs will also continue to increase.[1-3] More elderly patients will not accept tooth extraction unless there are no alternatives.[4,5] They have a high utilization rate of dental services.[6] The expectations for dental health parallel their demands for quality medical care. An even more important consideration is that these dentitions will continue to experience caries[7] and decades of dental disease, in addition to restorative[4] and periodontal procedures

(Fig. 25.1). These all have compound adverse effects on the pulp and periapical and surrounding tissues (Fig. 25.2). In other words, the more injuries inflicted, the greater the likelihood of irreversible disease and thus the greater the need for treatment. The number of elderly endodontic patients is increasing and will continue to do so.[8]

The combination of an increase in pathosis and dental needs, coupled with greater expectations, has resulted in more endodontic procedures among aging patients (Fig. 25.3). Furthermore, expanded dental insurance benefits for retirees and more disposable income have made complex treatment more affordable.[1] Other means will likely be available to finance the costs of oral health care in the future.[9]

Endodontic considerations in elderly patients include biologic, medical, and some psychologic differences from younger patients, in addition to treatment complications. These considerations are further discussed in this chapter.

441

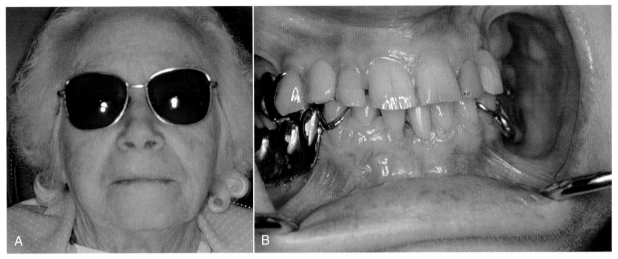

Fig. 25.1 **A,** This 87-year-old woman has Alzheimer's disease. **B,** Her dentition shows diverse problems caused by many years of disease, restorations, and oral and systemic changes. Diagnosis is challenging, and the dentition will be difficult to restore to acceptable function and esthetics, particularly in a patient with mental impairment.

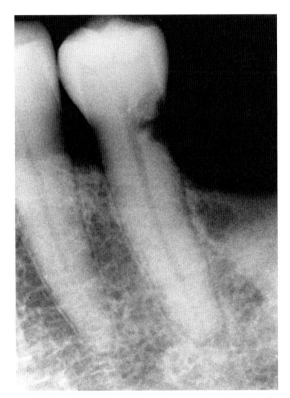

Fig. 25.2 Cervical external resorption exposing the pulp. A free-end removable partial denture has settled posteriorly, exerting pressure on the gingiva and inducing inflammation and root resorption. (From Walton RE: Endodontic considerations in the geriatric patient, *Dent Clin North Am* 41:795, 1997.)

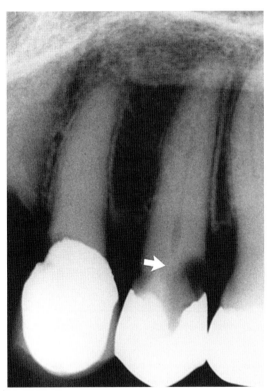

Fig. 25.3 Restorations, caries, and time have resulted in dentin formation. The first premolar shows calcific metamorphosis (a very small pulp space is present). The second premolar has dentin formation *(arrow)* in response to recurrent caries. Both are difficult to treat and restore. (From Walton RE: Endodontic considerations in the geriatric patient, *Dent Clin North Am* 41:795, 1997.)

BIOLOGIC CONSIDERATIONS

Biologic considerations are both systemic and local. The wide variety of systemic changes related to the patient's medical status are covered in other textbooks. In the older patient, systemic or local changes unique to endodontics are no different from those for other dental procedures. Similarly, the response of the pulp and periapical tissues is not markedly different.

PULP RESPONSE

Changes with Age

Two considerations are important in age-related changes in pulp response: (1) structural (histologic) changes that take place as a function of time and (2) tissue changes that occur in response to irritation from injury. These tend to have similar appearances in the pulp. In other words, injury may prematurely "age" a pulp. Therefore, an "old" pulp may be found in a tooth of a younger person (e.g., a tooth that has experienced caries, restorations, and so on). Whatever the etiology, these older (or injured) pulps react somewhat differently than do younger (or uninjured) pulps.

Chronologic Versus Physiologic
Does a pulp in an older individual react differently from an injured pulp in a younger individual? This question has not been answered definitively. Probably a previously injured pulp (from caries, restoration, and so on) in a younger person has *less* resistance to injury than an undamaged pulp in an older individual. At a histologic level, there are some consistent changes in these older pulps and in irritated pulps.

Structural
The pulp is a dynamic connective tissue. With age there are changes in cellular, extracellular, and supportive elements (see Chapter 1). There is a decrease in cells, including both odontoblasts and fibroblasts. There are also fewer supportive elements (i.e., blood vessels and nerves).[10,11] Fewer and smaller vessels result in a decrease in blood flow in the pulp[12]; the significance of this decrease is unknown. Capillaries show somewhat degenerative changes in the endothelium with age.[13] There is presumably an increase in the percentage of space occupied by collagen but less ground substance.[14]

Calcifications
Calcifications include denticles (pulp stones) and diffuse (linear) calcifications. These increase in the aged pulp[15] and in the irritated pulp.[16] Pulp stones tend to be found in the coronal pulp, and diffuse calcifications are found in the radicular pulp. It has been speculated that the nidi of calcification arise from degenerated nerves or blood vessels, but this has not been proved. Another common speculation is that pulp stones may cause odontogenic pain; however, this is not true.

Dimensional
In general, pulp spaces progressively decrease in size and often become very small,[17] a phenomenon known as *calcific metamorphosis.*[18] Dentin formation may be accelerated by irritation from caries, restorations, and periodontal disease and is not uniform. For example, in molar pulp chambers there is more dentin formation on the roof and floor than on the walls.[10] The result is a flattened (disklike) chamber (Fig. 25.4).

Nature of Response to Injury
The older patient does tend to have more severe pulpal reactions to irritation than the reactions that occur in the younger patient. The reason for these differences is not fully understood, but they probably result from a lifetime of cumulative injuries.

From Irritation
There are reasons for pulp pathosis after restorative procedures. First, the tooth may have experienced several injuries in the past. Second, the tooth is likely to have undergone more extensive procedures that involve considerable tooth structure, such as crown preparation. Multiple potential injuries are

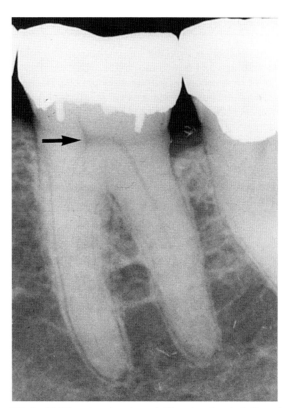

Fig. 25.4 Disklike chamber *(arrow)*. The chamber is flattened because of dentin formation on the roof and floor. These chambers and canals are a challenge to locate. (From Walton RE: Endodontic considerations in the geriatric patient, *Dent Clin North Am* 41:795, 1997.)

associated with a full crown, such as foundation placement, bur preparation, impressions, temporary crown placement (often these leak), cementation, and unsealed crown margins. The coup de grâce of a pulp that is already stumbling along may be that final restoration.

Age
The aging pulp may be less resistant to injury, although this has not been proven. Pulp responses to various procedures in different age groups have not shown differences, although the large number of variables in these types of clinical studies make it difficult to isolate age as a factor. This is not necessarily the case with the immature tooth (open apex) in which pulps have indeed been shown to be more resistant to injury. There is a theory that pulps in older teeth may in fact be *more* resistant because of decreased permeability of dentin.[19] Again, this resistance to injury in old teeth has not been proved.[20] The bottom line is that older pulps in older patients require more care in preparation and restoration; this is probably the result of a history of previous insults rather than age per se.

Systemic Conditions
There is no conclusive evidence that systemic or medical conditions directly affect (decrease) pulp resistance to injury. One proposed condition is atherosclerosis, which has been presumed to directly affect pulp vessels[21]; however, the phenomenon of pulpal atherosclerosis could not be demonstrated.[22]

PERIAPICAL RESPONSE

Little information is available on changes in bone and soft tissues with age and how these might affect the response to irritants or to subsequent healing after removal of those irritants. There is some indication that relatively little change occurs in periapical cellularity, vascularity, or nerve supply with aging.[23] Therefore, it is unlikely that there are significantly different periapical responses in older patients compared with younger individuals.

HEALING

A popular concept is that healing in older individuals is impaired, compromised, or delayed. This is not necessarily true. Studies in animals have shown remarkably similar patterns of repair of oral tissues in the young and the old, but with a slight delay in the healing response in the latter.[24] Radiographic evidence of healing in younger and older patients after root canal treatment demonstrated no apparent difference in success and failure.[25] No evidence exists that vascular or connective tissue changes in older individuals result in significantly slower or impaired healing. Overall, there is little difference in the nature of healing between the age groups, including healing of both bone and soft tissue. Vascularity is critical to healing, and in healthy individuals, periapical blood flow is not impaired with age.[26]

MEDICALLY COMPROMISED PATIENTS

Certainly, systemic problems tend to occur in the older patient more often and with greater severity. In general, medical conditions are no more significant for endodontic procedures in the older patient than for other types of dental treatment. In fact, there is little information on the relationship of medical conditions or medically compromised status to adverse reactions during or after endodontic procedures.

Some conditions tend to be more common in older patients and require particular consideration. These include hypertension, cardiovascular disease, osteoporosis (often accompanied by bisphosphonate administration) and joint prostheses. A recent controversy is whether to administer prophylactic antibiotics prior to dental procedures in patients with joint prostheses. A recent Medicare Current Beneficiary Survey indicated that antibiotics are *not* indicated.[27]

Both type I and type II diabetes make healing less predictable,[28] although this is true at any age. There is particular concern about the person with severe, uncontrolled diabetes, who may require additional precautions and careful monitoring.[29]

Another common condition is hypertension. Contrary to popular belief, using epinephrine in local anesthetics in hypertensive patients carries a very low risk of adverse effects.[30]

Evidence exists that osteoporosis, a rather common condition of postmenopausal women, is associated with a decrease in trabecular bone density in the jaws, particularly in the anterior maxilla and the posterior mandible.[31,32] However, it is not known whether patients with osteoporosis have impaired bony healing after root canal treatment or surgery. As related to diagnosis of periapical pathosis, osteoporotic changes are probably not of sufficient magnitude[33] to confuse pretreatment or post-treatment evaluation. Interestingly, analysis of optical density from periapical radiographs from the posterior mandible is an indicator of osteoporotic changes in the lumbar and femoral regions in the elderly.[34] Other considerations and the impact of bisphosphonate drug therapy, which is a co-factor in osteonecrosis of the jaws,[35,36] are reviewed in Chapter 5.

Anticoagulant therapy is common and tends to increase with age. These drugs are not a concern with conventional endodontic procedures. They are a consideration with surgery; there is ample opportunity for hemorrhage from both soft tissue and bone. The general recommendation is that anticoagulants not be altered before, during, or after these surgeries.

In summary, elderly medically compromised patients are generally at no more risk for complications than are other age groups. In fact, for a medically compromised patient, root canal treatment or other endodontic procedures are far less traumatic and damaging than extraction. A good example is the patient taking (or having taken) bisphosphonates. Root canal treatment and restoration are preferred to avoid the trauma of extraction.

Another important consideration is that older patients are more likely to be taking more and stronger medications.[37] Caution is required to avoid interactions, particularly when prescribing additional medications.

DIAGNOSIS

The same basic principles and diagnostic approaches apply for older patients as for younger ones. A difference is seen in the presence and level of responses.

Diagnostic Procedure

A routine sequence is applied to diagnosis, particularly with elderly patients. The most important findings are from the subjective examination to determine symptoms and the history. Careful questioning and allowing sufficient time for the older patient to recall and answer often yield valuable information.

Chief Complaint

The patient must be allowed to express the problem or problems in his or her own words. Not only does this divulge symptoms, but it also provides an opportunity to determine the patient's dental knowledge and ability to communicate. This ability may be impaired because of problems with sight, hearing, or mental status.

Medical History

The prudent diagnostician not only discusses positive responses marked on the medical history form, but also repeats important items that may not have been marked or were overlooked by the patient. Systemic conditions, medications, and related considerations should be discussed in depth. It is appropriate at this time to explain how medical conditions might affect diagnosis, treatment planning, treatment, and outcomes.

Dental History

In general, elderly patients have a lot of history to review and recall. Important dental occurrences may be only a dim memory and require prompting by the examiner. Examples include a history of traumatic injury, fractures, caries, or pain and swelling.

Subjective Findings

Subjective findings include information obtained by questioning the patient's description of current signs and symptoms. Many older patients are stoic, do not readily express adverse symptoms, and may consider them to be minor relative to other systemic problems or pains. A careful, concerned discussion about these seemingly minor problems also helps establish rapport and confidence.

Overall, symptoms of pulpitis are not as acute in the older patient. One reason may be that there is a reduced pulp volume and a decrease in sensory nerves,[38] particularly in dentin.

The *absence* of significant signs and symptoms is also very common, more so than their *presence*. Of course, the absence of significant signs and symptoms does not indicate the absence of significant disease; most irreversible pulpal and apical pathoses are asymptomatic at any age. Therefore, when pathosis is suspected, objective tests are required, regardless of whether significant signs and symptoms are present.

Objective Tests

Objective findings are primarily related to pulpal and periapical tests. Oral examination and transillumination are also commonly required.

1. *Pulp testing:* Although pulp testing is similar in older and younger patients, there are some differences. The pulp becomes less responsive to stimuli with age, particularly with calcific metamorphosis (Fig. 25.5).[8] Therefore, testing in older patients should be done slowly and carefully, with

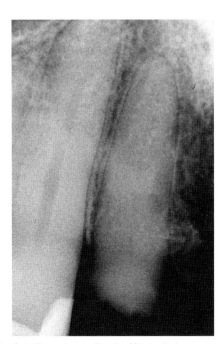

Fig. 25.5 Calcific metamorphosis. Although there usually is vital pulp tissue, the teeth in older adults often do not respond to pulp testing because of a decreased nerve supply and an increase in insulating dentin. (From Walton RE: Endodontic considerations in the geriatric patient, *Dent Clin North Am* 41:795, 1997.)

the use of different stimuli. It is common for a tooth with a vital pulp to be unresponsive to one form of testing (e.g., cold) but to respond to another stimulus (e.g., electrical stimulus). Also, teeth are less responsive with gingival recession and attachment loss.[39] These results must be correlated with other tests and findings and with radiographs.

The question has arisen of whether electrical pulp tests should be used in patients with pacemakers.[40] Although it is unlikely that these tests could cause a pacemaker to malfunction, other tests can be used safely to obtain information on pulp status. It is recommended that electrical tests *not* be used when a patient has a pacemaker.

A test cavity is often indicated but may not be as useful in the older patient because of reduced dentin innervation. A false-negative (no response/vital pulp) response is not unusual, even with a test cavity.

2. *Periapical testing:* Percussion (biting and tapping) and palpation tests indicate periapical inflammation but are not particularly useful unless the patient reports significant pain. These are most useful to confirm that such symptoms are indeed from a particular tooth and to determine the severity of response.

Radiographic Findings

Current, good-quality periapical films are always necessary, and the same principles apply for older patients as for younger ones. The techniques of making radiographs in the two age groups are similar, but some differences must be noted. In older patients, bony growths, such as tori and muscle attachments (frena), may affect film positioning. Also, the older patient may have difficulty placing the film; therefore, holders should be used. In general, a parallel film is preferred for diagnosis, with occasional supplementation with mesially or distally angled cone positioning or a Panelipse or occlusal view. Often, bitewing projections are helpful in showing chamber size and location and the relative depths of caries and restorations.

Apically, there may be some differences in the older patient. The incidence of nonendodontic pathosis of the jaws tends to increase with age; careful determination of pulp status is even more important in these situations when the nature of the pathosis is uncertain. If the pulp is vital, a lesion in the apical region is not endodontic.

Radiographs are studied for pulp size and for root and pulp anatomy. As mentioned, in older patients pulps tend to be smaller and may disappear radiographically (Fig. 25.6). It is important to note that nonvisualization of a pulp space does not mean that a pulp is not present. In fact, it has been demonstrated that there is always a pulp space,[41] even when it is not visible radiographically. Apical root and canal anatomy tends to be somewhat different in elderly patients because of continued cementum formation.[42,43] This may be further complicated by apical root resorption from pathosis.[44]

DIFFERENTIAL DIAGNOSIS

Differential diagnosis is the ultimate determination of whether there is an endodontic or other type of pathosis and, if an endodontic pathosis exists, the specific details of the pulp or periapical lesion.

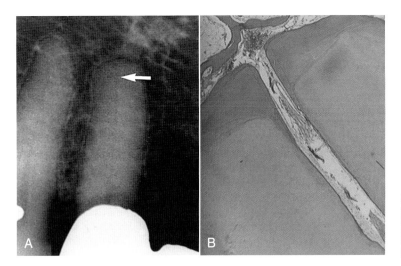

Fig. 25.6 **A,** Although the pulp is barely visible apically *(arrow)*, a corresponding histologic section of this region **(B)** shows a sizable pulp space containing vital tissue. (From Walton RE: Endodontic considerations in the geriatric patient, *Dent Clin North Am* 41:795, 1997.)

Endodontic Pathosis

Signs and symptoms, test results, and other observations in the older patient should follow a fairly consistent pattern. Other complications may include mind-altering medications and occasionally perceptive problems. Vague symptoms that cannot be localized or do not follow an identifiable pattern probably are not endodontic in origin. Other pathosis or non-pathologic entities must then be considered, including psychosomatic conditions.

Other Pathoses

Other soft and hard tissue pathoses include numerous entities; many are more common in the elderly. The lesion that commonly mimics endodontic pathosis is the periodontal lesion. Nonendodontic symptomatic disorders that may mimic endodontic pathosis include sinus infection, muscle spasm, headache, temporomandibular joint dysfunction, and neuritis and neuralgia. The incidence of these tends to increase somewhat with age, particularly in patients who have specific disorders, such as arthritis, that may affect the joints.

Differentiating periodontal from endodontic pathosis is a common problem because of the increasing incidence of both endodontic and periodontal disease. Usually the underlying problem is either periodontic or endodontic, with few true combined lesions (see Chapter 7). Radiographic changes, swelling, sinus tracts, and deep probing defects may be either endodontic or periodontic in origin. Although all findings should be considered, the ultimate indicator is pulp testing. If the pulp is indeed vital, the problem is periodontal. If the pulp is necrotic, the likelihood is that the problem is endodontic. Pulp tests are critical; therefore, a test cavity may be helpful.

TREATMENT PLANNING AND CASE SELECTION

After differential diagnosis, a definitive treatment plan is determined—usually root canal treatment, but additional procedures may be included. Everything should be considered (restorability, periodontal status, and overall treatment plan); this is the time to consider referral of the patient to an endodontist if the situation is deemed too complex.

Procedure

Whatever the treatment, procedures are generally more technically complex in older patients. Extensive restorations, a history of multiple carious insults, periodontal involvement, decreasing pulp size, tipping (Fig. 25.7), and rotation are all factors. An original treatment plan often has to be modified during the procedure because of unexpected findings. For example, root canal treatment may be initiated, only to find that a canal cannot be located or negotiated. Root-end (periapical) surgery then becomes a necessity (Fig. 25.8). These possibilities should be explained to the patient, preferably before treatment is begun.

Prognosis

Although periapical tissues heal as readily in elderly as in young patients,[45,46] there are many factors that reduce the rate of success. The same factors that complicate treatment may compromise ultimate success. An extensively restored tooth is more prone to coronal leakage. Canals that cannot be negotiated to length may contain persistent irritants. Tipped or rotated teeth restored with castings that are misaligned are more difficult to access and therefore more difficult to clean, shape, and obturate.

Each patient should have a pretreatment and post-treatment assessment of prognosis. The pretreatment assessment is the anticipated outcome, and the post-treatment assessment reviews what should happen according to modifiers determined during treatment. Many teeth are severely compromised and would be a problem to retain (Fig. 25.9). Extraction is often the preferred approach. A study on the outcome of not replacing a missing tooth showed that the consequences generally were not significant.[47] Therefore, when extraction is discussed as an option, the patient is informed that "filling the space" may be unnecessary.

Number of Appointments

Whether to treat in a single visit or in multiple visits has always been a subject of debate and conjecture. Studies have shown that there are no advantages overall to multiple appointments with regard to post-treatment pain or the prognosis.[48] However, with pulp necrosis, treatment in multiple

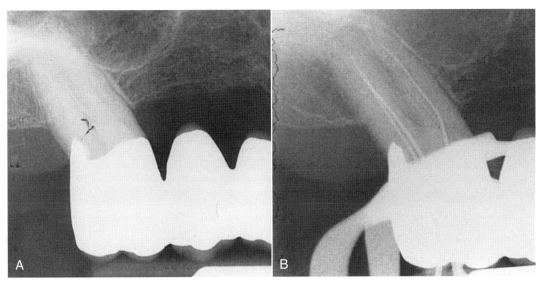

Fig. 25.7 **A,** Castings are frequently misoriented because of tipping and rotation. **B,** Access is more challenging. Observation before and caution during access are critical to avoid perforation. (From Walton RE: Endodontic considerations in the geriatric patient, *Dent Clin North Am* 41:795, 1997.)

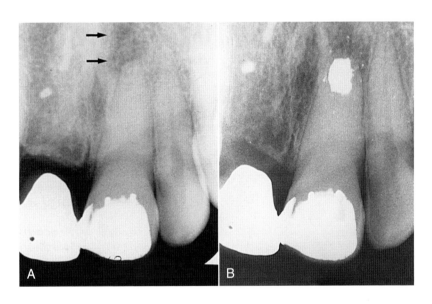

Fig. 25.8 **A,** Calcific metamorphosis and apical pathosis *(arrows)* after trauma. In this tooth, conventional access would be difficult and would jeopardize retention of the bridge. **B,** A surgical approach was used with the hope of sealing in irritants apically. (From Walton RE: Endodontic considerations in the geriatric patient, *Dent Clin North Am* 41:795, 1997.)

appointments and the use of calcium hydroxide as an intracanal medicament may speed healing[49] and possibly promote better long-term outcomes.[50,51]

Single-appointment procedures are often beneficial in elderly patients. Longer appointments may be less of a problem than several shorter appointments if the patient must rely on others for transportation or requires assistance to reach the office or to get into and out of the chair. At times the elderly patient may require special positioning of the chair; support of the back, neck, or limbs; or other such considerations (Fig. 25.10). Conversely, these problems may require shorter, multiple appointments.

Additional Considerations

In treatment planning for elderly patients, the tendency is to plan according to anticipated longevity.[52] It is natural to assume that procedures need not be as permanent because the patient may not live very long. The concept that treatment should not outlast the patient is not accepted by most elderly patients, who desire health care equivalent to that rendered to younger patients. Esthetic and functional concerns may be no different.

ROOT CANAL TREATMENT

Treatment Considerations
Time Required

On average, longer appointments are necessary to accomplish the same procedures in elderly patients, for the reasons discussed earlier.

Anesthesia
Primary Injections

The need for anesthesia is somewhat less in the older patient. It is necessary for vital pulps but is often unnecessary for pulp necrosis, obturation appointments, and retreatments. Older patients tend to be less sensitive and are more likely to prefer **447**

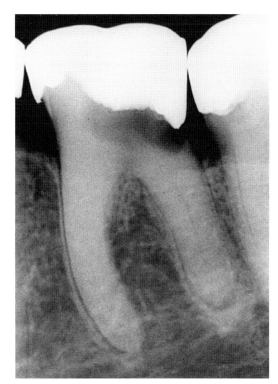

Fig. 25.9 Recurrent caries has created challenges in retaining this molar. Crown lengthening would be necessary for both restoration and isolation during root canal treatment. Crown lengthening may infringe on the furcation. Canals would be difficult to locate and negotiate. The tooth probably should be extracted. (From Walton RE: Endodontic considerations in the geriatric patient, *Dent Clin North Am* 41:795, 1997.)

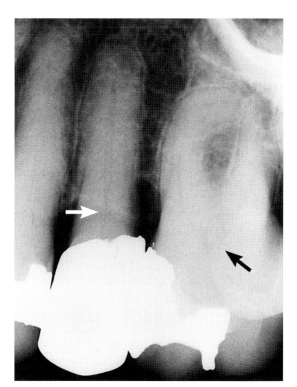

Fig. 25.11 Age, caries, and restorations have resulted in small chambers *(arrows)*. Either would be a challenge to access, and referral should be considered.

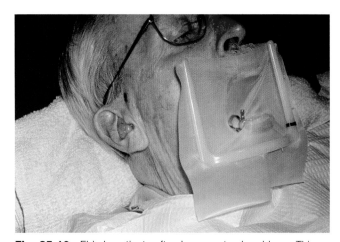

Fig. 25.10 Elderly patients often have postural problems. This patient is made comfortable with a rolled-up towel used to form a brace under his neck.

procedures without anesthetic. Also, they tend to be less anxious and therefore have a higher threshold of pain. Although there are no differences in effectiveness of anesthetic solutions, various systemic problems or medications may preclude the use of vasoconstrictors.

Supplemental Injections
Intraosseous, periodontal ligament (PDL), and intrapulpal forms of anesthesia are effective adjuncts if the primary

anesthesia is not adequate. Certain cardiac conditions may preclude the use of epinephrine, particularly with the intraosseous and PDL techniques. The duration of anesthesia is considerably decreased without a vasoconstrictor, and reinjection during the procedure may be required.

Procedures
Isolation
Isolation is often difficult because of subgingival caries or defective restorations. However, placement of a rubber dam is imperative and often requires ingenuity (see Chapter 15).

Access Preparation
Achieving good access that enables the clinician to locate and then negotiate canal orifices is challenging in older teeth because of the internal anatomy (Fig. 25.11). Radiographs are helpful. A slightly larger, rather than a too small, access opening is preferred, particularly through large restorations such as crowns. Magnification is also helpful, either from a microscope or from other visual aids.

A supraerupted tooth, as a result of caries or restoration, has a short clinical crown, requiring a less deep access preparation. The distance from the reference cusp to the chamber roof should be measured on the bur radiographically. A very small or invisible chamber may be an indication to begin the access without the rubber dam; this helps the clinician stay in the long axis of the tooth (Fig. 25.12). Once the canal has been located, the rubber dam is immediately placed, before working length radiographs are made.

Locating canal orifices is often fatiguing and frustrating for both the clinician and the patient. Although a reasonable time

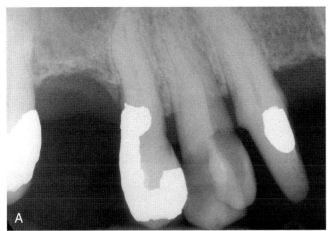

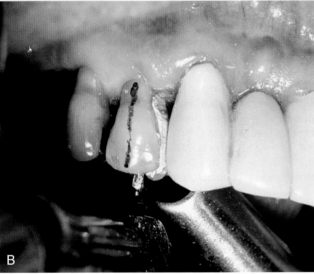

Fig. 25.12 **A,** The first premolar is tilted and has a "receded" pulp chamber. **B,** Aids in orientation during access. The preparation is initiated without the rubber dam in place. A pencil mark is placed on the crown to guide the bur in the long axis of the root. (From Walton RE: Endodontic considerations in the geriatric patient, *Dent Clin North Am* 41:795, 1997.)

should be allocated for this, there is a limit. It may be best to stop and have the patient return for another appointment. Often the canals are readily located at a subsequent visit. This also is a time to consider a referral because another procedure, such as surgery, may be indicated.

Working Length

There are some differences in working length in the older patient.[53] Because the apical foramen varies more widely (Fig. 25.13) than in the younger tooth and because of the decreased diameter of the canal apically, it is more difficult to determine the preferred length.[43] In teeth of any age, materials and instruments are best confined to the canal space. One to 2 mm short of the radiographic apex is the preferred working and obturation length[54]; this should be decreased if an apical stop is not detected. Electronic apex locators are also useful, particularly when there is difficulty obtaining adequate working length radiographs.[55]

Cleaning and Shaping

A common challenge is a much smaller canal that requires more time and effort to enlarge. A very small canal may be more easily negotiated and initially prepared with a lubricant, such as glycerin. This may be used through two or three smaller sizes of files to facilitate enlargement and to reduce the risk of binding and separation. The same principles of debridement and adequate shaping are followed.

Intracanal Medicaments

Intracanal medicaments are contraindicated, with the exception of calcium hydroxide. This chemical is antimicrobial, inhibits bacterial growth between appointments, and may reduce periapical inflammation.[56] It is indicated if the pulp is necrotic and the canal preparation is essentially complete.

Obturation

There is no demonstrated preferred approach, although cold-lateral and warm-vertical gutta-percha obturations are the most commonly used and the best documented.

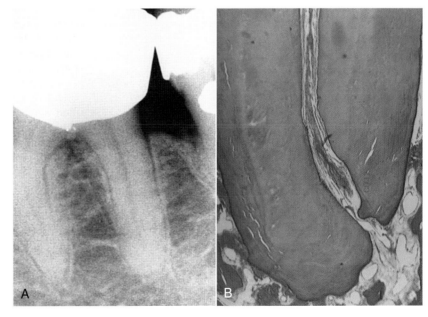

Fig. 25.13 Variability in apical foramen location. **A,** The foramen is not visible radiographically. **B,** Histologically, the distal root shows the foramen to be well short of the apex. (From Walton RE: Endodontic considerations in the geriatric patient, *Dent Clin North Am* 41:795, 1997.)

IMPACT OF RESTORATION

In general, the larger and deeper the restoration, the more complicated the root canal treatment. The old tooth is more likely to have a full crown. There are two concerns when there is a crown: (1) potential damage to retention or components of the crown and (2) blockage of access and poor internal visibility.

The porcelain-fused-to-metal (PFM) crown is more common than a full metal crown and creates additional problems. Porcelain may fracture or craze. This problem is minimized by using burs specifically designed to prepare through porcelain,[57] combined with slow cutting and copious use of water spray. Occlusal access is wide (Fig. 25.14). Metal should not be removed after the chamber has been opened to prevent metal shavings from entering and blocking canals. Access through a PFM or gold crown (either anterior or posterior) that is to be retained is best permanently repaired with amalgam. Anterior nonmetallic crowns may be repaired with composite.

RETREATMENT

Factors that lead to failure tend to increase with age; thus retreatment is more common in older patients. Retreatment at any age is often complicated and should be approached with caution; these patients should be considered for referral. Retreatment procedures and outcomes are similar in older and younger teeth (see Chapter 20).

ENDODONTIC SURGERY

Considerations and indications for surgery are similar in elderly and younger patients. These include incision for

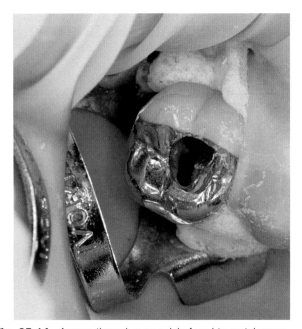

Fig. 25.14 Access through a porcelain fused to metal crown. The outline is large for visibility. Also, the preparation does not extend to the porcelain to avoid fracture of the porcelain. (From Walton RE: Endodontic considerations in the geriatric patient, *Dent Clin North Am* 41:795, 1997.)

drainage, periapical procedures, corrective surgery, root removal, and intentional replantation. Overall, the incidence of most of these increases with age. Small nonnegotiable canals, resorptions, and canal blockages occur more often with age. Perforation during access or preparation, ledging, and instrument separation are related to restorative and anatomic problems.

Medical Considerations
Medical considerations may require consultation and are a concern but generally do not contraindicate a surgical approach.[58] This is particularly true when extraction is the alternative; surgery is often less traumatic.

Excessive hemorrhage during or after surgery is a concern; many elderly patients are receiving anticoagulant therapy. Interestingly, recent studies examined bleeding patterns in oral surgery patients taking low-dose aspirin[59] and prescribed anticoagulants.[60,61] The findings were that anticoagulant therapy should not be altered and that hemorrhage was controllable by local hemostatic agents.

Biologic and Anatomic Factors
Bony and soft tissues are similar and respond the same in older and younger patients. There may be somewhat less thickness of overlying soft tissue; however, alveolar mucosa and gingiva seem to be structurally similar. Anatomic structures, such as the sinuses, floor of the nose, and location of neurovascular bundles, are essentially unchanged. Often, periodontal and endodontic surgery must be combined. Also, crown-to-root ratios may be compromised because of periodontal disease or root resorption.

Healing After Surgery
Hard and soft tissues heal as predictably in older patients as in younger ones, although somewhat more slowly.[62-64] Postsurgical instructions should be given both verbally and in writing to minimize complications. If the patient has cognitive problems, instructions are repeated to the person accompanying the patient. Even very elderly patients have good healing, provided they follow post-treatment protocols. Ice and pressure (in particular) applied over the surgical area reduce bleeding and edema and minimize swelling. Overall, older patients experience no more significant adverse effects from surgery than do younger patients. Outcomes depend more on oral hygiene than on age, as has been shown in periodontal surgery patients.[65]

One problem that seems to be more prevalent in older patients is ecchymosis after surgery. This is hemorrhage that often spreads widely through underlying tissue and commonly presents as discoloration (Fig. 25.15). Patients are informed that this may occur and should not be a concern. Normal color may take 1 to 2 weeks or longer to return. In addition, the discoloration may go through different color phases (purple, red, yellow, green) before disappearing.

BLEACHING

Both internal and external tooth discoloration occurs in older patients.[19] Internal discoloration is related to dental (restorative or endodontic) procedures or to an increase in dentin formation with a loss of translucency. External discoloration occurs from stains and also from restorative procedures (see Fig. 25.1). Overall, teeth tend to discolor with time and with age. Both external and internal bleaching procedures can be successful in these patients.

Internal Stains

Stains that are most amenable to internal bleaching are related to discoloration after root canal treatment or pulp necrosis.

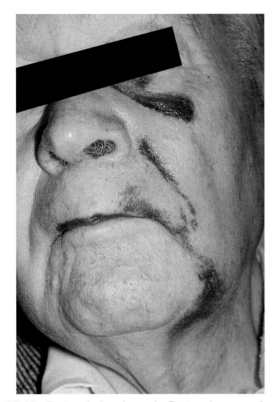

Fig. 25.15 Postsurgical ecchymosis. Root-end surgery of a maxillary lateral incisor resulted in widespread migration of hemorrhage into the tissues, with resultant discoloration. This is not an uncommon occurrence in elderly patients. No treatment is indicated, and the problem resolves in 1 to 2 weeks.

The considerations related to diagnosis, etiology, treatment planning, and prognosis for successful short-term and long-term internal bleaching are detailed in Chapter 24. Often, discolorations in these teeth can be significantly resolved, much to the satisfaction of the older patient.

Teeth that are discolored because of increased amounts of dentin formation and loss of translucency generally should not be considered for internal bleaching because these would require root canal treatment first.

RESTORATIVE CONSIDERATIONS

Overdenture Abutments

Overdenture abutments involve the reduction of a root to permit a removable partial or complete denture to rest on a restored or natural root face. An important consideration is that although a pulp space may not be evident on a radiograph (Fig. 25.16), small components of the pulp chamber usually extend into the crown.[41] Reduction would create a clinically undetectable exposure. If left untreated, this results in pulp necrosis. Teeth to be reduced for overdenture abutments should have root canal treatment, followed by an appropriate restoration to seal the access. Amalgam, composite resin, and glass ionomer are adequate materials.[66] Reduction of the crown and placement of a sealing material, without root canal treatment, is another approach (Fig. 25.17). Overdenture abutments, if properly prepared, restored, and maintained, have a very good long-term prognosis.[67]

Coronal Seal

In the elderly (as in the younger) patient, the coronal surface must be sealed from oral fluids forever to prevent failure. A concern for elderly patients is that the dentist may be less careful with the design and placement of a restoration or select less durable materials. In addition, the older patient is more susceptible to recurrent caries or abrasion, particularly on cervical root surfaces. These lesions do not have to penetrate as deeply to expose the obturating material. With such

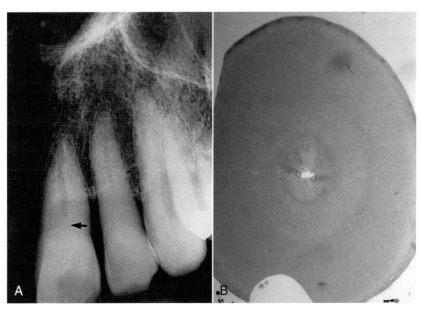

Fig. 25.16 **A,** This central incisor was cross-sectioned at the level of the arrow, where no pulp space is visible. **B,** Histologically, a small pulp space is apparent. Reducing such a tooth for overdentures would result in pulp exposure. (From Walton RE: Endodontic considerations in the geriatric patient, *Dent Clin North Am* 41:795, 1997.)

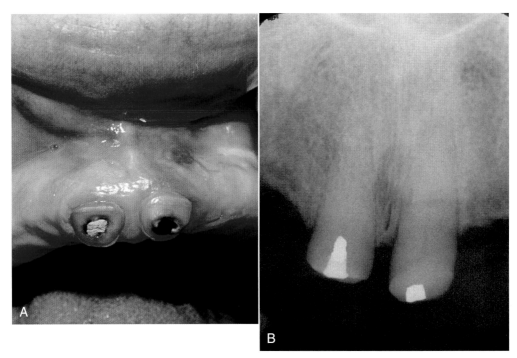

Fig. 25.17 Overdenture abutments must be restored **(A)** to seal a pulp space **(B),** which is always present. Root canal treatment is not necessary in some situations.

exposure, the obturating material becomes contaminated by saliva and bacteria, with resultant periapical pathosis. This is probably the number one cause of treatment failure and the primary reason for retreatment.

TRAUMA

Traumatic injuries occur in elderly patients with recreational activity and because of postural instability and loss of coordination. In general, the older patient who experiences facial trauma has different concerns and requires some different approaches from those used in younger patients.[68]

A major issue is that there may be cranial injuries that are masked by the obvious superficial facial trauma. Evidence of such injuries, as shown by in-office tests (see Chapter 11), requires an immediate visit to a hospital emergency department. Other concerns are similar to those discussed earlier in this chapter: medical status, cognitive factors, and the patient's expectations. With regard to these considerations, the actual management of the hard and soft tissues is similar to (and has an expected outcome much like) that for a younger patient.

With many elderly trauma patients, initial injury management may be performed by a generalist, who then refers the patient to an oral surgeon for facial injury assessment. Follow-up and long-term dentition care may be best managed by an endodontist.

REFERENCES

1. Berkey DB, Berg RG, Ettinger RL, et al: The old-old dental patient: the challenge of clinical decision-making, *J Am Dent Assoc* 127:321, 1996.
2. Chiappelli F, Bauer J, Spackman S, et al: Dental needs of the elderly in the twenty-first century, *Gen Dent* 50:358, 2002.
3. Meskin L, Berg R: Impact of older adults on private dental practices, 1988-1998, *J Am Dent Assoc* 131:1188, 2000.
4. Lloyd PM: Fixed prosthodontics and esthetic considerations for the older adult, *J Prosthet Dent* 72:525, 1994.
5. Marcus SE, Drury TF, Brown LJ, et al: Tooth retention and tooth loss in the permanent dentition of adults: United States, 1988-1991, *J Dent Res* 75(Spec No):684, 1996.
6. Warren JJ, Cowen HJ, Watkins CM, et al: Dental caries prevalence and dental care utilization among the very old, *J Am Dent Assoc* 131:1571, 2000.
7. Tan H, Lo E, Dyson J, et al: A randomized trial on root caries prevention in elders, *J Dent Res* 89:1086, 2010.

8. Goodis HE, Rossall JC, Kahn AJ: Endodontic status in older US adults: report of a survey, *J Am Dent Assoc* 132:1525, 2001.
9. Jones JA: Financing and reimbursement of elders' oral health care: lessons from the present, opportunities for the future, *J Dent Educ* 69:1022, 2005.
10. Bernick S, Nedelman C: Effect of aging on the human pulp, *J Endod* 1:88, 1975.
11. Fried K: Changes in innervation of dentine and pulp with age. In Ferguson DB, editor: *The aging mouth,* New York, 1987, Karger.
12. Ikawa M, Komatsu H, Ikawa K, et al: Age-related changes in the human pulpal blood flow measured by laser Doppler flowmetry, *Dent Traumatol* 19:36, 2003.
13. Espina AI, Castellanos AV, Fereira JL: Age-related changes in blood capillary endothelium of human dental pulp: an ultrastructural study, *Int Endod J* 36:395, 2003.
14. Stanley HR, Ranney RR: Age changes in the human dental pulp. I. The quantity of collagen, *Oral Surg Oral Med Oral Pathol* 15:1396, 1962.

15. Barkhorder R, Linder D, Bui D: Pulp stones and aging: changes in innervation of dentine and pulp with age (abstract 669), *J Dent Res* 69(Special Issue):192, 1990.
16. Sayegh FS, Reed AJ: Calcification in the dental pulp, *Oral Surg Oral Med Oral Pathol* 25:873, 1968.
17. Morse DR, Esposito JV, Schoor RS, et al: A review of aging of dental components and a retrospective radiographic study of aging of the dental pulp and dentin in normal teeth, *Quintessence Int* 22:711, 1991.
18. McCabe D: Pulp canal obliteration: an endodontic diagnosis and treatment challenge, *Int Endod J* 45:177, 2012.
19. Ketterl W: Age-induced changes in the teeth and their attachment apparatus, *Int Dent J* 33:262, 1983.
20. Stanley H: The factors of age and tooth size in human pulpal reactions, *Oral Surg Oral Med Oral Pathol* 14:498, 1961.
21. Bernick S: Age changes in the blood supply to human teeth, *J Dent Res* 46:544, 1967.

22. Krell KV, McMurtrey LG, Walton RE: Vasculature of the dental pulp of atherosclerotic monkeys: light and electron microscopic findings, *J Endod* 20:469, 1994.

23. Van der Velden U: Effect of age on the periodontium, *J Clin Periodontol* 11:281, 1984.

24. Hill M: Influence of age on the response of oral mucosa to injury. In Squier C, Hill M, editors: *Effect of aging on oral mucosa and skin*, Boca Raton, 1994, CRC Press.

25. Swift M, Wilcox L: Age and endodontic prognoses, *J Dent Res* 68(Special Issue):142, 1989.

26. Johnson G: Effects of aging on microvasculature and microcirculation in skin and oral mucosa. In Squier C, Hill M, editors: *Effects of aging in oral mucosa and skin*, Boca Raton, 1994, CRC Press.

27. Skaar D, O'Connor H, Hodges, et al: Dental procedures and subsequent prosthetic joint infections, *J Am Dent Assoc* 143(12):1343, 2011.

28. Fouad AF: Diabetes mellitus as a modulating factor of endodontic infections, *J Dent Educ* 67:459, 2003.

29. Murrah VA: Diabetes mellitus and associated oral manifestations: a review, *J Oral Pathol* 14:271, 1985.

30. Brown RS, Rhodus NL: Epinephrine and local anesthesia revisited, *Oral Surg Oral Med Oral Pathol Oral Radiol Endod* 100:401, 2005.

31. Dervis E: Oral implications of osteoporosis, *Oral Surg Oral Med Oral Pathol Oral Radiol Endod* 100:349, 2005.

32. Jeffcoat MK: Osteoporosis: a possible modifying factor in oral bone loss, *Ann Periodontol* 3:312, 1998.

33. Mohajery M, Brooks SL: Oral radiographs in the detection of early signs of osteoporosis, *Oral Surg Oral Med Oral Pathol* 73:112, 1992.

34. Lee BD, White SC: Age and trabecular features of alveolar bone associated with osteoporosis, *Oral Surg Oral Med Oral Pathol Oral Radiol Endod* 100:92, 2005.

35. Barasch A, Cunha-Cruz J, Curro F, et al: Dental risk factors for osteonecrosis of the jaws: a CONDOR case-control study, *Clin Oral Invest* (epub): December 2012.

36. Ruggiero SG, Gralow J, Marx R, et al: Practical guidelines of the prevention, diagnosis, and treatment of osteonecrosis of the jaw in patients with cancer, *J Oncol Pract* 2:7, 2006.

37. Miller CS, Kaplan AL, Guest GF, et al: Documenting medication use in adult dental patients: 1987-1991, *J Am Dent Assoc* 123:40, 1992.

38. Bernick S: Effect of aging on the nerve supply to human teeth, *J Dent Res* 46:694, 1967.

39. Rutsatz M, Baumhardt L, Feldens D, et al: Response of pulp sensibility tests strongly influenced by periodontal attachment loss and gingival recession, *J Endod* 38:580, 2012.

40. Woolley LH, Woodworth J, Dobbs JL: A preliminary evaluation of the effects of electrical pulp testers on dogs with artificial pacemakers, *J Am Dent Assoc* 89:1099, 1974.

41. Kuyk JK, Walton RE: Comparison of the radiographic appearance of root canal size to its actual diameter, *J Endod* 16:528, 1990.

42. Nitzan DW, Michaeli Y, Weinreb M, et al: The effect of aging on tooth morphology: a study on impacted teeth, *Oral Surg Oral Med Oral Pathol* 61:54, 1986.

43. Zander HA, Hurzeler B: Continuous cementum apposition, *J Dent Res* 37:1035, 1958.

44. Malueg LA, Wilcox LR, Johnson W: Examination of external apical root resorption with scanning electron microscopy, *Oral Surg Oral Med Oral Pathol Oral Radiol Endod* 82:89, 1996.

45. Barbakow FH, Cleaton-Jones P, Friedman D: An evaluation of 566 cases of root canal therapy in general dental practice. Part 2. Postoperative observations, *J Endod* 6:485, 1980.

46. Swartz D, Skidmore A, Griffin J Jr: Twenty years of endodontic success and failure, *J Endod* 9:198, 1983.

47. Shugars DA, Bader JD, Phillips SW Jr, et al: The consequences of not replacing a missing posterior tooth, *J Am Dent Assoc* 131:1317, 2000.

48. Figini L, Lodi G, Gorni F, et al: Single versus multiple visits for endodontic treatment of permanent teeth: a Cochrane Systematic Review, *J Endod* 34:1041, 2008.

49. Trope M, Delano E, Ørstavik D: Endodontic treatment of teeth with apical periodontitis: single vs multivisit treatment, *J Endod* 25:345, 1999.

50. Waltimo T, Trope M, Haapasalo M, et al: Clinical efficacy of treatment procedures in endodontic infection control and one year follow-up of periapical healing, *J Endod* 31:863, 2005.

51. Weiger R, Rosendahl R, Lost C: Influence of calcium hydroxide intracanal dressings on the prognosis of teeth with endodontically induced periapical lesions, *Int Endod J* 33:219, 2000.

52. Braun RJ, Marcus M: Comparing treatment decisions for elderly and young dental patients, *Geriodontics* 1:138, 1985.

53. Stein TJ, Corcoran JF: Anatomy of the root apex and its histologic changes with age, *Oral Surg Oral Med Oral Pathol* 69:238, 1990.

54. Wu MK, Wesselink PR, Walton RE: Apical terminus location of root canal treatment procedures, *Oral Surg Oral Med Oral Pathol Oral Radiol Endod* 89:99, 2000.

55. Gordon MP, Chandler NP: Electronic apex locators, *Int Endod J* 37:425, 2004.

56. Katebzadeh N, Sigurdsson A, Trope M: Radiographic evaluation of periapical healing after obturation of infected root canals: an in vivo study, *Int Endod J* 33:60, 2000.

57. Haselton DR, Lloyd PM, Johnson WT: A comparison of the effects of two burs on endodontic access in all-ceramic high Lucite crowns, *Oral Surg Oral Med Oral Pathol Oral Radiol Endod* 89:486, 2000.

58. Campbell JH, Huizinga PJ, Das SK, et al: Incidence and significance of cardiac arrhythmia in geriatric oral surgery patients, *Oral Surg Oral Med Oral Pathol Oral Radiol Endod* 82:42, 1996.

59. Ardekian L, Gaspar R, Peled M, et al: Does low-dose aspirin therapy complicate oral surgical procedures? *J Am Dent Assoc* 131:331, 2000.

60. Blinder D, Manor Y, Martinowitz U, et al: Dental extractions in patients maintained on oral anticoagulant therapy: comparison of INR value with occurrence of postoperative bleeding, *Int J Oral Maxillofac Surg* 30:518, 2001.

61. Wahl MJ: Myths of dental surgery in patients receiving anticoagulant therapy, *J Am Dent Assoc* 131:77, 2000.

62. Holm-Pedersen P, Loe H: Wound healing in the gingiva of young and old individuals, *Scand J Dent Res* 79:40, 1971.

63. Rapp EL, Brown CE Jr, Newton CW: An analysis of success and failure of apicoectomies, *J Endod* 17:508, 1991.

64. Stahl SS, Witkin GJ, Cantor M, et al: Gingival healing. II. Clinical and histologic repair sequences following gingivectomy, *J Periodontol* 39:109, 1968.

65. Lindhe J, Socransky S, Nyman S, et al: Effect of age on healing following periodontal therapy, *J Clin Periodontol* 12:774, 1985.

66. Keltjens HM, Creugers TJ, van't Hof MA, et al: A 4-year clinical study on amalgam, resin composite and resin-modified glass ionomer cement restorations in overdenture abutments, *J Dent* 27:551, 1999.

67. Ettinger R, Qian F: Postprocedural problems in an overdenture population: a longitudinal study, *J Endod* 30: 310, 2004.

68. Marciani RD: Critical systemic and psychosocial considerations in management of trauma in the elderly, *Oral Surg Oral Med Oral Pathol Oral Radiol Endod* 87:272, 1999.

Pulpal anatomy and access preparations

Lisa R. Wilcox

The illustrations in this appendix depict the size, shape, and location of the pulp space within each tooth and also the more common morphologic variations. Based on this knowledge of the shape of the pulp and its spatial relationship to the crown and root, the correct outline form for access preparation is presented from the occlusal, lingual, and proximal views. From these illustrations, the following features can be observed:

1. The *location* of access on posterior teeth relative to occlusal landmarks such as marginal ridges and cusp tips

2. The *size* and *appearance* of the access on anterior teeth as viewed from the incisal surface
3. The *approximate size* of the access opening
4. The *location of canal orifices* and their positions relative to occlusal landmarks and to each other
5. The *canal curvatures* and the location of the apical foramina
6. The *configuration of the chamber* and cervical portion of the canals after straight-line access preparation
7. The *root curvatures* that are most common

Each illustration gives the following information:

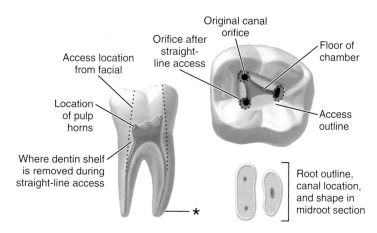

Access location from facial

Location of pulp horns

Where dentin shelf is removed during straight-line access

Orifice after straight-line access

Original canal orifice

Floor of chamber

Access outline

Root outline, canal location, and shape in midroot section

*Most common root curvatures

In addition, the percentages of the more common morphologic variations of the roots and canals are given. With many of the tooth groups, the percentages do not total 100%. The remaining percentage represents the less common variations not illustrated. Percentages are approximate to give general information, primarily to demonstrate relative occurrences. The more common root and canal curvatures are included. These are curvatures not readily identified on radiographs (i.e., toward the facial and lingual aspects).

Maxillary Right Central Incisor

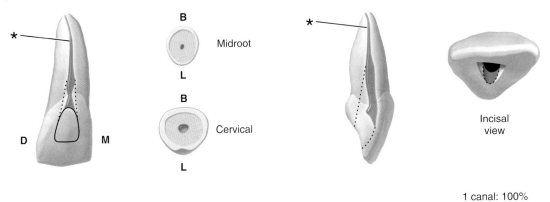

D   M

B
L   Midroot

B
L   Cervical

Incisal view

1 canal: 100%

*Most common root curvatures

Maxillary Right Lateral Incisor

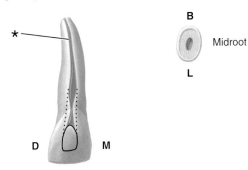

D   M

B
L   Midroot

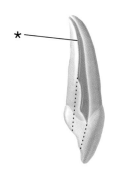

Incisal view

1 canal: 100%

*Most common root curvatures

Maxillary Right Canine

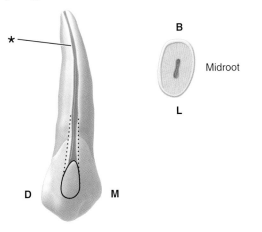

D   M

B
L   Midroot

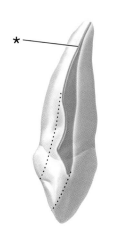

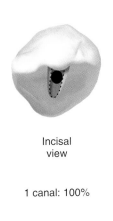

Incisal view

1 canal: 100%

*Most common root curvatures

Maxillary Right First Premolar

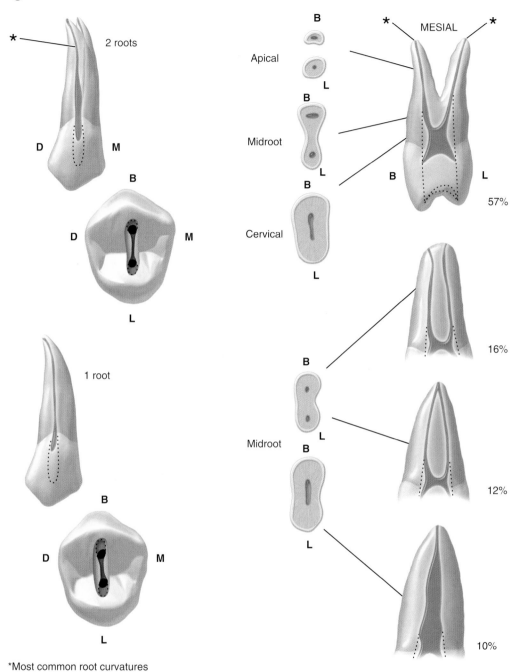

2 roots

1 root

*Most common root curvatures

57%

16%

12%

10%

Maxillary Right Second Premolar

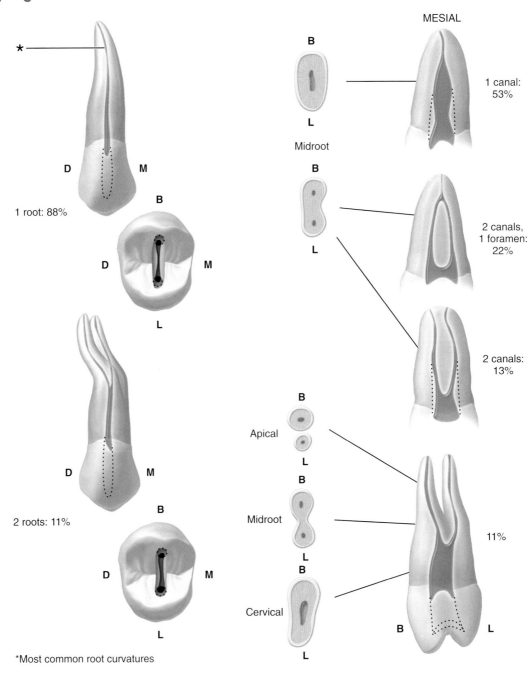

*

1 root: 88%

2 roots: 11%

*Most common root curvatures

MESIAL

B

L

Midroot

1 canal:
53%

B

L

2 canals,
1 foramen:
22%

2 canals:
13%

Apical

B

L

Midroot

B

L

Cervical

B

L

11%

B   L

Maxillary Right First Molar

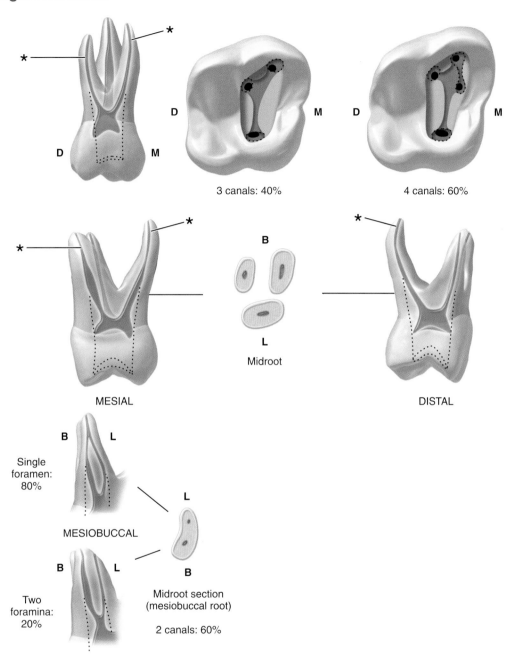

3 canals: 40%

4 canals: 60%

B

L

Midroot

MESIAL

DISTAL

B   L

Single
foramen:
80%

MESIOBUCCAL

L

B   L

Two
foramina:
20%

Midroot section
(mesiobuccal root)

2 canals: 60%

*Most common root curvatures

Maxillary Right Second Molar

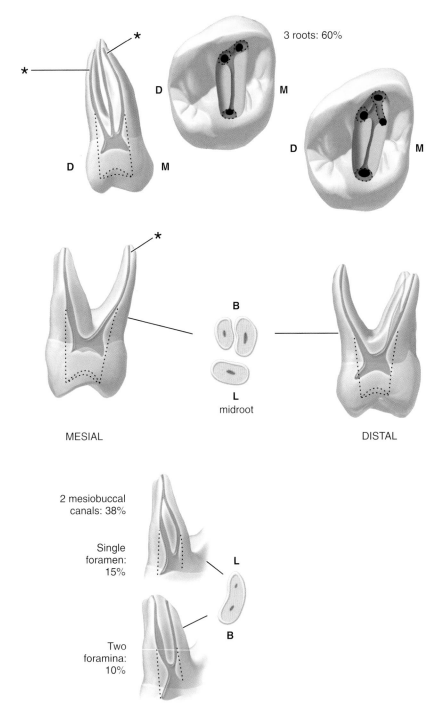

3 roots: 60%

D   M

D   M

D   M

*

*

*

B

L
midroot

MESIAL

DISTAL

2 mesiobuccal
canals: 38%

Single
foramen:
15%

L

Two
foramina:
10%

B

*Most common root curvatures

Maxillary Right Second Molar

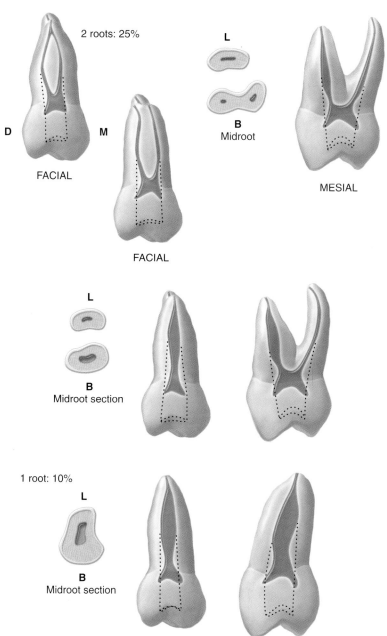

2 roots: 25%

L

B
Midroot

D M

FACIAL

FACIAL

MESIAL

L

B
Midroot section

1 root: 10%

L

B
Midroot section

*Most common root curvatures

Mandibular Right Central and Lateral Incisor

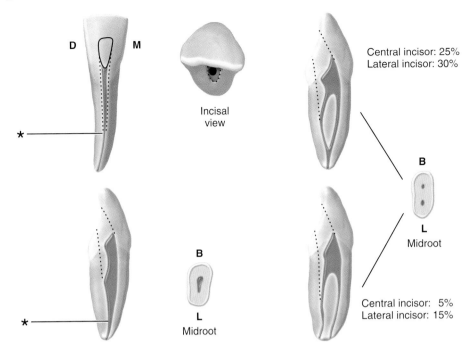

Central incisor: 25%
Lateral incisor: 30%

Central incisor: 5%
Lateral incisor: 15%

B

L
Midroot

B

L
Midroot

D   M

Incisal
view

*

*

B

L
Midroot

*Most common root curvatures

Mandibular Right Canine

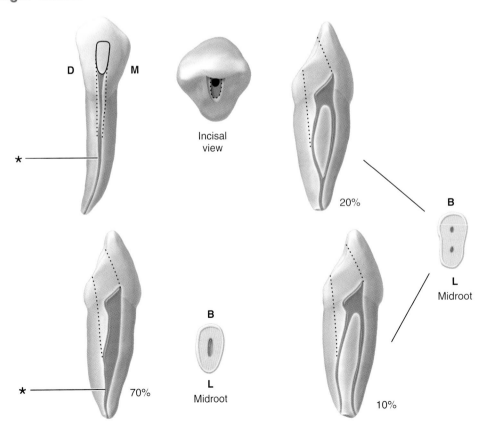

D   M

Incisal
view

*

*

B

L
Midroot

20%

10%

70%

B

L
Midroot

*Most common root curvatures

Mandibular Right First Premolar

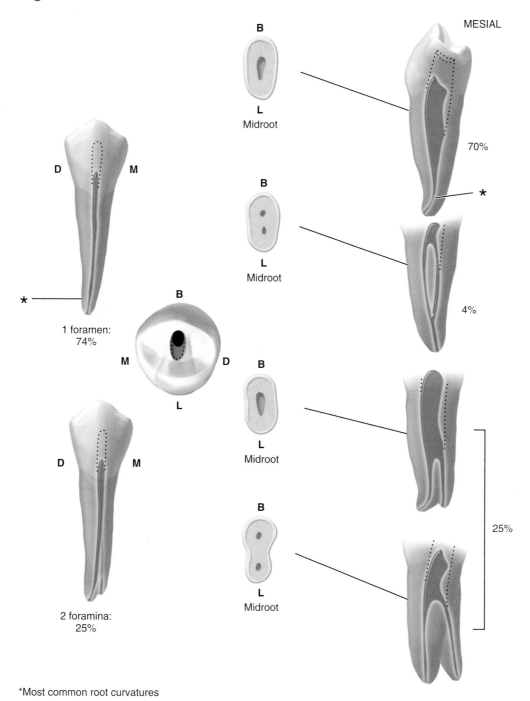

MESIAL

B
L
Midroot

B
L
Midroot

B
L
Midroot

B
L
Midroot

70%

4%

25%

*

D   M

*

1 foramen:
74%

B

M   D

L

D   M

2 foramina:
25%

*Most common root curvatures

Mandibular Right Second Premolar

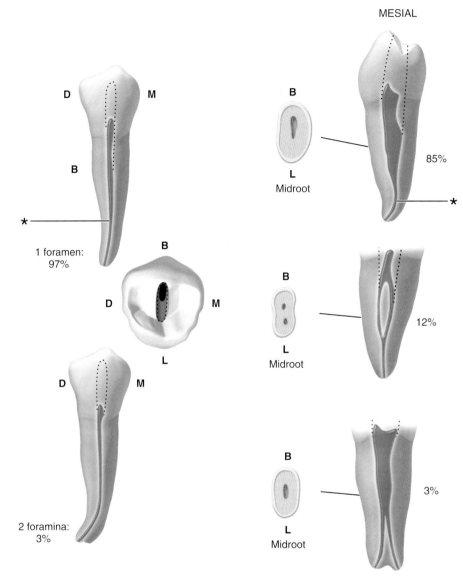

MESIAL

B
L
Midroot

85%

*

D   M

B

*

1 foramen:
97%

B

D   M

L

2 foramina:
3%

B
L
Midroot

12%

B
L
Midroot

3%

*Most common root curvatures

Mandibular Right First Molar

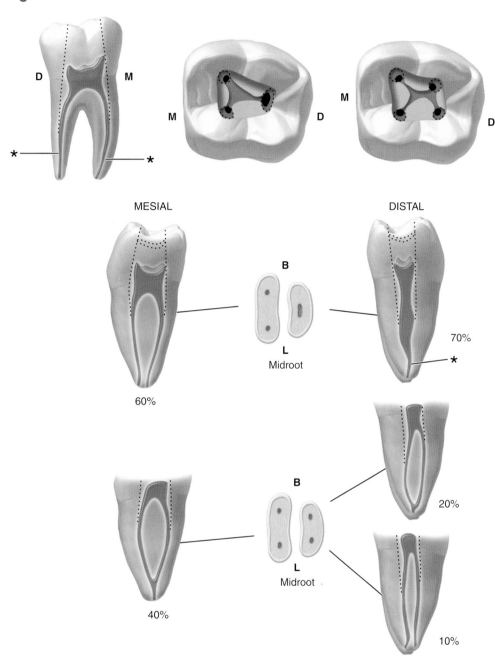

MESIAL

DISTAL

D   M

M   D

M   D

*

*

B

L

Midroot

60%

70%

*

B

L

Midroot

40%

20%

10%

*Most common root curvatures

Mandibular Right Second Molar

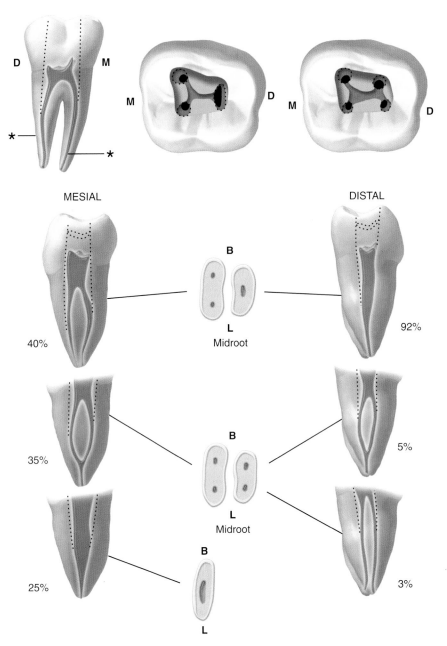

MESIAL

DISTAL

D   M

M   D   M   D

B
L
Midroot

40%

92%

B
L
Midroot

35%

5%

B
L

25%

3%

*Most common root curvatures

Mandibular Right Second Molar

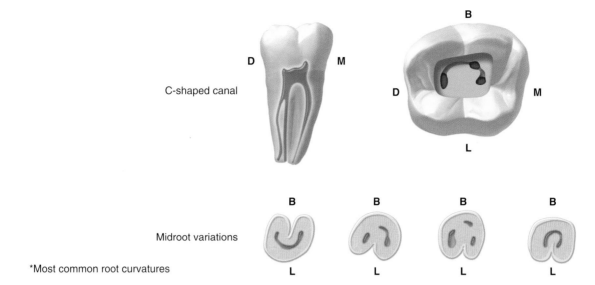

C-shaped canal

Midroot variations

*Most common root curvatures

Some Uncommon Variations

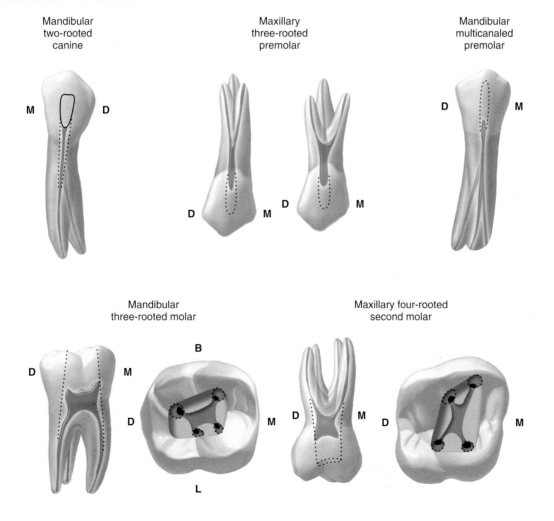

Mandibular
two-rooted
canine

Maxillary
three-rooted
premolar

Mandibular
multicanaled
premolar

Mandibular
three-rooted molar

Maxillary four-rooted
second molar

Examples of access openings prepared in extracted teeth are given here. It is important to recognize (1) the location of the access relative to occlusal or lingual landmarks (marginal ridge and cusp tips) and (2) the size and shape of the access relative to the size and shape of the occlusal or lingual surface.

1. Maxillary central incisor

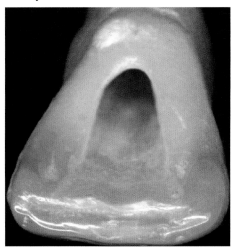

2. Maxillary canine

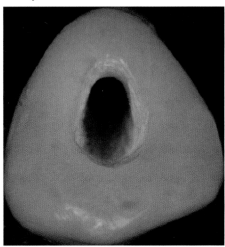

3. Maxillary first premolar

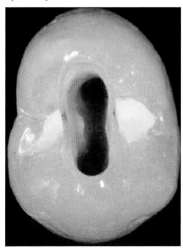

4A. Three-canal maxillary molar

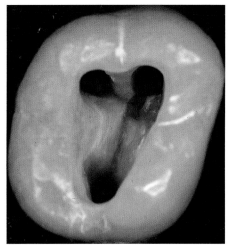

4B. Four-canal maxillary molar

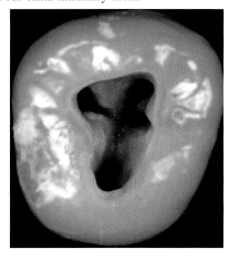

5. Mandibular incisor

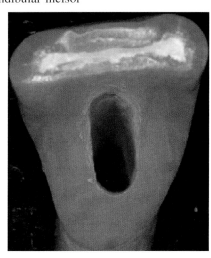

6. Mandibular canine

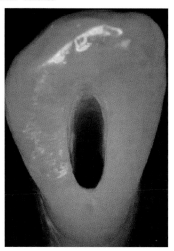

8A. Three-canal mandibular molar

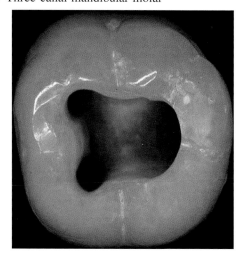

7. Mandibular premolar

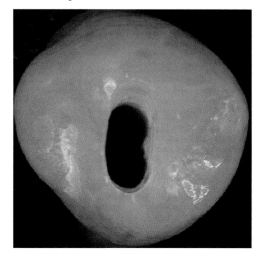

8B. Four-canal mandibular molar

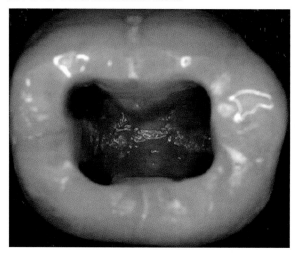

Index

Page numbers followed by "f" indicate figures, "t" indicate tables, and "b" indicate boxes.